Disease Management

Second edition

Disease Management

A guide to clinical pharmacology

Michael D Randall

MA, PhD
Associate Professor and Reader in Cardiovascular Pharmacology
University of Nottingham Medical School
Nottingham, UK

Karen E Neil

BPharm (Hons), PhD, MRPharmS
Pharmacist
Nottingham, UK

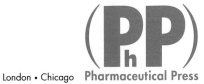

London • Chicago **Pharmaceutical Press**

Published by the Pharmaceutical Press

An imprint of RPS Publishing

1 Lambeth High Street, London SE1 7JN, UK
100 South Atkinson Road, Suite 200, Grayslake, IL 60030–7820, USA

© Michael D Randall and Karen E Neil 2009

$\left(\mathbf{P_hP}\right)$ is a trade mark of RPS Publishing

RPS Publishing is the publishing organisation of the
Royal Pharmaceutical Society of Great Britain

First edition published 2003
Second edition published 2009

Typeset by Type Study, Scarborough, North Yorkshire
Printed in Great Britain by Cambridge University Press, Cambridge

ISBN 978 0 85369 767 1

A catalogue record for this book is available from the British Library

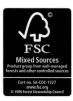

FSC
Mixed Sources
Product group from well-managed
forests and other controlled sources
Cert no. SA-COC-1527
www.fsc.org
© 1996 Forest Stewardship Council

This book is dedicated to our other halves, Clare and Geoff, and to Thomas and Tamsin Randall and Jenna Neil.

Contents

Preface xi
General reading xiii
Note to the reader xv
Acknowledgements xvi
About the authors xvii
Abbreviations xviii

Part A

The patient   1

1   Signs and symptoms   3

2   Clinical laboratory tests   15

3   Lifestyle   21

4   Herbal medicine and alternative remedies   37

Part B

Treatment   47

5   Adverse drug reactions and interactions   49

6   Clinical pharmacokinetics   73

Part C

Gastrointestinal diseases   83

7   Dyspepsia and peptic ulcer disease   85

8   Nausea and vomiting   97

9   Lower gastrointestinal problems   103

10   The liver patient   113

Part D

Cardiovascular diseases   117

11   Hypertension   119

12   Hyperlipidaemia   133

13   Obesity   147

14   Ischaemic heart disease   157

15   Heart failure   169

16   Thromboembolic prophylaxis   185

17   Anaemias   193

18   The renal patient   199

Part E

Respiratory diseases   207

19   Coughs and colds   209

20   Allergy   217

21   Respiratory diseases: asthma and chronic obstructive pulmonary disease   225

Part F

Central nervous system disorders   239

22   Migraine   241

23   Epilepsy   249

24	Affective disorders	259
25	Anxiety disorders	285
26	Insomnia	295
27	Schizophrenia	303
28	Parkinson's disease	317

Part G

Pain and palliation   325

29	Pain management	327
30	Musculoskeletal pain	347
31	The cancer patient: cancer and palliative care	361

Part H

Infections   375

32	Bacterial infections	377
33	Non-bacterial infections	397

Part I

Dermatology   405

34	Dermatology	407

Part J

Endocrine disorders   425

35	Diabetes mellitus	427
36	Thyroid disorders	441

Feedback on self-assessments   449

Appendices

1   Formulary of some important classes of drugs, commonly used examples,
     mechanisms of action and uses   455

2   Some important clinical measurements and therapeutic drug monitoring   463

     Index   467

Preface

OUR AIM IS TO PUT PHARMACOLOGY, which is being learnt or was learnt some time ago, into the context of clinical practice. We believe that this book will be of use to later-year pharmacy students who are encountering clinical pharmacy and pharmacology for the first time, and to pre-registration pharmacists who are putting their training into practice, and will be of general interest to pharmacists in practice. However, the prescribing role of other healthcare professions is likely to expand and we believe that *Disease Management* will also prove a useful resource for introducing and dealing with important issues associated with medicines management.

Disease Management has grown from a course in clinical pharmacy and pharmacology (Disease and the Goals of Treatment), with which we have been involved in the Master of Pharmacy course at the University of Nottingham. In that course, we have used a case study-based approach, coupled to summary lectures, to introduce important therapeutic areas. In doing this we have become aware of the value of a disease-based approach to learning. In *Disease Management* we have sought to build on the course by taking common diseases such as diabetes, hypertension, asthma, depression and peptic ulceration, and dealing with the therapeutic issues. The structure that we have adopted is to provide a brief outline of the disease characteristics and clinical features. We have generally worked on the basis that diagnosis is beyond the scope of this book but have provided clinical features, particularly in the context of alerting symptoms for referral. These are followed by brief accounts of the pharmacology of the agents used to manage the conditions. Where guidelines exist and are in widespread use, we have incorporated brief summaries. The reader is of course referred to the more detailed guidance available and should also recognize that there are currently a wealth of resources that provide clinical guidance, such as the National Institute for Health and Clinical Excellence (NICE).

We have focused on drug choice and taken a holistic approach to recognize that a patient may have several related or unrelated conditions, e.g. rational drug choice in hypertension should be based on managing the hypertension without affecting other concurrent conditions such as asthma. Similarly, drug interactions represent an important therapeutic challenge and here we have attempted to highlight important examples of interactions and how they may be dealt with. Given the plethora of information on drug interactions we have largely drawn on *Stockley's Drug Interactions* (Baxter 2008) for information, because this provides an evidence-based approach with considered advice.

The topics of drug choice are intended to enable the reader to appreciate the rationale behind logical prescribing and advice in medicines management. We have also considered the patient rather than the disease, and here we have produced some points in which patients should be counselled about their disease and their drug treatment.

Our initial concept was to produce a short textbook focused on primary care but we now believe that we have produced an introduction to the management of diseases that are commonly encountered in, but not exclusive to, primary care. As such, we believe that *Disease Management* will provide a useful generalist introduction to medicines management.

Michael D Randall and Karen E Neil,
September 2008

Reference

Baxter K, ed. (2008). *Stockley's Drug Interactions*, 8th edn. London: Pharmaceutical Press.

General reading

In producing this book we have used an extensive range of excellent standard textbooks and reference sources. These are listed here both as acknowledgement and to enable the reader to carry out further reading. More specific references, further reading and resources are provided in each chapter.

General medicine

Boon NA, Colledge NR, Walker BR *et al* (2006). *Davidson's Principles and Practice of Medicine*, 20th edn. Edinburgh: Churchill Livingstone.

Longmore M, Wilkinson I, Turmezei T *et al* (2007). *Oxford Handbook of Clinical Medicine*, 7th edn. Oxford: Oxford University Press.

Kumar P, Clark M (2005). *Clinical Medicine*, 6th edn. Edinburgh: WB Saunders.

Basic and clinical pharmacology

Bennett PN, Brown MJ (2003). *Clinical Pharmacology*, 9th edn. Edinburgh: Churchill Livingstone.

Grahame-Smith DG, Aronson JK (2002). *Oxford Textbook of Clinical Pharmacology and Drug Therapy*, 3rd edn. Oxford: Oxford University Press.

Hardman JG, Limbird LE, Goodman Gilman A, eds (2001). *Goodman & Gilman's The Pharmacological Basis of Therapeutics*, 10th edn. New York: McGraw-Hill.

Page C, Curtis M, Sutter M *et al* (2002). *Integrated Pharmacology*, 2nd edn. Edinburgh: Mosby.

Rang HP, Dale M, Ritter JM *et al* (2003). *Pharmacology*, 5th edn. Edinburgh: Churchill Livingstone.

Waller DG, Renwick AG, Hillier K (2005). *Medical Pharmacology and Therapeutics*, 2nd edn. Edinburgh: WB Saunders.

Clinical pharmacy

Baxter K, ed. (2008). *Stockley's Drug Interactions*, 8th edn. London: Pharmaceutical Press.

Blenkinsopp A, Paxton P (2002). *Symptoms in the Pharmacy*, 4th edn. Oxford: Blackwell Science.

Edwards C, Stillman P (2006). *Minor Illness or Major Disease? The clinical pharmacist in the community*, 4th edn. London: Pharmaceutical Press.

Greene RJ, Harris ND (2008). *Pathology and Therapeutics for Pharmacists*, 3rd edn. London: Pharmaceutical Press.

Harman RJ, ed. (2001). *Handbook of Pharmacy Health Education*, 2nd edn. London: Pharmaceutical Press.

Harman RJ, ed. (2002). *Handbook of Pharmacy Health-Care*, 2nd edn. London: Pharmaceutical Press.

Lee A, ed. (2005). *Adverse Drug Reactions*, 2nd edn. London: Pharmaceutical Press.

Lee A, Inch S, Finnigan D (2000). *Therapeutics in Pregnancy and Lactation*. Oxford: Radcliffe Medical Press.

McGhee M (2000). *A Guide to Laboratory Investigations*, 3rd edn. Oxford: Radcliffe Medical Press.

Rutter P (2004). *Community Pharmacy*. Edinburgh: Churchill Livingstone.

Walker R, Edwards C (2003). *Clinical Pharmacy and Therapeutics*, 3rd edn. Edinburgh: Churchill Livingstone.

Wills S (2005). *Drugs of Abuse*, 2nd edn. London: Pharmaceutical Press.

Dietary supplements and clinical nutrition

Barnes J, Anderson LA, Phillipson JD (2007). *Herbal Medicines*, 3rd edn. London: Pharmaceutical Press.

Kayne SB (2008). *Complementary and Alternative Medicine*, 2nd edn. London: Pharmaceutical Press.

Mason P (2000). *Nutrition and Dietary Advice in the Pharmacy*, 2nd edn. Oxford: Blackwell Science.

Mason P (2007). *Dietary Supplements*, 3rd edn. London: Pharmaceutical Press.

Morrison G, Hark L (1999). *Medical Nutrition and Disease*, 2nd edn. Blackwell Science.

Webster-Gandy J, Madden A, Holdsworth M (2006). *Oxford Handbook of Nutrition and Dietetics*. Oxford: Oxford University Press.

Online resources

Bandolier is an excellent site with extensive summaries of recent clinical trials and experiments and is at www.jr2.ox.ac.uk/bandolier (accessed May 2008).

British National Formulary may be accessed and interacted with at www.BNF.org.uk (accessed May 2008).

Clinical Knowledge Summaries (formerly known as PRODIGY) is at www.cks.library.nhs.uk which is an excellent site (accessed May 2008).

Cochrane Collaboration for access to systematic reviews of healthcare interventions at www.cochrane.org (accessed May 2008).

Department of Health is at www.doh.gov.uk (accessed May 2008).

Medicines and Healthcare products Regulatory Agency (MHRA) is at www.mhra.gov.uk and provides information on drug safety (accessed May 2008).

NICE is at www.nice.org.uk, which is the site of the National Institute for Health and Clinical Excellence, providing guidance on prescribing policies (accessed May 2008).

SIGN for access to Scottish evidence-based clinical guidelines via www.sign.ac.uk (accessed May 2008).

Note to the reader

In producing this book we have attempted to provide a logical background to disease management. Although we have summarized some key guidelines, this book is not intended to provide definitive guidance and the reader should of course consult appropriate national and local guidelines. The examples of drug interactions, adverse drug reactions and counselling points are not exhaustive and are included to illustrate common or important examples. Similarly, *Disease Management* is not intended to replace professional experience and the reader is reminded of the need to consult the latest information presented in the latest *British National Formulary*, summary of product characteristics and evidence-based resources for the latest drug information.

The case studies may deliberately contain less than ideal regimens and are intended to illustrate important therapeutic issues. Once again, the reader is reminded of the importance of consulting the *British National Formulary*.

Acknowledgements

In producing *Disease Management* we are grateful to a number of colleagues who have provided comments on our drafts for the first edition. In particular, we are indebted to Professor Tony Avery, Professor of Primary Health Care at the University of Nottingham Medical School and a general practitioner, who commented on much of the clinical content. We are also extremely grateful to Dr Guy Mansford, a Nottinghamshire GP, and to Mrs Katie Grundy, a community pharmacist, for the much appreciated comments on many of the chapters. We are grateful to Naresh Chauhan, a community pharmacist in Nottingham, who provided detailed feedback on the first edition of *Disease Management*.

We would like to thank Professor Dave Kendall and Dr Ivan Stockley for their encouragement and shared enthusiasm for pharmacology. We should also like to thank Dr Tony Short for introducing us to the value of case study-based teaching.

In addition we would like to thank the many colleagues within the University of Nottingham Medical and Pharmacy Schools who have also provided detailed comments and criticisms on individual chapters in the first edition: Professor Claire Anderson, Professor of Social Pharmacy; Sandra Beatty, Hospital Pharmacist; Dr Sue Chan, Lecturer in Cell Signalling; Dr Vicky Chapman, Associate Professor and Reader in Neuroscience; Dr Dick Churchill, general practitioner and Associate Professor in General Practice; Dr Jeff Fry, Associate Professor and Reader in Molecular Toxicology; Dr Katie Hewitt, Research Fellow; Dr Roger Knaggs; Professor Charles Marsden, Professor of Neuropharmacology; Dr Rob Mason, Senior Lecturer in Neuroscience; Dr Kishor Patel; Dr Nick Pierce, Consultant; Dr Gary Whitlock. We are also indebted to: Dr Anna Cadogan; Anne Lee, Principal Pharmacist, Glasgow Royal Infirmary; Dr Swaran P Singh, Senior Lecturer in Community Psychiatry, St George's Hospital, London; and Mrs Louise Walmsley, Health Visitor, Nottingham, for their most helpful comments and advice. We would also like to thank Karen's sister, Alison Devine, Professional Services Manager, Alliance Boots and brother, Paul Wallace, a final year pharmacy student, Liverpool John Moores University for their helpful and honest comments.

Karen would like to thank Ju-hee Kim (affectionately known as Sylvia), Rose Hindle, and both the Wallace and the Neil families for their support and encouragement.

We are indebted to the staff of the Pharmaceutical Press, and especially Paul Weller, Tamsin Cousins, Louise McIndoe, Linda Paulus, Mildred Davis and Christina DeBono, for their invaluable assistance and advice in the production of the first and second editions.

Despite the extensive help that we have received, any of the errors and omissions within *Disease Management* are the sole responsibility of the authors and we would very much appreciate any constructive comments directed to michael.randall@nottingham.ac.uk or k.neil@ntlworld.com.

About the authors

Michael D Randall read natural sciences at the University of Cambridge and specialized in pharmacology. After his first degree, he remained at Cambridge, carrying out research into the vascular actions of the endothelial factors, nitric oxide and the endothelins, and obtained a PhD in cardiovascular pharmacology. He was then a postdoctoral research fellow at the University of Wales College of Medicine (now Cardiff University's Medical School), continuing research into vascular pharmacology. In 1993 he was appointed to a lectureship, and is now an associate professor and reader in cardiovascular pharmacology at the University of Nottingham Medical School, teaching pharmacology to both medical and pharmacy students. He is also on the editorial board of the *British Journal of Pharmacology*.

Karen E Neil studied pharmacy at the University of Nottingham, before completing pre-registration training based at Broadgreen Hospital in Liverpool. She then returned to Nottingham to develop an interest in pharmacology gained during her final year as an undergraduate. She researched a variety of mechanisms involved in mediating second-messenger cross-talk, with particular interest in pathways associated with β-adrenoceptors, nitric oxide and phosphodiesterases, and achieved a PhD in molecular pharmacology. The application of pharmacology to clinical pharmacy beckoned and this developed from experience gained as a community pharmacist and researcher investigating adverse drug events and particularly drug interactions. She has been involved in teaching clinical pharmacy to pharmacy undergraduates, using problem-based learning, for a number of years. She has been a special lecturer in clinical pharmacology at the University of Nottingham Medical School.

Abbreviations

5ASA 5-aminosalicylate
5HT 5-hydroxytryptamine (serotonin)
ACE angiotensin-converting enzyme
ADH antidiuretic hormone
ADME absorption, distribution, metabolism, or
  excretion
ADP adenosine diphosphate
ADR adverse drug reaction
AED antiepileptic drug
AF atrial fibrillation
AIDS acquired immune deficiency syndrome
AIN acute interstitial nephritis
ALP alkaline phosphatase
ALT alanine transaminase
AMP adenosine monophosphate
ANP atrial natriuretic peptide
APTT activated partial thromboblastin time
ARDS adult respiratory distress syndrome
ASH Action on Smoking and Health
AST aspartate transferase
AT angiotensin
ATP adenine triphosphate
AUC area under the curve
AV atrioventricular
BCG bacille Calmette–Guérin
BHF British Heart Foundation
BMI body mass index
BNF *British National Formulary*
BP blood pressure
BTS British Thoracic Society
CABG coronary artery bypass grafting
CAD coronary artery disease
CAI cholesterol absorption inhibitors
cAMP adenosine cyclic 3′:5′-monophosphate
CAPD continuous ambulatory peritoneal
  dialysis
CAPP Captopril Prevention Project
CBT cognitive–behavioural therapy
CCK cholecystokinin

CDH chronic daily headache
CFC chlorofluorocarbon
cGMP guanosine cyclic 3′:5′-monophosphate
CGRP calcitonin gene-related peptide
CHAOS Cambridge Heart Antioxidant Study
CHD coronary heart disease
CHF chronic heart failure
CHM Commission on Human Medicines
CK creatine kinase
CL clearance
CL_{cr} creatinine clearance
C_{max} maximum concentration
C_{min} minimum concentration
CNS central nervous system
CO_2 carbon dioxide
CoA coenzyme A
COC combined oral contraceptive
COMA Committee on Medical Aspects of Food
  and Nutrition Policy
COMT catechol-*O*-methyltransferase
CONSENSUS Cooperative North Scandinavian
  Enalapril Survival Study
COPD chronic obstructive pulmonary
  disease
COX cyclo-oxygenase
CPK creatine phosphokinase
CRF corticotrophin-releasing factor
CRP C-reactive protein
CSM Committee on Safety of Medicines
C_{ss} steady-state concentration
CTZ chemoreceptor trigger zone
CVA cerebrovascular accident
DCCT Diabetes Control and Complications
  Trial
DCT distal convoluted tubule
DDT dichlorodiphenyltrichloroethane
DEET diethyltoluamide
  (diethylmethylbenzamide)
DEXA dual-energy X-ray absorptiometry

DHA docosahexanoic acid
DHEA dehydroepiandrosterone
DHP dihydropyridine
DIG Digitalis Intervention Group
DMARD disease-modifying antirheumatoid drug
DNA deoxyribonucleic acid
DSM-IV *Diagnostic and Statistical Manual of Mental Disorders*
DVLA Driver and Vehicle Registration Agency
DVT deep vein thrombosis
ECG electrocardiogram
ECT electroconvulsive therapy
EEG electroencephalogram
eGFR estimated glomerular filtration rate
EPA eicosapentaenoic acid
EPO erythropoietin; evening primrose oil
ESR erythrocyte sedimentation rate
ET endothelin
FBC full blood count
FDA (US) Food and Drug Administration
FEV_1 forced expiratory volume in the first second
FSH follicle-stimulating hormone
FVC forced vital capacity
GABA γ-aminobutyric acid
GAD general anxiety disorder
GFR glomerular filtration rate
GGT γ-glutamyl transferase (transpeptidase)
G6PD glucose-6-phosphate dehydrogenase
GI gastrointestinal
GLUT glucose transporter
GORD gastro-oesophageal reflux disease
GP general practitioner
GTN glyceryl trinitrate
Hb haemoglobin
HbA1c glycated haemoglobin
Hct haematocrit
HDL high-density lipoprotein
HIV human immunodeficiency virus
HMG hydroxymethylglutaryl
HOPE Heart Outcomes Prevention Evaluation
HOT Hypertension Optimal Treatment
HPA hypothalamic–pituitary–adrenal
HRT hormone replacement therapy
IARC International Agency for Research on Cancer
IBS irritable bowel syndrome
IBW ideal body weight

ICD-10 *International Statistical Classification of Diseases and Related Health Problems*, 10th edn
Ig immunoglobulin
IHD ischaemic heart disease
INR international normalized ratio
IONA Impact Of Nicorandil in Angina
IP_3 inositol triphosphate
JVP jugular venous pressure
K_{ATP} ATP-sensitive K^+ channels
K_m Michaelis–Menten constant
LDH lactate dehydrogenase
LDL low-density lipoprotein
LFT liver function test
LH luteinizing hormone
LIFE Losartan Intervention for Endpoint Reduction in Hypertension
LMWH low-molecular-weight heparin
LVH left ventricular hypertrophy
MAOI monoamine oxidase inhibitor
MCA Medicines Control Agency
MCH mean corpuscular haemoglobin
MCV mean corpuscular (cell) volume
MDI metered dose inhaler
MDMA 3,4-methylenedioxymethamfetamine or ecstasy
MHRA Medicines and Healthcare products Regulatory Agency
MI myocardial infarction
MMR measles, mumps and rubella
MODY maturity-onset diabetes of the young
MOH medication overuse headache
MRSA meticillin-resistant *Staphylococcus aureus*
MS multiple sclerosis
NACC National Association for Colitis and Crohn's Disease
NANC non-adrenergic non-cholinergic
NARI noradrenaline (norepinephrine) reuptake inhibitors
NaSSA noradrenergic and specific serotoninergic antidepressant
NHS National Health Service
NICE National Institute for Health and Clinical Excellence
NK neurokinin
NMDA *N*-methyl-D-aspartate
NO nitric oxide
NPA National Pharmaceutical Association
NPC National Prescribing Centre
NPY neuropeptide
NRT nicotine replacement therapy

NSAIDs non-steroidal anti-inflammatory drugs
NSF National Service Framework
NSP non-starch polysaccharide
OA osteoarthritis
OCD obsessive compulsive disorder
ORT oral rehydration therapy
OTC over-the-counter
PAF platelet-activating factor
PCV packed cell volume
PDEI phosphodiesterase inhibitor
PE pulmonary embolism
PEF peak expiratory flow
PG prostaglandin
PGRs prandial glucose regulators
PI phosphatidyl inositol
PLA_2 phospholipase A_2
PMR patient medication record
POM prescription-only medicine
POP progestogen-only pill
PPAR peroxisome proliferator-activated receptors
PPI proton pump inhibitor
PRISM Platelet Receptor Inhibition in Ischemic Syndrome Management
PROGRESS Perindopril Protection Against Recurrent Stroke Study
PSA prostate-specific antigen
PTCA percutaneous transluminal coronary angioplasty
PTH parathyroid hormone
PUFA polyunsaturated fatty acid
RA rheumatoid arthritis
RAAS renin–angiotensin–aldosterone system
RAS renin–angiotensin system
RBC red blood cell
REIN Ramipril Efficacy In Nephropathy
REM rapid eye movement
RICE rest, ice, compression and elevation
RIMA reversible inhibitor of MAO-A
RPSGB Royal Pharmaceutical Society of Great Britain
4S Scandinavian Simvastatin Survival Study
SACN Scientific Advisory Committee on Nutrition
SAD seasonal affective disorder

SERM selective oestrogen receptor modulator
SIADH syndrome of inappropriate secretion of antidiuretic hormone
SIGN Scottish Intercollegiate Guidelines Network
SLE systemic lupus erythematosus
SM smooth muscle
SMAC Standing Medical Advisory Committee
SNRI serotonin–noradrenaline (norepinephrine) reuptake inhibitors
SPC summary of product characteristics
SRM serotonin receptor modulator
SSRI selective serotonin reuptake inhibitor
τ tau dosage interval
T_3 triiodothyronine
T_4 thyroxine
TB tuberculosis
TCA tricyclic antidepressant
TDM therapeutic drug monitoring
TEN toxic epidermal necrolysis
TENS transcutaneous electrical stimulation
TFT thyroid function test
THC Δ^9-tetrahydrocannabinol
THR traditional herbal registration
TIA transient ischaemic attack
$TNF\alpha$ tumour necrosis factor-α
TPN total parenteral nutrition
tRNA transfer ribonucleic acid
TrT troponin T
TSH thyroid-stimulating hormone
TxA_2 thromboxane
U&Es urea and electrolytes
UKPDS UK Prospective Diabetes Study
UT urinary tract
UTI urinary tract infection
UV ultraviolet
V_d volume of distribution
V_{max} maximum rate of reaction
VLDL very-low-density lipoprotein
VSM vascular smooth muscle
VTE venous thromboembolism
WBC white blood cell
WFSBP World Federation of Societies of Biological Psychiatry
WHO World Health Organization

Part A
The patient

1

Signs and symptoms

Symptoms and patient histories in the pharmacy

Role

The pharmacist has a central role in assessing a patient's complaint or condition, with a view to providing information, recommending appropriate treatment or referring the patient to a general practitioner (GP). Indeed the pharmacist may be the first health professional consulted by many patients, especially as an appointment is not required.

The consultation

Unlike the hospital doctor or GP, the pharmacist is unlikely to have the luxury of carrying out a full medical history and may not have access to the patient's medical records or test results. Indeed, the consultation may well be happening in a busy shop. Hence, the pharmacist has to establish the relevant facts, to differentiate between minor complaints and potentially serious conditions, and make a judgement or even diagnosis 'on the spot'. First, the patient must be identified and once this is established the pharmacist might then ask the person to explain what he or she believes the problem to be; this should then prompt more specific questions related to the condition. Throughout the interview the pharmacist should take the opportunity to assess the patient to make a judgement about how ill he or she looks and also to examine the patient for any signs that may point to disease, e.g. the following might be revealed:

- Skin colour: signs of jaundice or changes in skin coloration.
- Coloration of the sclera (may reveal jaundice).
- Marks on the skin: e.g. a change in a mole, a rodent ulcer or spider naevi (see Chapter 34).
- Breathing: is the patient short of breath or having trouble completing a sentence?
- Digital clubbing: the fingers take on a 'drumstick' appearance and this can indicate chronic pulmonary, cardiac or liver diseases.
- Does the patient *appear* to have a fever?
- Does the patient appear anxious? Signs of anxiety might indicate how serious the patient feels that the problem is or reveal a hidden concern.

The pharmacist should also attempt to make a judgement about the educational background or medical knowledge of the person, so that the questioning and any subsequent counselling may be appropriately phrased. A patient volunteering specific facts or requesting a specific medicine may reveal their medical knowledge or lack of it.

Establishing the facts

The questioning should be directed towards aiding a diagnosis or making a judgement as to the need for referral or over-the-counter (OTC) treatment. Relevant lines of questioning might be related to the following:

- What the problem appears to be.
- How bad the symptoms are.
- How long the patient has been aware of the problem.
- The main presenting symptoms.
- Any accompanying symptoms.

- What makes the condition worse.
- What provides relief.
- Any relevant social factors.
- Does the patient have a previously diagnosed medical condition?
- A drug history with particular attention to the use of OTC treatments.

The above may be summarized by the popular mnemonic, WWHAM (Blenkinsopp and Paxton 2002):

Who is the patient?
What are the symptoms?
How long have the symptoms been present?
Action taken, medicines tried?
Medicines taken for other conditions?

The drug history may be relevant to the current symptoms or influence the recommendation for OTC medicines or referral. Patients may regard non-prescription medicines and herbal remedies as being less important and so they should be directly questioned about their usage. In addition, it is clearly important for the pharmacist to establish if the patient is suffering from a previously diagnosed chronic condition, such as diabetes mellitus, asthma, chronic obstructive pulmonary disease (COPD), epilepsy, liver disease, renal disease and cardiovascular disease, or receiving long-term treatment, e.g. corticosteroids. It may be that the presenting complaint is associated with this condition or its treatment but this may not be obvious to the patient. Chronic conditions will also influence the use of OTC medicines and the importance of referral.

Patients may also make direct requests for named OTC medicines. In such cases this may suggest that a patient has a previously diagnosed condition, for which an OTC medicine may be appropriate within the limitations of its licence, e.g. a patient may be requesting sumatriptan for previously diagnosed migraine (see Chapter 22). A request for simvastatin to reduce cholesterol (and cardiovascular risk) would prompt a full history to check that the patient fulfils the criteria to receive it as an OTC medicine (see Chapter 12), and also provides an opportunity to explore any health concerns and provide appropriate lifestyle advice

In the case of women of child-bearing age it is important to establish if the patient *could be* pregnant and it may be sensible to assume that the patient is pregnant until proven otherwise. This level of caution is essential because many drugs may damage the fetus, especially in the early stages of pregnancy when the patient may not herself be aware that she is pregnant.

Once the presenting complaint has been established, the pharmacist should use his or her professional skills to select relevant searching questions, e.g. if a patient complains of a cough, an open and open-ended question may be:

'Tell me about the cough'

and, depending on the response, detailed questioning may enable the pharmacist to determine the underlying nature of the complaint (and thus course of action), e.g. the questioning might proceed as follows.

What are the symptoms?

'Is there any sputum?'

'What colour is the sputum?'

'Have you noticed any blood in the sputum?'

Alternatively, ask the patient to describe the sputum.

Indeed the last question is a more indirect approach than the question 'Have you coughed up any blood?'. Using appropriate questions is important because patients may wish to deny to themselves sinister symptoms such as haemoptysis (coughing up blood) or by contrast they may not appreciate their importance.

How long?

'How long have you had the cough?'

Action taken, medicines tried?

'Are you taking any medicines prescribed by a doctor or bought from a pharmacy?'

This essential question enables the identification of iatrogenic problems such as drug-induced blood dyscrasias in patients prescribed immunosuppressants or a cough induced by an angiotensin-converting enzyme (ACE) inhibitor. It may also identify problems where a drug has already been prescribed but the treatment has failed. Medicines taken for other conditions should also be considered. A drug history is imperative when OTC medication is recommended, allowing the exclusion of contraindications and avoidance of drug interactions.

Additional relevant questions might be:

'Have you ever smoked?'

This is a more searching question than 'Do you smoke?' because the person may have given up yesterday (perhaps in response to the symptom) and the answer would be no! Alcohol consumption is also likely to be under-reported by patients.

'Are you having any difficulty in breathing?'

'Have you noticed a wheezing noise or rattle?'

The outcome

The interview should enable the pharmacist to make a reasonable attempt at identifying the condition and then to decide on the appropriate course of action, whether advice, treatment or referral. If the outcome is that the pharmacist believes that it is in the patient's best interests to consult a GP, the importance of this should be emphasized without unduly worrying the patient. It is, however, important to give an indication of the urgency of referral, e.g. a patient presenting with cystitis and systemic symptoms such as fever should be seen urgently rather than wait for the next available appointment. In all cases the pharmacist should ensure that the patient understands fully the course of action that you recommend.

Signs and symptoms

In dealing with responding to symptoms the reader is referred to *Minor Illness or Major Disease?* by Edwards and Stillman (2006), *Symptoms in the Pharmacy* by Blenkinsopp and Paxton (2002), and *Community Pharmacy* by Rutter (2004),

which deal with responding to a range of common symptoms (see end of chapter).

Symptoms

A symptom is a perceived change in well-being by the patient that may or may not be associated with significant illness. The patient complains of a symptom and it is different from 'normal'. Several symptoms may present together to suggest or exclude a disease; this forms part of differential diagnosis, e.g. a patient may report breathlessness and also notice swollen ankles, which may appear unrelated but to the pharmacist may point to chronic heart failure (see Chapter 15). The following are some examples of symptoms:

- cough
- tiredness
- aches
- chest pains
- breathlessness
- indigestion.

Signs

A sign is a clinical change in a person, which may be observed by a clinician and indicates a disease. The following are some common examples of signs:

- Changes in skin (colour, markings).
- Digital clubbing (fingers clubbed in lung and hepatic diseases).
- Heart murmurs.
- Sounds on listening to the lungs (wheezes [rhonchi], crackles [crepitations]).
- Dullness to percussion of thorax (changes in sound on tapping).
- Changes to the retina.
- Enlarged lymph nodes.

There is obviously some overlap between signs and symptoms as a patient might notice ankle oedema but not realize that it is a significant sign of heart failure.

Table 1.1   Some causes of a cough

Underlying condition	Comments
Coryza (cold) (Chapter 19)	Associated with cold symptoms
Acute bronchitis (Chapter 19)	Often following a cold: there may be production of sputum, with wheezing and a temperature
Tracheitis	A dry, rasping and painful cough which is often associated with a viral infection
Pneumonia (Chapter 19)	Infection of the alveoli which leads to sputum (which may be blood stained and is often rusty in appearance), breathlessness, pleuritic chest pains and fever
Chronic bronchitis (Chapter 21)	• COPD • Associated with exacerbations • The 'smoker's cough' may herald the onset of COPD
Asthma (Chapter 21)	• May be associated with wheezing and breathlessness • Often a nocturnal cough and this may be the only symptom in a child
Drug induced (Chapters 11 and 15)	For example, with ACE inhibitors
Anxiety	A long-term 'nervous cough'
Foreign body	Associated with recent inhalation of an object
Tuberculosis (Chapter 32)	Associated with tiredness, malaise, weight loss, fever and haemoptysis
Bronchiectasis	• Dilated bronchioles with persistent infections and mucus • Copious amounts of sputum which may be blood stained
Congestive heart failure (Chapter 15)	Associated with breathlessness and oedema
Lung cancer	A history of smoking associated with haemoptysis. A change in a 'smoker's cough' is a serious alerting symptom

ACE, angiotensin-converting enzyme; COPD, chronic obstructive pulmonary disease.

Important examples of signs and symptoms

Cough

A cough may be a trivial symptom, either reflecting a minor ailment or possibly pointing to a serious underlying disease (Table 1.1).

Chest pains

Once again, chest pains represent an important symptom, which might be due to a minor illness or a serious condition and some common causes are detailed in Table 1.2.

Given the above (Table 1.2) presentations and diverse conditions, questioning should be directed towards establishing the following:

• The location and nature of the pain and additional symptoms.
• What provokes the pain?

• What relieves the pain (including the use of OTC medicines and rest)?
• Recent activity? For example, exertion that may have strained a muscle.
• Past medical history.
• If GTN (glyceryl trinitrate) failed to control the symptoms, is it actually in date?

Breathlessness

Similarly, breathlessness may be due to a whole range of conditions and the possible aetiologies include:

• congenital: cystic fibrosis
• infection: chest infection, tuberculosis
• inflammatory: asthma, anaphylaxis
• neoplastic: carcinoma
• haematological: secondary to anaemia
• psychogenic: panic attacks

Table 1.2   Some causes of chest pains

Underlying condition	Comments
Musculoskeletal in origin (Chapter 30)	Pain may be worse on moving an arm or follows strenuous or unusual exercise. This is a common explanation and is often the default diagnosis
Respiratory (Chapter 21)	The pain is likely to be associated with breathing and to be due to an underlying respiratory disease, e.g. asthma
Pleuritic pains	This may be due to some form of respiratory disease but, if associated with calf swelling, haemoptysis or risk factors for thromboembolism, it may point to pulmonary embolism
Gastric origin: peptic ulceration, reflux	Here there may be a relationship to food, being either brought on by a meal (gastro-oesophageal reflux disease) or temporarily relieved by food (peptic ulceration) (Chapter 7). It should be relieved rapidly by antacids. In patients >55 years of age, if this symptom is of recent onset it raises the suspicion of carcinoma, which should be excluded
Angina (Chapter 14)	Angina has the following characteristics, which often allow it to be diagnosed by a history: • A crushing feeling in the chest • Often accompanied by pains down the arm (often left) • Pains may radiate to the jaw • Stable angina is induced by exercise, emotional stress, cold weather or a meal • Unstable angina may occur at rest • It should be relieved by rest (unless unstable) or GTN • Characteristic ECG changes
Myocardial infarction (Chapter 14)	• This must be differentiated from angina and is characteristically severe chest pains, which are not relieved by rest or GTN • May be accompanied by nausea, breathlessness, pallor, sweating and pains down the arms and/or jaw • Often diagnosed by ECG changes and so-called 'cardiac enzymes' • Some patients may experience a silent myocardial infarction, which does not cause chest pains

ECG, electrocardiogram; GTN, glyceryl trinitrate.

- degenerative: COPD
- cardiac: chronic heart failure, acute left ventricular failure, myocardial infarction
- thromboembolic: pulmonary embolism
- functional: in pregnancy, ascent to altitude, obesity
- iatrogenic: bronchospasm secondary to drug treatment (e.g. β blockers, non-steroidal anti-inflammatory drugs [NSAIDs]); chronic pulmonary damage (e.g. amiodarone). (See Chapter 5.)
- Traumatic: physical damage to the chest.

In all cases, the serious nature of the potential conditions should lead to a referral, and the key question is the degree of urgency required.

Pain

Pain affects many parts of the body and represents an interesting complaint as it may point to a range of trivial or serious conditions, e.g. an uncomplicated tension headache would be treated by simple analgesia but a severe headache typical of migraine (see Chapter 22) with accompanying symptoms such as nausea and photophobia would require referral. A headache that is severe and explosive (the patient might describe it as feeling like being 'hit on the back of the head with a brick') might point to a sub-arachnoid haemorrhage, which is a medical emergency. In taking a history of pain it may help ask the patient to describe the severity on a scale of 1–10, with 10 representing 'the worst ever'.

Pain affecting other systems in the body requires close questioning of the relevant system, e.g. musculoskeletal pain may be the response to a recent injury or due to a chronic condition such as arthritis – in which case a diagnosis might be suggested by the time course of onset and provoking factors.

Gastrointestinal pain similarly represents a challenge. The first issue is one of location, e.g. heartburn is an obvious indication of upper gastrointestinal problems such as gastro-oesophageal reflux disease and would be exacerbated by eating. Lower gastrointestinal pain, which is colicky in nature, might point to a visceral cause, whereas pain with bloating, which is relieved by defecation, would be consistent with irritable bowel syndrome (IBS).

A 'funny turn'

This symptom encompasses a range of events from dizziness to total loss of consciousness that may involve fitting. As one might imagine, the range of events has a wide number of possible causes including the following.

Cardiovascular
Cardiovascular events such as a cerebrovascular accidents (including a transient ischaemic attack), arrhythmias and postural hypotension, which is particularly prevalent in elderly people and those taking vasodilators or diuretics. Vaso-vagal syncope (fainting) may involve bradycardia with vasodilatation as a response to fear, pain, emotion or standing for a prolonged period and result in a faint.

Neurological
Neurological causes include epilepsy, cerebro-vascular accidents, migraine and infections including meningitis.

Endocrine
Endocrine causes include postural hypotension due to Addison's disease, thyrotoxicosis and diabetes with hypoglycaemia or hyperglycaemia.

Psychological
Psychological causes include panic attacks.

Iatrogenic
Iatrogenic causes include postural hypotension, in those taking vasodilators or diuretics as mentioned above or confusion with benzodiazepines. In response to a funny turn, the following questions may help to implicate or exclude certain causes:

- What provokes an attack? For example, flashing lights in certain forms of epilepsy.
- Were there any prodromal symptoms? For example, an aura in epilepsy.
- Was there loss of consciousness?
- Was there injury? Tongue biting would be consistent with epilepsy.
- Were there any unusual movements? This might implicate epilepsy.
- Was there incontinence? Incontinence of urine is common in epilepsy.
- What colour did the patient go? Extreme pallor during the episode and flushing after the attack might suggest a cardiac cause.
- How did the patient recover? With neurological causes there may be confusion.
- How long did it last?
- Does the patient have a current illness or is he or she receiving any drugs?

Given the potential seriousness of the above causes of a 'funny turn', it is likely that a referral would be made.

Referral

The pharmacist has a major role in responding to symptoms. Initially, the pharmacist should respond with advice and where necessary counter prescribe for 'minor' conditions that would respond to OTC medicines. Compliance problems with prescribed medicines can often be rectified by the pharmacist. Equally, the pharmacist should be able to recognize potentially

Table 1.3   Some important gastrointestinal referral points

Leading feature	Features and comments
Mouth ulcers	• Recurrent and/or failure of OTC therapy • Possible ADR • Associated with agents that may cause neutropenia such as carbimazole, carbamazepine and clozapine (Chapter 5)
Swallowing	• Dysphagia (difficulty in swallowing) • Odynophagia (painful swallowing) that is not simply due to a sore throat
Vomiting (Chapters 8 and 9)	• Haematemesis (vomiting blood) – any and urgent referral if profuse. Bleeding may be profuse or present as 'ground coffee' in appearance (Chapter 7) • Symptoms of dehydration such as decreased output of urine, headache and confusion – care in special groups; taking laxatives or diuretics (advise to omit doses) • Nausea of more than 3–4 days
Dyspepsia/'Indigestion' (Chapter 7)	• Indigestion persisting after 2 weeks of OTC histamine H_2-receptor antagonists or 4 weeks of OTC omeprazole • Pain consistent with peptic ulceration • Following use of NSAIDs • Prolonged indigestion, also new or changed symptoms in patients >45 years of age, or alerting symptoms including anorexia, weight loss, anaemia and upper abdominal masses
Bowel habits (Chapter 9)	• Sustained (>2 weeks) alteration in bowel habits (particularly in those over 45 years of age) • Passing blood (frank or melaena, black 'tarry' stools) – this may be due to gastrointestinal bleeding • Severe diarrhoea while taking antibiotics, especially clindamycin – antibiotics may lead to colitis • Steatorrhoea – significant if not explained by concomitant orlistat • Pale stools
Weight loss	• Weight loss or wasting that is unexplained
Liver problems (Chapter 10)	• Jaundice

ADR, adverse drug reaction; NSAIDs, non-steroidal anti-inflammatory drugs; OTC, over-the-counter.

serious symptoms and refer patients to their GP, NHS drop-in centres or, in an emergency, a hospital accident and emergency department. Consultation via telephone, publications or on-line resources with NHS Direct is also a valuable source of referral information, triage and algorithms for patients.

In general, referral should be made for patients with potentially serious symptoms, for persistent symptoms and high-risk patients such as:

• babies
• children
• elderly people
• patients with diabetes
• pregnant or breast-feeding mothers
• immunocompromised patients.

In addition, many other disease states representing high risk (e.g. ischaemic heart disease, epilepsy, COPD, asthma) and then deterioration in the condition might warrant referral.

One should also be mindful of patients who frequently request OTC medicines for symptomatic relief, because they may be used to hide symptoms, e.g. the use of OTC H_2-receptor antagonists in peptic ulceration. Another reason

Table 1.4   Some important cardiorespiratory referral points

Leading feature	Features and comments
Chest pain (Chapter 14)	• Chest pain at rest or on exertion • Chest pain suggesting a myocardial infarction and that is not relieved by nitrates should prompt emergency hospital referral. Consider administering aspirin (150–300 mg)
Breathlessness	• Any of new onset or deterioration • Including breathlessness at night while lying down (Chapter 15) • Breathlessness (often wheezy) with signs of anaphylaxis such as urticaria, angio-oedema with swollen lips or eyelids, should lead to urgent hospital referral (Chapter 20)
Wheezing	• Any
Cough	• Persistent cough of >2–3 weeks, or with a history of bronchitis or green sputum (Chapter 19) • A change in smoker's cough • Persistent dry nocturnal cough in a child, which may indicate asthma (Chapter 21) • Haemoptysis (coughing up blood) • Cough with ACE inhibitors (Chapters 11 and 15), if the cough is intolerable
Symptoms consistent with anaemia	• Any (Chapter 17) – identify possible cause, including use of NSAIDs and associated gastrointestinal bleeding
Dizziness on standing (postural hypotension)	• Especially in patients taking ACE inhibitors, diuretics, α blockers and antipsychotics
Painful unilateral calf swelling	• Especially if accompanied by breathlessness and/or pleuritic pain, this should lead to urgent referral to hospital (Chapter 16)
Ankle swelling	• Any – new or deterioration
Xanthomas	• Yellowish lipid deposits, especially on eyelids (xanthelasmas), cornea and tendons (Chapter 12)
Sore throat	• Persistent sore throat (Chapter 19) • Sore throat with rash, fever, enlarged lymph nodes or infected tonsils (Chapter 19) • Sore throat or rashes, especially in patients taking drugs known to cause neutropenia such as carbimazole, clozapine and carbamazepine (Chapter 5)
Sinusitis	• Sinus pain or discharge that does not resolve after 7 days (Chapter 19)

ACE, angiotensin-converting enzyme; NSAIDs, non-steroidal anti-inflammatory drugs.

to refer would be due to the failure of OTC medicines to control or relieve a condition or requests for OTC medicines that are not covered by their licence. In addition, the following examples of alerting symptoms should also prompt a referral.

Gastrointestinal

Some important gastrointestinal referral points are shown in Table 1.3.

Cardiorespiratory

Some important cardiorespiratory referral points are shown in Table 1.4.

Neurological and psychiatric

Some important neurological and psychiatric referral points are shown in Table 1.5.

Table 1.5   Some important neurological and psychiatric referral points

Leading feature	Features and comments
Headache (Chapter 22)	• Headache that is severe, follows injury or accompanied by other alerting signs • Recurrent or persistent migraine not relieved by OTC medicines
Seizures or loss of consciousness	• Any, including absences (Chapter 23)
Signs or behaviour pointing to psychiatric disorders	• Any (Chapters 24–27)
Insomnia	• With repeat requests (>2 weeks) for OTC sleeping remedies (Chapter 26)
Problems with movement or tremor	Refer for specialist opinion (Chapter 28)

OTC, over-the-counter.

Others

Some other important referral points are shown in Table 1.6.

This list of referrals is intended as a list of common examples that should prompt referral to the patient's GP or urgent referral to hospital. Obviously, if there is any doubt the patient should be referred and, as emphasized in Chapter 5, the pharmacist should be alert to the possibility of patients presenting with an adverse drug reaction (ADR). The list is clearly not exhaustive and local referral protocols may already be established with GPs.

Table 1.6   Some other important referral points

Leading feature	Features and comments
Symptoms suggestive of diabetes mellitus (Chapter 35)	• Including polydipsia (increased drinking), polyuria, recurrent thrush, frequent skin infections, ketone breath
Symptoms suggestive of hyperthyroidism (Chapter 36)	• Including tachycardia, palpitations, fine tremor, warm peripheries, bulging eyes
Symptoms suggestive of hypothyroidism (Chapter 36)	• Including tiredness, weight gain, cold intolerance, dry skin and hair, goitre, puffiness around the eyes
Cushingoid symptoms	• Features include moon face, thinning of the skin, easy bruising and central weight gain • Including patients taking corticosteroids
Problems with urination	• Difficulty in passing urine • Blood in urine • Recurrent thrush or cystitis • Urinary dysfunction suggestive of prostatic hypertrophy
Urogenital problems	• Vaginal bleeding; in pregnancy this should lead to urgent referral • Recurrent infections • Urinary dysfunction, including haematuria (passing blood) and prostate problems • Any renal problems

Continued

Table 1.6   (Continued)

Leading feature	Features and comments
Somatosensory problems	• Eye problems • Eye infections where OTC treatment is not appropriate or is ineffective. One should be mindful of the risk of serious eye conditions that require urgent referral • Hearing problems • Otitis media not responding to simple analgesia • Disturbances of balance
Dermatological problems (Chapter 34)	• Eczema for the first time • Infected eczema (bacterial infection, eczema herpeticum) • Impetigo • Use of OTC topical steroids for >1 week • Secondary infection of bites • Psoriasis • Rosacea • Acne after 2 months of OTC treatment or risk of scarring • Jaundice • Spider naevi • Changes in moles • Rodent ulcers • Chickenpox in patients taking steroids • Shingles • Rashes: especially after taking a drug. Non-blanching rashes where there is suspicion of meningitis should lead to immediate hospital referral • Burns larger than a thumbnail in size • Purpura (easy bruising), especially in patients taking either drugs associated with thrombocytopenia or warfarin
Lumps	Especially in: • breast • testicles • neck • armpit
Musculoskeletal	• Pain on weight bearing • Significant pain not relieved by simple analgesia • Any significant trauma at high speed or significant load • Any significant limb or motor dysfunction • Muscle pains with statins and/or fibrates (Chapter 12) • Tendon pain with certain drugs, including quinolones
Drugs	• Overdose of drugs (especially paracetamol) requires urgent referral to hospital, even in the absence of any symptoms
Travel	• Ill after foreign travel

OTC, over-the-counter

CASE STUDIES

Case studies on coughs

A cough may be trivial symptom, either reflecting a minor ailment or possibly associated with serious underlying disease. The following cases are intended to illustrate the possible causes.

Case 1

A 4 year old with a cough as the presenting symptom was taken to their pharmacist. The pharmacist asked the following questions:

- 'Is it nocturnal?' – this might point to asthma.
- 'How long has the child had a cough?' – this would identity chronic conditions such as asthma, whereas a shorter duration would be consistent with an infection.
- 'Is there a family history of asthma?' – a family history of asthma and/or atopy might suggest asthma.
- 'Is it productive?' – this might point to a bacterial chest infection.
- 'Is it productive of vast quantities of sputum?' – large amounts of sputum that may contain blood might point to bronchiectasis.
- 'Is it a dry cough?' – this might point to a simple upper respiratory tract infection.
- 'Is it associated with wheezing?' – this may point to bronchiolitis or asthma.
- 'Is he eating and drinking normally?' – this may give an indication as to how ill he is.

It was found that the cough was non-productive and of recent onset, and a diagnosis of a viral infection was made. Reassurance was given and paracetamol was recommended for any fever and the mother was advised to take the toddler to the GP if it was no better after 2 weeks or it worsened in that time.

Case 2

In the course of a morning, a number of 60 year olds present to their GP with coughs and additional questioning went along the lines of:

- 'Have you ever smoked?'
- 'Is it a dry or productive cough?'
- 'How long have you had it?'

Patient A: A productive cough of recent onset with green sputum.

- This is consistent with bacterial infection and a chest infection was diagnosed.

Patient B: A smoker with a productive cough over many years, which is worse in winter and the sputum is grey or sometimes green.

- Smoking is a major risk factor for respiratory diseases and a 'smoker's cough' is an early sign of COPD. His present condition is consistent with severe COPD with an infection. Haemoptysis (coughing up blood) may occur in other serious conditions such as tumour, which should be excluded. An exacerbation of COPD was diagnosed.

continued

CASE STUDIES (continued)

Patient C: Smoker with changes in cough characteristics or persistent dry cough and coughing up blood.

- This may be a presenting symptom of carcinoma and other signs (which may include: haemoptysis, digital clubbing, pleural pain, weight loss, signs of metastasis, central nervous system changes including fits) are all ominous symptoms of carcinoma. The suspicion of carcinoma was raised.

Patient D: Non-smoker with productive cough, haemoptysis, weight loss, night sweats and risk factor for tuberculosis (TB) (homeless).

- A productive cough is a major respiratory symptom and night sweats are consistent with TB and Hodgkin's disease. The suspicion of TB was raised.

Patient E: Cough and breathlessness on mild exertion and lying down in bed at night.

- The suspicion of chronic heart failure was raised.

Patient F: Cough while taking an ACE inhibitor for chronic heart failure.

- These might point to inadequate treatment or an ACE inhibitor-induced cough.

References

Blenkinsopp A, Paxton P (2002). *Symptoms in the Pharmacy*, 4th edn. Oxford: Blackwell Sciences.

Edwards C, Stillman P (2006). *Minor Illness or Major Disease? The clinical pharmacist in the community*, 4th edn. London: Pharmaceutical Press.

Rutter P (2004). *Community Pharmacy*. Edinburgh: Churchill Livingstone.

Online resources

www.nhsdirect.nhs.uk

The website of NHS Direct, with advice available on how patients should respond to symptoms.

2

Clinical laboratory tests

The following sections are intended as a guide to the most commonly used laboratory tests. Reference values are included as a guide and represent average population values. It should be noted that these values may alter according to the assay procedure, particularly when measuring enzymes, and local values should be sought when interpreting clinical data.

Clinical biochemistry

The monitoring of clinical biochemistry is used alongside clinical symptoms to diagnose disease, regulate drug therapy and identify adverse drug reactions. Biochemical blood tests include:

- urea and electrolytes (U&Es): a standard request may provide sodium, potassium, urea and creatinine levels
- liver function tests (LFTs)
- lipid profiles
- glucose and glycated haemoglobin (HbA1c)
- thyroid function tests (TFTs).

Urea and electrolytes

The plasma concentration of urea and the electrolytes sodium, potassium, calcium and magnesium in blood plasma is used to indicate renal function, dehydration and electrolyte disturbances caused by drugs or disease, e.g. the retention of electrolytes may indicate impaired renal function or electrolyte loss may occur due to diarrhoea and vomiting, or the overuse of diuretics.

Drugs and the monitoring of U&Es

The requirement for electrolyte monitoring is discussed in individual chapters. A summary of some important drug-related electrolyte disturbances is given in Table 2.1.

Renal function tests

Renal function is often predicted from the results obtained from U&E monitoring. The main indicators are urea and creatinine. Urea is produced by protein metabolism and levels are raised following high protein intake, renal impairment, tissue damage and/or catabolism. So, although levels may be elevated in renal disease, they do not provide a reliable estimate of renal function.

Creatinine is produced from creatine in the skeletal muscle at a fairly constant rate and in normal individuals is renally cleared, so plasma levels are an index of renal function. A more precise predictor of renal function is therefore calculated as an estimate of the glomerular filtration rate (GFR) calculated from the plasma creatinine levels (see Chapter 18) and adjusted for age, weight and sex. The ideal body weight (IBW) should be used if the patient's weight is more than 20% in excess of it. A more accurate GFR may be calculated by comparing the amount of creatinine collected in a 24-h urine sample to the blood plasma measurement, using the Cockcroft–Gault equation:

$$\text{Creatinine clearance (mL/min)} = \frac{1.23 \text{ (males) or } 1.04 \text{ (females)} \times 140 - \text{age (years)} \times \text{weight (kg)}}{\text{Serum creatinine (micromol/L)}}$$

Although creatinine levels and clearance have been used for many years as a measure of renal

Table 2.1   Examples of drugs causing electrolyte disturbances

Electrolyte disturbance	Symptoms	Drugs implicated
Hypokalaemia (reduced potassium)	Hypokalaemia due to fluid loss (consider diuretics, vomiting, diarrhoea); may occur in hepatic failure due to aldosterone release; may lead to neuromuscular disturbances, cramps, muscle weakness, and tetany leading to paralysis and respiratory failure. Arrhythmias may also occur, especially in patients at increased risk, e.g. taking digoxin	Especially thiazide and loop diuretics; β_2-adrenoceptor agonists, corticosteroids, lithium and theophylline
Hyperkalaemia (increased potassium)	Hyperkalaemia may lead to a limp paralysis, arrhythmias and sudden death, but is initially asymptomatic	ACE inhibitors, aldosterone receptor antagonists, analgesics, angiotensin II receptor antagonists, potassium salts (salt substitute, effervescent preparations, e.g. low-sodium cystitis products and potassium citrate mixture), potassium-sparing diuretics and heparin
Hyponatraemia (reduced sodium)	Symptoms of hyponatraemia include orthostatic hypotension, reduced skin turgidity, confusion and ultimately convulsions. Hyponatraemia due to excess water may present as anorexia, heart failure, muscle weakness and oedema	ACE inhibitors, aldosterone inhibitors, analgesics, antidepressants, carbamazepine, loop diuretics, omeprazole, potassium-sparing diuretics, thiazide diuretics, chlorpropamide and tolbutamide
Hypernatraemia (increased sodium)	Hypernatraemia occurs in renal failure, producing symptoms of confusion, drowsiness, lethargy, dry skin, hypotension, muscle twitching, peripheral vasoconstriction and ultimately coma	Corticosteroids, NSAIDs, lithium
Hypomagnesaemia (reduced magnesium)	Hypomagnesaemia increases the risk of arrhythmias	Aminoglycosides, bisphosphonates, immunosuppressants, loop diuretics and thiazide diuretics
Hypercalcaemia (increased calcium)	Symptoms of hypercalcaemia include abdominal pain, anorexia, constipation, fatigue, nausea and vomiting, polyuria with nocturia and thirst. Progression to confusion, delirium, psychosis, gallstones, renal impairment (due to calculi or stones), stupor and coma may occur	Androgens, antacids, calcium salts, fat-soluble vitamins, sex hormones, thiazide diuretics, vitamin A derivatives and vitamin D derivatives
Hypocalcaemia (decreased calcium)	Hypocalcaemia tends to be asymptomatic. Worsening hypocalcaemia may produce paraesthesia of the face, fingers and toes, tetany or prolonged tonic muscle spasms and ultimately convulsions and psychosis	Loop diuretics, bisphosphonates

ACE, angiotensin-converting enzyme; NSAIDs, non-steroidal anti-inflammatory drugs.

function, it is now recommended (by a National Service Framework) that it be assessed by estimated GFR (eGFR). This is based on a study by Levey and colleagues (1999) which indicated that the so-called modification of diet in renal disease (MDRD) formula gives a more reliable measure. The MDRD formula takes account of serum creatinine levels, gender, age, ethnic origin, serum nitrogen urea and albumin, and takes the form:

$$eGFR = 170 \times [Serum\ creatinine]^{-0.999} \times (Age)^{-0.176} \times (0.762\ if\ female) \times (1.180\ if\ patient\ black) \times [Serum\ urea\ nitrogen]^{-0.170} \times [Albumin]^{0.318}$$

and is reported in mL/min per 1.73 m^2 (where m^2 refers to body surface area).

This equation should not be used for children, malnourished patients, or in pregnancy, in acute renal failure or oedema. From the eGFR values, renal function is expressed as:

- eGFR >90 mL/min per 1.73 m^2: normal renal function
- eGFR 89–60 mL/min per 1.73 m^2: mild renal impairment
- eGFR 30–59 mL/min per 1.73 m^2: moderate renal impairment
- eGFR 15–29 mL/min per 1.73 m^2: severe renal impairment
- eGFR <15 mL/min per 1.73 m^2: established renal failure.

The use of drugs in renal impairment may involve the avoidance or reduction of doses, according to the extent to which the kidneys are involved in the elimination of drugs. Individual chapters should be consulted for more detail. Important examples of drugs to be used with caution, often at reduced doses and with regular monitoring, or avoided in renal failure include:

- non-steroidal anti-inflammatory drugs (NSAIDs)
- angiotensin-converting enzyme (ACE) inhibitors
- tetracycline
- metformin
- digoxin
- gold salts
- penicillamine

- ciclosporin
- lithium.

Liver function tests

Impaired liver function may be detected from alterations in the levels of bilirubin, the enzymes transaminase, alkaline phosphatase and/or γ-glutamyl transferase (transpeptidase; GGT), and albumin and coagulation factors (see Appendix 2). An assessment of the LFT can be used to identify liver disease. For further discussion of liver disease see Chapter 10 and for drug-related liver disease see Chapter 5.

Acute cellular damage

Damage to hepatocytes leads to hepatic enzymes leaking out of the liver cells and passing into the hepatic circulation. Therefore, blood plasma levels of the enzymes alanine transaminase (ALT) and aspartate transaminase (AST) are increased in patients with acute hepatocyte damage. However, they are somewhat non-specific and AST is also found in cardiac muscle and skeletal muscle and therefore blood levels may be raised following either damage to cardiac cells after a myocardial infarction or non-specific muscle damage.

The damaged liver also fails to clear bilirubin, a breakdown product from the haem component of red blood cells. The unconjugated form of bilirubin, termed 'free bilirubin', therefore builds up in the blood, causing a yellowing of the skin, together with pruritus (see Chapter 10).

Chronic cellular damage

Chronic cellular damage, such as alcohol-induced cirrhosis, results in the deposition of fibrous tissue in place of dysfunctional hepatocytes. Transaminase levels are often normal but synthetic activity of the liver may be impaired and this impacts on albumin and clotting factors, which are normally produced by the liver. Therefore patients may have hypoalbuminaemia and an increased prothrombin time (or international normalized ratio or INR: see Chapter 16) due to reduced clotting ability.

Cholestasis

In cholestasis, substances that are normally secreted by the liver build up due to impaired metabolism or excretion, e.g. in obstructive cholestasis the liver can no longer excrete bilirubin and alkaline phosphatase (ALP) also accumulates. The enzyme GGT is also elevated but is not a reliable indicator of cholestasis because it may be induced by drugs such as alcohol and anticonvulsants, thereby increasing levels in the absence of cholestasis. A drug history is useful in determining alternative causes of raised GGT levels.

Summary of LFT interpretation

In general, LFTs are considered abnormal when a value is more than double the maximum value of the normal reference range.

Acute hepatitis

- Large elevations of ALT and AST.
- Possible slight increases in ALP and GGT.
- Possible large elevation of bilirubin.
- Prothrombin time may occasionally be increased.
- No change in albumin levels.

Chronic cellular damage

- ALP, ALT and AST tend to be normal or only slightly increased.
- GGT levels may show an elevation.
- Albumin levels are low.
- Bilirubin levels may show marginal to large increases.
- Prothrombin time is prolonged.

Cholestasis

- ALP levels show a large increase.
- GGT is usually elevated.
- ALT and AST tend to be only marginally raised or normal.
- Bilirubin levels may show marginal to large increases.
- Albumin levels are normal.
- Prothrombin time may occasionally be increased.

Drugs requiring regular LFTs (see also individual chapters)

The requirement for monitoring LFTs when prescribing is indicated in individual chapters. Examples of drugs for which monitoring is appropriate include:

- statins
- fibrates
- amiodarone
- isotretinoin
- isoniazid
- methyldopa
- rifampicin
- rosiglitazone, pioglitazone
- sodium valproate
- sulfasalazine.

Herbal preparations should also be considered when patients present with signs of hepatic disease (see Chapters 4, 5 and 10).

Lipids

A full screen of lipids (see Chapter 12) from patients when fasting includes the measurement of:

- total cholesterol (ideal target <5.2 mmol/L)
- high-density-lipoprotein (HDL)-cholesterol (ideal: >0.9 mmol/L male, >1.2 mmol/L females and >20% of total cholesterol)
- low-density-lipoprotein (LDL)-cholesterol (<3.35–4.0 mmol/L)
- triglyceride (<2.1 mmol/L)
- ratio total cholesterol:HDL-cholesterol (<4.5).

Isotretinoin treatment may alter serum lipids and monitoring is recommended 1 month after treatment is initiated and again at the end of treatment (Chapter 5).

Glucose

See Chapter 35.

Thyroid function tests

Thyroid function is determined by comparing clinical features, as discussed in Chapter 36, with biochemical values of thyroid-stimulating hormone (TSH), free thyroxine (fT_4) and free tri-iodothyronine (fT_3). Drug treatments requiring regular monitoring of thyroid function include lithium and amiodarone (see Chapters 5 and 36).

Summary

Monitoring requirements are also considered within individual chapters. Further information can be found in the summary of product characteristics (SPCs), in the latest *British National Formulary* or direct from the drug manufacturer. It should be noted that requirements for monitoring change according to the clinical presentation of the patient, together with risk factors. For monitoring of drug levels in blood plasma, see Chapter 6 and Appendix 2.

Haematology

Haematological monitoring is used as a general screening test to aid the diagnosis of inflammatory conditions or drug-related blood dyscrasias, identify anaemias and monitor coagulation such as during warfarin therapy. Tests include (see Appendix 2):

- full blood count (FBC): standard request provides haemoglobin, white blood cell count (WBC), platelets, mean cell volume (MCV), mean corpuscular haemoglobin (MCH), red blood cell count (RBC), haematocrit (Hct) and estimates of differentiated types of white blood cells
- erythrocyte sedimentation rate (ESR)
- blood coagulation
- vitamin B_{12} and folate.

Full blood count

Appendix 2 summarizes some of the main haematological parameters measured. Drugs requiring a regular FBC include immunosuppressants, clozapine and methyldopa.

Monitoring of oral anticoagulants

See Chapter 16.

Immunological tests

These tests generally involve the detection of antibodies that may point to autoimmune disease or may indicate general immune status. The following tests are used:

- Autoantibody or autoimmune screening includes the detection of antibodies to preparations of thyroid cytoplasm, parietal cells, mitochondria, smooth muscle, and liver or kidney microsomes.
- Rheumatoid factor: a positive test confirms a diagnosis of rheumatoid arthritis/autoimmune rheumatoid disorders.
- C-reactive protein (CRP) is elevated during infection and/or severe inflammation and may be repeated to monitor the outcome of treatment. CRP is more specific for inflammation, necrosis or infection and changes more rapidly than ESR.
- Thyroid antibodies (Graves' disease: see Chapter 36).
- Immunoglobulins: patients presenting with epigastric pain may be tested for the presence of serum immunoglobulin G (IgG) against *Helicobacter pylori* infection (see Chapter 7).
- Paul–Bunnell test (infectious mononucleosis or glandular fever) in response to persistent sore throat, lethargy, fever, headache and cervical adenopathy.
- Prostate-specific antigen (PSA): a positive test provides an early indication of prostate cancer even when the patient is asymptomatic. This is, however, a relatively non-specific test, because only a proportion of patients who have a high value have malignancy.

Microbiology

Microbiology tests are performed on samples such as urine, sputum, cerebrospinal fluid, faeces, or swabs from the vagina or cervix, nose or eyes. These tests tend to be requested when treatment has failed, or sinister causes are suspected, e.g. in symptoms suggestive of meningitis or if there is a risk of sexually transmitted infections such as chlamydia infection, gonorrhoea or syphilis.

References

Levey AS, Bosch JP, Lewis JB *et al* (1999). A more accurate method to estimate glomerular filtration rate from serum creatinine: A new prediction equation. *Ann Intern Med* **130**: 461–70.

Martin J, ed. *British National Formulary*, latest edition. London: British Medical Association and Royal Pharmaceutical Society of Great Britain.

Further reading

Barber N, Wilson A, eds (1999). *Clinical Pharmacy Survival Guide*. London: Churchill Livingstone.

Harman RJ, Mason P, eds (2002). *Handbook of Pharmacy Health Care*, 2nd edn. London: Pharmaceutical Press.

Hoffbrand AV, Pettit JE, Moss PAH (2001). *Essential Haematology*, 4th edn. Oxford: Blackwell Science.

Lee A, ed. (2006). *Adverse Drug Reactions*, 2nd edn. London: Pharmaceutical Press.

McGhee M (2000). *A Guide to Laboratory Investigations*, 3rd edn. Oxford: Radcliffe Medical Press.

3

Lifestyle

Lifestyle interventions are essential to the prevention and treatment of almost all diseases. There is therefore a move towards greater emphasis on promoting healthy lifestyle in the management of disease. This is not an easy task as the harm caused by an unhealthy lifestyle may not be experienced for a number of years; conversely some benefits of improving lifestyle are not always observed immediately, thereby reducing motivation of patients to make these changes. Added to this, people do not respond well to being told to change their lifestyle and even those willing to change may find it difficult to change lifelong habits.

A useful approach is to provide education as to the benefits of pursuing a healthy lifestyle and regular support in implementing changes. This can take the form of poster campaigns, the provision of verbal and written advice, health clinics, and signposting to useful internet sites and health clubs.

The aim of this chapter is to emphasize the importance of providing lifestyle advice alongside drug treatment and highlight current recommendations. The effects of diet on drug treatment are also considered.

Clinical features

Typically an unhealthy lifestyle includes excessive calorific intake, particularly from saturated fat, sugar and alcohol. A vicious circle of weight gain, fatigue, low self-esteem and lack of motivation to exercise then develops and poor health will inevitably follow. The following are just some conditions caused or exacerbated by an unhealthy lifestyle:

- anxiety
- arthritis
- cancer
- depression
- diabetes mellitus
- dyspepsia
- ischaemic heart disease
- hypertension
- stroke
- liver disease
- osteoporosis.

A healthy diet

A healthy diet comprises an intake of calories appropriate for energy expenditure and from a variety of food groups, to include a balance of carbohydrate, non-starch polysaccharides (NSPs), protein, fats, water, and vitamins and minerals.

A useful way to explain the balance of food for a healthy diet is to display a picture of 'the wheel of good health', which shows a plate divided into segments with proportions relevant to a healthy intake of each food type. Fruit and vegetables and bread, cereals and potatoes therefore dominate the picture. Changes often required are a reduction in fat, particularly saturated fat, sugar and salt intake. Another important recommendation is the intake of five portions of a variety of fruit and vegetables daily (see Williams 1995). A diet rich in fruit and vegetables has been estimated to reduce heart disease, stroke and cancer by up to 20% (Department of Health 2000). The World Health Organization (WHO) estimates that up to 2.7 million lives worldwide could be saved each year with increased fruit and vegetable consumption (WHO 2003). The health benefits are due to complex interactions of vitamins, minerals and phytochemicals including flavonoids, glucosinilates and phyto-oestrogens, some of which have protective antioxidant properties. Fruit and vegetables are also an important source of NSPs.

A portion of fruit and vegetables including canned, frozen and dried products is defined as 80 g for adults and children over 5 years of age. A common misconception is that fruit and vegetables count only if they are fresh. Consuming five portions or more a day is therefore easier than many people think. Fruit juice (150 mL) may be counted once a day and baked beans also count. Potatoes are excluded because these represent a 'starchy staple'. It should be noted that intake should be appropriate to age, sex and activity. An approximate guide (Food Standards Agency or FSA 2001) is:

1 desert bowlful of salad
1 banana, apple or orange
1 cupful or handful of grapes, cherries or similar
½–1 tablespoonful of dried fruit.

The FSA (2005) has produced some guidelines for a healthy diet:

- The dominance of starchy food in a meal.
- A diet rich in fruit and vegetables.
- Increased consumption of oily fish (at least one portion per week, see Chapter 12).
- Reducing saturated fat and sugar.
- Reducing salt (maximum 6 g/day, see Chapter 11).
- Maintaining a healthy weight.
- Increasing water intake.
- The importance of breakfast for controlling weight.

Drug–food Interactions

A number of clinically significant interactions including food have been reported and the reader should consult *Stockley's Drug Interactions* (Baxter 2008). Food interactions may predictably involve absorption interactions but also effects on cytochrome P450 isoenzymes, leading to metabolic interactions. An important example is that constituents of grapefruit juice are inhibitors of CYP3A4 and so may inhibit drug metabolism by this isoenzyme, leading to increased plasma concentrations and the risk of adverse events. Examples of drugs that may be affected by consumption of grapefruit juice include amiodarone, felodipine, nisoldipine, verapamil (and possibly other calcium channel blockers), sildenafil, vardenafil and simvastatin. Table 3.1 includes other examples of clinically significant food–drug interactions.

Diet and mental health

Not surprisingly, mental well-being may be associated with diet. However, specific evidence for this relationship is limited, although the Mental Health Foundation (Cornah 2006) has sought to raise awareness of this area by drawing attention to the need for dietary considerations as part of mental health care. Mental disorders including depression, schizophrenia, neurodegenerative conditions and drug abuse are well known to be associated with poor nutritional status, possibly leading to a vicious cycle of decline.

The brain is composed largely of essential fatty acids, protein and water, and has a high energy demand. It is therefore not surprising that diets lacking in important nutrients such as essential fatty acids have been implicated in mental disorders including depression, schizophrenia and attention deficit hyperactivity disorder. Dietary amino acids such as tyramine and tryptophan are essential precursors of the monoamine neurotransmitters, important for mood control, and the depletion of dietary tryptophan precipitates relapse in depressed patients in remission. Tryptophan is present in meat, fish, eggs, milk, cheese, nuts, beans, lentils, vegetable protein and mycoprotein, and it is therefore important that at least one of these proteins forms part of each meal.

Poor eating habits result in large fluctuations in blood glucose levels, which have a deleterious effect on brain function and exacerbate conditions such as anxiety. Low blood sugar leads to low mood, irritability and fatigue, with the temptation to eat sugary food for a quick 'high'.

Table 3.1   Drug interactions with food

Interaction	Consequences	Comments
Aspirin with vitamin C	Reduced absorption of vitamin C	Aspirin reduces the absorption of vitamin C by approximately a third
Bisphosphonates with food, iron or zinc	Reduced absorption by polyvalent cations	Alendronate, ibandronic acid and risedronate should be taken at least 30 min before the first food of the day. Clodronate should be taken at least 1 h before or after food. Etidronate and tiludronate should be given at least 2 h before or after food. Timing should be similar for polyvalent cations, which are also present in antacids
Ciprofloxacin and norfloxacin with dairy products, zinc or iron	Reduced bioavailability	Avoid dairy products within 1–2 h of these antibiotics. Note that enteral feeds may also reduce absorption significantly. Quinolones should also be taken 2 h before zinc and iron
Colestyramine or orlistat with fat-soluble vitamins (A, D, E, K)	Reduced absorption of vitamins	Supplements may be required with long-term treatment. Supplements should be taken at least 2 h after orlistat or at bedtime and 1 h before or 4–6 h after colestyramine
Diuretics or lithium with sodium chloride (salt)	Excess salt increases excretion of lithium, reducing levels. Conversely, reducing salt intake increases lithium levels. Sodium chloride opposes beneficial effects of diuretics by increasing water retention by kidney	Patients prescribed lithium should be counselled about maintaining salt and fluid intake. Patients prescribed diuretics should avoid excess salt in their diet
Isoniazid	Reduced absorption. Histamine poisoning reaction may occur with mature cheese and some fish (e.g. salmon, tuna, mackerel)	Advise patients to take at least 30 min before or 2 h after food. Check diet if patients report chills, diarrhoea, flushing, itching, headache, tachycardia and/or wheeze
Isotretinoin with vitamin A (retinol)	A condition similar to vitamin A overdose may result from concurrent administration	High doses of vitamin A (>4000–5000 units) should be avoided with isotretinoin
Lansoprazole	Bioavailability reduced by up to 50%	Lansoprazole should be taken at least an hour before food
MAOIs	Risk of life-threatening hypertensive crisis with tyramine-rich foods such as cheese, salami, yeast extracts, pickled herrings and some beers and wines	Patients prescribed irreversible MAOIs such as phenelzine should avoid these foods. Large amounts of these foods may affect some patients taking the reversible MAOI moclobemide

Continued

Table 3.1   (Continued)

Interaction	Consequences	Comments
Methotrexate, phenobarbital, phenytoin primidone With folates, vitamin D	Methotrexate acts as a folate antagonist, the latter therefore affecting toxic and therapeutic effects Folate deficiency may occur with long-term phenobarbital, phenytoin or primidone treatment but supplements should be introduced with monitoring because serum levels of antiepileptics may fall Long-term phenytoin use can lead to osteomalacia, large doses of vitamin D supplementation may be required	Folic acid is given with methotrexate to reduce adverse effects
Tetracyclines with dairy products, iron and zinc	Milk and other dairy products and dietary calcium reduce the absorption of most tetracyclines significantly Zinc reduces absorption by up to 50%	Take 1 h before food or 2 h after Doxycycline and minocycline less affected by food 3 h separation between drug and iron or zinc may be required (see *Stockley's Drug Interactions* (2008))
Warfarin (and other coumarins)	Cranberry juice can produce potentially life-threatening increases in INR Vitamin K reduces the effects of warfarin, a vitamin K antagonist	The MCA/MHRA recommend that patients limit or avoid drinking cranberry juice or taking other cranberry products Large changes in consumption of vitamin K-containing foods, e.g. green vegetables, green tea and vitamin K supplements, should be avoided Less significant interactions may occur with supplements, e.g. fish oils, glucosamine, coenzyme Q10, vitamin E, though patients should have their INR checked when starting these preparations.

INR, international normalized ratio; MAOI, monoamine oxidase inhibitor; MCA, Medicines Control Agency; MHRA, Medicines and Healthcare products Regulatory Agency.

However, the relief is temporary due to insulin release, and low mood and fatigue soon return. The consumption of complex carbohydrate, described as low glycaemic index (GI) foods, is therefore important for the regulation of blood sugar levels, preventing mood swings and enabling optimum functioning of the brain. Examples of foods with a low or medium GI include porridge, sweet corn, pasta, baked beans and pitta bread, Excessive consumption of caffeine and alcohol can also be detrimental to mental health because they alter the structure and function of the brain.

Alcohol

The consumption of excess alcohol is associated with acute health risks (e.g. poisoning, accidents), and chronic disease such as cardiovascular disease, cancer, hepatic disease and mental health problems. The high calories associated with alcohol also contribute towards the risk of obesity and associated morbidity. Alcohol misuse continues to be a major health concern with binge drinking a particular problem that impacts on society and health service resources.

Pharmacists should be alert for patients presenting with effects of alcohol misuse and provide information of local services providing specialist help (Mason 2003). Symptoms include irritability, anxiety, insomnia, smelling of alcohol, self-neglect and unsteady gait. Signs of chronic alcohol abuse may include reddening of the palms and signs of alcoholic liver disease such as spider naevi (see Chapter 34) and jaundice (see Chapter 10).

Pharmacological activity

Alcohol has central nervous system (CNS)-depressant and disinhibitory effects through non-specific actions similar to those of general anaesthetics. Peripheral effects of alcohol include increased gastric acid secretions, resulting in chronic gastritis. Hormonal effects can include reduced synthesis of testosterone (which may lead to impotence), reduced release of anti-diuretic hormone (which causes diuresis and may lead to dehydration, which contributes to a 'hangover') and increased levels of corticosteroids.

Long-term effects

Long-term alcohol abuse is in some, but not all, patients associated with liver damage. Initial changes involve reversible fatty infiltration of the liver and may proceed to cirrhosis of the liver (see Chapter 10). Alcoholism is also associated with thiamine (vitamin B_1) deficiency, due to malnutrition and impaired metabolism, and this may lead to neurological problems such as Wernicke's encephalopathy. Excessive alcohol consumption is also associated with cancer of the mouth, larynx and oesophagus.

Current guidelines in the UK recommend that the safe limits of weekly alcohol consumption are 14 units for women and 21 units for men, where a unit is defined as one small glass of wine, a 'shot' of spirit or a half-pint of weak beer. However, there is confusion as to what constitutes a unit and, for example, generous self-measures of wine in large glasses may yield several units. For guidance, on average a bottle of wine contains approximately 10 units and one pint of strong lager contains 3 or more units. The recommendations also suggest that women should not consume more than 2–3 units and men 3–4 units per day to avoid binge drinking. It is also recommended to have 2 days a week without consuming alcohol. Despite these guidelines for safe drinking, consumption of alcohol in excess of these limits is widespread and some authorities regard consumption of more than 35 units per week as hazardous.

The recommendations for drinking in pregnancy have varied over the years but the most recent evidence suggests that there is no safe limit and current guidelines recommend that alcohol should not be consumed during pregnancy. If expectant mothers do drink, this should be limited to no more than 1–2 units and on no more than two occasions per week. Alcohol can also affect conception and so those wishing to conceive should limit alcohol consumption or stop drinking.

Drug interactions

The main interaction occurring between drugs and alcohol is with other drugs with CNS-depressant activity. This includes analgesics, anticonvulsants, antidepressants, sedating antihistamines, benzodiazepines and antipsychotics (also risk of postural hypotension), increasing side effects and the ability to perform skilled tasks such as driving. Other examples of drugs interactions with alcohol are detailed in Table 3.2.

Caffeine

Caffeine consumption has become increasingly fashionable and caffeine dependence, together with patients increasing their intake due to the development of tolerance, is more common although not easily defined. The effect of caffeine on health may be minimal compared with alcohol. However, it can be a neglected cause of symptoms that may be confused with other conditions. Patients presenting with the following

Table 3.2   Drug interactions with alcohol

Drug	Consequences	Comments
Antihypertensives	Reduced effect of antihypertensives Risk of additive effect of hypotension	Alcohol increases blood pressure (see text) so patients should be advised to reduce alcohol intake
Central nervous system depressants	See text	
Isoniazid	Increased effect on driving and risk of hepatitis Effects of isoniazid possibly reduced	Alcohol intake should be limited
Lithium	Impaired performance of skilled tasks such as driving	Patients should be advised accordingly
Methotrexate	Increased risk of hepatic cirrhosis and fibrosis	Manufacturers recommend that patients taking methotrexate avoid drugs, including alcohol, associated with hepatotoxicity
Metoclopramide	Increased absorption of alcohol	Patients should be advised of this and the possible effect on driving and other skilled tasks
Metronidazole	Disulfiram (flushing)-type reaction	Patients should be warned because this reaction is unpleasant and potentially frightening
Paracetamol	Increased risk of hepatotoxicity with heavy drinking	Close monitoring is recommended for heavy drinkers prescribed regular paracetamol
Phenytoin	Increased serum phenytoin levels	Dose increase may be required for heavy drinkers Note that dose may need to be reduced in hepatic impairment
Verapamil	Increased blood alcohol levels and prolonged effects	Patients should be warned

symptoms should therefore be asked about their caffeine intake: anxiety and/or panic, increased blood pressure, tremor, dyspepsia, dizziness, headaches, insomnia, palpitations, vertigo and tinnitus. Excess caffeine intake is also associated with withdrawal effects including headache, fatigue, anxiety, depression and poor concentration.

Pharmacology

Caffeine is a methylxanthine compound, therefore exhibiting similar pharmacology to other methylxanthines such as theophylline. These act as adenosine receptor antagonists, opposing the inhibitory effect of adenosine pathways in the CNS. Methylxanthines also inhibit phosphodiesterases and so augment the actions of catecholamines, leading to an increase in heart rate and bronchodilatation. Diuresis is thought to occur following renal vasodilatation, leading to an increase in glomerular filtration rate. Caffeine also stimulates gastrin production and may therefore exacerbate gastrointestinal disease.

Drug interactions

There appear to be few clinically significant interactions with caffeine, with the exception of reduced clearance in the presence of disulfiram. Increased levels of caffeine may produce symptoms similar to those of alcohol withdrawal and patients should therefore be advised to limit caffeine consumption. As caffeine stimulates the release of catecholamines, resulting in increased heart rate and blood pressure, caffeine intake should be limited by patients prescribed medication for cardiovascular disease and anxiety. Additional drug–disease interactions may include excessive intake of caffeine in patients taking medication for gastrointestinal disease.

Food supplements

Patients may request food supplements and advice given should be evidence based. In general, supplements such as vitamins and minerals should not replace a healthy balanced diet and high doses of single vitamins or minerals should be avoided. Indeed, a major conclusion from the Heart Protection Study (2002) was that antioxidant supplementation with vitamins A, C and E was not associated with an improvement in mortality of high-risk patients and that a balanced diet was more appropriate. Furthermore, some studies have now revealed harmful effects of these antioxidant supplements as highlighted by a recent Cochrane review (Bjelakovic *et al* 2008).

Despite concerns over indiscriminate use of certain vitamins, it is clear that special groups (such as pregnant and breast-feeding women, infants, children, adolescents, vegans, elderly people and those who are convalescing) benefit from and indeed require vitamin and mineral supplementation. Some examples of appropriate recommendations of supplements are summarized in Table 3.3. It should also be noted that vitamin and mineral supplements supplied within the EU are currently regulated by the Food Supplements Directive, which came into effect in the UK in 2005.

Exercise

It has long been known that physical activity is important for good health. However, scientific evidence is increasingly quantifying the contribution of physical activity to health and disease. A report commissioned by the British government found that physical activity reduces the risk of coronary heart disease, stroke and type 2 diabetes by 50% and premature death by 20–30% (Wanless 2004). There is also evidence for the therapeutic benefits for these diseases and also musculoskeletal disorders such as osteoarthritis. Communication of this information to patients can be an important motivator for increasing physical activity. Indeed, in 2004 the UK's Chief Medical Officer recommended that adults should exercise for at least 30 minutes each day for at least 5 days a week for health benefits. The 30 minutes may consist of an accumulation of 10-minute sessions, which may include simple changes such as walking for a bus instead of driving. This level of activity has been shown to reduce the risks highlighted above, together with improving mental health and reducing the risk of many cancers. Prolonged activity up to 45–60 minutes a day is recommended to prevent obesity and 60 minutes for young people and children, including exercise for bone health, muscle strength and flexibility.

Stress

Prolonged excessive stress is known to be detrimental to health, being associated with mental health problems, reduced immunity and cardiovascular disease, e.g. a recent study of over 10 000 civil servants found that stress at work increases the risk of the metabolic syndrome, a predictor for the development of cardiovascular disease and type 2 diabetes (Chandola *et al* 2006). Patients presenting with insomnia, changes in appetite, panic attacks, muscle pain, headaches, hypercholesterolaemia, gastrointestinal problems and low mood would particularly benefit from advice regarding stress reduction, such as taking regular exercise.

Tobacco smoke

Tobacco smoking is the single most harmful lifestyle activity and is clearly linked to cancers,

Table 3.3   Recommendation of food supplements

Special considerations for use of vitamins and minerals	Supplement	Comments
Alcohol misuse	Thiamine (vitamin B$_1$) and multivitamins	Risk of Wernicke's encephalopathy and Korsakoff's psychosis necessitates thiamine supplementation in chronic alcoholism. Multivitamins may also be recommended because diet is likely to be poor
Individuals who are elderly, housebound or have low exposure to sunlight	Vitamin D	Consider additional risk factors for osteoporosis and long-term treatment with drugs such as phenytoin
Preconception to first 12 weeks of pregnancy	Folic acid 400 micrograms	For the prevention of neural tube defects Patients prescribed proguanil or antiepileptic drugs, e.g. phenytoin require 5 mg on prescription
Ante- or postnatally, following surgery, menorrhagia, vegetarians, symptoms of deficiency, e.g. breathlessness on exertion	Iron	Patients may request iron supplements over-the-counter and it is important that appropriate questions are asked to assess the risk of anaemia. Some preparations do not contain adequate levels of iron salts and patients should be referred to their GP for a blood test and an appropriate dose prescribed
Vegetarians	Calcium, vitamin D, iron and vitamin B$_{12}$	Vegan vegetarians are particularly at risk of nutrient deficiency due to the absence of meat and dairy products in the diet (the Food Standards Agency and Vegan Society at www.vegansociety.com provide useful information)

respiratory disorders and cardiovascular disease. Smoking cessation may therefore be considered to be the most important intervention by health professionals in the treatment and prevention of disease. The powerful addictive nature of nicotine, however, makes this an extremely difficult task, although the availability of nicotine replacement therapy (NRT) has improved quit rates in combination with support and will power.

Pharmacological activity

Tobacco smoke contains nicotine, carcinogenic tars (polycyclic hydrocarbons) and carbon monoxide. Nicotine stimulates subtypes of nicotinic receptors leading to neuronal excitation. These receptors are distributed on neurons in the brain and on autonomic ganglia and neuromuscular synapses (mainly in the heart and lungs) in the periphery. Carbon monoxide reduces the oxygen-carrying capacity of haemoglobin, contributing further to the adverse cardiovascular effects outlined above. Irritant, carcinogenic and other toxic substances found in cigarette smoke include arsenic, benzene, lead, DDT (dichloro-diphenyltrichloroethane, an insecticide), nitric acid and toluene (methylbenzene). Carcinogenic tars may lead to chronic obstructive pulmonary disease (COPD) and cancer of the lungs, upper respiratory tract, oesophagus, pancreas and bladder.

Treatment of nicotine addiction

Patients who smoke more than 10 cigarettes a day may benefit from nicotine replacement, counselling and support. All preparations of NRT have been shown to be effective in smoking cessation, with cessation rates increased by 50–70% (Cochrane review by Stead *et al* 2007). The National Institute for Health and Clinical Excellence guidance (NICE 2002) recommends that NRT or bupropion should be prescribed only after the agreement of a target stop date with the smoker. Initial treatment is for 2 weeks for NRT or 3–4 weeks of bupropion. The dosage form is selected according to patient preference. Bupropion may also be used but current NICE (2002) guidelines do not recommend concurrent use with NRT.

Withdrawal symptoms include:

- dysphoric or depressed mood
- insomnia
- irritability, frustration or anger
- anxiety
- difficulty concentrating
- restlessness
- decreased heart rate
- increased appetite and weight gain.

Varenicline, a partial nicotinic receptor agonist, is a recent introduction to aid smoking cessation and is recommended for patients wanting to stop smoking and preferably in addition to behavioural support (NICE 2007). As a partial agonist, it will provide weak stimulation to reduce withdrawal reactions but oppose the actions of nicotine itself.

Concurrent disease

Some considerations of prescribing or recommending therapy for smoking cessation in concurrent diseases are detailed in Table 3.4.

Drug interactions and adverse effects

Tobacco smoke

Components of tobacco smoke, thought to be polycyclic hydrocarbons, induce cytochrome P450 enzymes in the liver, thereby increasing the metabolism of some drugs, e.g. the metabolism of theophylline is accelerated in smokers and so higher dosages are required. However, on cessation the induction of enzyme activity will be reduced and so the dosage should be decreased.

Increased insulin-opposing hormones caused by smoking necessitate greater insulin doses in people with diabetes who smoke and a reduced dosage on cessation of smoking (*Stockley's Drug Interactions* – Baxter 2008). Smoking also adds to the already increased cardiovascular risk of patients with diabetes mellitus. A further increased risk of thromboembolic disease occurs in women taking oral contraceptives if they also smoke.

Bupropion

The increased risk of seizures should be considered when co-prescribing drugs known to lower the seizure threshold (see Chapters 5 and 23). A maximum dose of 150 mg daily of bupropion is recommended when prescribed with other drugs that lower the convulsive threshold.

Bupropion also exhibits a number of metabolic interactions including with antipsychotics such as haloperidol and risperidone, antiepileptics (note that bupropion is contraindicated in epilepsy), selective serotonin reuptake inhibitors (SSRIs) and tricyclic antidepressants. The effects of these interactions should be monitored carefully. Adverse effects of bupropion may also occur in combination with drugs competing for the same metabolic enzymes, e.g. valproate, ritonavir, clopidogrel, paroxetine and fluoxetine. Note that the long half-life of drugs such as fluoxetine may also increase the risk of interactions after the cessation of treatment.

Varenicline

Drug–disease interactions are detailed in Table 3.4.

General counselling

For smoking cessation to be successful, patients must make the decision to stop. Health professionals therefore need to recognize the

Table 3.4   Concurrent disease and prescribing of smoking cessation aids (derived from the *British National Formulary* [BNF])

Disease	Cautions and contraindications	Comments
Cardiovascular disease, including peripheral vascular disease	Nicotine products are used with caution in severe cardiovascular disease such as: • severe arrhythmias • recent myocardial infarction, TIA or CVA Monitoring is appropriate for other conditions	These patients should be encouraged to stop smoking due to the adverse effects outlined in the text Monitoring for signs of deterioration is required. The harmful effects produced by toxic components of smoke are obviously removed but unwanted effects due to nicotine remain. This information may be useful for patients reluctant to stop using NRT
Depression, bipolar disorder	The use of bupropion is contraindicated Varenicline has been associated with depression (MHRA) and should be used with caution in patients with a history of psychiatric disease	Increased risk of precipitating or exacerbating the manic phase
Diabetes mellitus	NRT and bupropion should be used only with caution	See risk of seizures with bupropion use in diabetes mellitus The effects of nicotine may mask the signs of hypoglycaemia and increase the risk of damage to the microvascular circulation Smoking cessation is imperative in these patients due to the increased risk of diabetic complications (Chapter 35) and NRT may be useful in the short term with monitoring
Epilepsy, risk of seizures	Bupropion is contraindicated when there is a risk of seizures as follows: • a history of seizures or eating disorders • a CNS tumour • during acute withdrawal from alcohol or benzodiazepines	Buproprion may be used with caution and close monitoring when benefit exceeds risk in the following situations: • alcohol abuse • history of head trauma • diabetes • concurrent use of stimulants or anorectic drugs, which may lower the seizure threshold (e.g. antidepressants, antimalarials, sedating antihistamines, corticosteroids, theophylline, tramadol)
Hyperthyroidism	NRT should be used only with caution	Nicotine may exacerbate symptoms of hyperthyroidism and complicate its management
History of gastritis and peptic ulcer	NRT should be used with caution	Nicotine may worsen gastritis and peptic ulcer disease and patients should be monitored accordingly. Smoking cessation is, however, particularly important for these patients

Continued

Table 3.4   (Continued)

Disease	Cautions and contraindications	Comments
Pregnancy and breast-feeding	Bupropion is contraindicated. NRT should be used only when attempts to quit without it have failed	Smoking cessation should be strongly encouraged in pregnant women and those with young children Intermittent use of NRT is preferred and avoiding liquorice-flavoured products
Chronic generalized skin disease	Nicotine patches are contraindicated	NRT patches should not be used on broken skin
Renal and hepatic impairment	NRT, bupropion and varenicline should be used with caution	• Dose adjustment may be required (BNF appendices 2 and 3) • Avoid bupropion in severe hepatic cirrhosis

CNS, central nervous system; CVA, cerebrovascular accident; MHRA, Medicines and Healthcare products Regulatory Agency; NRT, nicotine replacement therapy; TIA, transient ischaemic attack.

different stages involved in arriving at this decision. This ranges from the patient who has never considered stopping smoking to the patient who is ready to stop. Information leaflets may be given to patients who smoke and encouragement to stop smoking given at every opportunity. A successful attempt to quit is more likely when the patient has actually made the decision and is ready to stop. The patient should be advised to set a date to stop smoking completely and discard all remaining cigarettes. The importance of willpower and the use of NRT to alleviate the symptoms of withdrawal should be stressed.

The following points may help the patient to be successful:

• Explain that chest symptoms such as increased secretions may occur initially on cessation but these should abate within 2–3 weeks.
• Try to avoid situations associated with smoking, e.g. take up a hobby in the evening if this is when most cigarettes are smoked.
• Encourage the patient to return with questions or difficulties.
• Avoid excess intake of caffeine because this may worsen the withdrawal effect of nicotine.
• A list of the benefits of smoking cessation may particularly help patients who are long-term smokers. Rapid improvements in taste and sense of smell, circulation and lung function

are experienced. The risk of a heart attack decreases rapidly on smoking cessation (Kenfield et al 2008).
• Other benefits include increased exercise capacity, reduced odour, avoiding premature ageing of the skin and tooth loss.

NRT (patches, gum, inhalator, lozenges, sublingual, nasal spray)

• The nasal spray should not be used when driving due to the risk of sneezing or watery eyes.
• Side effects include nausea, dizziness, headache, cold and influenza-like symptoms, palpitations, dyspepsia, insomnia and vivid dreams (particularly with the 24-h patch). The 24-h patch should be removed if these symptoms are troublesome: a 16-h patch may be more suitable.
• Patches should not be applied to broken skin.
• Patches are not appropriate for occasional smokers.

Bupropion

• Side effects include dry mouth, gastrointestinal disturbances, insomnia, tremor, tachycardia and hypertension.
• Blood pressure should be monitored weekly if bupropion is used with NRT. Patients who

relapse should be encouraged to self-refer due to the risk of increased blood pressure.

- Bupropion should be used with caution when driving or performing skilled tasks.
- Bupropion increases the risk of side effects with over-the-counter (OTC) cough preparations containing dextromethorphan.

Varenicline

- Start 1–2 weeks before target stop date.
- Avoid abrupt withdrawal.
- Side effects include gastrointestinal disturbances, changes to appetite, dry mouth, taste disturbance, headache, dizziness and sleep disorders.
- Report changes in mood to GP.
- May affect driving, so patients should not drive until they know they are not affected.

Over-the-counter medicines

OTC medicines are also prone to misuse and this may complicate diagnosis and use of prescribed medication that may interact. Examples of OTC drugs associated with abuse include the following:

- Sedative antihistamines, including those contained in cough medicines, may be used chronically for insomnia, leading to dependence (see Chapter 26).
- Laxatives may be misused for weight loss, particularly by female patients and those suffering from anorexia nervosa.
- Patients addicted to opioids may misuse codeine and other opioid-containing preparations, such as kaolin and morphine. The antihistamine cyclizine is also subject to misuse by these patients as it is thought to increase the effects of opioids.
- Sympathomimetics such as ephedrine and pseudoephedrine are used for their alerting and euphoric effects, for fatigue, improving athletic performance (see banned substances in the *British National Formulary*), for weight loss, to reduce craving for amphetamines and for the manufacture of amphetamines.
- Caffeine-containing products include some analgesics and preparations marketed for

increased energy, e.g. Pro Plus and drinks such as Red Bull (see Caffeine above).

Contraception

The choice of contraception is an important lifestyle decision for sexually active people and this is a critical area for health promotion. The transmission of sexually transmitted infections such as chlamydia infection is on the increase and some pharmacies are providing screening, treatment and sexual health promotion services as part of the National Chlamydia Screening programme. The prescribing of hormonal contraception is considered below in relation to the presence of concurrent disease and drug interactions.

Pharmacology

Hormonal contraception comprises a combination of oestrogen and a progestogen (combined oral contraceptive, COC) or a progestogen alone (POP). These agents modify the hormonal control of the menstrual cycle and in particular the oestrogens inhibit the release of follicle-stimulating hormone (FSH) from the anterior pituitary, preventing the development of ovarian follicles. Progestogens inhibit the release of luteinizing hormone (LH), preventing ovulation, and also alter the cervical mucus to prevent insemination. Both hormones affect the endometrium and oppose implantation.

Hormonal contraception may be administered as an oral tablet, dermal implant or injection. COCs are also prescribed to reduce symptoms of menstrual disorders such as dysmenorrhoea and reduce the risk of ovarian and endometrial cancers. Adverse effects, however, include an increased risk of venous thromboembolism, mood changes and mineralocorticoid effects that can lead to increases in blood pressure. Prescribing of COC therefore requires an initial risk assessment of concurrent diseases.

COCs pose a risk for cardiovascular disease and the *British National Formulary* specifies risk factors that either preclude the use of COCs or mean that they should be used with caution. These include:

- a family history of cardiovascular disease
- diabetes mellitus
- hypertension
- smoking
- age >35 years
- obesity
- migraine (Table 3.5).

COCs also pose a risk for venous thrombosis due to an increase in the levels of coagulation factors. Indeed, in the 1990s a new generation of COCs was withdrawn due to the increased risk. Current recommendations suggest that the presence of two or more risk factors should preclude the use of COCs, and cautious use is advised if any of the following risk factors are present:

- family history, e.g. first-degree relative <45 years (gestodene and desogestrel should be avoided)
- obesity
- immobility (e.g. after surgery)
- varicose veins

Other considerations are summarized in Table 3.5.

Choice of drugs

COCs are the most effective form of reversible contraception and are appropriate for patients who are sufficiently motivated to remember to take a dose within 12 hours every day. COCs have many advantages such as reducing dysmenorrhoea, symptoms of fibroids and ovarian cysts, benign breast disease, anaemia, premenstrual syndrome, and the risk of ovarian and endometrial cancer. Disadvantages, however, include an increased risk of thrombosis (see above), adverse effects such as nausea, weight gain and mood changes, and mineralocorticoid effect, which can increase blood pressure. There is also a small increase in risk of breast cancer and the MHRA (Medicines and Healthcare products Regulatory Agency) recently highlighted an increase in the risk of cervical cancer with long-term use of hormonal contraceptives. These risks need to be considered alongside the benefits and the availability of screening services.

POPs are often regarded as being more suitable for patients who cannot take COCs due to age, smoking status, cardiovascular risks or migraine. However, for most POPs they must be taken within 3 hours of the same time each day to maintain efficacy. POPs are considered the pill of

Table 3.5   Prescribing of oral contraceptives in the presence of concurrent disease

Condition	Effect on drug choice	Comments
Cardiovascular disease and venous thrombosis risk	See text	
Depression	COC used with caution in severe depression	Patients should report worsening mood associated with COC
Inflammatory bowel disease	COC used with caution	Increased risk of contraceptive failure due to reduced absorption
Migraine	COC contraindicated if: typical focal aura severe migraine >72 hours despite treatment treatment with ergot derivatives Cautious use of COC if treated with $5HT_1$-receptor agonists and for migraine without focal aura	Increased frequency and/or worsening symptoms should be reported by patients
Sex-steroid-dependent cancer	Use with caution	

COC, combined oral contraceptive.

choice in breast-feeding mothers as COCs may suppress lactation.

Drug interactions

The interaction of drugs with hormonal contraception involves reduced absorption of oestrogens by broad-spectrum antibiotics (see Chapter 32) or increased metabolism in the presence of enzyme inducers such as carbamazepine, phenobarbital, phenytoin, rifampicin, rifabutin and St John's wort (see Chapter 5). POPs, patches, implants or injectable contraceptives are not affected by reduced absorption in the presence of broad-spectrum antibiotics.

Patients prescribed potent enzyme inducers such as rifampicin and rifabutin are advised to use an intrauterine device or barrier methods. High doses of oestrogen or 'tricycling' whereby three cycles of pill are taken without the usual 7-day breaks are alternatives for less potent inducers but are not without risk.

Self-assessment

Consider whether the following statements in relation to advising patients about their lifestyle are true or false:

1. 30 minutes of moderate intensity exercise is recommended each day on 5 or more days a week to reduce obesity.
2. Norethisterone does not interact with antibiotics.
3. Grapefruit juice inhibits the metabolism of calcium channel blockers.
4. Vitamin K-containing foods may alter the actions of warfarin.
5. Varenicline tablets should be used with caution in patients with a history of depression.

Practice points

- Pharmacists should participate in health promotion campaigns; provide leaflets with information on healthy lifestyle and signpost to information sources, e.g. resources promoting healthy eating and the consumption of five portions of fruit and vegetables.
- *At least five a week* (Department of Health 2004) should be consulted for a useful summary of evidence of the benefits of physical activity in health and disease.
- The pharmacist has a major role in educating patients in relation to safe alcohol consumption and smoking cessation.

CASE STUDIES

1. A 36-year-old woman requests a blood pressure test in the pharmacy and you notice that her breath smells of tobacco smoke. Her patient medication record (PMR) reveals that she takes Microgynon tablets. You measure her blood pressure as 160/85 mmHg. You ask her if she smokes and she admits that she has recently increased to 40 cigarettes a day due to a period of stress. What course of action do you take?

   This patient has potentially three risk factors for cardiovascular disease and she should therefore be advised to see her GP for a review of her oral contraceptive. Her systolic blood pressure is elevated, though this would need to be repeated on a further two occasions and taking into consideration any recent caffeine consumption, smoking and anxiety. In addition she is aged over 35 years and a smoker. Combined hormonal contraception is not recommended if a patient has two or more risk factors for arterial disease. A referral for smoking cessation support and information about stress management would also benefit this patient. You should explain the risks, without causing alarm, to ensure that she does speak to her GP.

2. You receive a prescription for 350 micrograms norethisterone daily. You notice that the patient is purchasing products for her forthcoming holiday. How do you proceed?

   This case illustrates the importance of checking the indication for all prescribed drugs before dispensing. The above dose of norethisterone is appropriate for contraception. On further questioning, the patient was prescribed norethisterone to postpone menstruation during her holiday. The GP was contacted and the dose changed to 5 mg three times daily.

References

Baxter K, ed. (2008). *Stockley's Drug Interactions*, 8th edn. London: Pharmaceutical Press.

Bjelakovic G, Nikolova D, Gluud LL *et al* (2008). Antioxidant supplements for prevention of mortality in healthy participants and patients with various diseases. *Cochrane Database System Rev* issue 2: CD007176.

Chandola T, Brunner E, Marmot M (2006). Chronic stress at work and the metabolic syndrome: prospective study. *BMJ* **332**: 521–5.

Cornah D (2006). *Feeding Minds. The impact of food on mental health*. London: Mental Health Foundation.

Department of Health (2000). *The NHS Plan*. London: DH.

Department of Health (2004). *Physical Activity, Health Improvement and Prevention. At least five a week. Evidence on the impact of physical activity and its relationship to health*. London: DH.

Heart Protection Study (2002). MRC/BHF Heart Protection Study of antioxidant vitamin supplementation in 20 536 high risk individuals: a randomised placebo controlled trial. *Lancet* **360**: 23–33.

Kenfield SA, Stampfer MJ, Rosner BA *et al* (2008). Smoking and smoking cessation in relation to mortality in women. *JAMA* **299**: 2037–47.

Mason P (2003). Alcohol misuse – a case study. *Pharm J* **271**: 777–9.

Food Standards Agency (2001) *The Balance of Good Health*. Information for educators and communicators. London: FSA in consultation with the Department of Health.

Food Standards Agency (2005). *Eatwell. Your guide to healthy eating*. London: FSA.

National Institute for Clinical Excellence (2002). *Guidance on the use of nicotine replacement therapy (NRT) and bupropion for smoking cessation*. Technology appraisal guidance, No. 39. London: NICE.

National Institute for Health and Clinical Excellence (2007) *Varenicline for smoking cessation.* Technology appraisal guidance, No. 123. London: NICE

Stead LF, Perera R, Bullen C *et al* (2007). Nicotine replacement therapy for smoking cessation (Cochrane review). *Cochrane Database System Rev* issue 3: CD000146.

Wanless D (2004). *Securing Good Health for the Whole Population. Final report.* London: Department of Health.

World Health Organization (2003). *Fruit, Vegetables and NCD Disease Prevention. Global strategy on diet, physical activity and health.* Geneva: WHO

Williams C (1995). Healthy eating: clarifying advice about fruit and vegetables. *BMJ* **310**: 1453–5.

Online resources

www.foodstandards.gov.uk
The website of the Food Standards Agency; provides evidence-based advice and nutrition leaflets with advice for different age groups (accessed February 2008).

www.food.gov.uk/multimedia/pdfs/vitmin2003.pdf
A report by the Expert Group on Vitamins and Minerals provides useful, detailed characteristics, including risk assessments and safe upper levels for vitamins and minerals. This information is particularly important when patients request advice on the safety of combining multivitamin preparations with supplements such as cod liver oil, which contains vitamin A, or calcium and vitamin D tablets (accessed February 2008).

www.nutrition.org.uk
The website of the British Nutrition Foundation, a charity providing useful information and resources promoting healthy eating (accessed February 2008).

www.mentalhealth.org.uk
The website of the Mental Health Foundation for useful information on the diet and mental health including leaflets such as *Healthy Eating and depression* (accessed February 2008).

www.fpa.org.uk
The website of the Family Planning Association; provides information for both patients and health professionals (accessed February 2008).

4

Herbal medicine and alternative remedies

Herbal remedies are natural products largely of plant origin and may contain pharmacologically active compounds, which may be beneficial or have adverse effects. The use of certain natural products is established in medicine, e.g. by the use of digoxin from foxglove, but many remedies are poorly characterized in terms of efficacy and side-effect profile.

The use of herbal remedies is widespread, being particularly attractive due to the publicity of adverse effects associated with conventional medicine. Indeed the public perception that herbal medicines are safe has probably led to an under-reporting of adverse events and patients failing to report the use of herbal medicines alongside prescribed and over-the-counter (OTC) medicines. This problem is highlighted by the use of St John's wort, which has pharmacological actions similar to selective serotonin reuptake inhibitors (SSRIs) but has a range of significant interactions with conventional medicines (Table 4.1). Another issue is the lack of quality control, in that the composition of active ingredients may vary considerably between preparations.

Drug history-taking and responding to symptoms should involve active enquiry about herbal medicines. Any change in clinical outcome should be assessed for possible drug interactions or adverse drug reactions (ADRs) thought to result from concurrent use of conventional and herbal drugs. Suspected problems should be reported using the Yellow Card system.

Evidence

It is difficult for health professionals to recommend the use of many herbal preparations in the absence of sound evidence of safe efficacious use, particularly in combination with conventional medicines. Added to this, an extensive variety of preparations is available and doses and purity may vary. Some herbal preparations have a product licence or marketing authorization whereby safety, quality and efficacy, together with evidence for safe use, are provided. These products are identifiable by a PL number on the label. Most herbal preparations are, however, unlicensed products under the Medicines Act 1968. They are not therefore assessed for safety and quality and lack the rigorous testing of conventional drugs. The introduction of the Traditional Herbal Registration (THR) scheme by the MHRA (Medicines and Healthcare products Regulatory Agency) should help to improve patient safety when using these products. Those registered with the scheme are assessed by the MHRA for safety, quality and the provision of patient information. It should be noted, however, that indications are based on traditional uses rather than evidence of efficacy. Products are identifiable by a THR number on the label and those with marketing authorization will continue to display a PL number. *Professional Standards and Guidance for the Sale and Supply of Medicines by Pharmacists* (Royal Pharmaceutical Society of Great Britain 2007) recommends that pharmacists competent to supply complementary therapies, including herbal medicines are required to:

> ... assist patients in making informed decisions by providing them with necessary and relevant information; ensure any stock is from a reputable source; recommend a remedy only where you can be satisfied of its safety and quality, taking into account the MHRA registration schemes for homeopathic and herbal remedies.

Table 4.1   Examples of interactions between herbal and conventional medicines for which clinical evidence exists or potential interactions based on *in vivo* or *in vitro* pharmacological activity

Physiological effects	Implicated herbs and interactions with conventional drugs	Comments
Anticoagulant or antiplatelet activity	Danshen (Chinese herb), dong quai (Chinese), garlic, feverfew, ginkgo, ginger, ginseng (*Panax*), kangen-karyu (Chinese) and liquorice with warfarin or antiplatelet drugs (aspirin, dipyridamole, clopidogrel and ticlopidine)	• An isolated report of spontaneous bleeding from the iris in a patient taking low-dose aspirin and ginkgo biloba • A Canadian database reported 21 possible ADRs with ginkgo, most relating to bleeding abnormalities and including a fatal haemorrhage in a patient taking ginkgo with ticlopidine (*Stockley's Drug Interactions* – Baxter 2008). It may be sensible for patients prescribed antiplatelet treatment to avoid these herbal preparations • Case reports of significantly increased effects of warfarin with dansheen or dong quai • Patients reporting increased bleeding, e.g. bruising, should be asked about their use of herbal preparations • These products should also be avoided or discontinued at least 24–48 h before surgery and considered alongside an increased risk of bleeding with drugs such as NSAIDs and SSRIs
Cardioactive activity, e.g. antiarrhythmic, inotropic or calcium channel effects	Cola, coltsfoot, fenugreek, ginger, ginseng (*Panax*), motherwort, shepherd's purse and wild carrot with antiarrhythmics (amiodarone), digoxin and other cardioactive agents	Patients at increased risk include those with cardiovascular disease and/or taking drugs with cardiovascular activity
Diuresis	Dandelion, elder, java tea, nettle, saw palmetto, shepherd's purse and squill	• Potential to interact with concurrent diuretic and other antihypertensive treatment (Chapter 11) • Particular caution may be required with drugs associated with significant hypotensive effects such as ACE inhibitors, α-adrenoceptor antagonists and antipsychotics
Hormone activity	Dong quai (Chinese), vitex berry (*Agnus castus*), hops flower, ginseng root, black cohosh, saw palmetto with tamoxifen	• There is little evidence of a problem but these products demonstrate binding to oestrogen receptors and some physiological oestrogenic activity. The action of tamoxifen, and other drugs that reduce stimulation of oestrogen receptors, may therefore be opposed by these herbs. They may also stimulate the growth of oestrogen-sensitive tumours of the breast
	Saw palmetto with antiandrogens (finasteride)	• Saw palmetto has been reported to possess antiandrogen activity and this should be considered when prescribing antiandrogens for prostatic hyperplasia

Continued

Table 4.1   (Continued)

Physiological effects	Implicated herbs and interactions with conventional drugs	Comments
Hyperglycaemic	Ginseng (*Panax*), hydrocotyl, rosemary	Increased risk for patients with diabetes mellitus and also concurrent treatment with corticosteroids (Chapters 21 and 35)
Hypoglycaemic	Aloe vera, burdock, celery, corn silk, dandelion, garlic, ginger, ginseng, ispaghula, juniper, marshmallow, nettle, sage	Increased risk of hypoglycaemia in patients with diabetes due to possible additive effects
Immunomodulation	Cat's claw, camomile (German), echinacea, ephedra, ginseng (*Eleutherococcus*), mistletoe, saw palmetto with immunosuppressants (corticosteroids, azathioprine)	Risk of potentiation or antagonism of immunosuppressants
Increased levels of digoxin	Ginseng (Siberian) with digoxin	Siberian ginseng contains glycosides related to digoxin
Increased effects	Ginseng with MAOIs (phenelzine)	Increased side effects such as headache, insomnia and psychoactive effects
Increased effects	St John's wort with triptans, SSRIs	An increased risk of serotoninergic effects, so should be avoided
Decreased effects	St John's wort with anticonvulsants (phenytoin, phenobarbital), warfarin, digoxin, theophylline, ciclosporin, hormonal contraceptives	• St John's wort induces cytochrome P450 isoenzymes • Avoid concurrent use • Dose adjustment is not appropriate due to varying doses of St John's wort according to preparation
Laxative effects	Aloes, cascara, ispaghula, rhubarb and senna	• Risk of abuse by patients with anorexia nervosa • Increased risk of dehydration and electrolyte disturbances in patients taking drugs such as diuretics (Chapters 11 and 15)
Sedation	Celery, kava, camomile (German), ginseng, hops, nettle, sage, and valerian with opioids, antihistamines, alcohol, antidepressants, benzodiazepines	• Possibility of severe sedation with concurrent use of St John's wort with SSRIs (paroxetine) and other antidepressants; avoid concomitant use (see above) • It may be a sensible precaution to avoid concurrent use of St John's wort with all antidepressants due to the risk of additive pharmacological effects. • Increased effects of CNS depressants • Patients requesting herbal products for insomnia should be advised as for conventional hypnotics (Chapter 26) • As a precaution, patients should not take herbs such as valerian up to 2 h before driving or performing other skilled tasks

Continued

Table 4.1 (Continued)

Physiological effects	Implicated herbs and interactions with conventional drugs	Comments
Sympathomimetic activity	Aniseed, arnica, borage, capsicum, cohosh (black, blue), cola, ephedra, gentian, ginseng (*Panax*), nettle, parsley, valerian and vervain	• Reduced effect of antihypertensives
Thyroid effects	Kelp with amiodarone, thyroxine, lithium and antithyroid drugs	Iodine content of kelp may alter thyroid function (caution also with warfarin due to vitamin K content)
Urinary effects (see diuresis and hormone activity above)	Saw palmetto	Patients at risk include those with concurrent prostatic hyperplasia, incontinence or taking drugs such as diuretics If possible, patients requesting herbs for bladder problems should be asked about symptoms, which may indicate prostatic hyperplasia requiring referral to their GP, including: • a sensation of incomplete bladder emptying on urination • needing to urinate within 2 h of previous urination • frequent urination during the night • non-continuous urine flow • a weak urinary stream • difficulty starting urinating • difficulty postponing urination

Information obtained from *Stockley's Drug Interactions* (Baxter 2008), and *Herbal Medicines* by Barnes et al (2007).

ACE, angiotensin-converting enzyme; CHF, chronic heart failure; CNS, central nervous system; MAOIs, monoamine oxidase inhibitors; NSAIDs, non-steroidal anti-inflammatory drugs; SSRIs, selective serotonin reuptake inhibitors.

The most important role of health professionals in the use of herbal preparations is to advise patients of potential problems, particularly associated with concurrent use of conventional medicine (Table 4.1) and to help identify adverse effects, which should be reported as discussed above. When available, the evidence of efficacy and safety may be communicated to patients and this information is increasingly available in systematic reviews of current trials, e.g. Cochrane and Bandolier reviews.

Safety Issues

In 2002, the Medicines Control Agency or MCA (now part of the MHRA) produced a report on the *Safety of Herbal Medicinal Products*, concluding overall that these medicines did not pose a major threat to human health. A number of safety issues were, however, highlighted:

• licensing issues and particularly risks associated with unlicensed products
• addition of prescription medicines (sildenafil, glibenclamide, warfarin, alprazolam) and toxic heavy metals to herbal products; other examples are corticosteroids in herbal eczema

creams for children and fenfluramine in a slimming product

- interactions with conventional medicines
- hepatotoxicity with comfrey and coltsfoot
- hypersensitivity to herbs with allergenic potential, e.g. chamomile, feverfew
- contamination by microbes, pesticides, fumigants and toxic metals.

Attention was given to patient groups at risk of adverse reactions such as pregnant or breast-feeding mothers, elderly people, children, or with cardiovascular disease and those undergoing surgery, e.g. some herbs such as blue cohosh, burdock, fenugreek, hawthorn, nettle and raspberry were found to exert a stimulant effect on uterine smooth muscle, making them unsuitable for pregnant women. Herbal teas were also identified as a source of pharmacologically active herbal ingredients. A case was described in which hepatotoxicity occurred in a newborn baby after the consumption of a herbal tea by the mother during pregnancy. The tea contained pyrrolizidine alkaloids associated with hepatotoxicity.

Current safety issues are reported in regular Drug Safety Updates by the MHRA and the Herbal Safety News section of the MHRA website. Examples of reports include:

- interactions between conventional drugs and St John's wort (see Table 4.1)
- hepatotoxicity with kava-kava and black cohosh
- renal failure with certain Chinese herbs
- severe skin reactions with *Psoralea corylifolia* fruit in Chinese herbal remedies
- the substitution of plantain by digitalis, leading to serious cardiac arrhythmias.

Interactions between herbal and conventional medicines

Examples of interactions between herbal and conventional medicines, for which clinical evidence exists, are given in Table 4.1. The possibility of drug interactions extrapolated from *in vitro* and *in vivo* pharmacological activity is also considered. For further information the reader is referred to *Stockley's Drug Interactions* (Baxter 2008) and *Herbal Medicines* by Barnes *et al* (2007).

Homeopathy

To date, there is no proven scientific evidence for efficacy of homeopathy. However, these remedies continue to be available on the National Health Service (NHS) and many patients choose homeopathy. Healthcare professionals should be alert for a possible delay in consulting advice for serious symptoms (see Chapter 1) by patients choosing homeopathy. Advice should be provided only after adequate training. It should be noted that adverse effects involving an exacerbation of symptoms may be reported. Patients should discontinue treatment and consult a healthcare professional. There are no known interactions with conventional medicines.

The main principle of homeopathy is the treatment of 'like with like', as implied by the prefix 'homeo-', e.g. insomnia is treated with an extract from the green coffee bean (*Coffea*). Extremely small quantities of the homeopathic preparation are administered following serial dilution, agitation and formulation. A product is recommended according to the presenting complaint but also the individual, providing a holistic approach.

Nomenclature used to express potency uses centesimal and decimal systems. For the centesimal system, mother tincture is prepared from an extract of the source material, which may be plant, animal, insect, biological or chemical material, in a mixture of alcohol and water. One drop of mother tincture is then added to 99 drops of diluent (20–60% triple-distilled alcohol and water). The resulting solution is shaken vigorously (a process known as succussion) and then serial dilutions are made, indicated by a multiple of 'c' representing the number of successive dilutions of 1 in 100, e.g. a potency of 6c gives a concentration of 10^{-12}. It is the process of serial dilution and claims of increased therapeutic potency (potentization) with each dilution that many people find difficult to accept.

The decimal system involves the addition of one drop of mother tincture to nine drops of diluent and is represented as a multiple of 'x'. The letters M and CM are used to represent greater dilution levels of 1000 and 10 000, respectively. If one compares the two systems for denoting potency, therefore, 6c is equivalent to 12x.

The following points of advice may be given to patients taking homeopathic preparations. The active ingredient is placed on the surface of the dosage form and absorbed through the oral mucosa. Inappropriate handling is therefore thought to inactivate the product. Patients should be counselled as follows:

- The product should be kept in its original container.
- Homeopathic medicines should not be handled but transferred to the mouth via the container cap.
- Take at least 30 min before or after food.
- Suck or chew tablet before swallowing.
- Mother tincture should be diluted in a mouthful of water, gargled and then swallowed.
- Highly flavoured or aromatic foods should be avoided, e.g. peppermints.
- Avoid the inhalation of aromatic products containing eucalyptus and camphor, as well as smoking and coffee or tea.
- Stop the treatment when the condition improves.

Homeopathy and pregnancy

Highly diluted homeopathic remedies are considered safe for use during pregnancy but should not delay referral to exclude serious conditions.

Practice points

- Health professionals should enquire routinely about the use of herbal remedies by patients.
- Herbal remedies should be avoided in pregnancy and lactation, due to the absence of safety data.
- The risk of ADRs caused by herbal preparations is increased, as for conventional drugs, with polypharmacy, long-term use, high doses, history of allergy, patients at extremes of age and impaired renal and hepatic function.
- Safety information produced by the MHRA should be communicated to patients.

Self-assessment

Consider whether the following statements about herbal medicines are true or false:

1. These are natural products and therefore unlikely to be associated with side effects.
2. All herbal preparations should have a THR number.
3. Suspected adverse events should not be reported on a Yellow Card as these are not drugs.
4. They are unlikely to cause a problem for people undergoing surgery.
5. St John's wort should not be taken with hormonal contraceptives, antidepressants, anticonvulsants (phenytoin, phenobarbital), warfarin, digoxin, theophylline or ciclosporin.

CASE STUDIES

Case 1
A 25-year-old woman has recently been diagnosed with Crohn's disease. She has been given dietary advice and her symptoms have improved. Her symptoms have, however, worsened in the last 24 h and she does not understand why. She says that she feels very low and is tearful. She has started taking St John's wort. She is also complaining of a sore throat and chest infection. Should she take echinacea? She is very keen on taking herbal remedies, as they are natural. She gives you her prescription:

venlafaxine 75 mg twice daily
azathioprine 50 mg three times daily
prednisolone 5 mg enteric coated tablets as directed
mesalazine 400 mg enteric coated tablets two three times daily.

While you dispense her medication, she starts to tell you about a party that she went to the previous night.

Is it appropriate for this patient to take St John's wort with echinacea? What general advice would you give to this patient about herbal medicines?

There were a number of issues to consider from this case:

- Was she taking a calcium supplement to reduce the risk of osteoporosis due to her prednisolone treatment, particularly in view of malabsorption as a result of her Crohn's disease (see Chapter 9)?
- How much alcohol was she consuming? Alcohol is a central nervous system depressant and may therefore worsen her depression (assumption that patient has depression because of prescription for venlafaxine) and could also exacerbate her Crohn's disease. The corticosteroid may also contribute to her low mood (see Chapter 5).
- St John's wort should not be given with antidepressant therapy. She should be referred back to her GP if her antidepressant treatment is not effective. Perhaps check first how long she has been taking the venlafaxine, because there may be a delay in efficacy at the start of treatment.
- Hopefully her sore throat is the result of too much singing the night before. However, in view of her immunosuppressant therapy, she should be referred to her GP for a full blood count.
- Echinacea may interfere with immunosuppressive therapy because it is thought to have immunomodulatory activity.
- It may be wise to advise this patient to avoid herbal medicine in view of her drug treatment.

Case 2
A 21-year-old woman asks what you think about kelp tablets for weight loss. Her gym instructor recommended them.

What further questions would you ask?

- It is important to establish if the patient is overweight and to consider her lifestyle and diet (see Chapter 3). Her medical history and any current medication should also be considered.
- Further questioning reveals a history of thyroid dysfunction and excessive calorie intake from lager.

Continued

CASE STUDIES (continued)

Are kelp tablets suitable for this patient?

No. Kelp tablets contain iodine, which could exacerbate her thyroid problem (see Chapter 36). There is also a risk of the presence of toxic heavy metals. Possible mechanisms for the weight-loss effect of kelp tablets include increased thyroid activity and/or laxative effects and are not, therefore, a healthy option for weight loss. General lifestyle factors should be considered and the patient advised that the best way to lose weight is to increase exercise and reduce her calorie intake (see Chapter 3). This patient was only marginally overweight and this was corrected by avoiding lager and continuing her exercise routine.

Case 3

A 56-year-old woman informs you that she has been taking a herbal remedy containing ginseng root to relieve her menopausal symptoms. She has found that her symptoms have improved and thought that you would like to know so that you could recommend them to other patients. You notice from her computer records that she is currently taking tamoxifen 20 mg/day for breast cancer.

Are you happy for the patient to continue with the herbal remedy?

No. In view of her tamoxifen treatment and the absence of sufficient safety data, the ginseng root is not recommended because it has been shown to possess oestrogen receptor-binding activity. There is a risk that the herbal preparation could interfere with her tamoxifen treatment. This case illustrates the importance of asking patients about their use of herbal preparations, as the information is not always volunteered.

Case 4

A patient asks your advice on the use of karela (*Momordica charantia*) for diabetes. She says that she has found good evidence on the internet for its blood sugar-lowering effect and is worried she is at risk of diabetes. How do you respond?

Initially, the patient's risk factors should be assessed and blood glucose measured. Referral to her GP may be required or to a local pharmacy providing this service. On inspection of the internet site that she found it reveals claims such as 'lower blood sugar naturally' and advertising to buy on-line. The next place to look might be the MHRA website to check for any current safety warnings. This reveals a warning in 2005 regarding the presence of heavy metals in some preparations of karela. The patient should be advised to avoid these products. Diabetes UK has also provided a warning (www.diabetes.org.uk) regarding concerns over the advertising of karela to lower blood sugar and the absence of good evidence for safe use in diabetes. Karela cannot therefore be recommended. As karela is widely available it is important to be aware that patients may take it alongside other medicines for diabetes. *Stockley's Drug Interactions* (Baxter 2008) warns of the potentiation of antidiabetic drugs and that unexplained changes in blood sugars may be attributed to the use of karela, including as a cooking ingredient added to curries.

References

Barnes J, Anderson LA, Phillipson JD (2007). *Herbal Medicines,* 3rd edn. London: Pharmaceutical Press.

Baxter K, ed. (2008). *Stockley's Drug Interactions,* 8th edn. London: Pharmaceutical Press.

Medicines Control Agency or MCA (2002). *Safety of Herbal Medicinal Products.* London: Department of Health. Available at: www.mhra.gov.uk/home/groups/es-herbal/documents/websiteresources/con009293.pdf (accessed April 2008).

Royal Pharmaceutical Society of Great Britain (2007). *Professional Standards and Guidance for the Sale and Supply of Medicines.* London: Royal Pharmaceutical Society of Great Britain.

Further reading

Barnes J (2002). Herbal therapeutics (1). An introduction to herbal medicinal products. *Pharm J* **268**: 804–6.

Barnes J (2002). Herbal therapeutics (2). Depression. *Pharm J* **268**: 908–10.

Barnes J (2002). Herbal therapeutics (3). Cognitive deficiency and dementia. *Pharm J* **269**: 160–2.

Barnes J (2002). Herbal therapeutics (4). Hyperlipidaemia. *Pharm J* **269**: 193–5.

Barnes J (2002). Herbal therapeutics (5). Insomnia. *Pharm J* **269**: 219–21.

Barnes J (2002). Benign prostatic hyperplasia. *Pharm J* **269**: 250–2.

Fugh-Berman A (2000). Herb–drug interactions. *Lancet* **355**: 134–8.

Kayne SB (2008). *Complementary and Alternative Medicine,* 2nd edn. London: Pharmaceutical Press.

Online resources

www.cfsan.fda.gov
The website for the US Food and Drug Administration, information relating to dietary supplements, including warnings and safety information on the use of herbal preparations (accessed April 2008).

www.mhra.gov.uk
The website of the MHRA with policy information for the use and licensing of herbal medicines and the latest safety information (accessed 20 April 2008).

Royal Pharmaceutical Society of Great Britain (2002). *Homeopathy, Useful Information for Pharmacists.* London: RPSGB. Available at: www.rpsgb.org.uk.

www.nimh.org.uk
The National Institute of Medical Herbalists provides information and research relating to herbal medicines and access to suitably trained herbalists (accessed May 2008).

Part B
Treatment

5

Adverse drug reactions and interactions

Adverse drug reactions (ADRs) and drug interactions are related topics, e.g. a drug interaction results in a change to the expected treatment outcome and occurs as a result of concurrent exposure to another drug, food or chemical. The result may be an adverse event but this is not always the case. In either event ADRs and drug interactions tend to be more important for drugs that exhibit a narrow therapeutic window, which is the margin between a therapeutic dose and a toxic dose. However, this is not always the case and some drugs may cause severe adverse reactions at low or therapeutic doses. A thorough knowledge of these topics is essential for safe prescribing and drug safety, in both prevention of events and recognition of adverse outcomes. A key element of prescribing is that the benefits of a drug treatment must always outweigh its drawbacks, of which ADRs are the major component.

The purpose of this chapter is to explore the nature and mechanisms, when known, resulting in ADRs and interactions. For a more comprehensive coverage of these topics the reader is referred to Lee's *Adverse Drug Reactions* (2006), the *British National Formulary* and *Stockley's Drug Interactions* (Baxter 2008).

Adverse drug reactions and side effects

These terms are difficult to distinguish and in practice are often used interchangeably. It may be helpful to consider side effects of a medicine as predictable secondary effects that may be beneficial (e.g. sedation with antihistamines when used as an over-the-counter [OTC] sleep medicine) or undesirable (e.g. sedation with antihistamines used for allergy relief). By contrast, ADRs are side effects that are always deleterious.

Recent evidence indicates that the magnitude of ADRs with significant morbidity and mortality is substantial, with 6.5% of hospital admissions being ADR related, leading to a mortality rate of 0.15% (Pirmohamed *et al* 2004). Of these, non-steroidal anti-inflammatory drugs (NSAIDs) were associated with the greatest proportion of admissions (29.6%) and the causes included peptic ulceration, renal impairment, cerebrovascular accident and wheezing. Based on this study and other work the following are associated with the greatest burden of ADRs and their use should always ring alarm bells:

- NSAIDs (e.g. peptic ulceration, asthma, renal dysfunction)
- diuretics (e.g. electrolyte disturbances, postural hypotension)
- warfarin (e.g. bleeding)
- angiotensin-converting enzyme (ACE) inhibitors and angiotensin receptor antagonists (e.g. electrolyte disturbances, renal dysfunction)
- antidepressants (e.g. cardiac toxicity with tricyclic antidepressants)
- lithium (e.g. renal impairment)
- β blockers (e.g. bronchospasm)
- opioids (e.g. constipation)
- digoxin (e.g. toxicity)
- oral steroids (e.g. adrenal suppression)
- oral hypoglycaemic agents (e.g. hypoglycaemia).

ADRs are often divided into type A (augmented response) and type B (bizarre or idiosyncratic reactions).

Table 5.1   Examples of adverse drug reactions that may be predicted from the pharmacology of the drug class; further information is given in the relevant chapters

Drug class	Side effect	Pharmacological mechanism	Possible solutions
β Blockers	Cold extremities	Antagonism of peripheral β_2-adrenoceptors	• Choose a more cardioselective agent such as atenolol, which has less affinity for agent β_2-adrenoceptors • Choose a β blocker with vasodilator actions, e.g. nebivolol
β Blockers	Bradycardia	Antagonism of chronotropic cardiac β_1-adrenoceptors	• Withdraw β blockers gradually to prevent rebound tachycardia
β Blockers	Bronchospasm	Antagonism of bronchial β_2-adrenoceptors	• All β blockers are contraindicated in asthma. A cardioselective one may be used with extreme caution under specialist supervision Cardioselective β blockers should be used with caution in COPD
α Blockers, diuretics, ACE inhibitors	Postural hypotension	Impairment of blood pressure regulation	• Caution on standing • Take first dose of α blocker or ACE inhibitor on retiring to bed
Thiazide and loop diuretics	Hypokalaemia	Activation of the renin–angiotensin–aldosterone system See Chapter 15	Potassium levels should be monitored
Nitrates	Flushing, headache	Vasodilatation	• Headache relieved by paracetamol • Sublingual tablets may be discarded by spitting them out
Oral anticoagulants	Increased bleeding	Plasma concentration too high or increased bleeding tendency	• Monitoring of INR required and dose adjustment may be required
Opioids	Constipation	Inhibition of lower GI tract motility	• Use a laxative such as lactulose or senna
Tricyclic antidepressants; certain older antihistamines (e.g. promethazine)	Antimuscarinic effects such as dry mouth, blurred vision, constipation and urinary retention	Antagonism of muscarinic receptors	• Consider an SSRI for depression • Choose a newer antihistamine with less muscarinic binding, e.g. loratadine
Sulphonylureas	Hypoglycaemia	Augmented pharmacological effect	• Careful monitoring with dose adjustment • Use short-acting agents

Continued

Table 5.1   (Continued)

Drug class	Side effect	Pharmacological mechanism	Possible solutions
Broad-spectrum antibiotics	Diarrhoea	Alterations of lower GI flora	• Caution: severe diarrhoea should alert one to the risk of pseudomembranous colitis. Otherwise a short course of loperamide may be used with caution
NSAIDs	Gastric damage	Inhibition of the production of cytoprotective prostaglandins	• Use a less irritant NSAID such as ibuprofen • Consider a COX-2 inhibitor. • Combine NSAID with misoprostol or a PPI
NSAIDs	Bronchospasm	Inhibition of the production of prostaglandins, favouring the production of leukotrienes	• Avoid in patients with asthma who are sensitive to NSAIDs
Cytotoxic agents	Myelosuppression	Cytotoxic effects on bone marrow	• Prophylactic antibacterial and antifungal agents • Use of transfusions or colony-stimulating factors to increase white blood cell counts

ACE, angiotensin-converting enzyme; COPD, chronic obstructive pulmonary disease; COX-2, cyclo-oxygenase 2; GI, gastrointestinal; INR, international normalized ratio; NSAIDs, non-steroidal anti-inflammatory drugs; PPI, proton pump inhibitor; SSRI, selective serotonin reuptake inhibitor.

Type A: augmented response

This type of ADR can be explained or predicted on the basis of the drug's pharmacology. Type A reactions are often dose dependent and may often be managed by dose reduction. If they are anticipated, measures may be taken to ameliorate or prevent the problem, e.g. the use of anti-emetics in patients receiving chemotherapy, or laxatives with opioid analgesics.

Type B: bizarre or idiosyncratic reactions

These ADRs are unrelated to the known pharmacology of the drug, which makes them less common and unpredictable; they may also be severe. This group of ADRs is often related to genetics or immunology, which means that certain individuals may be at a higher risk than others.

Risk factors for developing ADRs

When considering ADRs there are a number of risk factors that may predispose a patient to adverse responses:

- extremes of age
- gender
- concurrent drug usage
- concurrent disease, e.g. respiratory disease and β blockers
- pharmacokinetic variables, e.g. renal or hepatic function
- pharmaceutical factors, e.g. nature of dosage form or excipients

- genetics, e.g. glucose-6-phosphate dehydrogenase (G6PD) deficiency.

Mechanisms of adverse reactions

The effects of a drug may be enhanced by various pharmacodynamic or pharmacokinetic factors, leading to enhanced side effects or adverse reactions.

Pharmacological mechanisms

These represent the most straightforward examples that may be predicted from a sound knowledge of a drug's pharmacology. The best example is β-adrenoceptor antagonists which, to varying degrees, will block β_2-adrenoceptors on the bronchial smooth muscle, opposing the actions of circulating adrenaline (epinephrine), which may lead to bronchoconstriction, and it is for this reason that they are contraindicated in asthma. Other examples are given in Table 5.1. These predictable responses are dose dependent and so increases in plasma concentration, which may occur as a consequence of pharmacokinetic mechanism (as outlined below) or drug interactions (see later), necessarily increase their likelihood and impact.

Pharmacokinetic mechanisms
Pharmacokinetic ADRs result from impaired **a**bsorption, **d**istribution, **m**etabolism or **e**xcretion (ADME). The first potential site is absorption and this might be delayed if, for example, gastric emptying is slowed and the consequences might be retarded absorption, leading to failure of therapy, which is itself an ADR. Metabolism and elimination are far more important, e.g. a reduced rate of elimination, often due to impaired renal function, is likely to increase plasma concentrations, leading to augmented effects. These are common causes of ADRs and may often be prevented by careful prescribing and patient monitoring. Impaired renal function is common in elderly people and neonates, and should be measured so that drug doses or dosage intervals are adjusted as appropriate to prevent an ADR. An important example of this is digoxin, which is predominantly (about two-thirds) cleared by

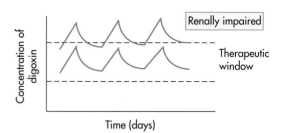

Figure 5.1 A schematic graph illustrating the variation of plasma concentration of digoxin over time. In patients the ideal is to maintain the plasma concentration within the therapeutic window. However, in the renally impaired patient, without a dose reduction, the plasma concentration rises to toxic levels.

the kidneys, and in renally impaired patients the plasma concentration may reach toxic levels (Figure 5.1). Accordingly, when using digoxin the dose should be determined in relation to renal function.

The alternative strategy that is used with aminoglycosides such as gentamicin is to increase the dosage interval in renally impaired patients.

Important examples where serious toxicity may arise as a consequence of renal impairment are:

- digoxin
- lithium
- NSAIDs
- metformin
- ACE inhibitors
- aminoglycoside antibiotics.

Differences in hepatic metabolism
Alterations in drug metabolism may also lead to increased plasma concentrations. Metabolism may be altered at the extremes of age, such that neonates conjugate drugs at a relatively slow rate, whereas microsomal enzyme activity in the liver by cytochrome P450 isoenzymes decreases variably with age. An example of this is the prolonged half-life of diazepam with age, and hence the increased propensity to side effects, including oversedation. Hepatic metabolism may be impaired in liver disease and this may lead to the enhanced effects of drugs that are usually cleared by the liver.

Genetic differences in the expression of cytochrome P450 isoenzymes may also contribute to variations in metabolism. Approximately 10% of the population express a defective P450 isoenzyme, CYP2D6, which slows down the metabolism of a range of drugs including flecainide, metoclopramide and some antidepressants. Accordingly, patients may vary in the way that they handle drugs.

Disorders of metabolism

These include a lack of G6PD in erythrocytes and porphyria. G6PD is an enzyme present in red blood cells, which provides reducing power, thereby maintaining glutathione in the reduced form. This prevents oxidative damage to the cells. The absence of G6PD therefore leads to fragile red blood cell membranes and haemolysis, resulting in anaemia. G6PD deficiency is prevalent in the Mediterranean population and patients are sensitive to the effects of oxidative drugs such as antimalarials, sulphonamides, quinolones, nalidixic acid, nitrofurantoin, sulfasalazine and aspirin (refer to Section 9.1.5. of the *British National Formulary*), leading to oxidative damage with haemolysis and anaemia.

Individuals with porphyria lack one of the enzymes for haemoglobin synthesis and there is an accumulation of porphyrin precursors, leading to gastrointestinal (GI), neurological and behavioural disturbances. Cytochrome P450 inducers including barbiturates, carbamazepine, griseofulvin and hormonal contraceptives (refer to Section 9.8.2 of the *British National Formulary*) tend to provoke an attack by inducing amino laevulinic acid synthase, giving rise to porphyrins.

Immunological responses

Drugs are foreign molecules and some may induce an immunological response. These reactions may be delayed and tend not to be dose related, occurring with the smallest doses of drug. They are usually reversible on cessation of the causative agent. Patients at risk of these responses tend to have a predisposition to allergic disorders and the responses may vary from simple skin rashes to life-threatening anaphylaxis (see Chapter 20). Important examples of

causative agents are penicillins and streptokinase.

Penicillins couple to proteins, forming immunogens, which may precipitate hypersensitivity reactions. Management includes stopping the drug and treating the patient with antihistamines, adrenaline and/or parenteral steroids according to severity (see Chapter 20). In the case of penicillins, the allergic reaction is a class effect resulting from the presence of the β-lactam ring in the drug molecule and approximately 10% of penicillin-allergic patients are also sensitive to chemically similar cephalosporins. It is therefore appropriate that non-penicillin, non-cephalosporin antibiotics are chosen for patients with a history of penicillin allergy.

In the case of streptokinase, once patients have been treated with this agent for thrombolysis they are likely to develop antibodies against it. This means that on a subsequent exposure the antibodies may either prevent it from acting or lead to an allergic reaction. It is for this reason that patients do not generally receive streptokinase a second time and usually receive an alternative clot-busting agent for a second heart attack.

The increasing use of monoclonal antibodies (e.g. in immunological diseases and anticancer chemotherapy) is also likely to be associated with increased instances of immunological responses. These drugs are likely to be used in specialist settings and the patient should be observed for the period immediately after administration for hypersensitivity reactions, which might involve skin reactions, breathing problems and hypotension. In some cases corticosteroids and anthistamines are given prophylactically.

Withdrawal responses

The withdrawal of certain drugs may lead to predictable symptoms and patients should be counselled appropriately. This type of reaction tends to result from physiological adaptation during the course of treatment, e.g. chronic treatment with β blockers leads to receptor upregulation, i.e. an increase in the number of β-adrenoceptors occurs in response to the blockade of existing receptors. Sudden withdrawal of β blockade may therefore result in over-stimulation of β-adrenoceptors. In the heart this may predispose to arrhythmias and is associated with increased mortality. Common examples of drugs where abrupt withdrawal may lead to adverse reactions are given below.

Alcohol

Delirium tremens and seizures occur after chronic excessive alcohol intake. Treatment includes short-term chlordiazepoxide or clomethiazole (inpatients only) (*British National Formulary*, Section 4.10).

Antidepressants

Selective serotonin reuptake inhibitors (SSRIs, particularly paroxetine), tricyclic antidepressants and monoamine oxidase inhibitors (MAOIs) of 8 weeks' use or more should be withdrawn gradually over at least 4 weeks (up to 6 months after long-term maintenance). Monitor for withdrawal symptoms such as nausea, vomiting, anorexia, headache and panic anxiety (see Chapter 24 and the *British National Formulary*, Section 4.3).

Benzodiazepines

Withdrawal from benzodiazepines requires a gradual reduction of dose to prevent symptoms of confusion, toxic psychosis, convulsions or those similar to delirium tremens following alcohol withdrawal. These symptoms may take from a few hours to 3 weeks to develop with longer-acting agents. Milder symptoms include insomnia, loss of appetite, anxiety, weight loss, tremor, sweating, tinnitus and disturbances of perception. Patients are transferred to the equivalent dose of diazepam (*British National Formulary*, Section 4.1.1). The dose is then reduced by increments of approximately one-eighth of the daily dose (or 2–2.5 mg) every 2 weeks, maintaining the new dose for a longer period if withdrawal symptoms occur. The time taken to withdraw completely from long-term benzodiazepine use can be from 4 weeks to a year or occasionally longer. Specialist counselling may benefit some patients, including education about the risks and benefits of withdrawing from these drugs.

It should be noted that antipsychotics aggravate the symptoms of benzodiazepine withdrawal and should not be used (see the *British National Formulary*, Section 4.1).

Anticonvulsants

See Chapter 23.

Opioids

'Cold turkey' may be experienced after opioid addiction but is rare when opioids are prescribed for pain relief. Debilitating diarrhoea may occur; this may be treated with loperamide.

Baclofen

There is a risk of serious withdrawal reactions. The dose should be reduced gradually over at least 1–2 weeks, or longer if symptoms develop (*British National Formulary*, Section 10.2.2).

Corticosteroids

Prolonged use of corticosteroids results in the suppression of endogenous production and treatment should therefore be withdrawn gradually according to the recommendations of the Committee on Safety of Medicines or CSM (*British National Formulary* Section 6.3.2; the CSM is now called the Commission for Human Medicines or CHM).

The gradual withdrawal is recommended for patients whose disease is unlikely to relapse and who have:

- recently received repeated courses
- taken a short course within 1 year of stopping long-term therapy
- other possible causes of adrenal suppression
- received more than 40 mg prednisolone (or equivalent) daily
- repeat doses given in the evening
- received more than 3 weeks' treatment.

Sympathomimetics

Prolonged use of topical decongestant vasoconstrictors causes tolerance and rebound congestion, probably due in part to down-regulation of α-adrenoceptors.

Antipsychotics

Withdraw gradually after long-term therapy and monitor closely for acute withdrawal syndromes or rapid relapse (*British National Formulary*, Section 4.2.1).

Type A ADRs

In the simplest case, one may predict many common type A ADRs on the basis of the known pharmacology of the drugs. Some common examples are given in Table 5.1.

Gastrointestinal ADRs

ADRs can occur throughout the GI system and, as indicated above, NSAID-induced damage represents the most significant of all ADRs.

Oral problems

The mouth may be the site of ADRs leading to unpleasant side effects, e.g. drugs with significant antimuscarinic activity (e.g. tricyclic antidepressants, older antihistamines) may lead to a dry mouth, which is a minor problem and may be resolved by selecting an alternative (e.g. an SSRI for depression). Alternatively artificial saliva might be recommended. More significant problems include tooth discoloration with tetracycline (which should be avoided in pregnant patients and in children under 12 years) and gingival hyperplasia with phenytoin and calcium channel blockers.

Oesophageal disorders

These may be induced by the local effects of drugs such as aspirin, tetracycline, doxycycline and bisphosphonates on the oesophagus, leading to irritation, or by drug-induced relaxation of the gastro-oesophageal sphincter producing reflux (e.g. opioids, calcium channel antagonists, nitrates). Symptoms include dysphagia or odynophagia (difficult or painful swallowing, respectively), heartburn, substernal chest pain or the feeling of something lodged in the throat (see Chapter 7).

Bisphosphonates pose a significant risk of oesophagitis and, in the case of alendronic acid, ibandronic acid and risedronate sodium, patients should be counselled to take the tablets with a full tumbler of water in the sitting or standing position and not to lie down for 30 minutes afterwards. These measures are to prevent the tablet becoming lodged in the oesophagus. When a patient is affected then cessation of the particular drug may be appropriate or, in the case of ulceration and/or reflux, a proton pump inhibitor (PPI) might be prescribed.

NSAID gastrotoxicity

NSAID-induced gastrotoxicity represents the most important ADR and is discussed in Chapter 7.

Antiplatelet drugs and gastrotoxicity

The adenosine diphosphate (ADP) receptor antagonist clopidogrel is used as an alternative antiplatelet agent to low-dose aspirin for patients with aspirin sensitivity. Clopidogrel has been shown to exhibit comparable efficacy and fewer adverse GI effects when compared with low-dose aspirin but may cause GI bleeding in patients at risk and should not be used for patients at risk of GI bleeding (see Chapter 14; Harker *et al* 1999).

Diarrhoea

Drug-induced diarrhoea is discussed in Chapter 9.

Nausea and vomiting

Drug-induced nausea and vomiting are discussed in Chapter 8.

Constipation

Drug-induced constipation is discussed in Chapter 9.

Malabsorption

As the major role of the GI tract is the digestion and absorption of food, alterations in absorption can arise from adverse drug effects, e.g. the pancreatic lipase inhibitor, orlistat, reduces the absorption of fat and consequently the absorption of fat-soluble vitamins. In some cases it may be appropriate to give vitamin supplements (in particular vitamin D), which should be given at least 2 hours after orlistat. Another example are the bile-binding agents such as colestyramine which also reduce the absorption of fat-soluble vitamins, and supplementation with vitamins A, D, E and K might be appropriate.

Hepatic ADRs

Liver function may be altered by drugs to varying degrees, ranging from mild, reversible and asymptomatic changes identified by routine liver function tests (LFTs) to severe damage, leading to hepatic failure. Drug types and classes associated with altered liver function through to liver failure include:

- antiepileptic drugs
- halothane
- paracetamol
- methotrexate
- amiodarone
- flucloxacillin
- clavulonic acid in co-amoxiclav.

Risk factors for developing drug-induced hepatic dysfunction:

- pre-existing liver disease
- female sex
- age
- genetic variations in the expression of cytochrome P450 isoenzymes
- concurrent treatment with enzyme inducers (see Drug interactions below)
- polypharmacy
- concurrent disease: diabetes mellitus predisposes patients to methotrexate-induced damage
- nutritional status: fasting patients lack glutathione required in the non-toxic pathway of paracetamol metabolism
- alcohol consumption.

Clinical features

The presentation of liver impairment may vary but key features that should raise the suspicion of liver dysfunction include anorexia, nausea, vomiting, jaundice, itching, pale stools and dark urine. Patients who are prescribed drugs that are known to cause liver dysfunction should be counselled to report these symptoms if they occur. Diagnosis may be based on a drug history, clinical features, an LFT and a biopsy.

Paracetamol-induced hepatotoxicity and patient counselling

Paracetamol is the most common cause of drug-induced hepatotoxicity. This is partly due to a lack of awareness of the potential toxicity of paracetamol or its presence in different medicines taken together, leading to accidental ingestion of excessive doses (see Chapter 29).

Monitoring

The monitoring of liver function is discussed in Chapter 2. It should be noted that elevated LFTs are not always followed by hepatic injury. Generally an increase of two to three times any baseline value would indicate possible drug-induced hepatotoxicity and the need to stop the drug.

Cardiovascular ADRs

Drug-induced cardiovascular disorders are common and often predictable type A reactions, particularly in patients with pre-existing heart disease. Additional risk factors include undisclosed self-medication with OTC drugs, electrolyte disturbances and impaired renal function.

Drugs used to manage cardiovascular diseases may have predictable cardiovascular consequences, e.g. volume depletion with diuretics or inhibition of autonomic homeostatic mechanisms (e.g. α blockers) are very commonly associated with orthostatic or postural hypotension. This is especially prominent in elderly patients and associated with a high risk of falls. Obviously judicious prescribing might reduce this risk by choosing safer alternative agents and counselling patients to take care when changing posture. In the case of ACE inhibitors and α blockers they also pose a risk of first-dose hypotension (especially if the patient is already taking a diuretic) when the initiation of treatment may lead to a precipitous drop in blood pressure. When these drugs are used the patient should be counselled initially to take the drug when retiring to bed to reduce the problems posed by first-dose hypotension.

Drugs may themselves exacerbate or increase cardiovascular risk. Long-term NSAID usage can be associated with increased risk of coronary disease (Kearney *et al* 2006), whereas the fluid-retaining properties of NSAIDs may exacerbate chronic heart failure or lead to hypertension. Similarly there has been concern that the antidiabetic rosiglitazone might increase cardiovascular risk, and this is especially important because patients with diabetes are already at increased risk (Nissen and Wolski 2007). Obviously assessing a patient's overall cardiovascular risk is important when deciding on a treatment and identifying drug-induced cardiovascular effects as appropriate.

Reduction in heart rate or slowing of atrioventricular conduction is the aim of using β blockers, rate-limiting calcium channel blockers or digoxin. However, at high doses or if the patient has conduction problems, this may lead to bradycardia with a reduction in cardiac output. Hence, patients taking digoxin are counselled to ensure that their heart rate does not drop below 60 beats/min and all negative chronotropic drugs should be used with caution in patients with conduction problems.

The prolongation of the Q–T interval, as revealed by electrocardiogram (ECG), and subsequent risk of life-threatening torsade de pointes arrhythmias, have led to the withdrawal of drugs such as cisapride, terfenadine, thioridazine and astemizole. The CSM/CHM has advised against the co-prescribing of two or more drugs known to prolong the Q–T interval. Drugs associated with Q–T prolongation include:

- amiodarone
- sotalol
- disopyramide
- macrolide antibacterial agents
- azole antifungal agents
- tricyclic antidepressants (amitriptyline and imipramine)
- antipsychotic agents (including chlorpromazine, haloperidol, sertindole).

Risk factors for developing this ADR include:

- female sex
- family history of coronary heart disease
- smoking
- high stress levels
- substance misuse, particularly alcohol or cocaine
- renal or hepatic impairment or slow metabolizers
- metabolic-type drug interactions (due to increased drug levels)
- electrolyte disturbance such as hypokalaemia or hypomagnesaemia, e.g. with laxatives or diuretics
- high doses, particularly of antipsychotics
- polypharmacy and particularly concurrent diuretic treatment
- bradycardia
- cardiovascular disease: hypertension, congestive heart failure
- a history of Q–T interval prolongation.

For further information and a list of drugs that prolong the Q–T interval, see Haddad and Anderson (2002) and www.torsades.org.

Patient counselling

Patients prescribed drugs with the potential to prolong the Q–T interval should be advised to report urgently symptoms of arrhythmia such as dizziness, light-headedness, irregular pulse, palpitations and fainting. Drugs should be stopped immediately and the ECG monitored.

Renal ADRs

The kidneys are responsible for the elimination of many drugs and are common targets for drug-induced toxicity, particularly in elderly patients with age-related renal impairment. Drugs implicated commonly include ACE inhibitors, diuretics and NSAIDs, commonly prescribed for the ageing patient with cardiovascular disease and chronic inflammatory conditions such as rheumatoid arthritis. Common mechanisms for drug-induced renal impairment include:

- reduced renal perfusion, e.g. volume depletion during diuretic therapy

- altered glomerular filtration due to altered tone of renal arterioles in the presence of ACE inhibitors or NSAIDs, which inhibit the effects of angiotensin II or prostaglandins respectively
- damage to renal tubules due to inflammatory reactions triggered by many drugs, including NSAIDs.

Additional risk factors for renal ADRs include dehydration, cirrhosis or heart failure (due to sodium retention), diabetes, polypharmacy (particularly of nephrotoxic drugs), high doses of the causative agent, hypotension, sepsis and shock.

Clinical features

See Chapter 18.

Patient counselling

- Patients with risk factors for renal disorders as outlined above should report nausea, vomiting and muscle cramps. Urinalysis should be undertaken to check for the presence of protein.
- Patients taking diuretics and/or laxatives are at risk of prerenal failure due to reduced renal perfusion and should therefore report fatigue, postural hypotension and muscle cramps. This is particularly important in elderly patients and those taking additional nephrotoxic drugs. Patients should be referred to their general practitioner (GP) and/or a dose of diuretic omitted when suffering from conditions that may result in dehydration, e.g. excess sweating, diarrhoea and/or vomiting.

Haematological ADRs (Table 5.2)

Drugs such as cytotoxic agents cause predictable suppression of bone marrow and could therefore be considered type A reactions. Many drugs may, however, unpredictably affect the bone marrow and blood cell production. With the exception of cytotoxics, drug-induced blood dyscrasias are rare but potentially fatal, and therefore health professionals should be aware of drugs known to

cause these effects. Drugs can cause aplastic anaemia in which typically all cells lines are affected; they can cause neutropenia (agranulocytosis) with white cells affected and thrombocytopenia in which there is a reduction in platelets. Alerting symptoms include sore throat, mouth ulcers, bruising or bleeding, rash, malaise and fever, or non-specific illness.

Other drug-induced haematological problems include haemolytic anaemia (as discussed above in patients with G6PD deficiency) and megaloblastic anaemia through impaired metabolism of either vitamin B_{12} or folic acid. In this latter case methotrexate's pharmacological action is to interfere with DNA synthesis by acting as a folate antagonist and so megaloblastic anaemia is a dose-dependent ADR. To avoid this, patients may receive folate supplements.

Respiratory ADRs

The most significant respiratory ADR is bronchospasm with β blockers and is discussed in detail in Chapter 21. Other examples include anaphylaxis with bronchospasm, which may be life threatening (see Chapter 20), and ACE inhibitor-induced cough (see Chapter 11). Long-term lung damage may also occur and examples of this include amiodarone leading to pulmonary fibrosis and pneumonitis, and methotrexate also causing pneumonitis. In both cases patients should report any change in respiratory function.

Psychiatric ADRs

These are relatively common and consist mainly of type A reactions predictable from pharmacological activity. Psychiatric and cognitive problems occur with a range of drugs and can be exacerbated by alcohol abuse, liver disease or a history of depression. A number of drugs can induce depression and these include isotretinoin, rimonabant (for weight loss), varenicline (for smoking cessation) and the antimalarial mefloquine, which is contraindicated in neuropsychiatric disorders, including depression, or convulsions. SSRIs have been implicated in inducing suicidal thoughts (Fergusson *et al*

Table 5.2   A summary of adverse drug reactions involving the haematological system

Haematological disorder	Important examples of causative drugs	Comments
Aplastic anaemia (total or partial failure of the bone marrow)	**Antidiabetic** (chlorpropamide, tolbutamide) **Antiepileptics** (carbamazepine, phenytoin, lamotrigine) **Anti-inflammatory** (diclofenac, gold, indometacin, penicillamine, piroxicam, sulindac, sulfasalazine) **Antimicrobials** (chloramphenicol, co-trimoxazole, sulphonamides) **Antipsychotics** (chlorpromazine) **Antithyroid agents** (carbimazole, propylthiouracil)	• Reduced red cell (anaemia), white cell (leukopenia) and platelet (thrombocytopenia) counts • Often irreversible despite drug withdrawal
Neutropenia (profound reduction of granulo-cytes with neutrophil count <0.5×10^9/L)	**Antibiotics** (e.g. co-trimoxazole) **Antidepressants** (e.g. imipramine, mianserin) **Antiepileptics** (e.g. carbamazepine, phenytoin) **Anti-inflammatory** (e.g. gold, penicil-lamine, lefunomide, sulfasalazine, NSAIDs) **Antipsychotics** (e.g. chlorpromazine, clozapine) **Antithyroid drugs** (carbimazole, propylthiouracil)	• Recovery usually 2–3 weeks after drug is withdrawn • Repeat exposure to causative drug not recommended due to sensitization
Thrombocytopenia (reduced platelets to <150×10^9/L)	**Antimicrobials** (e.g. chloramphenicol, co-trimoxazole) **Antiepileptics** (e.g. sodium valproate) **Anti-inflammatory** (e.g. gold, NSAIDs, penicillamine) **Diuretics** (thiazides, furosemide) **Others** (tolbutamide, digitoxin, methyldopa, heparin [less likely with low-molecular-weight heparin], quinidine)	• May present as easy bleeding, bruising or purpura • Prolonged bleeding time but INR remains normal • Usually occurs 7–10 days after drug started • Avoid future exposure to the causative agent • Aspirin and NSAIDs reduce the effects of remaining platelets and therefore should be avoided during thrombocytopenia
Pure red cell aplasia (total or partial failure of red cell production)	Azathioprine, phenytoin, isoniazid, penicillamine, chlorpropamide, chloramphenicol, erythropoietin	Anaemia with a marked reduction in reticulocytes (immature red cells)

NSAIDs, non-steroidal anti-inflammatory drugs; INR, international normalized ratio.

2005), especially in children, and it is for this reason that they are no longer recommended for use in patients under 18 years of age. Many centrally acting drugs cause sedation and this is particularly true of tricyclic antidepressants, benzodiazepines, barbiturates, opioids, antipsychotic agents and sedating antihistamines. Although this can be an advantage when sedation is required, e.g. depression with insomnia, it can be a particularly debilitating side effect and may lead to a lack of patient compliance. When prescribing, this might be avoided by choosing a safe alternative, e.g. an SSRI for depression. When sedating drugs are used it may help to counsel the patient to take the drug when retiring to bed to reduce the side effect, and in all cases the patient should be counselled about the sedating effects.

Neurological ADRs

Neurological disorders encompass disorders of the nervous system, including the brain, spinal cord and all peripheral nerves. Common examples include the following.

Drug-induced movement disorders

Drugs with antidopaminergic actions (such as antipsychotics and metoclopramide) may lead to a drug-induced form of Parkinson's disease (see Chapter 28). The general approach to the management of this ADR is to withdraw the offending drug and use a safer alternative.

Decreased seizure threshold

Some drugs may reduce the threshold for seizure and increase the risk of convulsions. These drugs include antidepressants, bupropion, mefloquine, chloroquine, sedating antihistamines, tramadol, theophylline and quinolone antibiotics. The risk of convulsions is greatest in patients with a history of epilepsy, brain tumours or trauma, and the drug should be used with caution.

Endocrine ADRs

ADRs may also affect a variety of endocrine control systems such as the thyroid and adrenal glands.

Glucose control

See Chapter 35.

Thyroid dysfunction

See Chapter 36.

Adrenal function

Cushing's syndrome
Cushing's syndrome is caused by prolonged treatment with corticosteroids. Clinical signs include 'moon face', weight gain, excess growth of facial and body hair, raised blood pressure, raised blood glucose levels, osteoporosis, psychiatric symptoms, including depressed mood, and skin thinning.

Adrenal insufficiency
Abrupt withdrawal of corticosteroids following prolonged treatment may lead to headache, dizziness, joint pain, weakness and emotional changes. Abrupt withdrawal from long-term treatment may be more severe and potentially fatal.

Drugs that themselves can precipitate adrenal insufficiency include the antifungal agent ketoconazole and rifampicin.

Hyperprolactinaemia

Prolactin is synthesized and stored in the anterior pituitary gland, being released following childbirth, stimulating milk production and progesterone production by the corpus luteum in the ovary. Drug-induced hyperprolactinaemia may occur in patients taking drugs that increase serotonin (5-hydroxytryptamine or 5HT) or reduce dopamine effects (e.g. phenothiazines), leading to galactorrhoea (abnormal milk production), amenorrhoea, impotence or infertility. The condition is usually reversible on cessation of treatment.

Syndrome of inappropriate secretion of antidiuretic hormone (SIADH)

Some drugs can cause an inappropriate secretion of the antidiuretic hormone (ADH or vasopressin) from the pituitary gland, leading to increased reabsorption of water in the kidneys and an increase in extracellular volume with dilute plasma. Symptoms include confusion, weakness, lethargy, weight gain, headache, nausea and vomiting, and ultimately convulsions, coma and death. Monitoring of baseline serum sodium levels is prudent in patients prescribed drugs known to cause SIADH, particularly antipsychotics, carbamazepine and antidepressants (particularly SSRIs), especially if co-prescribed with other drugs that may cause hyponatraemia (see Chapter 2).

Dermatological ADRs (Table 5.3)

The skin a major site of ADRs, from trivial rashes right through to life-threatening reactions. Any drug, chemical, herb or pharmaceutical excipient has the potential to cause a dermatological reaction. The mechanisms involved are often unknown but tend to result from an allergic or toxic reaction or exacerbation of a pre-existing inflammatory condition. Allergic reactions such as urticaria may persist for a long time after a drug is stopped or may occasionally fail to develop for up to a week after a drug is withdrawn. The drugs most commonly implicated in ADRs include penicillins, NSAIDs, phenytoin, gold, chlorpromazine and cytotoxic agents.

Identification of the causative agent of a dermatological reaction can be difficult, as rechallenge is not appropriate, with the possible exception of fixed drug eruptions. When making a diagnosis, it is important to consider the information included in summaries of product characteristics (SPCs), previous case reports, the pattern of eruption, together with consideration of a temporal relationship between drug administration and ADR development. A temporal relationship may be apparent in some cases but in others a reaction may take anything from hours to years to develop. Any serious skin reaction should be reported to the CHM/MHRA on a Yellow Card, particularly angio-oedema, bullous eruption, epidermal necrolysis and generalized exfoliation. In addition, any dermatological reactions suspected to result from new drugs should be reported.

Some important dermatological skin reactions are summarized in Table 5.3.

Table 5.3   A summary of adverse drug reactions involving the skin

Dermatological disorder	Important examples of causative drugs	Comments
Urticaria	Penicillins, NSAIDs, ACE inhibitors	Itchy, weal-and-flare rash. Should respond to oral antihistamines
Erythematous eruptions	Penicillins, NSAIDs	Reddening, may resemble measles as a maculopapular rash
Stevens–Johnson syndrome	Co-trimoxazole, phenytoin, lamotrigine	May be preceded by a flu-like illness. Large fluid-filled mucosal blisters. May develop into toxic epidermal necrolysis
Toxic epidermal necrolysis	Co-trimoxazole, carbamazepine, phenytoin	Rare but may be fatal with blistering and skin peeling off
Psoriasis	β Blockers, chloroquine, lithium	These drugs may exacerbate the condition
Photosensitivity	Thiazides, isotretinoin, amiodarone	Patients should avoid direct sunlight or wear sunblock

ACE, angiotensin-converting enzyme; NSAID, non-steroidal anti-inflammatory drug.

Patient counselling

- Educate patients to avoid direct sunlight and sunbeds, wear protective clothing and use high-protection factor sunscreen during and for a few months after receiving photosensitizing drugs.
- Patients should be aware of previous allergic reactions to drugs and encouraged to report them to health professionals. The distinction between traditional side effects and allergy should be made to avoid confusion.

Musculoskeletal ADRs

Drugs may adversely affect muscles, bone and connective tissues in a number of ways, from fluid retention in muscle producing mild aches and pains, to debilitating osteoporosis or life-threatening rhabdomyolysis. It is important to be aware of drugs causing musculoskeletal pathology because early recognition and cessation of the drug can prevent unnecessary suffering and uncertainty, while improving the outcome for patients.

Rhabdomyolysis

This is the breakdown of skeletal muscle leading to the release of myoglobin, which has the potential to block renal tubules and result in renal failure. Rhabdomyolysis may follow myopathy and so it is important that patients reporting muscle pain associated with drug therapy are investigated. Important examples of drugs causing myopathy include fibrates and statins. The co-prescribing of these drugs increases the risk of myopathy. Indeed cerivastatin was withdrawn in 2001 because it was associated with high instances of myopathy, especially when used with fibrates.

Patient counselling

- Patients taking statins and/or fibrates should report muscle weakness, pain or tenderness.
- To prevent drug-induced osteoporosis, patients prescribed long-term steroid courses should be advised to stop smoking, limit alcohol consumption, take regular weight-bearing exercise, and ensure an adequate calcium and vitamin D intake.
- Patients should stop taking quinolone antibiotics at the first sign of tendon damage such as pain or inflammation. The affected limb should be rested until tendon symptoms have resolved.
- Young patients prescribed minocycline for more than 6 months should report symptoms such as arthralgia, fever, rash and pleuritic pain, which may indicate systemic lupus erythematosus (SLE).

Monitoring for ADRs

- ECG monitoring should be considered for patients taking tricyclic antidepressants and other drugs that prolong the Q–T interval, and particularly in the presence of additional risk factors such as coronary heart disease. Consider also regular monitoring of potassium levels and the avoidance, if possible, of drugs known to cause hypokalaemia, such as high-dose β_2-adrenoceptor agonists or diuretics (see Chapter 2).
- Patients prescribed treatment long term should be monitored regularly for adverse effects, e.g. patients taking minocycline for longer than 6 months should be monitored for hepatotoxicity, pigmentation and SLE.
- Consider drugs for which regular blood tests are recommended. Common tests include LFTs, full blood counts, renal function or thyroid function tests (see Chapter 2). Monitoring of renal and hepatic function is particularly important for elderly patients taking prescribed drugs.

Reporting of suspected ADRs

Doctors, dentists, coroners, pharmacists and nurses may submit Yellow Cards to the CHM/MHRA for all suspected ADRs produced by new (black triangle) drugs and serious ADRs for all other drugs.

The lessons from rofecoxib

Rofecoxib is a selective cyclo-oxygenase-2 (COX-2) inhibitor that was introduced in the late 1990s to selectively inhibit this 'pathological' isoform of the enzyme associated with inflammation, and leave the 'physiological' isoform responsible for gastroprotection unaffected, so reducing the incidence of peptic ulceration. Indeed it was hailed as a 'wonder drug'. However, in 2000 the VIGOR trial indicated that rofecoxib was associated with increased cardiovascular events compared with the naproxen control (Bombardier *et al* 2000). One interpretation at the time was that naproxen was, in comparison, actually protective and that rofecoxib was safe. This resulted in further studies which indicated that rofecoxib increased cardiovascular risk by 1.5- to 3.6-fold and that between 1999 and 2004 this may have led to 88 000–140 000 excess cases of severe coronary artery disease in the USA (Graham *et al*

2005). Consequently rofecoxib was immediately withdrawn form the market. Although this adverse safety profile appeared confined to rofecoxib, patients should be assessed for cardiovascular risk when using COX-2 inhibitors such as celecoxib. Further work has also indicated a small but significant increase in cardiovascular risk for NSAIDs when used long term and at high doses (low dose and occasional use being regarded as safe) (Kearney *et al* 2006). The risk is greatest for diclofenac with naproxen being regarded as safe.

The clear lesson learnt from the rofecoxib story is to exercise caution in all areas of drug safety, especially with new drugs, even if their introduction to the market appears to be a landmark in therapeutics. The second lesson is that careful analysis can reveal safety issues with well-established drugs, hence the need to use NSAIDs with appropriate caution.

Practice points

- Health professionals should always consider the adverse effects of drugs, including OTC and herbal supplements when making a diagnosis. Early identification of ADRs may improve the outcome for the patient and prevent unnecessary treatment and intervention.
- Always check the medication history when presented with a rash. Consider drugs stopped recently.
- Take care to identify drug allergies because reintroduction may be more severe. Drug allergies should be recorded prominently on all patient medication records.
- Prescribe a drug only when there is a good indication.
- NSAID-induced gastric damage is a major ADR. To reduce the risk:
  - only one NSAID should be prescribed at any one time
  - a less toxic agent such as ibuprofen should be used first line
  - the lowest effective dose is recommended
  - the maximum daily dose should not be exceeded
  - patients at risk should be prescribed prophylaxis (Chapter 7)
  - long term, repeat prescriptions should be reviewed
  - patients should be counselled to report warning symptoms (see above).
- Ideally, NSAIDs should be avoided in patients with coronary heart disease and particularly congestive heart failure and hypertension, due to an increase in fluid retention and potential for increased cardiovascular risk. If essential, the lowest effective dose should be prescribed and drugs with a long elimination half-life avoided.
- The greatest bone loss induced by corticosteroid therapy occurs during the first 6–12 months. Early preventive steps are therefore important. Patients taking prednisolone 7.5 mg or more daily for 3 months or more, particularly if aged over 65 years, should be assessed for prophylaxis with hormone replacement therapy, bisphosphonate or calcitriol as appropriate (see Chapter 30).
- Always use the lowest effective dose of all drugs.
- Withdraw drugs associated with withdrawal symptoms gradually.
- Increased monitoring and education of patients to improve the recognition and reporting of suspected ADRs are important issues for preventing ADRs (Avery *et al* 2002).

Drug interactions

Drug interactions may simply be thought of as the actions of one drug being enhanced or inhibited by the presence or actions of another drug or exogenous substance. These may be adverse or beneficial. In addition to recognizing the potential for prescribed medicines to interact, one must always bear in mind the potential for OTC medicines, foods and the constituents of herbal remedies to interact with them.

Although the number of established interactions is extremely large, their importance varies from trivial to potentially life threatening. On the face of it, it is difficult to predict straightforwardly the importance of an interaction but this comes with clinical experience. How does one deal with interactions? Clearly there are a small number of life-threatening combinations that should be avoided. Other interactions require vigilance and careful monitoring, e.g. measuring the international normalized ratio (INR) with warfarin when co-prescribed with an interacting drug and responding with appropriate dosage alterations. In other cases, an interaction may be extremely rare but established in the literature, and in such cases vigilance is important because being over-cautious might result in a patient not receiving a drug when the likelihood of an interaction is very small. As with all drug usage, it is the balance between the beneficial and the adverse effects.

In practice, drug interactions are continually being identified by automated systems and databases and it is often difficult to differentiate between clinically significant and trivial interactions. The BNF is also a valuable resource for interactions but does not necessarily indicate the likelihood of an interaction or how to deal with it. The reader is referred to *Stockley's Drug Interactions* (Baxter 2008) for evidence-based information presented in a user-friendly reference with a concise summary of reported drug interactions. In the following chapters an attempt is made to highlight common, serious and clinically significant drug interactions relevant to each section.

Mechanisms of drug interactions

When considering drug interactions the following, in particular, may alert the practitioner to potential problems, which may predispose towards an interaction:

- drugs with a narrow therapeutic window: anticoagulants, anticonvulsants, digoxin, lithium, theophylline and cytotoxic agents
- metabolic enzyme inducers and inhibitors
- drugs with similar pharmacological effects
- extremes of age.

As with ADRs, the mechanisms of interactions are often pharmacological or pharmacokinetic. In one sense the pharmacological interactions are the easiest ones to predict and respond to, e.g. one would expect the actions of a β_2-adrenoceptor agonist for asthma to be opposed by the concurrent use of a β blocker. This is one reason why β blockers are avoided in asthma. Other examples of pharmacological interactions are given in Table 5.4.

Pharmacokinetic interactions

These follow the established pattern of ADME.

Absorption
Absorption reactions may result in a change in either the rate of drug absorption or the total amount of drug absorbed. The following are some key mechanisms.

Acid suppression
Drug absorption occurs best with the uncharged form, which is determined by the individual pK_a for a drug. Accordingly, changes in pH (e.g. rises in the presence of antacids and acid suppressors) may influence the absorption of other drugs. The importance of other interactions resulting from changes in gastric pH is uncertain due to the involvement of additional mechanisms affecting absorption. It is therefore advisable to separate in time the administration of drugs such as antacids, H_2-receptor antagonists and PPIs from other drugs (see Chapter 7).

Table 5.4   Examples of pharmacodynamic interactions

Interacting drugs	Consequences	Explanation
β-Adrenoceptor agonists and ß blockers Adrenaline (epinephrine) and ß blockers	Antagonism Antagonism	These agents will oppose each other • Adrenaline used in anaphylaxis treatment will be opposed by β blockers • Risk of hypertensive crisis (especially with non-selective β blockers) as the vasoconstrictor activity of adrenaline via α-adrenoceptors will no longer be opposed by $β_2$-adrenoceptor-mediated vasodilatation
β Blockers and verapamil	Addition of actions	The combined negative inotropic and chronotropic effects may lead to asystole
Nitrates and sildenafil, tadalafil or vardenafil	Potentiation, leading to severe hypotension	Nitrates act via cGMP, the metabolism of which is prevented by the phosphodiesterase inhibitors. These drugs should be avoided in combination
Antihypertensives	Potentiation, leading to a severe hypotension or used clinically for more effective blood pressure control	Summation of actions (see Chapter 11)
Antihypertensives and oral sympathomimetic decongestants	Opposing actions	Avoid sympathomimetics in hypertension, particularly if poorly controlled
SSRIs and $5HT_1$-receptor agonists	Serotonin syndrome (Chapter 24)	SSRIs will prevent the breakdown of endogenous 5HT, leading to over-stimulation of serotoninergic system
Betahistine and antihistamines	Antagonism	Betahistine is a histaminergic agent with actions opposed by antihistamines
Warfarin and vitamin K	Antagonism	Warfarin is a vitamin K antagonist
Hypoglycaemic drugs and corticosteroids	Antagonism	Corticosteroids have a diabetogenic effect
Alcohol and sedative agents (including sedative antihistamines)	Potentiation	Potentiation
Potassium-sparing diuretics, ACE inhibitors and potassium	Potentiation, leading to hyperkalaemia	All cause potassium retention
Levodopa activity and some antipsychotic and antiemetic drugs	Antagonism	Some antipsychotic drugs may induce parkinsonism
Drugs that cause Q–T prolongation (e.g. amiodarone, sotalol), macrolide antibacterial agents, azole antifungal agents, tricyclic antidepressants (amitriptyline and imipramine), antipsychotic agents (including chlorpromazine, haloperidol, sertindole)	Potentiation	Risk of torsade de pointes, arrhythmia and potentially fatal ventricular fibrillation
Drugs with antimuscarinic side effects (e.g. tricyclic antidepressants; certain older antihistamines, e.g. promethazine, see above)	Enhanced antimuscarinic side effects	Side effects include blurred vision, urinary retention, dry mouth and possibly cardiac effects

5HT, 5-hydroxytryptamine or serotonin; ACE, angiotensin-converting enzyme; cGMP, guanosine cyclic 3′5′-monophosphate; SSRI, selective serotonin reuptake inhibitor.

Binding of drugs

The chemical binding of co-prescribed drugs or drugs with metals in the diet may prevent the drug from being absorbed. A classic example of this is the chelation of tetracyclines with metallic cations, e.g. calcium in diary products or iron in iron replacement therapy. The simple solution to preventing an interaction is to separate the doses of tetracycline from iron administration or dairy products consumption by 2–3 h. Another example is colestyramine, which binds to and reduces the absorption of digoxin (see Chapters 10 and 12) and once again concurrent drugs should be taken 1 h before or 4–6 h after colestyramine.

Altered gastric motility

Gastric emptying determines the rate of movement of drugs into the small intestines, the site at which many drugs are absorbed. Accordingly changes in gastric emptying may influence the rate of drug absorption, e.g. metoclopramide accelerates gastric emptying and is used to enhance the rate of onset of action of paracetamol in some compound antimigraine preparations.

Altered bacterial flora

Broad-spectrum antibiotics often alter the balance of gut bacteria and this may also lead to indirect drug interactions, e.g. the use of erythromycin may inhibit the production of vitamin K by gut bacteria and, if the patient is taking the vitamin K antagonist warfarin, this can enhance the actions of warfarin leading to toxicity.

Drugs excreted in the bile may undergo metabolism by gut flora to active metabolites, which are then reabsorbed. This is thought to underlie a potential interaction between oral contraceptives and some broad-spectrum antibiotics, where alterations in gut flora may interrupt this cycle and reduce the amount of oestrogens. This can lead to a failure of contraception and so patients are advised to use barrier methods of contraception when receiving broad-spectrum antibiotic regimens of less than 3 weeks.

Distribution

Protein-binding interactions

This type of interaction typically involves two drugs competing for plasma protein or tissue binding. The resulting interaction may lead to displacement from binding sites and increased plasma concentrations. However, the rise in plasma concentration is often offset by enhanced elimination. Accordingly, the clinical significance of this type of interaction tends to be limited. An example of this is the interaction occurring between valproate and phenytoin, where phenytoin may be displaced from plasma protein binding by the former.

Metabolism

Although drug metabolism occurs at a range of sites, hepatic metabolism, and particularly that involving cytochrome P450-dependent mechanisms, represents the most common site of interaction. Alterations in drug metabolism can occur via the induction or inhibition of cytochrome P450-dependent enzymes. As this family comprises a range of isoenzymes, there is added complexity because some forms will be affected by specific inhibitors or inducers and others will not. Accordingly it is difficult to predict which drugs will interact in this way. Having said that, as indicated below certain drugs are established as either enzyme inhibitors or inducers and should ring alarm bells for potential interactions.

Enzyme inhibition

Some drugs inhibit cytochrome P450 enzymes, resulting in reduced metabolism of other drugs. These are dose dependent and interactions generally develop relatively rapidly with an increase in plasma concentrations (Figure 5.2) and pharmacological effects of the affected drug. Important examples of drugs that may inhibit the various isoenzymes include:

- cimetidine
- ciprofloxacin
- erythromycin
- clarithromycin
- metronidazole
- fluoxetine
- ketoconazole
- fluconazole

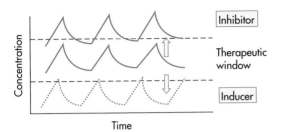

Figure 5.2 A graph of plasma concentration–time for a theoretical drug with a narrow therapeutic window. Enzyme inhibitors may increase the plasma concentrations leading to toxic levels and inducers may reduce concentrations to subtherapeutic levels.

- itraconazole
- grapefruit juice
- verapamil
- omeprazole.

Enzyme induction

This forms an extremely common mechanism for drug interactions and leads to increased metabolism of the affected drug, reducing plasma concentrations (Figure 5.2) and therapeutic effects. The result may be failure of treatment and an important example of this occurs with oral contraceptives when used with inducing agents such as rifampicin or carbamazepine. An increased dose may be required due to the increased metabolism of a co-prescribed drug.

In addition, autoinduction occurs, whereby a drug enhances its own metabolism, so that the doses need to be built up. Important examples of this include barbiturates and carbamazepine. Enzyme induction involves an increase in the amount of microsomal enzymes and cytochrome P450 levels in liver cells. Such interactions take from days to 2–3 weeks to develop and also to reverse when a drug is stopped. Good monitoring is essential, particularly as any change in dose may need to be corrected on cessation of the enzyme inducer to prevent overdose.

Agents associated with induction include:

- barbiturates
- rifampicin
- omeprazole
- phenytoin
- ethanol

- carbamazepine
- St John's wort
- tobacco and cannabis smoke (polycyclic hydrocarbons).

Renal excretion

The weak acid and weak base transporters in the proximal convoluted tubules may be the site of drug interactions, where there is competition for excretion. One very important example of this occurs between methothrexate and certain NSAIDs, and this may result in methotrexate toxicity as its excretion is reduced. Hence, patients taking methotrexate should not take NSAIDs, even as OTC medicines, without the advice of their doctor.

Excretion of drugs via the weak acid and weak base transporters is also pH dependent, such that alkaline urine enhances the excretion of weak acids and vice versa. This is generally of minor significance but can lead to differences in excretion rate between individuals and was previously employed to enhance drug elimination in overdose when alkaline diuresis was used to enhance the elimination of salicylates.

Conclusions

The management of ADRs and drug interactions remains central to the prevention of drug-related problems. Key issues include the implementation of updated computer warning systems to support health professionals in interpreting the ever-increasing number of potential drug interactions, together with the avoidance of polypharmacy, particularly in elderly patients.

Summary of some key interactions

As indicated above there are numerous drug interactions of varying importance and some key drug interactions include:

- NSAIDs and warfarin: leading to enhanced bleeding
- NSAIDs and methotrexate: leading to methotrexate toxicity
- warfarin and erythromycin: leading to enhanced bleeding

- ACE inhibitors and potassium/potassium-sparing diuretics: risk of hyperkalaemia
- verapamil and β blockers: risk of asystole
- digoxin and amiodarone: risk of digoxin toxicity

- digoxin and verapamil: risk of digoxin toxicity
- oral contraceptives and certain inducing agents (e.g. rifampicin, carbamazepine and phenytoin): risk of failure of contraception.

Practice points

- The key point is clearly vigilance to any changes in a patient's condition that may point to an ADR or interaction.
- Become familiar with clinically significant interactions.
- Warfarin, lithium, theophylline and digoxin therapy should always alert practitioners to be vigilant for ADRs or interactions.
- The change to a patient's therapy that involves a drug known to influence metabolism should prompt a review of all concurrent drugs, whether prescribed, OTC or herbal remedies.
- Consider the pharmacology of drugs when prescribing to allow for the prediction of pharmacodynamic reactions. Avoid using drugs with similar pharmacology.
- It is good practice to be familiar with common interactions as current computer systems have been found to be lacking in the management of drug interactions.
- Patients should always be questioned about their use of OTC and herbal medicines.

 CASE STUDIES

Case 1
A man returning from 6 months in India reports a scaly rash on his knees and elbows.

What is the most likely cause of this rash?
Possibly drug-induced psoriasis if the patient took chloroquine for malaria prophylaxis.

Case 2
A man prescribed a prolonged course (more than 14 days) of co-amoxiclav for a persistent chest infection reports vomiting, general malaise and pruritus.

What is the likely cause of his symptoms?
Clavulanic acid-induced cholestatic hepatitis should be suspected.

Case 3
A woman requests that her GP give her a prescription for antibiotics to treat cystitis. On further questioning the symptoms include polyuria, loin pain and blood-stained urine. There is no pain on urination and no clouding or offensive smell. The only medication that the woman takes are painkillers that she buys from the supermarket for headaches.

These symptoms may point to analgesic nephropathy because cystitis normally presents with a burning pain on urination and/or clouding and an offensive smell. Cystitis is more common, but, in view of the symptoms, together with the chronic use of painkillers, further investigation is required. Antibiotics may not be appropriate.

continued

Case 4
A middle-aged man requests aspirin tablets to treat pain.

What further questions should be asked?

• Has he taken it before?

This real but hard-to-believe case turned out to be a request for analgesia to treat stomach pain. On further questioning about the nature of the pain, the patient reported a past history of peptic ulcer disease, which he thought had returned.

Case 5
A 65-year-old woman presents with a chesty cough of 2–3 weeks' duration. She takes ibuprofen and methotrexate.

This case includes a possible interaction between ibuprofen and methotrexate, leading to reduced clearance of methotrexate with an increased risk of methotrexate toxicity. The combination of methotrexate and ibuprofen is, however, often used without problems but patients should be closely monitored. Signs of infection may indicate a methotrexate-induced blood dyscrasia. In this example, a full blood count is required. The cough may also suggest pulmonary toxicity with methotrexate.

Case 6
A 41-year-old woman has been taking imipramine since the birth of her baby, now 2 years old. She has been troubled with a persistent sore throat and has white spots on the back of her tongue and is feeling tired and run-down.

On checking the SPC for imipramine, you are alerted to the possibility of agranulocytosis and order a full blood count to be carried out. This is a sensible precaution.

Case 7
A 44-year-old woman prescribed nifedipine for Raynaud's phenomenon reports palpitations. She has been drinking grapefruit juice recently.

This case illustrates a possible interaction between nifedipine and grapefruit juice. The mechanism is thought to involve inhibition of cytochrome P450 isoenzymes by components of grapefruit juice and therefore increased levels of nifedipine.

Case 8
A man has been taking timolol tablets long term for the treatment of hypertension. A colleague prescribed an adrenaline injection for emergency treatment of peanut allergy over the last few years. The patient has administered a single dose in the last year without apparent problems.

In this case, the blockade of β-adrenoceptors will render the adrenaline less effective but could lead to unopposed α-adrenoceptor vasoconstriction. A number of antihypertensives are available, and the timolol should be gradually withdrawn.

continued

CASE STUDIES (continued)

Case 9
A 22-year-old woman requests some medicine for a dry cough. The counter assistant asks the pharmacist if it is appropriate to sell a product containing dextromethorphan to this woman. Her records indicate that she is taking paroxetine.

   This is a rare but potentially serious drug interaction, due to the risk of the patient developing a serotonin-like syndrome (see Chapter 24). Symptoms include tremor, confusion, tachycardia, hypertension and abnormal movements. It would therefore not be appropriate to recommend this product with paroxetine.

References

Avery AJ, Sheikh A, Hurwitz B *et al* (2002). Safer medicines management in primary care. *Br J Gen Pract* **52**(suppl): S17–S22.

Baxter K, ed. (2008). *Stockley's Drug Interactions*, 8th edn. London: Pharmaceutical Press.

Bombardier C, Laine C, Reicin A *et al* (2000) Comparison of upper gastrointestinal toxicity of rofecoxib and naproxen in patients with rheumatoid arthritis. VIGOR Study Group. *N Engl J Med* **343**: 1520–8.

Fergusson D, Doucette S, Glass KC *et al* (2005). Association between suicide attempts and selective serotonin reuptake inhibitors: systematic review of randomised controlled trials. *BMJ* **330**: 396–9.

Graham DJ, Campen D, Hui R *et al* (2005). Risk of acute myocardial infarction and sudden cardiac death in patients treated with cyclo-oxygenase 2 selective and non-selective non-steroidal anti-inflammatory drugs: nested case-control study. *Lancet* **365**: 475–81.

Haddad PM, Anderson IM (2002). Antipsychotic-related QTc prolongation, torsade de pointes and sudden death. *Drugs* **62**: 1649–71.

Harker LA, Boissel JP, Pilgrim AJ *et al* (1999). Comparative safety and tolerability of clopidogrel and aspirin. Results from CAPRIE. *Drug Safety* **21**: 325–35.

Kearney PM, Baigent C, Godwin J *et al* (2006). Do selective cyclo-oxygenase-2 inhibitors and traditional non-steroidal anti-inflammatory drugs increase the risk of atherothrombosis? Meta-analysis of randomised trials. *BMJ* **332**: 1302–8.

Lee A, ed. (2006). *Adverse Drug Reactions*, 2nd edn. London: Pharmaceutical Press.

Martin J, ed. *British National Formulary*, latest edition. London: British Medical Association and Royal Pharmaceutical Society of Great Britain.

Nissen SE, Wolski K (2007). Effect of rosiglitazone on the risk of myocardial infarction and death from cardiovascular causes. *N Engl J Med* **356**: 2457–71.

Piromhamed M, James S, Meakin S *et al* (2004). Adverse drug reactions as cause of admission to hospital: prospective analysis of 18 820 patients. *BMJ* **329**: 15–19.

Further reading

Bhatia P, O'Reilly JF, Li-Kam-Wa E (2001). Adverse reactions and the respiratory system. *Primary Care Respir J* **10**: 39–43.

Dean T (2000). Withdrawing drugs not the solution. *Prescriber* **11**: 11.

Merlo J, Liedholm H, Lindblad U *et al* (2001). Prescriptions with potential drug interactions dispensed at Swedish pharmacies in January 1999: cross sectional study. *BMJ* **323**: 427–8.

Sipilä J, Klaukka T, Martikainen J *et al* (1995). Occurrence of potentially harmful drug combinations among Finnish primary care patients. *Int Pharm J* **9**: 104–7.

Stockley IH (2000). Interaction warnings. *Prescriber* **11**: 120.

Online resources

www.torsades.org
The website of the Arizona Center for Education and Research on Therapeutics which maintains a list of drugs associated with Q–T prolongation (accessed April 2008).

6

Clinical pharmacokinetics

Pharmacokinetics is the study of how the body handles a drug from absorption, distribution and metabolism to excretion (ADME). The interaction of these processes determines both the plasma concentration and how long a drug persists in the blood. Clinical pharmacokinetics is the application of this area of pharmacology and is used to construct dosage regimens and, in the context of therapeutics, it takes account of the variations between individual patients.

Basic pharmacokinetic principles

Absorption and bioavailability

Drugs are administered by various routes, including orally, intravenously, intramuscularly, subcutaneously, by inhalation and rectally. Clearly, the oral route is the most convenient and preferred by patients but it can be less predictable compared with the intravenous route, because absorption can be affected by the presence of food in the stomach, acidic pH, gastric emptying and 'first-pass' metabolism. This last complication is due to absorbed drugs passing straight to the liver where they may be extensively metabolized and their entrance to the systemic circulation is limited. Common examples of drugs undergoing first-pass metabolism include morphine, propranolol and glyceryl trinitrate (GTN); indeed GTN is given as a sublingual spray to overcome this problem. Interestingly, in the case of statins, first-pass metabolism is an advantage because it limits the actions of statins to the liver (see Chapter 12).

The above processes limit the amount of drug administered reaching the systemic circulation.

To account for this, the bioavailability of the drug is considered. This is the fraction of drug administered that reaches the systemic circulation, i.e. the fraction absorbed. Bioavailability (*F*) is calculated from the ratio of the area under the curve (AUC) of the oral dose to the AUC of an intravenous dose:

$$F = \frac{\text{AUC oral}}{\text{AUC i.v.}}$$

For example, the *F* for digoxin tablets is 0.70 (i.e. 70% is absorbed) and so if 250 micrograms are given orally then 70% of the dose (0.70 × 250 = 175 micrograms) enters the circulation. This can then be applied to determine the amount of a drug required. So:

$$\text{Dose given} = \frac{\text{Amount needed}}{F}$$

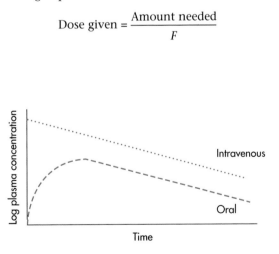

Figure 6.1 A comparison of the log plasma concentration–time plot for a drug via the intravenous and the oral routes. The oral route shows a rising phase as the drug is absorbed. As the drug has a bioavailability <1, the area under the curve (AUC) under the oral plot is proportionally less than under the intravenous plot.

Salt factor

In addition to bioavailability, some medicines are made up of active drug and inert salts. The best example is aminophylline, which is the salt of theophylline, so 80% of the amount of aminophylline is theophylline. This fraction is termed the 'salt factor' or S. So:

$$\text{Amount} = S \times \text{Dose}$$

Amount of drug administered

To take account of F and S the following is applied:

$$\text{Amount} = \text{Dose} \times F \times S$$

Volume of distribution

The volume of distribution (V_d) of a drug is the apparent volume in which a drug is dissolved in the body to give the plasma concentration measured:

$$V_d = \frac{\text{Amount in body}}{\text{Concentration}} = \frac{\text{Dose}}{\text{Concentration at } t = 0}$$

where t is time.

The volume of distribution and (therefore) plasma concentration are determined by where the drug goes in the bodily fluids. A widely distributed drug (e.g. one that moves into fat or other tissues) or one that has extensive protein binding has a high V_d and one that is largely retained in the plasma or has low binding has a low value. A commonly encountered drug with a high V_d is digoxin and this reflects wide tissue distribution. In the case of digoxin, a population average V_d is 7.3 L/kg body mass, so for a 70-kg person this would equate to a V_d of 511 L. This value clearly greatly exceeds body volume and is due to the plasma concentration being lower as a result of wide sequestration in the tissues. The V_d is not merely of scientific interest because it is applied clinically in determining loading doses (see later).

Elimination

Elimination is the removal of the active drug from the body and is largely made up of hepatic metabolism and renal excretion. Generally speaking, it is the sum of these two components, the contributions of which vary greatly. Indeed, knowledge of the routes of elimination is essential for drug choice in renal and hepatic impairment, e.g. digoxin is cleared predominantly (about two-thirds) by the renal route and so doses of digoxin are determined in relation to renal function. The dihydropyridine drug amlodipine is cleared via the hepatic route and is therefore a suitable antihypertensive for patients with renal disease because its elimination is not impaired.

Clearance

Clearance (CL) is a measure of the rate of elimination and is largely made up of renal and hepatic clearance. It is defined as the volume of plasma cleared of a drug in unit time and usually expressed in litres per hour or day. The clearance of drug determines the amount of drug required in a maintenance regimen (see later).

Kinetics of elimination

Most drugs illustrate first-order kinetics and the plasma concentration undergoes an exponential decay (analogous to radioactive decay), so there is a logarithmic relationship between plasma concentration and time (Figure 6.2).

Due to first-order kinetics, the rate of elimination is proportional to the concentration of drug:

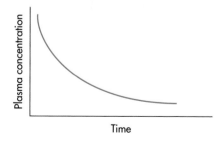

Figure 6.2   The plasma concentration–time plot for a drug illustrating exponential decay due to first-order kinetics.

$$C_t = C_0 e^{-kt}$$

where C_t is the concentration at time t, C_0 the concentration at $t = 0$ and k the rate constant (/min or /h).

This equation is applied to predict plasma concentrations when the concentration at time 0 is known; it may also be used to estimate the time to reach a safe concentration from a toxic level, e.g. if the plasma concentration of a drug such as digoxin is too high, it enables the time for withholding doses to be calculated to reach safe levels.

Rate constant

First-order kinetics involves a rate constant (k) and this is simply the fraction of drug eliminated per unit time, when k is 0.1/day, 10% is eliminated per day. This can be applied mathematically as the clearance per unit time is the fraction of V_d that is cleared per unit time. So:

$$k = \frac{CL}{V_d}$$

or

$$CL = k \times V_d$$

Half-life

This is simply the time for the plasma concentration to decrease by 50%. Therefore at the half-life ($t_{1/2}$):

$$C_t = 0.5\, C_0$$

So:

$$0.5\, C_0 = C_0 e^{-kt}$$

$$\ln 0.5 = -kt$$

$$-0.693 = -kt$$

So $t_{1/2} = \dfrac{0.693}{k}$

Regimens

Pharmacokinetics is applied in the construction of dosing regimens, the purpose of which is to maintain the plasma concentration within the

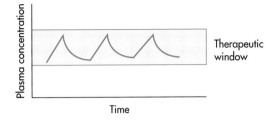

Figure 6.3 The plasma–concentration–time plot for a drug regimen to illustrate the usual approach of maintaining the peaks and troughs within the therapeutic window, to maintain clinical effectiveness and prevent toxicity.

therapeutic window, which is the desired range between toxicity and sub-therapeutic levels. The aim is also to limit the differences between peaks and troughs (Figure 6.3).

In order to achieve a steady state within the therapeutic window regimens are generally based on:

- once daily
- twice daily
- three times daily, often based around 'breakfast, lunch and dinner'
- four times daily.

A once-daily interval is favoured as the most convenient and is likely to achieve the best compliance. However, the above applies to a stable regimen, and at the start of therapy it will take time to achieve steady-state concentration (C_{ss}). A general rule is that it takes 5 half-lives to reach steady state (Figure 6.4).

The explanation to this rule of thumb is provided in Table 6.1, in which the amount

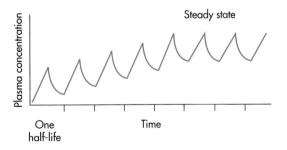

Figure 6.4 The plasma–concentration–time plot for a drug at the start of an oral regimen, when it takes approximately 5 half-lives to reach steady-state concentration.

Table 6.1   Demonstration that steady state is reached after approximately 5 half-lives

Dose	Amount present in the body after one $t_{1/2}$ from dose (%)	Percentage of C_{ss}
First	50	50
Second	50 + 25	75
Third	50 + 37.5	87.5
Fourth	50 + 43.8	93.8
Fifth	50 + 46.9	96.9

present after each half-life is added cumulatively until the amount approaches 100%.

Loading doses

This rule is clinically significant because drugs with a short half-life will soon reach C_{ss}. However, for drugs with long half-lives the time to attain C_{ss} will be prolonged, e.g. digoxin has a half-life of 40 h and will therefore take 200 h or over 8 days to reach C_{ss}. Digoxin is widely used to control ventricular rate in atrial fibrillation and the therapeutic effect is required urgently. Therefore, to overcome the delay, drugs with long half-lives or drugs that require immediate action (e.g. lidocaine in ventricular ectopic beats) are often given as a loading dose to take the plasma concentrations quickly up to a desired level (Figure 6.5).

To calculate a loading dose, the amount required is determined by the desired (safe) plasma concentration multiplied by the volume of distribution:

Amount required = target concentration $\times V_d$.

The dose required must then take account of F and S as follows:

$$\text{Loading dose} = \frac{\text{Amount required}}{F \times S}$$

Maintenance doses

Many therapies involve a maintenance dose to maintain the C_{ss} within the therapeutic window. The maintenance dose equals the amount of drug eliminated per dosage interval and maintains the steady state. Therefore the rate of input equals the rate of output. To consider maintenance dosing, the pharmacokinetics are analogous to a continuous infusion, which involves an increase in plasma concentration followed by a plateau at the steady state where input equals output (Figure 6.6).

So the maintenance dose equals the amount removed. Therefore, we have the relationship:

Infusion rate = CL $\times C_{ss}$

This can then be applied to the oral dosing and the 'infusion' rate equates to the dose per dosage interval (tau or τ). Therefore for an oral regimen there is the important equation:

$$\text{Dose} = \frac{[\text{CL} \times C_{ss} \times \tau]}{F}$$

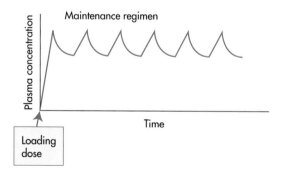

Figure 6.5   The plasma–concentration–time plot for a drug following a loading dose to raise the plasma concentration to therapeutic levels, before the maintenance regimen.

For drugs that display first-order kinetics, the relationship between dose and plasma concentration is clearly linear, so doubling the dose will

3 EXAMPLE 1

A patient requires digoxin to manage atrial fibrillation. For this patient, his V_d is 511 L, the therapeutic range is 0.8–2 micrograms/L and the F value for digoxin tablets is 0.7.

Solution: the target plasma concentration is chosen as 1.5 micrograms/L, therefore the amount required is 1.5 micrograms $\times$ 511 = 767 micrograms. To take account of F, 767 is divided by 0.7, so the dose needed is 1.096 mg. To take account of the tablets available (62.5, 125, 250 micrograms), the patient might receive 1062.5 micrograms in divided doses over 24 h. This would give a C_{ss} of 1.46 micrograms/L which is acceptable.

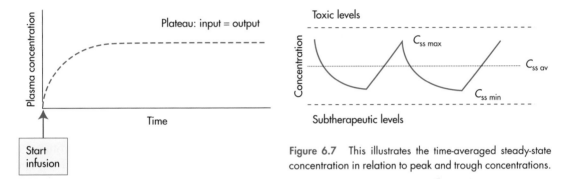

Figure 6.7 This illustrates the time-averaged steady-state concentration in relation to peak and trough concentrations.

Figure 6.6 The plasma–concentration–time plot for a drug administered by intravenous infusion. At plateau the rate of input equals the rate of output and the steady-state plasma concentration is achieved.

double the concentration, whereas halving the dose will halve the concentration.

Peak and trough concentrations

The steady-state plasma concentration is the time-averaged concentration i.e. the mean plasma concentration. For drugs with a wide therapeutic window C_{ss} is appropriate but, for drugs with a narrow therapeutic window, it is important to consider the maximum (C_{max}) or peak and minimum (C_{min}) or trough concentrations (Figure 6.7). In many instances C_{max} and C_{min} should be maintained within the therapeutic window, usually by altering the dose or the dosage interval.

The following equations are used to determine peak and trough plasma concentrations (Winter 2004):

$$\text{Peak } C_{ss} = \frac{F \times \text{Dose}}{V_d(1 - e^{-k\tau})}$$

$$\text{Trough } C_{ss} = \frac{F \times \text{Dose}}{V_d(1 - e^{-k\tau})} \times e^{-k\tau}$$

Dosage interval (tau)

As indicated above, the dosage interval determines the peaks and troughs. For drugs with a long half-life the dosage interval is 24 h and the dose required equals the amount eliminated in 24 h. However, for drugs with a relatively short half-life and a narrow therapeutic window, the dosage interval may be determined from the half-life in relation to the magnitude of the therapeutic window, e.g. for theophylline, the C_{max} is 20 mg/L and the C_{min} is 10 mg/L, so the width of

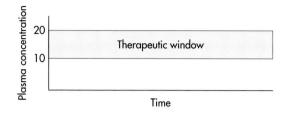

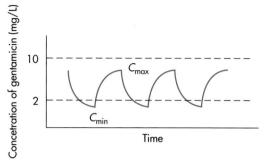

Figure 6.8   A plasma concentration–time plot to illustrate the therapeutic window in relation to dosage intervals. In the case of theophylline, the maximum concentration is 20 mg/L and the minimum 10 mg/L. The time to drop from 20 mg/L to 10 mg/L is logically one half-life. Therefore, to maintain a plasma concentration within the therapeutic window, the dosage interval should be less than one half-life.

the therapeutic window is 10 mg/L and it would take one half-life for the plasma concentration to drop from C_{max} to C_{min}. Therefore, the dosage interval chosen is less than one half-life and this will ensure that the plasma concentration remains within the safe area (Figure 6.8).

An exception to this approach is the aminoglycosides, such as gentamicin, where, although the peak plasma concentration is within the therapeutic window, the trough concentration is chosen to be subtherapeutic to avoid toxicity, e.g. the trough concentration for gentamicin is <2 mg/L and the peak is in the range 5–10 mg/L. Once again the dosage interval is determined by the half-life, e.g. if the peak plasma concentration after an intravenous dose were 8 mg/L then the time to decrease to 2 mg/L would be two half-lives, so the dosage interval would be chosen to be over two half-lives (Figure 6.9).

Real life clinical pharmacokinetics

In spite of the precise science surrounding pharmacokinetic models, patients do not always conform to mathematical equations and this is a result of individual variations that may alter pharmacokinetics, including:

- renal function
- hepatic function
- drug metabolism
- disease
- drug interactions.

Figure 6.9   The plasma concentration–time plot for the aminoglycoside gentamicin, where the peak (C_{max}) is usually between 5 and 10 mg/L for clinical effects, but the trough (C_{min}) is subtherapeutic to prevent adverse effects. If the peak is 8 mg/L, a dosage interval of two times the half-life will mean that the trough is 2 mg/L or less.

Population variables

To take account of individual variation, in terms of renal function and weight there are empirical population-based equations that enable one to calculate a reasonable estimate of volume of distribution and clearance for a drug. The population-based equations are specific to a drug and are useful for recommending a regimen for a patient, the V_d (Example 2) helping to determine the loading dose and CL (Example 3) the maintenance dose.

Applications of population-based equations

Population-based equations are used to predict pharmacokinetics and may be used to recommend dosages, e.g. given the patient below, (Example 2), we now know that his V_d is 415 L. Therefore to determine his loading dose, we can carry out the following:

$$\text{Loading dose} = \frac{C_{ss} \times 415}{F}$$

$$\text{So loading dose} = \frac{1.5 \times 415}{0.7}$$

Loading dose = 889 µg and using available tablets one might recommend the loading dose as 7 × 125 µg tablets and a 62.5 µg tablet = 937.5 µg.

EXAMPLE 2

The V_d for digoxin is given by the equation (Winter 2004):

$$Vd\ (L) = (3.8)\ (\text{weight in kg}) + (3.1)\ (CL_{cr}\ \text{in mL/min})$$

As digoxin is largely eliminated by the renal route, an estimate of renal function, i.e. creatinine clearance (CL_{cr}) is used to estimate CL. This is obtained from the Cockcroft–Gault equation:

$$CL_{cr} = \frac{[1.23(140 - \text{Age}) \times \text{Weight}]}{[\text{Serum creatinine}]}$$

In females, 1.04 replaces 1.23.

So for a 70-year-old man, who weighs 70 kg and has a plasma creatinine = 125 μmol/L, his V_d for digoxin is given by:

$$V_d\ (L) = (3.8)\ (\text{weight in kg}) + (3.1)\ (CL_{cr}\ \text{in mL/min})$$

(Note that, although the CL_{cr} is given in mL/min, the calculated V_d is in litres).

$$V_d\ (L) = (3.8 \times 70) + 3.1\ (CL_{cr})$$

$$CL_{cr} = \frac{[1.23(140 - 70) \times 70]}{125} = 48.2\ \text{mL/min}$$

Therefore V_d = 266 + 3.1(48.2) = 415 L.

EXAMPLE 3

For digoxin the clearance (CL) is given by the equation (Winter 2004):

$$CL\ (\text{mL/min}) = (0.8\ \text{mL/kg per min})\ (\text{weight in kg}) + CL_{cr}\ (\text{mL/min})$$

So for a 70-year-old man, who weighs 70 kg and has a plasma creatinine = 125 μmol/L, his CL for digoxin is given:

$$CL_{dig} = (0.8) \times (70) + CL_{cr}$$

$$CL_{dig} = 56 + \frac{[1.23(140 - 70) \times 70]}{125}$$

$$CL_{dig} = 104.2\ \text{mL/min} = 6.25\ \text{L/h}$$

Population-based equations may also take account of disease states and drug interactions, e.g. in chronic heart failure the clearance for digoxin is reduced and the population-derived equation is:

$$CL\ (\text{L/h}) = (0.33 \times \text{Weight in kg}) + 0.9\ CL_{cr}\ (\text{mL/min})$$

In hyperthyroidism the CL for digoxin is increased by 1.3 fold, and in hypothyroidism it is reduced by 0.7 (Winter 2004).

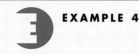 **EXAMPLE 4**

The patient in Examples 2 and 3 was receiving 312.5 µg digoxin/day and his plasma digoxin concentration was found to be 2.5 µg/L. In practice the digoxin would be stopped until therapeutic levels (<2 µg/L) returned but the data allow for a dosage alteration. Given:

$$\text{Dose rate} = C_{ss} \times CL.$$

$$\text{Then } 312.5 \times F = C_{ss} \times CL \text{ (per day)}$$

$$312.5 \times 0.7 = 2.5 \times CL$$

$$\text{Therefore } CL = \frac{218.8}{2.5} = 87.5 \text{ L/day}$$

Therefore the new daily dose to attain a C_{ss} of 1.5 should be:

$$\text{Daily dose} \times F = C_{ss} \times CL$$

$$\text{Daily dose} = \frac{[1.5 \times 87.5]}{0.7} = 187.5 \text{ µg/day}$$

and so he could be given a new regimen of 125 µg plus 62.5 µg tablets, which equals 187.5 µg/day.

Similarly, using the CL one can calculate the maintenance dose given:

$$\text{Dose rate} = C_{ss} \times CL$$

From Example 3, dose rate = 1.5×6.25 (L/h) = 9.375 µg/h. As digoxin is given daily the patient requires 24×9.375 µg/day = 225 µg/day. To take account of F the oral dose must be 225/0.7 = 321 µg, and to account for available tablets he should receive 250 mg and 62.5 µg tablets, as a dose of 312.5 µg/day.

Revising a regimen

Once a patient has been prescribed a regimen based on population data, he or she may actually handle the drug in a different manner and this will result in a different plasma concentration from predicted. The difference is due to the clearance being at a different rate. If clearance is greater than predicted then C_{ss} will be lower and if it is less than predicted then the C_{ss} will be higher. An actual measurement of the C_{ss} for this patient can be used to determine the revised dosage. If the C_{ss} is measured then, as we know the dose rate (Example 4, above), we can calculate the patient's actual clearance. This actual (as opposed to population-based) value enables the new maintenance dose to be determined.

Zero-order kinetics

Most drugs show first-order kinetics with the rate of elimination being proportional to the concentration of the drug. However, for some drugs, notably the antiepileptic drug phenytoin and ethanol, the enzymes responsible for their elimination become saturated, so the rate of elimination is no longer proportional to the drug's concentration. This means that these drugs exhibit zero-order kinetics with the rate of elimination not being proportional to the drug concentration, so small changes in their dosage leads to disproportionate increases in plasma concentrations. Controlling the dose of phenytoin is

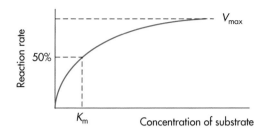

Figure 6.10 The Michaelis–Menten enzyme kinetics plot of reaction rate against concentration of substrate, where V_{max} relates to the maximum rate of elimination and K_m is analogous to the affinity of the metabolizing enzymes.

therefore difficult to achieve. The pharmacokinetics of phenytoin are described by the Michaelis–Menten enzyme kinetics (Figure 6.10), where V_{max} relates to the maximum rate of elimination and K_m is analogous to the affinity of the metabolizing enzymes for phenytoin.

The consequence of the zero-order kinetics is a dose–plasma concentration profile that varies between individuals due to variability in V_{max} (Figure 6.11).

In constructing regimens for phenytoin the loading dose is calculated in the usual way by ($C_{ss} \times V_d$), because this is independent of metabolism. However, the maintenance dose is calculated from a modified form of the Michaelis–Menten equation:

$$\frac{[S \times F \times \text{Dose}]}{\tau} = \frac{[V_{max} \times C_{ss}]}{K_m + C_{ss}}$$

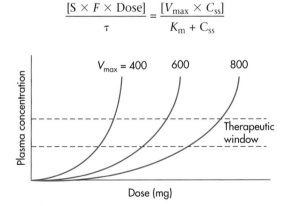

Figure 6.11 These are the plasma concentration–time plots for three different patients (with different V_{max} values) and demonstrates the variation between individuals. The zero-order kinetics means that increases in dosage cause a disproportionate rise in plasma concentration.

where V_{max} and K_m are obtained from population averages. When adjusting regimens (i.e. once the plasma concentration is known in relation to the dosage), one can calculate the patient's individual V_{max}, assuming that this is more variable and the population K_m is fixed.

Therapeutic drug monitoring (Appendix 2)

The major clinical application of pharmacokinetics is in therapeutic drug monitoring (TDM), which involves taking a blood sample and measuring the concentration of a specific drug. This enables a dosage regimen to be altered in relation to a patient's individual clearance and also detects toxic dosing, subtherapeutic dosing and non-compliance. The sample is taken at a specific time point post-dose (to allow the drug to distribute) or immediately pre-dose. Therapeutic drug monitoring is generally used for drugs with a narrow therapeutic window such as:

- theophylline
- lithium
- phenytoin
- gentamicin
- ciclosporin.

In the case of drugs that show first-order kinetics the dose may be adjusted:

$$\text{New dose} = \frac{\text{Target } C_{ss}}{\text{Measured } C_{ss}} \times \text{Current dose}$$

Practice points

- When determining oral doses, one should take account of the salt factor and bioavailability.
- Population-based equations are used to estimate V_d and CL.
- V_d is used to calculate loading doses.
- Clearance is used to calculate maintenance doses.
- A patient's actual data can be used to determine actual parameters.
- Regimens are generally based on 6-, 8-, 12- and 24-hourly dosing.
- The $t_{1/2}$ determines the dose interval.

Reference

Winter ME, ed. (2004). *Basic Clinical Pharmacokinetics*, 4th edn Philadelphia: Lippincott, Williams & Wilkins.

Part C
Gastrointestinal diseases

7

Dyspepsia and peptic ulcer disease

Dyspepsia describes upper gastrointestinal symptoms, including heartburn, acidity, nausea, discomfort and wind, and may be referred to as 'indigestion' by the patient.

Disease characteristics

The major problem is one of acidity, in the form of increased acid secretion, reflux of corrosive gastric contents or gastric damage. Clinically, upper gastrointestinal problems encompass simple to serious diseases:

- Gastro-oesophageal reflux disease (GORD) is reflux of the gastric contents into the oesophagus, which leads to erosion (reflux oesophagitis). Contact oesophagitis also occurs and is induced by contact with certain drugs (Chapter 5).
- Gastritis: inflammation of the stomach.
- Peptic ulceration: gastric and duodenal.
- Drug-induced peptic damage (largely non-steroidal anti-inflammatory drugs [NSAIDs] and oral steroids).
- Zollinger–Ellison syndrome: a rare gastrin-secreting tumour of D-cells of the pancreas.

A patient presenting with symptoms of dyspepsia ('indigestion'), which may include upper abdominal or epigastric pain, requires differential diagnosis from cardiac problems (see Chapter 1). In the context of primary care, there may be alerting clinical features that may suggest more serious underlying pathology, such as carcinoma, which must be excluded and these include:

- age (patients aged >45 years of age with new or changed symptoms or aged >55 years)

- weight loss
- anaemia
- dysphagia (difficulty in swallowing)
- haematemesis (vomiting blood)
- melaena (tarry stools)
- upper abdominal masses
- persistent symptoms with repeat requests for over-the-counter (OTC) remedies
- onset of new or changed symptoms.

Gastro-oesophageal reflux disease

As the name implies, this is due to the reflux of gastric contents into the oesophagus, causing erosion, which leads to pain, experienced as 'heartburn', although sometimes there may be back or shoulder pain. There may occasionally be wheezing and a cough or an exacerbation of asthma. This condition must be distinguished from oesophageal carcinoma, although dysphagia is also a leading feature of the latter. GORD may be caused or exacerbated by an increase in abdominal pressure (due to over-eating, obesity or pregnancy) or incompetence of the gastro-oesophageal sphincter as a result of a hiatus hernia or drugs (e.g. nitrates, antimuscarinic agents, theophylline, opioids and calcium channel blockers). Reflux oesophagitis may lead to Barrett's oesophagus, a premalignant condition.

Contact oesophagitis

This is caused by local damage resulting from drugs (see Chapter 5).

Table 7.1   Regulation of gastric acid production

Increase acid release	Reduce acid release
Histamine via H$_2$-receptors	Prostaglandins E$_2$ and I$_2$ (which are also cytoprotective via mucus and bicarbonate release). Their production is inhibited by NSAIDs
Gastrin via CCK receptors Acetylcholine via M$_3$-receptors and histamine release	

NSAIDs, non-steroidal anti-inflammatory drugs; CCK, cholecystokinin

Peptic ulceration

Peptic ulceration includes both gastric and duodenal ulceration and is characterized by erosion of the inner lining, which may perforate as a serious complication or erode a major blood vessel, causing haematemesis (vomiting of blood). The leading clinical features of peptic ulceration include:

- epigastric pain, which may be precisely located by the patient by pointing
- hunger pain, which is relieved by eating
- night pain, which is relieved by food, milk or antacids
- waterbrash, which is the appearance of saliva in the mouth
- nausea and, less frequently, vomiting.

It may also present as anaemia (see Chapter 17) due to chronic blood loss or as melaena (tarry stools) due to bleeding.

It is now well established that infection with the Gram-negative bacterium *Helicobacter pylori* is the cause of up to 95% of cases in duodenal ulceration and 70–80% of gastric ulceration. The infection leads to chronic inflammation and gastric damage, leading to ulceration. There is no evidence that emotional stress or eating spicy foods leads to peptic ulceration. Indeed in 2005 the Nobel Prize for medicine was awarded to two Australian doctors (R Marshall and B Warren) who made the controversial proposal in the 1980s that ulceration was associated with this bacterium.

The other leading cause of ulceration is the use of NSAIDs and, to a much lesser extent, oral steroids, generally with concomitant NSAID therapy. The explanation for the ulcerogenic effect of NSAIDs is that prostanoids synthesized in the stomach are cytoprotective by inhibiting acid release and stimulating the production and release of protective mucus and bicarbonate (Figure 7.1 and Table 7.1). These cytoprotective prostanoids are produced by the constitutive cyclo-oxygenase 1 (COX-1), which is inhibited by NSAIDs, so NSAIDs alter the balance in favour of increased acid activity, predisposing towards gastric damage. This important adverse drug

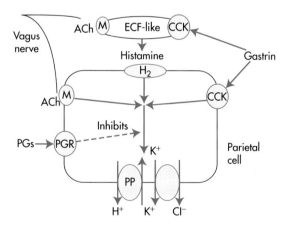

Figure 7.1   A schematic diagram of the parietal cell and the regulation of acid release. ACh is acetylcholine; CCK is cholecystokinin; ECF is the enterochromaffin-like cell; M indicates the muscarinic receptor; H$_2$ indicates the histamine H$_2$-receptor; PGs are prostanoids; PGR is a prostanoid receptor; CCK is the cholecystokinin receptor on which gastrin acts; PP is the proton pump. This figure is based on diagrams in Rang *et al* (2003) and Hardman *et al* (2001).

reaction led to the development of selective COX-2 inhibitors ('coxibs': celecoxib; etodolac and meloxicam), which inhibit COX-2, associated with inflammation, but leave COX-1 largely unaffected. However, these agents still appear to cause some gastric damage and their early promise was not fully realized.

Goals of treatment

Depending on the conditions, the general goals are symptomatic relief or cure. Symptomatic relief may involve lifestyle changes, avoidance of causative drugs, suppression of acid release or activity, and mucosal protection. Cure may involve suppression of acid release to allow natural healing and, if appropriate, eradication of *H. pylori* infection. This latter goal is also aimed at reducing the possibility of developing gastric carcinomas, because *H. pylori* is regarded as a carcinogen.

Pharmacological basis of management

Control of acid secretion

In order to understand the mechanisms of drug action, the control of acid secretion must be considered. Figure 7.1 and Table 7.1 show that the release of protons via the proton pump is regulated physiologically.

Antacids

As the name implies, antacids are anti-acid. A variety of preparations is available that raise pH:

Sodium bicarbonate: $HCO_3^- + H^+ \rightarrow CO_2 + H_2O$

with the 'belching' of CO_2, which makes it less suitable in patients who have flatulence.

Magnesium hydroxide $(Mg(OH)_2)$ and aluminium hydroxide $(Al(OH)_3)$ are also used:

$$Al(OH)_3 + 3HCl \rightarrow AlCl_3 + 3H_2O$$

$$Mg(OH)_2 + 2HCl \rightarrow MgCl_2 + 2H_2O.$$

To complicate matters, aluminium compounds are constipating and magnesium salts are laxative, and so they are often used in combination to negate these effects. The use of calcium salts (including ingestion of milk) may in fact stimulate gastrin release and so increase acid secretion, leading to an exacerbation of ulceration.

Antacids provide rapid relief of dyspepsia, removing the symptoms, but they do not lead to a cure. Liquid preparations have a faster onset of action.

Alginates

These are mucopolysaccharides and may be combined with antacids (e.g. Gaviscon preparations). The alginic acid, when combined with saliva, forms a viscous foam that floats on the gastric contents, forming a raft that protects the oesophagus during reflux.

H$_2$-receptor antagonists, e.g. *Cimetidine, famotidine, ranitidine*

These are competitive antagonists at the histamine H_2-receptor and inhibit histamine-induced gastric acid secretion. Accordingly, they provide symptomatic relief and in the long term promote ulcer healing, but, if *H. pylori* infection has not been eliminated, then relapse on discontinuation is common. They are most active against basal, as opposed to stimulus-evoked, acid release and are most effective when given at night. Ranitidine and famotidine have fewer interactions than cimetidine. Low doses are available over-the-counter for short-term relief of dyspepsia (<2 weeks) and higher doses are prescription-only medicines (POMs).

Proton pump inhibitors, e.g. *Lansoprazole, omeprazole (esomeprazole as its S-isomer), pantoprazole, rabeprazole*

These newer drugs are widely used and act via irreversible inhibition of the proton pump (H^+/K^+ ATPase) and hence suppress proton secretion. This leads to a greater than 90% inhibition of acid secretion which is long lasting (24 h). The proton pump inhibitors (PPIs) are converted to active drugs at acid pH, which means that their actions are largely confined to the gastric mucosa, leading to selectivity. Omeprazole is now available over-the-counter for a maximum of 4 weeks.

Prostaglandin analogues, e.g. *Misoprostol*

This is a stable prostaglandin analogue E_1, which inhibits the release of acid and is also cytoprotective by stimulating the release of mucus and bicarbonate.

Bismuth chelate

Bismuth chelate kills *H. pylori*, coats the ulcer, absorbs pepsin, increases prostaglandin production and increases bicarbonate secretion, thereby bringing about ulcer healing.

Prokinetic drugs, e.g. *Domperidone, metoclopramide*

These agents facilitate the movement of gastric contents from the stomach to the duodenum. Domperidone closes the gastro-oesophageal sphincter and promotes gastric emptying, and this is of benefit in reflux oesophagitis. Metoclopramide acts locally to increase gastric motility and promote emptying. Both agents will provide symptomatic relief of 'bloating'.

Choice of drugs (Figure 7.2)

This is related to the disease and goals of treatment, because occasional heartburn may be effectively relieved by simple antacids or low-dose H_2-receptor antagonists, with the antacids having immediate effects. In more serious disease, the first issue is to establish the nature of the complaint because the diagnosis will determine the most appropriate treatment. In the meantime symptomatic relief with antacids, alginates, H_2-receptor antagonists or PPIs is appropriate, depending on the severity. Diagnosis may involve breath ([^{13}C]urea) tests, serological tests for antibodies to *H. pylori* (these may give false-positive results because they indicate

past and not necessarily current infection) or stool antigen testing for *H. pylori* infection, and possibly gastroscopy and barium contrast radiology.

The urea breath test involves administering a tablet containing isotope ^{13}C-labelled urea, because *H. pylori* possesses urease activity, which leads to the production of labelled ^{13}CO$_2$ in the presence of infection. The ^{13}CO$_2$ readily and rapidly passes across the stomach wall and is absorbed into the bloodstream and appears in the breath, where it may be detected by mass spectroscopy, indicating infection. Before the breath test or gastroscopy, H_2-receptor antagonists, PPIs and antibiotics should be withheld for at least 2 weeks to prevent the symptoms being masked.

Gastro-oesophageal reflux disease

The initial approach is lifestyle changes such as reducing overeating, weight reduction if appropriate, reducing the intake of fatty foods and chocolate (which may lubricate the gastro-oesophageal sphincter), smoking cessation, reducing alcohol intake and avoiding tight clothes. If lifestyle changes are inadequate, antacids and then antacids plus alginates will provide rapid relief but limited healing. H_2-receptor antagonists may be used to provide relief in mild-to-moderate disease but are much less effective than PPIs. If symptoms persist, then PPIs are the most effective agents; they remove symptoms and allow healing. They may initially be used for 4–8 weeks, after which a lower maintenance dose should be tried. Prokinetic drugs may also be used, especially when the symptoms include postprandial bloating, nausea and belching.

Non-*H. pylori* dyspepsia

In the absence of proven *H. pylori* infection, the logical approach to dyspepsia, due to gastritis or ulceration, is a stepped approach, stepping up or down as appropriate:

* Step 1: antacid or alginate and antacid.
* Step 2: H_2-receptor antagonist.
* Step 3: PPI.

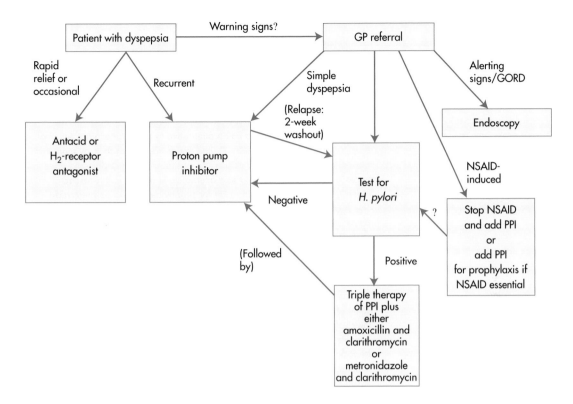

Figure 7.2   A flow diagram of the principles of the management of dyspepsia. The summary indicates the role of over-the-counter medicines and the need for GP referral with appropriate investigations. The diagram takes account of National Institute for Health and Clinical Excellence (2004) guidance but full guidance should be consulted for details of patient management. GORD, gastro-oesophageal reflux disease; NSAID, non-steroidal anti-inflammatory drug; PPI, proton pump inhibitor.

PPIs are the most effective agents and current National Institute for Health and Clinical Excellence (NICE) guidelines (2004) indicate that PPIs should be used empirically in uninvestigated dyspepsia.

H. pylori infection

In patients who are infected with *H. pylori* or those with duodenal ulceration who are assumed to be infected, eradication is the logical course. This may be achieved by a number of different regimens, which involve antibiotics and antisecretory agents ('triple therapy'), and these are associated with 90% eradication rates. Typically, triple therapy involves a PPI (or sometimes ranitidine or ranitidine bismuth citrate) plus two antibacterial agents from either clarithromycin

and amoxicillin or clarithromycin and metronidazole for 1 week. There is significant resistance to metronidazole: patients who have recently received this for other conditions may be harbouring resistant organisms and so this agent should be avoided. Eradication is confirmed by a urea breath test; serology is inappropriate because antibodies to *H. pylori* may persist in the plasma. After eradication, PPIs may be required for 4–8 weeks after triple therapy to promote further healing, especially if the ulcer was associated with bleeding or NSAID usage.

NSAID-induced ulceration

After *H. pylori* infection, NSAID use is the next most common cause of ulceration. Gastric damage due to NSAIDs is highest in older

Table 7.2   Considerations of drug choice for dyspepsia in concurrent conditions

Condition	Implications for treatment
Heart failure	Patients should avoid antacids with a high sodium content, especially if they are also receiving diuretics
Prophylaxis of myocardial infarction and stroke with antiplatelet drugs	Low-dose aspirin is associated with gastric bleeding. Clopidogrel is an antiplatelet drug that is used as an alternative to low-dose aspirin. Although it is used when aspirin is contraindicated, there is evidence that, by inhibiting platelet aggregation, it may also cause gastric bleeding and should not necessarily be regarded as a safe alternative to aspirin in this respect. Indeed, low-dose aspirin with a PPI for prophylaxis would be preferred
Women of child-bearing age	This is a contraindication for misoprostol, a prostaglandin agonist that may cause uterine contractions and subsequent abortion. If misoprostol must be used then effective contraceptive measures should be taken
Pregnancy	This is associated with an increase in GORD due to increases in intra-abdominal pressure. Alginates are the first-line drugs with efficacy and are safe. If alginates fail, then ranitidine or cimetidine is indicated if essential
Breast-feeding	Antacids, ranitidine or nizatidine is preferred. The BNF should be consulted: some of the other agents are not recommended by their manufacturers until their safety has been established
Renal impairment	Patients should avoid antacids with a high sodium content
Liver disease	Most agents require dose reductions; the BNF should be consulted. Ranitidine is often used for gastroprotection
Parkinson's disease	Avoid metoclopramide and domperidone due to extrapyramidal effects (although domperidone is recommended for levodopa-induced nausea). Metoclopramide may antagonize levodopa
Depression	SSRIs may impair blood clotting, leading to excess bleeding. Accordingly, they should be used with care in patients with gastric damage or with drugs that also impair clotting

BNF, *British National Formulary*; GORD, gastro-oesophageal reflux disease; PPI, proton pump inhibitor; SSRIs, selective serotonin reuptake inhibitors.

patients and is more often associated with certain NSAIDs, such as azapropazone, aspirin, naproxen and piroxicam, whereas ibuprofen, etodolac and nabumetone appear to cause fewer gastric side effects. It should be recognized that low-dose aspirin (75 mg) for antiplatelet therapy is also associated with a significant incidence of gastric side effects.

For NSAID-induced damage, the initial approach is to stop the NSAID if this is possible and switch to paracetamol for pain relief if this is required. Healing may be brought about by using either an H_2-receptor antagonist, as a cheap first-choice drug, or a PPI.

If the patient must continue with the NSAID or is initially identified as being at a high risk (>65 years, previous ulcer, concomitant oral steroids, concomitant anticoagulants, selective serotonin reuptake inhibitors [SSRIs] or venlafaxine) then prophylaxis is required, for which omeprazole, lansoprazole and misoprostol are currently licensed. According to Yeomans *et al* (1998), ranitidine is less effective than omeprazole at preventing and healing NSAID-induced ulceration. Furthermore, cimetidine has been shown to be ineffective at preventing NSAID-induced ulceration (Roth *et al* 1987). Misoprostol carries the compliance problem of being required two to four times daily and often causes diarrhoea, but is available in combination with either naproxen or diclofenac. Misoprostol should not be given to women of child-bearing age because it may cause uterine contractions and leads to abortions in pregnancy.

Other considerations

Other considerations concerning drug choice are detailed in Table 7.2.

Significant drug interactions

Cimetidine inhibits cytochrome P450 and therefore the metabolism of other drugs, resulting in important drug interactions. Similarly, omeprazole and lansoprazole also inhibit some isoforms of hepatic cytochrome P450. In addition, by altering gastric pH, many drugs used in dyspepsia may alter the absorption of other drugs and their administration should be separated. Examples of some important interactions of drugs used in dyspepsia and the management of peptic ulceration are detailed in Table 7.3.

Over-the-counter considerations

OTC antacids, low doses of H_2-receptor antagonists and low-dose omeprazole have important roles in the symptomatic relief of dyspepsia but their use is limited (to 2 weeks with H_2-receptor antagonists and to 4 weeks for omeprazole), after which time referral should be made if symptoms persist. Antacids and H_2-receptor antagonists are recommended for occasional symptoms and omeprazole is used for recurrent dyspepsia.

Counselling

In patients with dyspepsia general counselling should be directed at lifestyle advice. Altering the diet to avoid large meals, fatty foods and hot spicy food, and reducing alcohol consumption and smoking cessation should reduce provoking factors. Patients with GORD may (or may not) benefit from raising the head of the bed. Patients taking NSAIDs and other drugs such as doxycycline, tetracycline and bisphosphonates, which may cause contact oesophagitis, should be advised to take their medicine while standing or sitting with a glass of water; NSAIDs may be best taken after food but the effectiveness of this is debatable.

Patients taking NSAIDs should be instructed to tell their general practitioner (GP) and pharmacist that they are taking these agents, even if purchased over-the-counter. Of course they should be avoided if possible in patients with dyspepsia or with a risk of peptic ulceration.

Patients should be advised to report alerting symptoms such as:

- unexplained weight loss
- vomiting blood (with a ground-coffee appearance)
- melaena – black tarry stools that contain blood
- dysphagia (difficulty in swallowing).

Antacids

- These will cause immediate relief but normal doses are unlikely to lead to ulcer healing.
- These are most effective when taken 1 h after food. If they are taken earlier they may be emptied from the stomach.
- Magnesium salts alone may cause diarrhoea.
- Aluminium salts alone may cause constipation.
- Calcium salts will actually stimulate acid release.
- Their administration should be separated in time from a range of other drugs.

Alginates

These should be taken after food and when retiring to bed.

H_2-receptor antagonists

- When used over-the-counter for occasional dyspepsia, H_2-receptor antagonists should not be used for more than 2 weeks without consulting the GP.
- They should be taken regularly for prevention and not just for symptomatic relief.
- For ulceration, they are most effective when taken at night; a daily dose taken at night is effective at ulcer healing.
- Their actions may be suppressed by food, which stimulates acid secretion.

Table 7.3   Examples of some important interactions of drugs used for upper gastrointestinal disease

Interacting drugs	Consequences	Comments
Cimetidine with warfarin, phenytoin, theophylline, carbamazepine tricyclic antidepressants, diltiazem and nifedipine; antiarrhythmics (including amiodarone, flecainide, lidocaine and quinidine) and erythromycin	Cimetidine has been shown to increase the plasma concentration of a number of different drugs, leading to clinically significant interactions	• Monitoring the effects is appropriate and dose reductions may be required for the drug affected • With carbamazepine there are transient increases in the first few days • Generally speaking, these interactions are confined to cimetidine. Other H_2-receptor antagonists do not interact in this way, and so they should be regarded as safe alternatives
Cimetidine or ranitidine with ketoconazole and itraconazole	Reduced absorption of the imidazoles	• Separate dosing by 2–3 h • Fluconazole appears unaffected
Antacids with ACE inhibitors, chlorpromazine, ciprofloxacin, digoxin, ketoconazole, itraconazole, H_2-receptor antagonists, iron, rifampicin and tetracyclines	Antacids may reduce the absorption of these drugs	Their administration should be separated by 1–3 h and in the case of ciprofloxacin by 2–6 h
Sodium-containing antacids with lithium	Sodium may decrease lithium levels	Magnesium or aluminium salts would be appropriate
Omeprazole with benzodiazepines, ciclosporin, digoxin, phenytoin and warfarin	Evidence points to omeprazole having, on occasion, increased the concentration of these drugs	• Omeprazole may inhibit isoforms of cytochrome P450 • Monitoring is appropriate, especially when starting or finishing treatment
Omeprazole with macrolides	Clarithromycin increases the plasma concentration of omeprazole, which may be beneficial. Erythromycin may reduce the effects of omeprazole	
Lansoprazole with amoxicillin; clarithromycin with metronidazole	Glossitis, stomatitis and black tongue coloration have been reported	Monitoring is appropriate
Metronidazole with alcohol	Disulfiram reaction	Alcohol should be avoided with metronidazole

ACE, angiotensin-converting enzyme.

- Cimetidine may inhibit the metabolism of warfarin, phenytoin and theophylline, and it may increase their plasma concentrations.
- Cimetidine may occasionally cause impotence and gynaecomastia in males due to anti-androgenic actions.

Proton pump inhibitors

- PPIs should be taken regularly for prevention and not just for symptomatic relief.
- Relief may take several days for full effects; in the meantime a simple antacid might be used.

- Low dose (10 mg) omeprazole is available over-the-counter for the relief of recurrent dyspepsia.
- If OTC omeprazole is required for more than 4 weeks the patient should be referred to their GP.
- OTC omeprazole should not be used alongside H_2-receptor antagonists.
- They may cause diarrhoea (sometimes secondary to campylobacter infection).

Misoprostol

- Diarrhoea is a common side effect.
- Misoprostol should not be taken by women of child-bearing age who may be pregnant or become pregnant.

Bismuth chelate

- This may blacken stools and tongue.
- Bismuth chelate should be taken on an empty stomach, avoiding milk and antacids because they prevent the drug coating the ulcer.

Triple therapy for *H. pylori* eradication

- Eradication of the bacteria causing an ulcer is the most effective treatment to prevent a relapse.
- The course should be completed for eradication.
- The course is associated with a high incidence of side effects, including diarrhoea.
- Is the patient allergic to any antibiotics?
- Avoid alcohol with metronidazole, as there is a risk of a disulfiram-type reaction.

Guidance should be given for when to take the drugs, because this may appear complicated in triple therapy.

Self-assessment

Consider whether the following statements are true or false. In the management of dyspepsia:

1. Proton pump inhibitors are the most effective acid suppressors.
2. Proton pump inhibitors act via inhibition of the sodium pump (Na^+/K^+ ATPase).
3. The use of the H_2-receptor antagonist cimetidine is limited by its range of drug interactions due to inhibition of cytochrome P450.
4. Due to gastro-oesophageal reflux disease, lifestyle measures such as weight reduction, avoiding offending foods and eating smaller meals should be recommended alongside drug therapy.
5. Associated with bloating, prokinetic drugs such as metoclopramide may be beneficial.

In peptic ulceration:
6. The ^{13}C urea breath test is best carried out after 2 weeks treatment with a proton pump inhibitor.
7. A positive ^{13}C urea breath test indicates active *H. pylori* infection.
8. Triple therapy involves a regimen of three antibiotics.
9. The patient may present with anaemia.
10. Due to NSAIDs, this represents the most prevalent and important adverse drug reaction.

Practice points

- Frequent requests for OTC remedies for dyspepsia should prompt referral.
- Peptic ulceration is largely due to *H. pylori* infection (which should be eradicated).
- NSAID-induced peptic damage is a very important adverse drug reaction. Patients should be asked about their use of OTC NSAIDs and it should be recognized that low-dose aspirin may cause ulceration.
- Cyclo-oxygenase 2 (COX-2) inhibitors may cause gastric damage and should not be used in active ulceration.
- Drugs that alter gastric pH may alter the absorption of other drugs. Cimetidine inhibits hepatic cytochrome P450, with a range of important interactions.
- If PPIs are used, the cheapest agent should be chosen.

CASE STUDIES

Case 1

A 64-year-old woman who has recently been prescribed celecoxib (200mg/day) for osteoarthritis complains to her community pharmacist that she has recently developed stomach pains.

1. Explain the likely cause of her new complaint: COX-2 inhibitors may cause gastric bleeding. Despite being COX-2-selective, they may inhibit COX-1, which is responsible for the production of cytoprotective prostaglandins in the stomach, altering the balance in favour of gastric damage
2. How would you respond? The patient should discuss the dyspepsia with her GP.
3. What steps may be taken to overcome this new problem? Withdrawal of the coxib seems logical, and paracetamol may be used as a substitute. Acid suppression may be required for healing.

Case 2

A 25-year-old man has developed 'indigestion' and his GP has prescribed cimetidine (400 mg twice daily). He does not smoke, rarely uses NSAIDs and consumes fewer than 21 units of alcohol per week. The GP decides to carry out a $[^{13}C]$urea breath test before starting the cimetidine.

1. What is the purpose of this test? To test for urease in the stomach, which indicates the presence of *H. pylori*.
   The $[^{13}C]$urea breath test proves positive.
2. What is the likely cause of the patient's gastric symptoms? Peptic ulceration due to *H. pylori*. Several weeks later the patient visits his GP for the results of the test and receives the following prescription:
   lansoprazole 30 mg twice daily
   clarithromycin 500 mg twice daily
   metronidazole 400 mg twice daily
   for 7 days.
3. What is the purpose of this new prescription?
   – acid suppression to relieve symptoms and allow healing
   – eradication of *H. pylori*.
4. How should you counsel the patient?
   – lifestyle advice regarding food and avoidance of NSAIDs
   – to complete the course
   – the tablets should be taken together in the morning and evening to aid compliance
   – to avoid alcohol, because there is an interaction with metronidazole
   – to take the metronidazole with food and plenty of water
   – not to take indigestion remedies at the same time as lansoprazole
   As the patient leaves the pharmacy, he asks you whether he should continue to take the cimetidine as well
5. What advice should you give him? He should not take cimetidine as he already has acid suppression. In addition, cimetidine interacts with metronidazole and clarithromycin, increasing their plasma concentrations, although this interaction is probably not significant.

References

Hardman JG, Limbird LE, Goodman Gilman A, eds (2001). *Goodman & Gilman's The Pharmacological Basis of Therapeutics*. New York: McGraw-Hill.

Martin J, ed. *British National Formulary*, latest edition. London: British Medical Association and Royal Pharmaceutical Society of Great Britain.

National Institute for Health and Clinical Excellence (2004). *Dyspepsia – management of dyspepsia in adults in primary care*. NICE Clinical Guideline no. 17. London: NICE. Available at: via www.nice.org.uk.

Rang HP, Dale M, Ritter JM *et al* (2003). *Pharmacology*, 5th edn. Edinburgh: Churchill Livingstone.

Roth SH, Bennett RE, Mitchell CS *et al* (1987). Cimetidine therapy in nonsteroid antiinflammatory drug gastropathy. Double-blind long-term evaluation. *Arch Intern Med* **147**: 1798–801.

Yeomans N D, Tulassay Z, Juhasz L *et al* (1998). A comparison of omeprazole with ranitidine for ulcers associated with nonsteroidal antiinflammatory drugs. *N Engl J Med* **338**: 719–26.

8

Nausea and vomiting

Clinical characteristics

Nausea (the desire to vomit) and vomiting are common occurrences and may reflect simple disease, e.g. after exposure to bacterial toxins, be associated with motion as occurs in travel sickness or reflect more serious underlying pathology. Causes of nausea and vomiting include:

- alcohol (the most common)
- viral and bacterial gastrointestinal infections
- motion sickness
- drugs (such as anticancer drugs, digoxin, erythromycin, levodopa, opioids, selective serotonin reuptake inhibitors [SSRIs], non-steroidal anti-inflammatory drugs [NSAIDs], theophylline, iron salts)
- peptic ulceration
- renal failure with uraemia
- myocardial infarction
- pregnancy
- migraine
- vestibular disorders including Ménière's disease
- head trauma.

Given the range of causative factors, there are several mechanisms of nausea, including local irritation of the stomach involving visceral afferent fibres, the central effects of toxins on the chemoreceptor trigger zone (CTZ), and the conflict between visual and balance information, which is thought to occur in motion sickness. The vomiting pathway is under common, central control, leading to a highly coordinated physiological response, involving respiratory, salivary and gastric control, and resulting in the expulsion of gastric contents. Vomiting is under the control of the vomiting centre, which receives a direct input from visceral afferent nerves and is also regulated by the CTZ. The CTZ is, in turn, sensitive to circulating drugs and toxins, and receives input from the vestibular nuclei, which is linked to the labyrinth of the inner ear. The centres involved in vomiting and their receptors are summarized in Table 8.1.

In the context of gastrointestinal infections, the vomit response may be appropriate for removal of the infective agents, whereas drug-induced nausea may lead to a lack of compliance and failure of treatment. Prolonged vomiting may lead to electrolyte disturbances (including hyponatraemia, hypokalaemia and alkalosis) and dehydration.

Pharmacological basis of management

When vomiting is undesirable removal of any precipitating factors is the first approach and antiemetic agents may be appropriate. Antiemetic drugs encompass a range of different drug classes, with different sites of action. The site of action determines the circumstances in which an agent is effective.

Histamine H_1-receptor antagonists, e.g. *Cinnarizine, cyclizine, promethazine (a phenothiazine)*

These older, sedative antihistamines also have appreciable antimuscarinic activity, which contributes towards their use as antiemetics. This is shown by the fact that the 'old antihistamine', chlorphenamine, which lacks antimuscarinic

Table 8.1   Summary of the different stimuli, pathways and receptors in vomiting

Stimuli	Site	Receptors
Toxins, irritation, drugs and mechanical	Visceral afferent nerves in the gastrointestinal tract and pharynx	$5HT_3$ Dopamine D_2
Toxins and drugs	Chemoreceptor trigger zone	$5HT_3$ Dopamine D_2 Opioid
Motion	Labyrinth and vestibular nuclei	Histamine H_1 Muscarinic
Inputs from visceral afferents, vestibular apparatus, chemoreceptor trigger zone	Vomiting centre	Muscarinic Histamine H_1 $5HT_3$

5HT, 5-hydroxytryptamine (serotonin).

activity, is not antiemetic. They act on the vestibular nuclei and are effective in motion sickness.

Antimuscarinic agents, e.g. *Hyoscine* (but also including other groups such as antihistamines and prochlorperazine)

Antimuscarinic agents act in both the vomiting centre and the vestibular apparatus, making them highly effective in motion sickness. They will also reduce gastrointestinal motility. However, substantial antimuscarinic side effects limit their usefulness.

Histamine analogues, e.g. *Betahistine*

This is a histamine H_1-receptor partial agonist and H_2-receptor antagonist, which has been suggested to increase blood flow to the inner ear and/or decrease endolymph pressure. It is used in vertigo and Ménière's disease.

Dopamine receptor antagonists, e.g. *Domperidone, metoclopramide, phenothiazines such as prochlorperazine*

These act in the CTZ but some may have unwanted central nervous system (CNS) effects (less so with domperidone), which may include extrapyramidal effects and drug-induced parkinsonism. Metoclopramide may also act at

5-hydroxytryptamine (serotonin) $5HT_3$-receptors when used at high doses. The prokinetic effects of domperidone and metoclopramide may increase gastric emptying, reducing any feelings of fullness and nausea. They are effective against anticancer drug-induced emesis.

5-Hydroxytryptamine receptor antagonists, e.g. *Ondansetron (also metoclopramide)*

These block 5HT, acting at $5HT_3$-receptors in the gut and CNS, and are particularly effective against anticancer drugs, which may cause the release of 5HT in the gastrointestinal tract, and also in postoperative nausea and vomiting.

Steroids, e.g. *Dexamethasone*

The mechanism of antiemetic actions of steroids is unknown.

Nabilone

This is a cannabinoid receptor agonist with effects that may be mediated via opioid receptors in the CTZ.

Choice of drugs

The initial approach is to remove, if possible, any stimuli that may provoke nausea and vomiting.

Table 8.2 Some drug choices in nausea and vomiting

Condition	Drug choice	Comment
Motion sickness	Antimuscarinic agents/antiemetic antihistamines	Hyoscine is the most effective but its use is limited by the antimuscarinic side effects
Vestibular disorders	Prochlorperazine or cinnarizine for acute attacks of vertigo. Betahistine is indicated for prophylaxis of Ménière's disease	Prolonged use of cinnarizine in Ménière's disease may render it less effective. Diuretics have been used but evidence supporting their effectiveness is absent
Anticancer drugs	$5HT_3$-receptor antagonists, domperidone, metoclopramide, nabilone and dexamethasone	The effects of $5HT_3$-receptor antagonists are enhanced by high doses of dexamethasone. The benzodiazepine lorazepam is also used; it may induce a degree of amnesia, reducing the anticipatory nausea associated with subsequent treatment
Use of 5HT-related drugs such as triptans and SSRIs	$5HT_3$-receptor antagonists	$5HT_3$-receptor antagonists will oppose the serotoninergic effects of triptans and SSRIs that are associated with transient nausea
Migraine	Metoclopramide, domperidone, prochlorperazine and buclizine	The prokinetic effects of metoclopramide and domperidone may enhance the rate of onset of concomitant analgesics. They should also be taken as early as possible in an attack before gastrointestinal motility is reduced
Radiotherapy	$5HT_3$-receptor antagonists and dopamine receptor antagonists are used	
Postoperative nausea and vomiting (due to surgical procedures and the use of opioids)	$5HT_3$-receptor antagonists, phenothiazines and cyclizine	
Myocardial infarction	Cyclizine, prochlorperazine or metoclopramide	Cyclizine should be used only if left ventricular function is satisfactory
Head trauma	Dexamethasone	
Renal failure with uraemia	Dopamine receptor antagonists	
Peptic ulceration	Treat the ulcer (see Chapter 7) with proton pump inhibitors or H_2-receptor antagonists	
Pregnancy	Antihistamine or a phenothiazine; promethazine is widely used	Vomiting in pregnancy that is potentially life threatening requires rehydration and may need short-term drug treatment under expert supervision
Levodopa-induced nausea in Parkinson's disease	Domperidone	Domperidone does not extensively penetrate the blood–brain barrier and so will not reduce the effectiveness of levodopa in Parkinson's disease

5HT, 5-hydroxytryptamine (serotonin); SSRIs, selective serotonin reuptake inhibitors.

In the case of infection or alcohol intoxication vomiting may be considered an appropriate response to eliminate the noxious agents. Not all antiemetics are effective for all conditions, e.g. $5HT_3$- and dopamine-receptor antagonists are ineffective in motion sickness. Some logical drug choices are summarized in Table 8.2.

Other considerations

In addition to selecting the most appropriate antiemetic to suit a specific cause other considerations are as follows.

- Asthma and peptic ulceration are relative contraindications to using betahistine, which is a histamine analogue and may worsen these conditions through the stimulation of histamine H_1- and H_2-receptors, respectively.
- Antimuscarinic side effects such as blurred vision, urinary retention and constipation of the antihistamines (and of course the antimuscarinic drugs) may be unacceptable, especially if a patient already has, for example, problems of micturition or constipation. Closed-angle glaucoma is a contraindication to using hyoscine. They should also be avoided if there is a risk of dementia in elderly people.
- Sedation may be a desired or undesired side effect of the antihistamines and hyoscine, which would preclude driving. Of the antihistamines, cinnarizine is the least sedating.
- Extrapyramidal effects may occur with phenothiazines (including prochlorperazine), cinnarizine and metoclopramide. These agents may uncover or worsen existing

Parkinson's disease. These effects are far less common with domperidone, which does not extensively penetrate the blood–brain barrier. The phenothiazines will antagonize and reduce the effects of levodopa in patients being treated for Parkinson's disease.

- Young children represent a particular group at risk from vomiting and may require referral at an early stage to prevent dehydration. Projectile vomiting in the first 2 months of life may be caused by pyloric stenosis and requires investigation. Motion sickness is common in children and the following over-the-counter (OTC) availabilities should be noted:
  - promethazine hydrochloride: 2 years and over
  - hyoscine: 4 years and over
  - cinnarizine: 5 years and over.
- Promethazine hydrochloride (Phenergan) is available as a syrup and has the advantage of convenient administration to a toddler but may be misused for sedation in children.
- Timing and duration of antiemetics for motion sickness: in choosing an antihistamine for motion sickness the timings shown in Table 8.3 may be helpful.
- Severe vomiting may preclude effective oral administration and transdermal, intramuscular or rectal administration may be preferred.
- Patients receiving diuretics and who are vomiting are at particular risk of dehydration and should be advised to seek advice at an early stage, which may include withholding the diuretic, the use of oral rehydration therapy and the prescription of appropriate antiemetic drugs.

Table 8.3   Dosage timings for drugs used in motion sickness

Antiemetic	Time of dose before travel	Dosage interval
Promethazine hydrochloride	Night before travel and also on the morning of travel if required	6–8 h as required
Hyoscine	30 min	6 h
Cinnarizine	2 h	8 h

Information in this table was derived from Goodyer (2001), Blenkinsopp and Paxton (2002) and the *British National Formulary*.

Important interactions

The interactions with antiemetics are reasonably logical. As indicated above, the dopamine receptor antagonists, except domperidone, may antagonize levodopa in Parkinson's disease. The antihistamines that are antiemetic are all sedating and so will synergize with other CNS depressants. In addition, their antimuscarinic actions (and those of hyoscine) will be enhanced by other drugs with pronounced muscarinic binding (e.g. tricyclic antidepressants). The combination of betahistine with antihistamines is not appropriate as the former is a histamine analogue.

Counselling

If the patient is taking other drugs for unrelated conditions, attention should be paid to ensure that measures are taken to overcome the problems of a missed or vomited dose.

Travel sickness

- Any medication should be taken before the journey (promethazine may be taken the night before).
- Measures that may help to reduce motion sickness include looking at the horizon and not reading.
- Patients taking antimotion-sickness preparations should be informed of their sedating properties and duration of action. This may be important as a patient may take an antiemetic for a sea crossing or a flight and may wish to drive on arrival at the destination.

Hyoscine

- This may cause drowsiness, dry mouth, blurred vision and constipation.
- The effects of patches may persist for up to 24 h after removal.
- Avoid alcohol while taking hyoscine.
- Patients should wash their hands after handling patches.

Antihistamines

- Some antihistamines are associated with antimuscarinic side effects.
- Patients taking sedating antihistamines or prochlorperazine should be advised that their ability to drive or operate machinery may be impaired. The sedation will be enhanced by alcohol.

Ondansetron

Zofran melts should be placed on the tongue and allowed to disperse before swallowing.

Nabilone

Patients should be warned of the possible adverse effects such as euphoria, hallucinations and difficulties in concentrating.

Herbal remedies

Ginger is advocated in the prevention of nausea and vomiting in a range of conditions including pregnancy, motion sickness and chemotherapy, but not postoperatively. There is evidence to support its use with effects significantly better than placebo (Ernst and Pittler 2000; Vutyavanich *et al* 2001).

Over-the-counter considerations

OTC antiemetics play a major role in the management of motion sickness. The pharmacist should be mindful of potential misuse, such as using them for sedation.

Practice points

- Antiemetics should be used only when they are essential.
- Antiemetics have different sites of action. Each class is effective only against certain forms of nausea and vomiting.

References

Blenkinsopp A, Paxton P (2002). *Symptoms in the Pharmacy*, 4th edn. Oxford: Blackwell Sciences.

Ernst E, Pittler MH (2000). Efficacy of ginger for nausea and vomiting: a systematic review of randomized clinical trials. *Br J Anaesth* **84**: 367–71.

Goodyer L (2001). Health problems associated with air and sea transport. *Pharm J* **267**: 464–9.

Martin J, ed. *British National Formulary*, latest edition. London: British Medical Association and Royal Pharmaceutical Society of Great Britain.

Vutyavanich T, Kraisarin T, Ruangsri RA (2001). Ginger for nausea and vomiting in pregnancy: randomized, double-masked, placebo-controlled trial. *Obstet Gynecol* **97**: 577–82.

Further reading

Veysey M, McNair A (2001). Drug treatment of nausea and vomiting. *Prescriber* **12**: 41–50.

9

Lower gastrointestinal problems

Diarrhoea

Diarrhoea is characterized by the passing of soft or watery stools at an increased frequency (more than three times a day). It is a common and debilitating condition, and in extreme circumstances can be life threatening, with some 5 million deaths annually worldwide due to dehydration. Prolonged diarrhoea, altered bowel habits or the passing of blood should all warrant referral (see Chapter 1). Diarrhoea may be acute, e.g. due to infection, or chronic, e.g. associated with other gastrointestinal pathologies.

Causes

Acute diarrhoea is often the result of bacterial or viral infections. In this regard, rotaviruses cause damage to small-bowel villi and adhesive enterotoxigenic bacteria (such as cholera, *Escherichia coli*, *Yersinia enterocolitica*) adhere to the brush border, and increase epithelial adenosine cyclic 3':5'-monophosphate (cAMP) levels, leading to Cl⁻ and Na⁺ secretion, which are followed by water secretion from the lower gastrointestinal tract. Other agents such as *Shigella* species release cytotoxins, causing ulceration of the mucosa. Additional pathogens that may cause diarrhoea include amoebae and *Giardia* spp.

Other causes of diarrhoea include the following:

- Broad-spectrum antibiotics may alter the natural gut flora, leading to superinfection. An important example of this is pseudomembranous colitis, which is a rare but serious complication of treatment with broad-spectrum antibiotics, especially clindamycin.

It involves the growth of *Clostridium difficile*, which may lead to colitis, with the possibility of toxic megacolon and perforation of the bowel.

- Proton pump inhibitors (PPIs) may suppress acid secretion sufficiently to cause achlorhydria (an absence of hydrochloric acid), which may allow infection, e.g. by *Campylobacter* spp.
- Orlistat, an anti-obesity drug, inhibits pancreatic lipases to prevent the breakdown of fat and this may lead to steatorrhoea (fatty diarrhoea), which may be part of its therapeutic action by ensuring that the patient avoids fatty food.
- Misoprostol activates prostanoid receptors in the intestines, increasing cAMP, which may lead to secretory diarrhoea.

Other drug-induced causes include non-steroidal anti-inflammatory drugs (NSAIDs), magnesium salts, withdrawal in opioid dependence, digoxin toxicity, acarbose, metformin and iron salts.

Chronic diarrhoea may be associated with:

- irritable bowel syndrome (IBS): see later
- ulcerative colitis: see later
- Crohn's disease: see later.

Pharmacological basis of management

The first step in the management of acute diarrhoea, where a simple cause such as an adverse drug reaction can be identified, is to remove the cause and the condition may resolve. The patient should continue normal feeding with simple foods such as boiled rice, and infants should continue with breast or formula milk feeds. The first active measure is oral rehydration therapy (ORT).

Oral rehydration therapy

The major adverse effect of diarrhoea is dehydration with electrolyte disturbances (which may increase the risk of adverse drug reactions [ADRs] with drugs such as diuretics, lithium and digoxin), and rehydration is an important goal. This may be achieved by ORT using an approved and specific mixture of electrolytes and glucose. ORT should be considered for all patients. Soft drinks do not substitute for ORT because they do not have the correct composition. The ORT must be made up to the correct osmolality, because a hyperosmotic mixture may promote further water loss from the gastrointestinal tract. The presence of glucose in ORT is to allow sodium to be co-transported with glucose by a specific transporter on the epithelial cells and this will be followed by water, leading to rehydration.

Antibiotics

Many simple gastrointestinal infections, especially in children, are viral and antibiotics are of no value. If a bacterial causative organism is identified by stool cultures then an appropriate antibiotic can be used. In the case of travellers' diarrhoea (associated with foreign travel and ingestion of contaminated food or water), ciprofloxacin is often effective and is sometimes provided to travellers to take at the start of an attack of diarrhoea. In the case of pseudomembranous colitis, metronidazole and vancomycin are indicated. Giardiasis and amoebic dysentery may be treated with metronidazole, and *Salmonella* spp. with ciprofloxacin and cholera with tetracycline.

Antimotility agents

Opioids (codeine and loperamide) and antimuscarinic agents

These agents provide symptomatic relief by reducing the motility of the lower gastrointestinal tract, allowing reabsorption of fluid and reducing the passage of watery stools. The relief allows bowel control and prevents diarrhoea

from interfering with daily activities. They should be used in addition to ORT. The use of antimotility agents does not alter the time course of the diarrhoea; indeed, diarrhoea may serve to eliminate the causative organisms from the body. Antimotility agents should not be used in children or in adults with severe inflammatory bowel disease where they may cause obstruction, leading to megacolon.

Opioids reduce tone and peristaltic movements of gastrointestinal muscle by presynaptic inhibition of acetylcholine release from the parasympathetic nerves and this is mediated via μ-opioid receptors. Loperamide is an opioid that is widely used and its efficient enterohepatic cycling means that it is largely retained in the gastrointestinal tract, which limits its systemic action. Furthermore, it does not penetrate the blood–brain barrier, and therefore does not have central opioid effects. Codeine and morphine (in kaolin and morphine mixture) are also available but their use is limited by the potential for central opioid effects. Kaolin may also absorb water and interfere with rehydration or increase the risk of obstruction with opioids.

Atropine is present in co-phenotrope and will reduce peristalsis through inhibition of muscarinic receptors on the gastrointestinal muscle. Its use is limited by the obvious widespread antimuscarinic effects.

Probiotics

Antibiotic-associated diarrhoea is due to alterations in gastrointestinal flora, allowing the outgrowth of pathogenic bacteria. A recent trial in elderly patients has indicated that a course of preventive treatment with probiotic drinks containing lactobacilli reduces the incidence of antibiotic-associated diarrhoea, including *C. difficile* infections (Hickson *et al* 2007). A similar trial in young children has also indicated that some but not all probiotic preparations reduce the duration of acute diarrhoea (Canani *et al* 2007).

Counselling

Patients taking diuretics are at increased risk of dehydration and electrolyte disturbances, and may be advised to consult their general practitioner (GP) or omit doses. In patients with diarrhoea it is worth enquiring about drug use and asking about the use of laxatives.

Oral rehydration therapy

- This should be made up with the correct amount of freshly boiled and cooled water.
- The amount required depends on the number of watery stools passed.
- Once reconstituted, ORT may be stored refrigerated for 24 h.

Antibiotics

- Many cases of diarrhoea are viral, so antibiotics are unlikely to be effective.
- Patients who are taking antibiotics (especially clindamycin) and then develop diarrhoea that is severe or bloody should consult their GP immediately.

Opioids

These are effective at symptomatic relief but will not shorten the course of the diarrhoea.

Constipation

Once again, this is a condition with a range of causes and is defined as altered bowel habits with reduced frequency (e.g. fewer than three motions per week) and the passing of hardened faeces. In the simplest case, constipation may reflect a diet lacking adequate roughage. Other causes may be: psychological; result from painful defecation associated with haemorrhoids or anal fissure, irritable bowel syndrome (IBS); pregnancy; postoperative (secondary to immobility, dehydration or constipating drugs); associated with ageing; caused by serious bowel pathology such as carcinoma of the bowel; secondary fluid restriction in renal failure (see Chapter 18); or induced by drug treatment. Drugs that may cause constipation include:

- opioids – when used as analgesics, antitussives or antidiarrhoeal agents
- tricyclic antidepressants
- antimuscarinic agents, including phenothiazines and older antihistamines
- aluminium salts, as antacids and also when used as phosphate binders in renal failure
- iron
- diuretics
- calcium channel blockers
- lithium.

The explanation for the constipating effects of opioids is straightforward: the effects result from the presynaptic inhibition of the parasympathetic nerves responsible for gastrointestinal motility, which underlies their use as antidiarrhoeal agents, as discussed above. The constipating action of antimuscarinic agents, including tricyclic antidepressants, is through postsynaptic inhibition of parasympathetic activity, as mentioned above. Diuretics may cause constipation secondary to dehydration and calcium channel blockers may cause direct relaxation of the gastrointestinal smooth muscle.

In the absence of an obvious cause, constipation, especially in older patients, should warrant referral resulting from the possibility of carcinoma of the bowel.

Management

The best approach to constipation is a balanced diet with non-starch polysaccharides (NSPs) and fluid or adding bulking agents (e.g. methylcellulose, ispaghula husk) to the diet. Exercise might also help. Otherwise laxatives may be indicated.

Osmotic laxatives: lactulose, magnesium salts

Lactulose is a disaccharide of galactose and fructose and enters the colon unchanged, where it is converted by bacteria to lactic and acetic acids, which osmotically raise the fluid volume. This increase in fluid volume leads to larger and softer stools.

Magnesium salts also have an osmotic effect, resulting in a laxative action; this occurs when magnesium is used as an antacid. Magnesium salts release cholecystokinin, which increases gastrointestinal motility.

Stimulant laxatives: dantron, senna extracts

These provide rapid relief of symptoms. Senna extracts enter the colon and are metabolized to anthracene derivatives which stimulate gastrointestinal activity by irritation. Dantron and sodium picosulphate are also irritants that stimulate lower gastrointestinal activity. Dantron is a carcinogen in animal tests and its use is limited to elderly people and terminally ill patients.

Counselling

- Patients should not expect to pass a motion every day – once every 3 days is within the normal range; it is change in bowel habits that is significant.
- A diet rich in NSPs and with plenty of water is likely to prevent constipation.
- Lactulose will take 2 days to have an effect.
- Stimulant laxatives given orally take approximately 8–12 h for an effect; when given as suppositories their action is more rapid.

Irritable bowel syndrome

This is a common, long-standing bowel disorder (present for at least 3 days per month in the last 3 months) with pain, discomfort (both of which may be relieved by defecation), and episodes of diarrhoea and/or constipation; diagnosis is based on the Rome III criteria (see Spiller *et al* 2007). The cause of IBS is poorly understood but may have a psychological basis and be associated with depression and stress. It is not thought to be associated with altered gastrointestinal motility but there may be a change in sensitivity of visceral nerves; there is also the concept of a 'brain–gut' interaction. Detailed guidance on IBS and its management has been produced by the British Society of Gastroenterology (Spiller *et al* 2007).

Pharmacological management

For constipating symptoms

Currently IBS is managed by adding NSPs (such as ispaghula) to the diet when constipation is a leading feature. In this respect, bran fibre is avoided because its fermentation may exacerbate any distension. Lactulose is also used for persistent symptoms.

For bloating and pain

Antispasmodic agents such as antimuscarinic agents and mebeverine are used for the relief of the pain and distension as required. Mebeverine is the most widely used agent and is appropriate for disease with pain and bloating. It causes direct relaxation of gastrointestinal smooth muscle and this is thought to be due to phosphodiesterase inhibition. Dicycloverine is an antimuscarinic agent and inhibits parasympathetic activity, so reducing smooth-muscle tone in the lower gastrointestinal tract. Peppermint oil is also widely used but there is no evidence to support its effectiveness.

Tricyclic antidepressants, such as amitriptyline, are used at low doses and may be effective through their constipating antimuscarinic effects and analgesic effects. They may potentially improve depression (although as the dose is low this may be unlikely) and alter visceral nerve activity. The British Society of Gastroenterology guidelines point to tricyclic antidepressants as being the most effective drugs in the management of IBS. In addition, selective serotonin reuptake inhibitors (SSRIs) are of proven benefit for improving quality of life in patients with IBS.

For diarrhoeal symptoms

Any diarrhoea may be managed by loperamide as required.

New treatments

Recent developments in drug therapy have focused on the use of the 5-hydroxytryptamine (serotonin) $5HT_3$-receptor antagonists, to reduce discomfort and gastrointestinal transit, and

$5HT_4$-receptor agonists for prokinetic effects. The benefits of probiotics are also under investigation.

Counselling

- Patients should be reminded of the importance of a healthy diet that is low in fat but with plenty of fruit combined with exercise (see Chapter 3).
- Exclusion of agents that exacerbate the condition may help. Avoidance of excessive caffeine and lactose in milk may help.
- Mebeverine should be taken 20 min before meals.
- If a tricyclic antidepressant is used, it should be pointed out that it is being used for its benefits in IBS as opposed to antidepressant actions (which require higher doses).

Ispaghula

- Ispaghula husk (Fybogel) should be taken with water and not at bedtime.
- Maintain adequate fluid intake.
- Flatulence and abdominal bloating may be worse on starting the treatment. The dose may be reduced to once daily for a few days if necessary.

Inflammatory bowel disease

This condition encompasses both ulcerative colitis and Crohn's disease, distinct inflammatory conditions that represent a high degree of morbidity and run relapsing–remitting courses. In both cases the causes are unclear and possibilities include genetics, microbial and environmental aetiologies, perhaps with an altered or inappropriate immune response to antigens in the gastrointestinal tract.

Clinical features of ulcerative colitis and Crohn's disease

These may include:

- diarrhoea
- faecal incontinence
- rectal bleeding, bloody diarrhoea
- passing of mucus
- cramping pains
- weight loss
- in Crohn's disease there may also be mouth ulcers and anal skin tags
- in Crohn's disease there may be malabsorption, leading to deficiencies of folate, vitamin B_{12} and iron associated with megaloblastic and iron-deficiency anaemia respectively; blood loss in ulcerative colitis may also lead to iron-deficiency anaemia (see Chapter 17)
- inflammatory bowel disease (IBD) may also occasionally be associated with arthritis, iritis, uveitis and an increased risk of thromboembolism.

Ulcerative colitis

Ulcerative colitis is characterized by inflammation that involves the rectum and spreads to the colon. In ulcerative colitis the inflammation tends to be superficial, affecting the mucosa.

Crohn's disease

Crohn's disease may affect any part of the gastrointestinal tract but mostly the ileum and/or colon are involved. The features of Crohn's disease and any associated deficiencies reflect the region of the gastrointestinal tract affected. In Crohn's disease T lymphocytes are activated, leading to transmural inflammation, and the extensive involvement may lead to the formation of fistulae.

Pharmacological basis of management

Drugs used in IBD are intended to suppress or prevent the inflammatory response. Guidelines for the management of IBD have been produced on behalf of the British Society of Gastroenterology (Carter et al 2004).

5-Aminosalicylates: balsalazide, mesalazine, olsalazine and sulfasalazine

5-Aminosalicylates yield 5-aminosalicylic acid (5ASA), which is the mainstay of therapy for ulcerative colitis, especially in milder disease. Although widely used in Crohn's disease, their effectiveness in maintenance therapy is less clear and a meta-analysis that examined the prophylactic use of mesalazine concluded that it was less effective at maintaining remission but was most effective in postsurgical patients (Camma *et al* 1997). Sulfasalazine (5ASA joined to sulfapyridine), olsalazine (two joined molecules of 5ASA) and balsalazide (a prodrug) are metabolized in the colon by gut flora to 5ASA, whereas mesalazine undergoes pH-sensitive cleavages of its enteric coat to yield 5ASA. The liberated 5ASA is thought to act via the inhibition of leukotriene and prostanoid formation, scavenging free radicals and decreasing neutrophil chemotaxis.

Sulfapyridine, derived from sulfasalazine, is a sulphonamide and is unsuitable for patients who are intolerant of sulphonamide: it leads to side effects that include reversible male infertility. Alternative agents such as mesalazine do not affect fertility. The sulfasalazine-derived sulphonamide is a risk factor for megaloblastic anaemia due to its antifolate properties. The release of 5ASA renders all of these agents unsuitable for patients who cannot tolerate salicylates, e.g. patients with asthma who are sensitive to aspirin. They may also cause interstitial nephritis and should be avoided in renal impairment.

The *British National Formulary* recommends that, for patients taking sulfasalazine, a full blood count and a liver function test should be carried out every month for 3 months at the start of treatment.

Significant interactions of 5-aminosalicylates are summarized in Table 9.1.

Corticosteroids

Corticosteroids are used in order to induce a remission in ulcerative colitis and Crohn's disease, especially in more severe disease. Steroid-induced side effects limit their long-term use for maintenance therapy. Oral prednisolone is widely used and more recently enteric-coated budesonide has been developed: this has poor absorption and extensive first-pass metabolism, both of which will limit its systemic side effects. Oral budesonide is intended for Crohn's disease, affecting ileal and ascending colonic regions. Enemas (prednisolone, budesonide and hydrocortisone) are used in more distal or rectal inflammation. The beneficial effects of corticosteroids are via their well-established anti-inflammatory and immunosuppressive actions.

Table 9.1   Some important drug interactions of 5-aminosalicylates

Drugs	Consequences	Comments
Mesalazine, olsalazine or sulfasalazine with azathioprine	5ASA may reduce the clearance of azathioprine with enhanced side effects such as bone marrow suppression	Their concurrent use should be monitored and the dose of azathioprine may need to be reduced
Sulfasalazine with antibiotics	Ampicillin and rifampicin have been shown to eradicate gut bacteria and reduce the release of 5ASA from sulfasalazine	The effectiveness of sulfasalazine may be reduced by concurrent antibiotics. Metronidazole does not appear to interact with sulfasalazine
Sulfasalazine with digoxin	The plasma levels of digoxin may be reduced	The levels or effectiveness of digoxin should be monitored

5ASA, 5-aminosalicylic acid.

Immunosuppressants: azathioprine, ciclosporin, methotrexate

The role of immunosuppressants in IBD is less clear but they may have a role in refractory disease and for steroid sparing. In this regard both azathioprine and intravenous ciclosporin are used for inducing remissions. If ciclosporin is given there is an increased risk of *Pneumocystis jiroveci* and prophylaxis may be required. Methotrexate is also effective in Crohn's disease for inducing a remission or maintenance but not in ulcerative colitis.

Infliximab

This is a monoclonal antibody that neutralizes the proinflammatory cytokine, tumour necrosis factor α (TNF-α), which is implicated in the pathology of Crohn's disease, possibly via leukocyte recruitment. The ACCENT I trial (ACCENT I Study Group 2002) has indicated that patients who show an initial response to a single dose of infliximab are likely to benefit from repeated doses of this agent, leading to remission and discontinuation of corticosteroids. Infliximab has been identified as a risk factor for developing tuberculosis.

The National Institute for Health and Clinical Excellence (NICE) guidelines released in 2002 recommended that infliximab can be used by experienced gastroenterologists for patients with severe Crohn's disease that is refractory to immunosuppressants and corticosteroids, where the disease is not fistulating and when surgery is not possible.

Loperamide

This may be of some use in diarrhoea associated with mild IBD but should be used with caution in more severe disease due to the risk of toxic megacolon.

Colestyramine

Colestryramine binds bile salts and may reduce diarrhoea due to malabsorption of bile salts in Crohn's disease.

Fish oils

Fish oils may be of benefit in maintaining a remission in addition to standard treatments in ulcerative colitis and Crohn's disease. Any potential benefit may be via interference with leukotriene synthesis.

Nutritional therapy

In Crohn's disease it is well established that parental nutrition allows the gastrointestinal tract to recover ('bowel rest') and results in patients entering remission without the need for steroids. Similarly, elemental feeding with simple, predigested foods is also effective in the management of Crohn's disease.

Probiotics

A small-scale trial has reported that non-pathogenic *Escherichia coli* (Nissle 1917) was as effective as mesalazine in maintaining a long-term remission in patients with ulcerative colitis (Rembacken *et al* 1999). The authors' explanations for the beneficial effects of *Escherichia coli* were that it may have blocked the binding of adhesive bacteria, produced toxins against pathogenic bacteria or altered the local environment. There is no evidence that probiotics are of benefit in Crohn's disease.

Vitamins and minerals

As IBD may be associated with malabsorption of iron, folate and vitamin B_{12}, leading to anaemia, it may be necessary to give appropriate oral or parenteral supplements of these nutrients. Patients taking corticosteroids are at risk of osteoporosis and may benefit from calcium supplementation.

Counselling

- The National Association for Colitis and Crohn's Disease (NACC) provides patient information and support. It produces a 'Can't Wait' card, which is recognized by many shops and is intended to help patients gain access to a toilet in an emergency.

- Smoking makes Crohn's disease (but not ulcerative colitis) worse.
- IBD may be exacerbated by NSAIDs.
- IBD may be exacerbated by alcohol.
- The effectiveness of dietary modifications is less clear but patients may identify by trial and error which foods exacerbate their condition. Wheat and dairy products may be implicated.
- Patients taking aminosalicylates should report any sore throats, fevers, easy bruising or bleeding due to the risk of blood dyscrasia.
- Aminosalicylates are associated with side effects including rashes, headaches and diarrhoea.
- Sulfasalazine may colour urine orange and discolour soft contact lenses.
- Mesalazine and balsalazide tablets should be swallowed whole.
- Patients should be maintained on the same brand of enteric-coated mesalazine.

Self-assessment

Consider whether the following statements are true or false. In a patient with altered bowel habits:

1. The time course of acute diarrhoea is reduced by loperamide.
2. Antibiotic-associated diarrhoea due to clindamycin should raise the suspicion of pseudomembranous colitis.
3. Constipation is a common side effect of opioid therapy.
4. Constipation is a major adverse effect of serotonin selective reuptake inhibitors (SSRIs).
5. A diagnosis of irritable bowel syndrome is likely if there is bloody diarrhoea and cramping.

Practice points

- Changes in bowel habits, including rectal bleeding, should lead to referral to the GP.
- ORT plays a major role in the treatment of diarrhoea.
- Antidiarrhoeal agents provide symptomatic relief but do not alter the course of the diarrhoea.
- Diarrhoea is an important side effect of antibiotic treatment and, if severe (especially with clindamycin), should lead to prompt referral.
- Constipation is best managed by a healthy diet, adequate fluid intake and exercise.
- Patients receiving chronic opioid treatment should receive a laxative.
- Be vigilant of laxative abuse in eating disorders.
- IBS is poorly defined and is managed according to its leading symptoms.
- Ulcerative colitis and Crohn's disease are distinct relapsing–remitting diseases with high morbidity.
- 5-Aminosalicylates are associated with blood dyscrasias.

 CASE STUDY

A husband requests senna tablets for his wife who has just been discharged from hospital. Suggest further questions that you may need to ask before making a sale.

The cause of her admission should be established. Constipation may result from a long stay in hospital with inevitable reduction in physical activity. Dehydration, poor diet and opioid analgesia may also be factors leading to constipation in the convalescing patient. It may appear strange that no laxatives were prescribed at discharge. This patient had received bowel surgery for an obstruction. The constipation could possibly be due to a new obstruction and senna could cause severe abdominal pain if given to this patient. Referral should be made to the GP in the first instance.

References

ACCENT I Study Group (2002). Maintenance infliximab for Crohn's disease: the ACCENT I randomised trial. *Lancet* **359**: 1541–9.

Camma C, Giunta M, Rosselli M *et al* (1997). Mesalamine in the maintenance treatment of Crohn's disease: a meta-analysis adjusted for confounding variables. *Gastroenterology* **113**: 1465–13.

Carani RB, Cirillo P, Terrin G *et al* (2007). Probiotics for treatment of acute diarrhoea in children: randomised clinical trial of five different preparations. *BMJ* **335**: 340–5.

Carter MJ, Lobo AJ, Travis SPL (2004). Guidelines for the management of inflammatory bowel disease in adults. *Gut* **53**(suppl V): v1–v16.

Hickson M, D'Souza AL, Muthu N *et al* (2007). Use of probiotic *Lactobacillus* preparation to prevent diarrhoea associated with antibiotics: randomised double blind placebo controlled trial. *BMJ* **335**: 80–4.

Martin J, ed. *British National Formulary*, latest edition. London: British Medical Association and Royal Pharmaceutical Society of Great Britain.

National Institute for Clinical Excellence (2002). *Guidance on the use of infliximab for Crohn's disease*. Technology appraisal no. 40. London: NICE. Available at: via www.nice.org.uk.

Rembacken BJ, Snelling AM, Hawkey PM *et al* (1999). Non-pathogenic *Escherichia coli* versus mesalazine for the treatment of ulcerative colitis: a randomised trial. *Lancet* **354**: 635–9.

Spiller R, Aziz Q, Creed F *et al* (2007). Guidelines for the management of irritable bowel syndrome: mechanisms and practical management. *Gut* **56**: 1770–98.

Further reading

Camilleri M (2001). Management of irritable bowel syndrome. *Gastroenterology* **120**: 652–68.

Farrell RJ, Peppercorn MA (2002). Ulcerative colitis. *Lancet* **359**: 331–40.

Forbes A (2002). Crohn's disease – the role of nutritional therapy. *Aliment Pharmacol Ther* **16**(suppl 4): 48–52.

Ghosh S, Shand A, Fergusson A (2000). Ulcerative colitis. *BMJ* **320**: 1119–23.

Jones J, Spiller R (2001). IBS: current approaches to management. *Prescriber* **12**: 93–102.

Meeman J (2001). IBD: a guide to ulcerative colitis and Crohn's disease. *Prescriber* **12**: 43–59.

Rampton DS (1999). Management of Crohn's disease. *BMJ* **319**: 1480–5.

Scribano ML, Prantera C (2002). Medical treatment of active Crohn's disease. *Aliment Pharmacol Ther* **16**(suppl 4): 35–9.

Shanahan F (2002). Crohn's disease. *Lancet* **359**: 62–9.

Online resource

www.nacc.org.uk
The website of the National Association for Colitis and Crohn's Disease (NACC), which provides patient information and support (accessed April 2008).

10

The liver patient

Hepatic impairment may result from infection (e.g. hepatitis), may be drug-induced (see Chapter 5) or associated with chronic alcohol abuse. Liver disease may be acute or chronic and ranges from hepatic impairment through to liver failure. Liver disease may have the following clinical features:

- Jaundice: impaired excretion of bilirubin into the bile by the liver leads to hyperbilirubinaemia, resulting in yellow coloration of the skin and sclera of the eyes.
- Hypoproteinaemia: the ability of the liver to synthesize proteins, including clotting factors, is impaired and leads to a reduction in plasma proteins.
- Decreased clotting: this occurs as a consequence of impaired synthesis of clotting factors, and may lead to easy bruising and bleeding.
- Ascites: this is the accumulation of fluid in the peritoneal cavity and in part is due to oedema secondary to hypoproteinaemia and sodium retention caused by secondary hyperaldosteronism, and also portal hypertension.
- Spider naevi: this is a sign of chronic liver failure and may be an early sign of alcoholic liver disease.
- Pruritus: hyperbilirubinaemia of jaundice leads to itching.
- Nausea.
- Digital clubbing: this may be a non-specific sign in chronic liver failure and its cause is unknown. There may also be white nails due to hypoalbuminaemia.
- Portal hypertension: this is associated with chronic liver failure due to liver fibrosis altering the haemodynamics and may result in bleeding oesophageal varices.

- Gynaecomastia: breast development, possibly due to reduced metabolism of oestrogens.
- Hypoglycaemia: reduced glucose output from the liver's glycogen stores.
- Encephalopathy: this is associated with both acute and chronic liver failure, leading to neuropsychiatric symptoms including changes in personality, disorientation, confusion and drowsiness. The causes of encephalopathy are not fully established but nitrogenous products and false neurotransmitters are believed to contribute. The gut flora are believed to produce many nitrogenous products, including ammonia, which are normally cleared by the liver. In liver failure these toxins are not adequately cleared and may exert neurological effects

The effects of hepatic impairment

As the liver represents a major site of drug metabolism and elimination, hepatic impairment has significant implications for drugs that are extensively cleared by the liver. On the basis of liver function tests (see Chapter 2) it is difficult to predict systematically how a patient will handle various drugs. Appendix 2 of the *British National Formulary* deals with prescribing issues associated with hepatic impairment and details which drugs are affected and how to alter or choose drug treatment. Measures include avoiding certain drugs, selecting alternative drugs that are not extensively eliminated by the liver and reducing doses.

In addition to the role of the liver in drug elimination, its other metabolic activities will be disrupted. In particular, the liver synthesizes a number of clotting factors and so their synthesis will be reduced, leading to an increased bleeding tendency. This will have important implications for the use of the oral anticoagulant warfarin, which is also metabolized by the liver. In patients with hepatic impairment receiving warfarin their international normalized ratio or INR (which may be elevated before treatment) should be closely monitored and the dose altered accordingly. Hypoproteinaemia will also reduce the plasma protein binding of certain drugs, increasing their free plasma concentration.

Pharmacological management of liver failure

Ascites

In addition to paracentesis (draining off the fluid), patients should have a sodium-restricted diet to limit sodium retention and fluid accumulation. Given the role of aldosterone in secondary hyperaldosteronism, the aldosterone receptor antagonist and potassium-sparing diuretic spironolactone is also used. However, spironolactone may cause gynaecomastia and in liver patients who already have gynaecomastia an alternative potassium-sparing diuretic such as amiloride should be used. Additional diuresis may be provided by loop diuretics. Fluid-retaining drugs such as corticosteroids and non-steroidal anti-inflammatory drugs (NSAIDs) should be avoided. A complication of ascites is spontaneous bacterial peritonitis, for which antimicrobial agents may be used.

Hepatic encephalopathy

To limit the production of nitrogenous products, protein in the diet may be restricted. To limit the production of these toxins, gut flora are eradicated with antibacterial agents such as neomycin or metronidazole. The osmotic laxative lactulose (see Chapter 9) is also routinely used in high doses and its beneficial effects may be via regular clearing of the bowel of toxins and/or alterations in the environment for the gut flora.

Sensitivity to centrally acting drugs

Patients with liver disease are especially sensitive to centrally acting drugs such as benzodiazepines, antipsychotic agents and opioids. These drugs should be used with great care, as there is a risk of precipitating a coma.

Hyperbilirubinaemia

Increased levels of bilirubin in the plasma give rise to jaundice and associated pruritus. In order to enhance the removal of bilirubin from the body, colestyramine is used as a bile-binding agent (see Chapter 12). Colestyramine binds bile in the intestines and so prevents the reabsorption of excreted bile and leads to enhanced overall excretion. This should limit the jaundice and associated symptoms. However, as discussed in Chapter 12, the binding nature of colestyramine gives rise to a range of interactions with other drugs and those affected should be given at different times.

Pruritus

As commented above, colestyramine reduces bilirubin levels and limits pruritus. Other measures to limit pruritus are the use of menthol in aqueous cream for its local cooling effect and oral antihistamines for patients with mild liver disease. Sedating antihistamines are used with caution especially at night if itching is preventing the patient from sleeping. Non-sedating antihistamines can also be of benefit. The 5-hydroxytryptamine (serotonin) $5HT_3$-receptor antagonist ondansetron has been shown to have a small beneficial effect in managing pruritus associated with jaundice (Muller *et al* 1998).

Gastric bleeding

An increased bleeding tendency means that gastric bleeding is more common in liver impairment and to this end antisecretory agents such as ranitidine may be prescribed to reduce the production of gastric acid.

Bleeding oesophageal varices

The bleeding from oesophageal varices is a medical emergency. To limit bleeding, vaso-pressin is infused and causes vasoconstriction. Octreotide, a somatostatin analogue, is also widely used (unlicensed indication) and is thought to cause vasoconstriction. A β blocker may be used in prophylaxis against bleeding varices and this may be secondary to lowering portal pressure.

Impaired clotting

The impaired clotting, secondary to the impaired synthesis of clotting factors, may be managed by parenteral vitamin K. The patient should of course avoid drugs that may inhibit clotting (anticoagulants, antiplatelet drugs) or cause bleeding (NSAIDs).

Hypoglycaemia

This may require intravenous glucose to correct hypoglycaemia.

Considerations in alcoholic liver disease

In addition to caution with the use of drugs when there is liver impairment, patients with alcohol dependence may receive drugs to control their addiction (such as disulfiram, acamprosate) and seizures associated with withdrawal reactions (benzodiazepines, principally chlordiazepoxide, and alternatively clomethiazole). Alcoholism is also associated with deficiencies of thiamine (vitamin B_1) and this may lead to Wernicke's encephalopathy with drowsiness, disorientation, nystagmus and ataxia. To prevent this, alcoholic patients are given vitamin B complex.

Over-the-counter considerations

Obviously greater caution should be exercised when using drugs in liver impairment and failure. Other considerations are the salt content in over-the-counter (OTC) preparations (e.g. antacids, effervescent preparation) if the patient is on a salt-restricted diet. The increased bleeding tendency also means that patients are at increased risk of gastric bleeding with aspirin and ibuprofen. NSAIDs may also lead to fluid reten-tion. These increased risks mean that low-dose paracetamol is a safer alternative for pain relief.

Counselling

- Colestyramine should be mixed with water or a drink and can be used in cooking.
- Colestyramine can interfere with the absorp-tion of other drugs, so other drugs should be taken at least 1 h before or 4–6 h after the colestyramine.

Practice points

- Liver function should always be taken into consideration when using drugs.
- Blood clotting is impaired in liver failure with increased bleeding tendencies and the actions of warfarin will be potentiated.
- Jaundice may be managed by colestyramine, ascites with spironolactone, and encephalopathy by neomycin and lactulose.

References

Martin J, ed. *British National Formulary*, latest edition. London: British Medical Association and Royal Pharmaceutical Society of Great Britain.

Muller C, Pongratz S, Pidlich J *et al* (1998). Treatment of pruritus in chronic liver disease with the 5-hydroxytryptamine receptor type 3 antagonist ondansetron: a randomized, placebo-controlled, double-blind cross-over trial. *Eur J Gastroenterol Hepatol* **10**: 865–70.

Further reading

North-Lewis P, ed. (2008). *Drugs and the Liver.* London: Pharmaceutical Press.

Part D
Cardiovascular diseases

11

Hypertension

Disease characteristics

The cause of essential hypertension is not known but may be multifactorial. Indeed, rather than a disease in its own right, we may view hypertension as blood pressure (BP) that is associated with significant cardiovascular risk. The cut-off point between normal BP and hypertension is arbitrary, and is now generally regarded as a sustained diastolic BP >90 mmHg or systolic BP >140 mmHg.

Over the years alterations in many cardiovascular control mechanisms (nitric oxide, endothelins, renin–angiotensin system and sympathetic nervous system) have been proposed as causing essential hypertension but there is no convincing evidence to support a 'universal cause'. Far less commonly, however, hypertension (<10%) may be secondary to another condition: renal disease, renovascular disease, Conn's syndrome (primary hyperaldosteronism), polycythaemia, Cushing's syndrome, hyperthyroidism, phaeochromocytoma and pregnancy, and these should be excluded. Drugs that may cause hypertension include:

- oral contraceptives
- sympathomimetics
- corticosteroids
- non-steroidal anti-inflammatory drugs (NSAIDs)
- ketoconazole
- moclobemide
- erythropoietin
- ciclosporin
- venlafaxine
- sibutramine.

Clinical features

Hypertension is almost always asymptomatic and often detected by routine measurement. The main complications are due to end-organ damage, principally left ventricular hypertrophy, ischaemic heart disease, renal failure, retinopathy and peripheral vascular disease. Ultimately, hypertension is a major risk factor for stroke (especially), myocardial infarction and the development of chronic heart failure, hence the need to treat this condition effectively.

Goals of treatment

The clear goal is a reduction in BP and, when this involves drug treatment, this should be with as few side-effects as possible. The joint guidelines of the National Institute for Health and Clinical Excellence (NICE) and British Hypertension Society (BHS) specify a target systolic BP of <140 mmHg and a target diastolic BP of <90 mmHg (80 mmHg in people with diabetes), whereas the Hypertension Optimal Treatment (HOT) trial (HOT Study Group 1998) indicated that there is little benefit from lowering BP further.

As a consequence of treatment the following are ideal goals:

- reduction in cardiovascular damage
- preservation of renal function
- limitation or reversal of left ventricular hypertrophy
- prevention of coronary artery disease and chronic heart failure
- reduction in mortality due to stroke and myocardial infarctions.

Pharmacological basis of management

Diuretics: thiazides and related agents, e.g. bendroflumethiazide, indapamide, metolazone

Diuretics are first-line drugs in the management of hypertension and cause a reduction in circulating volume, thus reducing preload and afterload, and hence cardiac work. In addition, they may have direct vascular effects leading to vasodilatation, which further reduces preload and/or afterload.

Thiazides act in the distal convoluted tubule to inhibit Na^+/Cl^- reabsorption, leading to diuresis. Loop diuretics, which are occasionally used when thiazides (except metolazone) are likely to be ineffective in renal impairment, act via inhibition of the $Na^+/K^+/Cl^-$ transporter in the thick ascending limb of the loop of Henle.

It should be noted that, with bendroflumethiazide, the most widely used agent, there is no benefit from increasing the dose above the optimum of 2.5 mg, because there is little additional antihypertensive effect and side effects are substantially increased.

The effectiveness of thiazide diuretics has been established over many years and was confirmed by the ALLHAT trial (2002), which demonstrated that they were effective at preventing cardiovascular disease and supported their use as first-line antihypertensives.

ACE inhibitors, e.g. captopril, enalapril, lisinopril, perindopril, ramipril

Angiotensin-converting enzyme (ACE) inhibitors are now recognized as having an important role in hypertension but are no more effective than other agents (CAPP Study Group 1999). By inhibiting ACE, they lead to reductions in angiotensin II, which in turn leads to:

- reductions in arterial and venous vasoconstriction (reduced total peripheral resistance)
- reduced aldosterone production, which leads to reductions in salt and water retention, hence reduced circulating volume (reduced cardiac output).

Clinical use

ACE inhibitors may cause pronounced first-dose hypotension and are best given initially on retiring at night. A low starting dose should be used and titrated up to the maximum effective and tolerated dose.

The renin–angiotensin system is activated in renovascular disease (atheroma of the renal artery) in order to maintain renal perfusion and filtration. Hence, ACE inhibitors may cause deterioration of renal function in pre-existing renal disease and these patients should be identified by measuring plasma creatinine and should not receive an ACE inhibitor.

A build-up of bradykinin, usually broken down by ACE, may produce a troublesome dry cough in some patients (10%) treated with ACE inhibitors.

Angiotensin II receptor antagonists, e.g. candesartan, irbesartan, losartan, valsartan

This new class of drugs blocks the action of angiotensin II at the angiotensin (AT_1) receptor. Hence these agents have similar consequences to ACE inhibitors but do not give rise to a cough. The Lifestyle Intervention for Endpoint Reduction in Hypertension (LIFE) trial (2002) reported that losartan was more effective than atenolol at reducing mortality in hypertensive patients, largely through a reduction in the incidence of stroke. In patients with diabetes with hypertension, the effects of losartan were even more impressive at reducing overall mortality, cardiovascular mortality and the development of heart failure. In both classes of hypertensive patients, losartan was also more effective than atenolol at reversing left ventricular hypertrophy. Current guidelines recommend that AT_1-receptor antagonists be used when ACE inhibitors are indicated but not tolerated, e.g. due to a cough.

Calcium channel blockers, e.g. diltiazem, felodipine, nifedipine, verapamil

There are three main classes of calcium channel blockers: (1) verapamil; (2) dihydropyridines –

nifedipine, nicardipine, amlodipine, lacidipine, nisoldipine; and (3) diltiazem. Verapamil exerts most of its effects on the heart compared with dihydropyridine effects, which target arteriolar smooth muscle. The activity of diltiazem is between class 1 and 2. Worldwide, calcium channel blockers are currently the most widely used antihypertensives and they act principally to inhibit voltage-operated calcium channels on vascular smooth muscle, leading to vasodilatation and a reduction in BP.

β Blockers: acebutolol, atenolol, bisoprolol, metoprolol, nadolol, pindolol, propranolol

β Blockers were once viewed as first-line drugs and have been widely used over many years. Their precise antihypertensive effect is unclear but it is thought to involve a reduction in sympathetic drive to the heart, reducing cardiac output, and a reduction in sympathetically evoked renin release from the kidneys. However, in 2006 joint guidance from NICE and the BHS recommended that they should no longer be used as first-line antihypertensives, based on their reduced effectiveness at reducing cardiovascular outcomes compared with other antihypertensives, as established by the ASCOT trial (2005).

α Blockers, e.g. doxazosin, prazosin

These should generally be regarded as agents of last choice, being added to therapy that has not achieved target BP. They are competitive receptor antagonists, inhibiting sympathetic activation of α_1-adrenoceptors on vascular smooth muscle, leading to vasodilatation and a drop in BP. As a result of this non-selective action, they lead to widespread side effects, making them poorly tolerated. They may, however, be useful for patients with diabetes or a lipid disorder (when diuretics or β blockers are sometimes avoided) or in older men with prostatic symptoms.

Centrally acting agents, e.g. clonidine, α-methyldopa, moxonidine

These agents are occasionally used, e.g. α-methyldopa in pregnancy or when other treatments have failed. Their action is on central vasomotor centres and they lead to a decrease in sympathetic output, causing a fall in BP. The interference with the sympathetic nervous system leads to widespread side effects. In the case of clonidine and moxonidine (an imidazoline receptor agonist), they should not be withdrawn suddenly, because there is a risk of a hypertensive crisis. For withdrawal, if moxonidine is used together with a β blocker, then the β blocker should be withdrawn slowly, several days before the centrally acting agent.

The beneficial pharmacological targets of cardiovascular drugs are listed in Table 11.1. Consideration of the distribution in the body of the sites of action for these drugs also explains some of the unwanted but predictable type A adverse drug reactions (Table 11.1).

Management of hypertension

Lifestyle measures play an important role both before and alongside drug therapy. Lifestyle modifications may involve weight reduction, reducing fat and salt intake, increasing fruit and oily fish in the diet, increasing exercise and stopping smoking. It has been reported that a sustained weight loss of 4.5 kg was associated with an 8–9 mmHg drop in diastolic and systolic BP (Stevens et al 2001) and made a significant contribution to blood pressure reduction. Particular attention should be paid to alcohol consumption, because excessive alcohol intake is closely associated with hypertension. In many patients the initial treatment will involve lifestyle changes to see whether these bring about a reduction in BP. During this process the patient's BP should be measured on several occasions to determine whether hypertension is established and to exclude 'white-coat' hypertension.

Table 11.1   Examples of principal type A adverse reactions of drugs used in hypertension

Drug	Pharmacological activity	Unwanted clinical effects
Thiazides	Act on the Na^+/Cl^- transporter of the renal distal convoluted tubule to cause diuresis and reduce circulating volume. May also have vasodilator actions	• Postural hypotension • Adversely alter lipid profile • May induce diabetes
Calcium channel blockers	Vascular smooth muscle: arteriolar relaxation (mainly dihydropyridines)	Headache, facial flushing, peripheral oedema (ankles), postural hypotension, gum hyperplasia
	CNS	Depression, extrapyramidal symptoms
(1) Verapamil	Smooth muscle: GI tract	Constipation
	Sinus or AV nodes: negative inotrope	Bradycardia or heart block
	Myocardium	Reduced cardiac output
(2) Dihydropyridines	Reflex sympathomimetic stimulation	Tachycardia or palpitations
(3) Diltiazem	Sinus or AV nodes: negative inotrope	Bradycardia or heart block
	Smooth muscle: GI tract	Constipation
β Blockers Hydrophilic (atenolol, acebutolol)	Myocardium: sympathetic drive mediated by β_1-adrenoceptors	Bradycardia, cardiac failure, conduction disorders
	Smooth muscle: bronchoconstriction	Bronchoconstriction
	Reduce lacrimation	Dry eyes
	Peripheral vascular smooth muscle: constriction	Raynaud's phenomenon, impotence
	Lipids	Adversely affect lipid profile: increase LDL and decrease HDL
	Liver and pancreas	Decrease glycogenolysis, and decrease secretion of insulin
Sotalol (hydrophilic)	As above + prolongation of Q–T interval	No longer licensed for hypertension
Lipophilic (propranolol, timolol, metoprolol, labetalol)	As above + CNS effects	Lethargy, depression, nightmares

AV, atrioventricular; CNS, central nervous system; GI, gastrointestinal; HDL, high-density lipoprotein; LDL, low-density lipoprotein.

Choice of drugs

If lifestyle measures do not bring about a satisfactory reduction in BP, the joint NICE and BHS guidelines (2006a, 2006b) suggest that drug treatment should be initiated in patients with BP that is consistently >160/100 mmHg or when the BP is 140/90 mmHg and cardiovascular disease is present, in patients with elevated cardiovascular risk (>20% over 10 years) or end-organ damage (such as left ventricular hypertrophy or renal damage).

The management of hypertension has been the subject of controversy with clinical trials giving different results regarding drug choice and the existence of conflicting guidelines. In 2006 the NICE and the BHS produced consensus guidelines that attempted to resolve these issues. The so-called Cambridge AB/CD rules were modified and adopted as 'A/CD' guidelines. These guidelines divide patients into groups under and over 55 years of age, with black patients of any age being treated as the latter group. The rationale for this is that younger patients are deemed to have high renin hypertension and respond best to ACE inhibitors (A) whereas older patients or black patients are initially treated with calcium channel blocker (C) or diuretic (D).

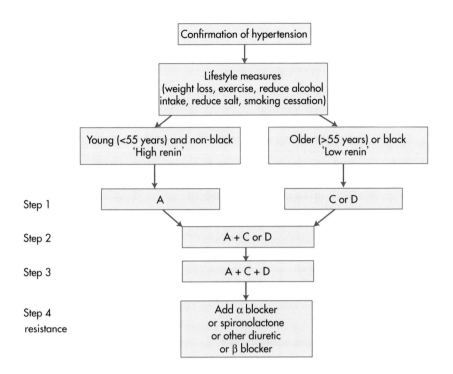

Figure 11.1   This is a summary of guidance from the National Institute for Health and Clinical Excellence (NICE 2006b) on the management of hypertension using the A/CD rules where A = ACE (angiotensin-converting enzyme) inhibitor, C = calcium channel blocker and D = diuretic. The stepwise care is shown and, once lifestyle measures have failed to control confirmed hypertension, patients are treated on the basis of age and ethnicity.

It is then acknowledged that most patients require more than one drug, so drug treatment is stepped up using an agent from the other group, e.g. patients who are younger than 55 years would normally be initiated on a ACE inhibitor and, if this failed to control their BP, they would then be additionally prescribed either a calcium channel blocker (C) or a diuretic (D) (step 2). After this the third step would involve adding the remaining class of drug. In cases of resistance (step 4), an additional diuretic, β blocker or α blocker should be added to therapy. In some cases, the aldosterone antagonist spironolactone is effective because the patient may have un-diagnosed Conn's syndrome with high aldosterone. β Blockers are also reserved for patients who are intolerant to ACE inhibitors and used in pregnancy.

Concurrent illnesses

In addition to the A/CD rules, concurrent illnesses also influence drug choice, for example asthma is a reason to avoid β blockers. Some reasons to favour or avoid certain antihypertensives are summarized in Table 11.2.

Hypertension is a major risk factor for cardiovascular disease, so the patient may have other related conditions. Hyperlipidaemia is common in the population at risk of hypertension and should be managed, usually with a statin (see Chapter 12). The NICE guidelines point to using a statin in patients with a 20% or greater 10-year risk of coronary artery disease. In addition, evidence from small-scale studies has also suggested that statins may themselves cause modest reductions in BP and, when used in combination with antihypertensives, may augment the regression of left ventricular hypertrophy, an effect

Table 11.2 Compelling indications and contraindications for antihypertensives

Condition	Drug indicated	Drugs contraindicated or used with caution
Ischaemic heart disease	β Blockers; diltiazem verapamil, long-acting dihydropyridines	Short-acting dihydropyridines – associated with increased mortality
Heart failure	ACE inhibitors and AT$_1$-receptor antagonists; diuretics; β blockers with caution (see Chapter 15)	Diltiazem and verapamil – due to negative inotropic effects
Left ventricular hypertrophy (LVH)	The AT$_1$-receptor antagonist, losartan, has been shown to be particularly effective at reversing LVH (LIFE trial)	
Diabetes mellitus	ACE inhibitors – they are renally and vasoprotective in diabetes (HOPE trial). The AT$_1$-receptor antagonist, losartan, reduces mortality more than atenolol in diabetic patients with hypertension (LIFE trial). Centrally acting agents and calcium channel blockers are also suitable	Thiazides and β blockers may cause hyperglycaemia. Thiazides may adversely affect the lipid profile. β Blockers may also mask signs of hypoglycaemia (e.g. tachycardia; see Chapter 35)
Elderly people	Thiazides	
Chronic obstructive pulmonary disease (COPD) and asthma	Centrally acting agents are safe	β Blockers are contraindicated in asthma, although in the absence of an alternative, β$_1$-receptor antagonists may be used with extreme caution. In COPD, cardioselective agents are used with caution
History of stroke	Perindopril and indapamide reduce the risk of stroke in both hypertensive and normotensive patients (PROGRESS trial); this may apply to any ACE inhibitor plus a thiazide	
Renal impairment		Thiazides less effective. Dose reduction of hydrophilic β blockers (atenolol, celiprolol, nadolol) may be necessary. Caution with ACE inhibitors. ACE inhibitors and AT$_1$-receptor antagonists should not be used in renovascular disease
Prostatic hypertrophy	α Blocker	Diuretics
Pregnancy	Methyldopa; β blockers (third trimester)	Consider all other agents
Gout	Centrally acting agents safe	Thiazides
Migraine	β Blocker; clonidine	
Resistant hypertension	α Blocker; minoxidil, hydralazine, sodium nitroprusside	
Depression		Side effect of β blockers, calcium channel blockers, clonidine and methyldopa
Parkinsonism		Indoramin has extrapyramidal side effects

ACE, angiotensin-converting enzyme; AT$_1$, angiotensin; HOPE, Heart Outcomes Prevention Evaluation; LIFE, Losartan Intervention for Endpoint Reduction in Hypertension; PROGRESS, Perindopril Protection Against Recurrent Stroke Study.

that is independent of lipid lowering (Glorioso *et al* 1999; Borghi *et al* 2000; Su *et al* 2000). The concurrent use of a statin would have no bearing on the choice of antihypertensive regimen.

Diabetes mellitus often coexists with hypertension and, as indicated above, may be a compelling reason to use an ACE inhibitor. Clinical trials certainly suggest that ACE inhibitors are less likely to cause diabetes and many clinicians favour them in patients with diabetes to reduce the chances of renal nephropathy. Both thiazides and β blockers may worsen glucose tolerance, so their use in combination is often avoided in diabetes and patients at risk of developing diabetes.

Heart failure is often a consequence of untreated hypertension and, as reviewed in Chapter 15, may well be treated with an ACE inhibitor, diuretic, β blocker or spironolactone, all of which are also indicated for hypertension. In the case of a β blocker, a very low dose would be introduced in heart failure, initially under the supervision of an appropriately experienced clinician.

Drug interactions

Given the diversity of drugs used in the treatment of hypertension there is a range of drug interactions. Some important interactions of antihypertensive drugs are summarized in Table 11.3.

General counselling

As outlined earlier, lifestyle changes (including weight reduction, increased exercise, smoking

Table 11.3 Summary of important interactions within drugs used in hypertension

Interacting drugs	Consequences	Comments
β Blockers with β agonists	Pharmacological antagonism	Bronchoconstriction may occur due to inhibition of bronchial β₂-adrenoceptors
α Antagonists with calcium channel blockers or β blockers	Hypotension	Additive effects require close monitoring and counselling
Calcium channel blockers with β blockers	Some combinations are safe (e.g. felodipine and β blockers). Bradycardia and heart block with verapamil or diltiazem and β blockers (avoid combination or monitor closely); dihyropyridines with β blockers are usually safe but should be monitored	Additive negative inotropic effects. Increased plasma levels of β blockers metabolized by the liver
ACE inhibitors with NSAIDs	Risk of renal impairment	Both associated with renal toxicity
Grapefruit juice with nifedipine (and possibly nicardipine, amlodipine)	Increased effects of calcium channel blockers	Inhibition of cytochrome P450, therefore reduced metabolism
Alcohol with antihypertensives	• Chronic: increase in blood pressure • Acute: postural hypotension and dizziness	• Evidence of reduced blood pressure when moderate-heavy drinkers taking antihypertensives; reduce alcohol intake • Acutely, alcohol causes vasodilatation

ACE, angiotensin-converting enzyme; NSAIDs, non-steroidal anti-inflammatory drugs.

cessation, a low salt diet and reduction in alcohol consumption) should be advocated. Failure of lifestyle changes alone would then indicate drug treatment. In talking to patients about drug treatment it should be stressed that the purpose is to lower their BP and this should reduce their risk of having a heart attack, stroke or kidney problems. Although hypertension has no symptoms and the drugs may have side effects, it is important to take the drugs; however, if they find the side effects intolerable, they may find that changing their drug is beneficial.

Diuretics

- Diuretics (or 'water tablets') will cause an increase in urine flow, which may subside after a couple of weeks.
- It is best to take the diuretic in the morning to limit sleep disturbance. A dose may be taken later in the day to avoid the need for urination interfering with social engagements during the day.
- Diuretic use in elderly people is associated with increased incidence of falls.
- Diuretics may cause impotence and this should be discussed with the patient.

ACE inhibitors

- Patients may experience pronounced first-dose hypotension that may be worse if the patient is also taking diuretics; it is best to take the ACE inhibitor on retiring to bed at night. Discuss any cough with their GP. Patients should be encouraged to persist with the ACE inhibitor, because this is an effective treatment.
- Consult a pharmacist before purchasing other medicines or supplements, e.g. avoid the use of potassium salts (salt substitute, effervescent preparations, cystitis treatments) and use NSAIDs with caution.
- If patients experience any lip, facial or tongue swelling (angio-oedema), they should stop taking the ACE inhibitor and seek immediate medical advice.

Calcium channel blockers

- Calcium channel blockers may cause flushing, constipation and ankle swelling. Gentle exercise or elevation of the foot may reduce ankle swelling. These side effects should improve after a few weeks. If the side effects become troublesome, patients should discuss this with their general practitioner.
- Avoid grapefruit juice if taking a dihydropyridine.

β Blockers

- Male patients may experience impotence.
- Report any additional breathlessness (due to worsening of symptoms or blockade of bronchial β_2-adrenoceptors); cold extremities or peripheral weakness may reflect blockade of vasodilator β_2-adrenoceptors.
- Do not stop taking the tablets suddenly (because this may increase the risk of myocardial infarction). β Blockers should be withdrawn gradually over at least a week.

α Blockers

- Patients should be alert to first-dose hypotension.
- Patients may also experience urinary incontinence.
- Take care when driving, because of possible drowsiness.

Centrally acting drugs

- Take care when driving, because of possible drowsiness.
- Do not stop taking the tablets suddenly (particularly clonidine).

Monitoring

Home and pharmacy blood pressure measurements

Automated devices are available for home monitoring by the patient. These devices measure BP on different principles from auscultation with a sphygmomanometer. Indeed, some devices measure at the wrist rather than the brachial artery and very few of these are accurate. Hence, they may give differing absolute values and only a few of the devices have been validated: further details may be obtained from the BHS. The machine should be calibrated annually. Other sources of inaccuracy in home measuring may be poor technique such as cuff placing and inadequate resting before measurement.

'White-coat' hypertension is a well-recognized clinical phenomenon whereby the patient's BP is significantly higher when recorded by a doctor, and is thought to be induced by anxiety. In a proportion of cases, 'white-coat' hypertension is so pronounced that patients who are normotensive under normal conditions may be classed and treated as hypertensive on the basis of measurements made by a doctor. However, 'white-coat' hypertension may be eliminated by nurses or patients themselves measuring BP. Similarly, the BHS (O'Brien *et al* 2000) has produced guidelines regarding the use of ambulatory BP monitoring, which also overcomes the problems of 'white-coat' hypertension.

Prior to treatment

The following may be assessed:

- An electrocardiogram (ECG) to test for left ventricular hypertrophy, because up to a third of people with hypertension have left ventricular hypertrophy. There may also be the need for an echocardiogram.
- Electrolytes, especially potassium, because a reduced level may reflect hyperaldosteronism. This is particularly important when initiating diuretics and ACE inhibitors.
- Plasma lipids and glucose: these may be adversely affected by β blockers and diuretics.
- Renal function; plasma creatinine: this will influence drug choice because thiazides, except metolazone, are ineffective in moderate renal failure and ACE inhibitors may make renal impairment worse. Dose reduction with close monitoring is required if glomerular filtration rate (GFR) is <50 mL/min.
- Uurinalysis, because protein and/or blood might indicate renal damage.
- Full blood count.

- Liver function test, with mean corpuscular volume to assess for excess alcohol consumption.
- Thyroid function test.

During treatment

- Measurement of BP.
- Monitor renal function and proteinuria (annually).
- Monitor electrolytes, especially potassium, with diuretics and ACE inhibitors.

Over-the-counter considerations

Most patients should be considered for low-dose aspirin therapy because this has been shown to reduce the incidence of myocardial infarction in hypertensive patients. Although NSAIDs should not generally be used with ACE inhibitors or thiazides, low-dose aspirin (75 mg) appears to be safe. Indeed, the HOT trial indicated that low-dose aspirin reduced cardiovascular events but not stroke. The BHS recommends that low-dose aspirin be used in primary prevention in people with hypertension who are aged over 50 years and have controlled BP (<150/90 mmHg), and those with end-organ damage, diabetes or a 15% or greater risk of coronary artery disease over 10 years. Even low-dose aspirin is associated with gastric damage and bleeding, to which the patient should be alerted. Ibuprofen may oppose the beneficial effects of aspirin (see Chapter 14).

There is some evidence that fish oil supplementation may cause a modest reduction in BP, although this has not been universally reported. None the less, fish oil supplementation appears a sensible approach to reducing overall cardiovascular risk and is advocated by the American Heart Association (Kris-Etherton *et al* 2002).

Some considerations of over-the-counter (OTC) medicines and their use in hypertension are detailed in Table 11.4.

Alternative remedies

Consideration should be given to herbal preparations and supplements with sympathomimetic

Table 11.4   Summary of the use of over-the-counter (OTC) medicines in hypertension

OTC medicine	Effects	Comments
Low-dose aspirin	Reduces risk of myocardial infarction and stroke	Need to select high-risk patients due to the risk of gastric damage associated with even low doses. Proton pump inhibitor may be used for prophylaxis
Aspirin or ibuprofen	May reduce effects of captopril	Caution: blood pressure should be monitored
	Aspirin (300 mg) may reduce the effects of enalapril	Paracetamol is a safe alternative analgesic
Antacids	Interaction with ACE inhibitors to reduce their absorption	Separate doses
Cimetidine	May increase plasma concentrations of diltiazem and nifedipine	Ranitidine may be used as an alternative
Systemic sympathomimetic decongestants	Weak pressor effects	Use topical agents (if not swallowed), steam or saline drops

ACE, angiotensin-converting enzyme.

activity (see Chapter 4). Diuretic effects of herbal preparations may also increase side effects in combination with antihypertensives.

There has been recent interest in non-pharmacological treatment using devices that aim to lower BP by guiding patients to control their breathing to a rate of 10 breaths/min for a short period each day. However, the effectiveness of these devices requires confirmation in large trials, although small studies have reported modest BP responses. There is also evidence for a lack of efficacy in patients with diabetes and hypertension (Logtenberg *et al* 2007). It could be that these devices may be of benefit in cases of selected patients with mild hypertension or as an adjunct to dug treatment.

Future developments

The currently available drug treatments for hypertension are extensive and, in the absence of a single identifiable cause, future directions are limited. Having said that, renin inhibitors are under investigation as possible novel antihypertensives.

Practice points

- The BHS and NICE have produced joint guidelines. The guidelines recommend the A/CD algorithm. β Blockers are no longer recommended as first-line antihypertensives.
- Most patients do not have their BP adequately controlled by the first drug used.
- Patients should be warned about first-dose hypotension with ACE inhibitors and α blockers (extra caution in combination with diuretics) due to the risk of falls.
- Monitor patients for hypertension secondary to drug treatment, e.g. NSAIDs, oral contraceptives, sympathomimetics, corticosteroids, ketoconazole, moclobemide, venlafaxine and ciclosporin.
- In treatment failure consider OTC drugs, alcohol consumption and compliance.
- The aim of antihypertensive treatment is to reduce cardiovascular risk, reduce/limit end-organ damage, especially kidneys, left ventricular hypertrophy, and reduce the risk of heart failure.
- Aim for BP control without unacceptable side effects, because hypertension is generally asymptomatic.
- Always enquire about side effects, particularly impotence.

Self-assessment

Consider whether the following statements are true or false. In the management of hypertension:

1. ACE inhibitors are associated with causing first dose hypotension.
2. Thiazide diuretics are most effective at lowering blood pressure in patients with moderate-to-severe renal impairment.
3. β Blockers should be avoided in concurrent ischaemic heart disease.
4. Most patients require more than one drug to control their BP to target levels.
5. AT_1-receptor antagonists are usually used in combination with ACE inhibitors.

CASE STUDY

Mr AH was found by his GP during a routine check-up to have a BP of 180/100 mmHg. Mr AH is 58 years old, smokes 20 cigarettes a day, drinks 'several pints each night', has a body mass index (BMI) of 28, but is otherwise healthy. His father died of 'heart trouble' in his 50s.

1. What would be the first steps in the management of Mr AH?
   - 180/100 mmHg is moderate hypertension; there is a need to confirm that this is sustained on several occasions (typically, three readings over 2 months). There is also a need to exclude 'white-coat' hypertension. In the meantime this is not a medical emergency. It is important to encourage the patient to 'own' the problem and to change his risks, rather than simply leave it as a problem to be solved with tablets. He should be advised to reduce alcohol intake (a risk factor for essential hypertension), reduce his BMI to <25 (risk factor), cease smoking (although not a risk factor for hypertension, smoking greatly enhances the cardiovascular risk from hypertension; smoking is a major risk factor for ischaemic heart disease) and increase exercise.

   Two months later Mr AH's BP was 170/98 mmHg.
2. Suggest clinical tests that might be carried out:
   - if not carried out at the initial appointment, physical examination: retina for vascular damage, auscultation of heart (and kidneys for renal bruits?)
   - ECG to test for left ventricular hypertrophy (up to a third of people with hypertension have left ventricular hypertrophy)
   - echocardiogram to determine his ejection fraction
   - electrolytes – especially potassium (a reduced level may reflect hyperaldosteronism; Conn's syndrome)
   - plasma lipids, cholesterol, glucose
   - renal function: plasma creatinine (this may influence drug choice; thiazides, except metolazone, are ineffective in moderate renal failure)
   - urine: protein/blood may indicate renal damage
   - the above would be the ideal, but monitoring may be poor in the community, which may lead to increased hospitalization, e.g. hypokalaemia.

continued

CASE STUDY (continued)

3. What active treatment is he likely to receive?
   - According to the A/CD rules he should be prescribed a thiazide or calcium channel blocker as a first pharmacological step.
   Following 2 months of treatment with 2.5 mg bendroflumethiazide tablets every morning his BP is now 166/96 mmHg.
4. Why was the bendroflumethiazide every morning?
   - The diuresis would interfere with sleep if taken at night.
5. Given the poor response to bendroflumethiazide, should the dose be increased to 5 mg?
   - With thiazides, increasing the dose has no additional benefit and increases the side effects. Also, thiazides become ineffective in moderate renal failure – this could of course be the explanation for the failure of the thiazide, and so it may be worth measuring creatinine levels.
6. Draw up a plan with the various steps to continue the patient's management:
   - step 1: thiazides as a first pharmacological step. Cheap and effective. Potassium supplements are not normally needed but plasma potassium should be checked after 3–4 weeks
   - step 2: add an ACE inhibitor as step 2 of the A/CD rules
   - step 3: add a long-acting calcium channel blocker
   - step 4: consider an α blocker, a β blocker or additional diuretic.
7. What counselling is appropriate for Mr AH if he subsequently receives lisinopril (2.5 mg/day) in addition to bendroflumethiazide?
   - He may experience a dry cough, which he should report to his GP. He should take the first dose of lisinopril at night and the diuretic in the morning due to the risk of first-dose hypotension.
9. What are the goals of treatment for Mr AH?
   - target BP of systolic <140 mmHg and diastolic <90 mmHg; lowering diastolic BP by 5 mmHg reduces the risk of ischaemic heart disease by 21%
   - reduce cardiovascular risk (both stroke and myocardial infarction)
   - reduce/limit end-organ damage, especially the kidneys
   - reduce the risk of heart failure
   - BP control without unacceptable side effects, because hypertension is generally asymptomatic.

References

ALLHAT Trialists (2002). Major outcomes in high-risk hypertensive patients randomized to angiotensin-converting enzyme inhibitor or calcium channel blocker vs diuretic. *JAMA* **288**: 2981–97.

ASCOT Investigators (2005). Prevention of cardiovascular events with an antihypertensive regimen of amlodipine adding perindopril as required versus atenolol adding bendroflumethiazide as required, in the Anglo-Scandinavian Cardiac Outcomes Trial-Blood Pressure Lowering Arm (ASCOT-BPLA): a multicentre randomised controlled trial. *Lancet* 366: 895–906.

Borghi C, Prandin MG, Costa FV *et al* (2000). Use of statins and blood pressure control in treated hypertensive patients with hypercholesterolaemia. *J Cardiovasc Pharmacol* 35: 549–55.

CAPP Study Group (1999). Effect of angiotensin-converting-enzyme inhibition compared with conventional therapy on cardiovascular morbidity and mortality in hypertension: the Captopril Prevention Project (CAPPP) randomised trial. *Lancet* **353**: 611–16.

Glorioso N, Troffa C, Filigheddu F *et al* (1999). Effect of the HMG-CoA reductase inhibitors on blood pressure in patients with essential hypertension and primary hypercholesterolaemia. *Hypertension* **34**: 1281–6.

HOT Study Group (1998). Effects of intensive blood-pressure lowering and low-dose aspirin in patients with hypertension: principal results of the Hypertension Optimal Treatment (HOT) randomised trial. *Lancet* **351**: 1755–62.

Kris-Etherton PM, Harris WS, Appel LJ (2002). Fish consumption, fish oil, omega-3 fatty acids and cardiovascular disease. *Circulation* **106**: 2747–57.

LIFE (Losartan Intervention for Endpoint Reduction in Hypertension) Study Investigators (2002). Cardiovascular morbidity and mortality in the Losartan Intervention for Endpoint reduction in hypertension study (LIFE): a randomised trial against atenolol. *Lancet* **359**: 995–1003.

Logtenberg SJ, Kleefstra N, Houweling ST *et al* (2007). Effect of device-guided breathing exercises on blood pressure in hypertensive patients with type 2 diabetes mellitus: a randomized controlled trial. *J Hypertens* **25**: 241–6.

Martin J, ed. *British National Formulary*, latest edition. London: British Medical Association and Royal Pharmaceutical Society of Great Britain.

National Institute for Health and Clinical Excellence (2006a). *Statins for the Prevention of Cardiovascular disease*. Technology Appraisal 94. London: NICE.

National Institute for Health and Clinical Excellence (2006b). *Hypertension: Management of hypertension in adults in primary care*. Clinical Guideline 34. London: NICE.

O'Brien E, Coats A, Owens P *et al* (2000). Use and interpretation of ambulatory blood pressure monitoring: recommendations of the British Hypertension Society. *BMJ* **320**: 1128–34.

Stevens VJ, Obarzanek E, Cook NR *et al* (2001). Long-term weight loss and changes in blood pressure: results of the trials of hypertension prevention, phase II. *Ann Intern Med* **134**: 1–11.

Su SF, Hsiao CL, Chu CW *et al* (2000). Effects of pravastatin on left ventricular mass in patients with hyperlipidaemia and essential hypertension. *Am J Cardiol* **86**: 514–18.

Further reading

Brown MJ (2001). Matching the right drug to the right patient in essential hypertension. *Heart* **86**: 113–20.

HOPE (Heart Outcomes Prevention Evaluation) Study Investigators (2000). Effects of an angiotensin-converting-enzyme inhibitor, ramipril, on cardiovascular events in high-risk patients. *N Engl J Med* **342**: 145–53.

LIFE Study Investigators (2002). Cardiovascular morbidity and mortality in patients with diabetes in the Losartan Intervention for Endpoint reduction in hypertension study (LIFE): a randomised trial against atenolol. *Lancet* **359**: 1004–10.

McInnes G (2001). Explaining hypertension and its risks to patients. *Prescriber* **12**: 19–26.

PROGRESS Collaborative Group (2001). Randomised trial of a perindopril-based blood pressure-lowering regimen among 6105 individuals with previous stroke or transient ischaemic attack. *Lancet* **358**: 1033–41.

Online resources

www.bhf.org.uk
The website of the British Heart Foundation, providing patient information (accessed April 2008).

www.bpassoc.org.uk
The website of the Blood Pressure Association, providing patient information (accessed April 2008).

www.bhsoc.org
The website of the British Hypertension Society, providing professional guidance, including the validation of BP-measuring devices (accessed April 2008).

12

Hyperlipidaemia

Disease characteristics

Hyperlipidaemia represents hypercholesterolaemia and/or hypertriglyceridaemia and is a major risk factor for atherosclerotic plaque formation on the inner surface of arteries, leading to ischaemic heart disease (IHD), cerebrovascular and peripheral vascular diseases. The cause may be genetic (primary or familial hypercholesterolaemia) or secondary to disease such as liver disease, renal failure, hypothyroidism or poorly controlled diabetes mellitus, or may be induced by drugs including:

- β blockers
- corticosteroids
- thiazide diuretics
- anabolic steroids
- retinoids
- oral contraceptives containing levonorgestrel.

A number of modifiable risk factors may contribute towards or exacerbate this condition:

- hypertension
- smoking
- obesity
- high-fat diet
- excess alcohol consumption
- hyperglycaemia
- reduced physical activity
- infection?

and should be considered in relation to the lipid profile.

Hypercholesterolaemia

Increased plasma cholesterol or hypercholesterolaemia is a major risk factor for atherosclerosis and is present when cholesterol exceeds the desirable level of <5 mmol/L. However, it is increasingly recognized that it is not necessarily the absolute level of cholesterol that is important, but the level in relation to other risk factors (composition of total cholesterol, blood pressure, gender, smoking status, diabetes), and how these give rise to the overall cardiovascular risk. Indeed decisions to use antihyperlipidaemic agents are now based on the patient's cardiovascular risk rather than absolute levels of total cholesterol.

The transport of lipids and cholesterol through the blood is carried out by one of four main classes of lipoprotein: high-density lipoprotein (HDL), low-density lipoprotein (LDL), very-low-density lipoprotein (VLDL) and chylomicrons. These lipoproteins, each with a different role, comprise a central core of hydrophobic lipid, encased in phospholipid, cholesterol and apolipoproteins. Classification is determined by differences in density, size and proportion of core lipid.

Lipoproteins

In the context of atherogenesis, it is the balance between LDL and HDL that plays a major role:

- LDL ('bad cholesterol') is cholesterol rich and taken up by the liver and tissues, and this involves the LDL receptor. LDL provides cholesterol for cell membranes, steroid synthesis and the production of bile acids. Its uptake into arterial walls is associated with atherogenesis.
- HDL ('good cholesterol') takes up cholesterol from cellular breakdown and prevents its deposition.

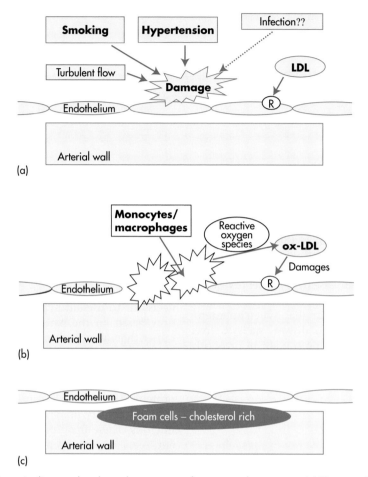

Figure 12.1   A schematic diagram that shows the sequence of events in atherogenesis. (a) Various risk factors may cause damage (b) resulting in the generation of reactive oxygen species, which may oxidize the low-density lipoprotein (ox-LDL), damaging the LDL receptor (R), and these changes may lead to (c) foam cells accumulating between the endothelium and arterial wall.

Atherogenesis

Especially important in atherosclerosis is a high LDL component or low levels of HDL. Indeed, the ratio LDL:HDL is of clinical importance (ideally <3). Blood vessels express LDL receptors for cellular uptake. However, when injury occurs or in the presence of risk factors (such as smoking), the activated monocytes and macrophages generate reactive oxygen species, which oxidize the LDL, and this damages the LDL receptor so that modified LDL is taken up by macrophages. In turn, these macrophages form foam cells that collect beneath the endothelium,

leading to fatty streaks. In the special case of familial hypercholesterolaemia, the LDL receptor is defective and thus LDL is cleared less rapidly and accumulates in the plasma. In contrast to the above role of LDL in atherogenesis, HDL binds cholesterol and removes it from local sites, taking it to the liver. Hence HDL is viewed as 'good cholesterol' and protects against atherogenesis. Accordingly, low levels of HDL will offer less protection and are viewed as an important cardiovascular risk.

The process of atherogenesis is regarded as an inflammatory response to injury and the release of inflammatory mediators leads to altered smooth muscle activity and growth. Over time the changes in the blood vessel lead to the formation of atherosclerotic plaques that are lipid rich and become calcified. This long-term process leads to stenosis or the narrowing of large arteries (e.g. the coronary arteries), whereas rupture of a plaque leads to platelet adhesion and aggregation, which may cause thromboembolic occlusion.

There is currently some suggestion, which is not universally accepted, that atherosclerosis may be encouraged by chronic infection. One agent to be implicated is *Chlamydia pneumoniae*, which is believed to be transported from the lungs by macrophages to the vascular smooth muscle, with local infection leading to damage and inflammation. Other evidence has shown that dental bacteria correlate with carotid artery thickening, which is a risk for atherosclerosis (INVEST Trial 2005). However, despite the potential involvement of chronic infection, the CLARICOR Trial in 2006 demonstrated that clarithromycin treatment actually increases mortality in patients with stable ischaemic heart disease.

Hypertriglyceridaemia

This is elevated plasma triglyceride levels, which may or may not coexist with hypercholesterolaemia. Elevated levels of triglycerides are often associated with other conditions such as obesity, diabetes mellitus, high doses of thiazides (transiently) and high alcohol intake. Its association with atherosclerosis is less strong compared with that for hypercholesterolaemia, but at very high levels it is associated with pancreatitis.

Clinical features

The patient may have few obvious symptoms and hyperlipidaemia may become apparent only after determination of plasma lipid levels. In severe hyperlipidaemia there may be physical signs such as xanthomas, which are yellowish lipid deposits, especially on the eyelids, cornea and tendons. Coronary artery disease presenting

as angina or myocardial infarction (MI) is a secondary manifestation of hyperlipidaemia.

Hyperlipidaemia may be associated with diabetes mellitus, renal failure and hypothyroidism, so blood glucose levels and renal and thyroid functions should be determined to exclude possible contributions from these conditions.

Goals of treatment

The primary objective of treating hyperlipidaemia is to bring about reductions of plasma cholesterol (improving the HDL:LDL ratio) and/or reducing triglyceride levels. This should lead to a reduction in risk of MI and stroke. The ideal goal would be regression of atherosclerotic lesions. If diet and lifestyle modification fail, the following pharmacological interventions may be considered in addition.

Pharmacological basis of management

HMG-CoA reductase inhibitors or 'statins', e.g. atorvastatin, fluvastatin, pravastatin, rosuvastatin, simvastatin

The statins inhibit the hepatic enzyme, hydroxymethylglutaryl coenzyme A reductase (HMG-CoA reductase), which catalyses the first committed step of cholesterol synthesis in the liver. Statins are hepatoselective with extensive first-pass metabolism, which is advantageous because the liver is the main site of cholesterol synthesis, with extrahepatic sites synthesizing essential cholesterol.

Fibrates, e.g. bezafibrate, fenofibrate, gemofibrozil

Fibrates are activators of peroxisome proliferator-activated receptor α (PPAR-α) and lead to alterations in lipoprotein metabolism. This results in the stimulation of peripheral lipoprotein lipases, which promotes the breakdown of VLDL (with small reductions in LDL and increases in HDL)

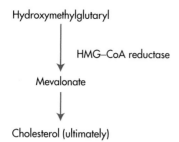

Hydroxymethylglutaryl

HMG–CoA reductase

Mevalonate

Cholesterol (ultimately)

Figure 12.2 Cholesterol synthesis in the liver. HMG-CoA, hydroxymethylglutaryl coenzyme A.

and also leads to reductions in triglycerides. The increased biliary excretion of cholesterol predisposes the patient to gallstones and fibrates are therefore contraindicated in gallbladder disease. Their use is associated with a reduction in cardiovascular events but not overall mortality (VA-HIT Trial Study Group 1999).

Cholesterol absorption inhibitors: ezetimibe

These agents, which may be used alone or in addition to a statin or fibrate, inhibit the absorption of exogenous and biliary cholesterol in the gastrointestinal tract, bringing about a reduction in total cholesterol and LDL. They may be ideal as an addition to statin therapy, instead of increasing the dose of statin that may be associated with side effects.

Bile acid-binding resins, e.g. colestyramine

These agents bind bile salts in the intestines, preventing both their reabsorption and their cycling. This interruption in bile cycling leads to incorporation of endogenous cholesterol to form bile salts and there is an increase in the number of LDL receptors, which favours the cellular uptake of cholesterol.

Colestyramine is generally used in addition to other agents and can cause a modest fall in plasma cholesterol, which may lead to a reduction in coronary artery disease. However, the binding nature of these agents will reduce the absorption of fat-soluble vitamins (A, D, E and especially K) and other drugs (including warfarin,

digoxin, thiazides, levothyroxine and paracetamol), which should not be given at the same time of day. Changes in the absorption of vitamin K may lead to increased effects of warfarin.

Nicotinic acid (niacin)

Vitamin B_3 or its derivatives inhibit hepatic triglyceride production and VLDL secretion. This results in a reduction in LDL and increase in HDL. Nicotinic acid is rarely used due to troublesome adverse effects such as headache and flushing (caused by prostaglandin production, which may be reduced by taking aspirin half an hour before the dose), palpitations, pruritus, hyperglycaemia and gout.

Fish oils

Fish oils rich in omega-3 fatty acids (eicosapentaenoic acid and docosahexaenoic acid) are used for hypertriglyceridaemia, although they do increase levels of LDL.

The low incidence of coronary artery disease in Eskimos is attributed to their high dietary intake of omega-3 fatty acids in oily fish. A fish-rich diet following an MI has been demonstrated to reduce mortality and reinfarction significantly. The consumption of at least two portions of oily fish per week or supplementation with fish oils is recommended by the American Heart Association (Kris-Etherton *et al* 2002). Fish oils should be used with caution in diabetes, haemorrhagic disorders, anticoagulant treatment and aspirin-sensitive asthma.

Antioxidants

The process of atherogenesis involves the production of reactive oxygen species and it was previously thought that antioxidants such as vitamin E might be protective. However, in patients with a high risk of death from cardiovascular disease (diabetes mellitus, ischaemic heart disease, hypertension or arterial disease), the Heart Protection Study Collaborative Group

(2002b) found that supplementation with anti-oxidants, β-carotene, vitamin C or vitamin E did not reduce mortality.

Sitostanol

This is a functional food that is added to certain brands of margarine and prevents the absorption of cholesterol. Additions of sitostanol to the diet reduce LDL by 10–15% and may be helpful as an addition to dietary restrictions or statin therapy.

Hormone replacement therapy

The apparent protective effect of oestrogen in premenopausal women has, for a long time, implicated a role for hormone replacement therapy (HRT) in the prevention of ischaemic heart disease (IHD) in postmenopausal women. One of the effects of oestrogen was thought to be in reducing plasma cholesterol levels. However, a large-scale trial involving HRT was stopped in 2002 when there was an increase in both heart attacks and strokes in patients receiving HRT. After this trial, HRT is no longer used to reduce cardiovascular risk in postmenopausal patients.

Ispaghula

Supplementation with non-starch polysaccha-rides (NSPs) reduces the absorption of bile acids and therefore leads to a reduction in LDL. It has no effect on triglyceride levels and is used to treat patients with mild-to-moderate hypercholestero-laemia who have not responded to dietary changes alone. Contraindications include intestinal obstruction, faecal impaction and colonic atony.

Choice of drugs

The number of patients who may potentially benefit from treatment with a lipid-lowering drug is enormous. Hence there is a need to identify those patients who would benefit most. The National Institute for Health and Clinical

Excellence (NICE 2006) recommends that statin therapy be initiated in patients with cardio-vascular disease and for primary prevention in patients with a 20% or greater risk of cardio-vascular disease over the next 10 years, as identified by risk tables. Where these tables are not appropriate, it is based on clinical judgement (e.g. in diabetes).

The Heart Protection Study Collaborative Group (2002a) found that treatment of patients at high risk of death from cardiovascular disease (diabetes mellitus, IHD, hypertension or arterial disease) with 40 mg simvastatin reduced cardio-vascular events by a quarter to a third. This effect was irrespective of cholesterol levels and was additive with other protective drugs such as angiotensin-converting enzyme (ACE) inhibitors, β blockers and aspirin.

Hypercholesterolaemia and reduction of cardiovascular risk

In hypercholesterolaemia, once dietary changes have been tried, and in patients who have cardio-vascular disease or who are at a high risk, statins are the drugs of choice. Statins are of benefit in types IIa and IIb hyperlipoproteinaemia (elevated LDL and LDL/VLDL respectively). They cause a reduction in plasma cholesterol, whereas the reduction in hepatic cholesterol synthesis leads to an upregulation of hepatic LDL receptors, pro-moting LDL uptake. However, with the exception of atorvastatin, they are less effective in homo-zygous familial hypercholesterolaemia, a very rare condition where the LDL receptor is lacking.

The 4S trial (Scandinavian Simvastatin Survival Study Group 1994) reported that simvastatin, in patients who had previously had an MI or had angina, caused a 35% reduction in LDL (increased HDL), and over 5 years this was associated with a 30% reduction in mortality. The WOSCOPS trial (Shepherd *et al* 1995) also confirmed the effectiveness of pravastatin in primary prevention, with a 20% reduction in cholesterol and a 28% reduction in mortality from coronary artery disease in patients with hypercholestero-laemia. Statins also reduce the progression of carotid artery disease and so reduce the risk of stroke. The Heart Protection Study Collaborative Group (2002a) has reported substantial benefits

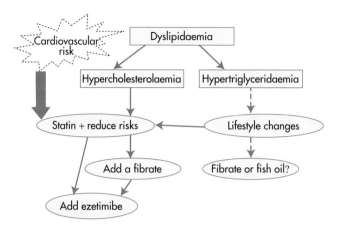

Figure 12.3 A flow diagram indicating approaches to manage dyslipidaemia and reduce cardiovascular risk. Hyper-cholesterolaemia and high cardiovascular risks (or disease) are reasons to use a statin, with fibrates and ezetimibe being added as appropriate. In the case of hypertriglyceridaemia, lifestyle changes can play a significant role. If drug therapy is required then statins are often used first line whereas fibrates have the greatest effect on triglyceride levels.

of simvastatin in high-risk patients, with marked reductions in events and mortality, and the protection was related to the level of risk rather than plasma lipid level. The PROSPER study (Shepherd *et al* 2002) has also demonstrated that pravastatin is effective at reducing mortality from coronary artery disease in elderly patients (70–84 years) with a history of, or risk factors for, cardiovascular disease.

The beneficial effects of statins may be due to regression of atherosclerosis, because there is some evidence that not only do they slow down atherosclerosis but they may also cause regression with lipid depletion, leading to stabilization of lesions. The large-scale ASTEROID (2006) trial has established that high doses of rosuvastatin actually cause regression of coronary atherosclerosis. This is a major goal in the management of cardiovascular disease and it remains to be established whether this is unique to rosuvastatin or due to high intensity therapy.

In severe disease it may be necessary to add a fibrate, although this increases the risk of myopathy.

Hypertriglyceridaemia

As a first step, care should be taken in patients with hypertriglyceridaemia to exclude and modify causes such as excess alcohol intake, obesity and diet. Treatment of hypertriglyceridaemia is less compelling but fibrates would be the agents of choice for severe disease (>10 mmol/L) because they are most effective. In this respect bezafibrate has been shown to lower triglycerides and raise HDL in patients with IHD and this was accompanied by a trend in the reduction of fatal and non-fatal MI (BIP Study Group 2000). Gemfibrozil was also shown to lower triglycerides and raise HDL in secondary prevention and reduced cardiovascular events, although not overall mortality (VA-HIT Trial Study Group 1999). Statins may also cause a modest reduction in plasma triglycerides and be considered first-choice agents in moderate hypertriglyceridaemia or combined hyperlipidaemia, although only atorvastatin and simvastatin are licensed for this indication. Fish oils are also effective in hypertriglyceridaemia. Anion-exchange resins may aggravate hypertriglyceridaemia.

Homocysteinaemia

This condition is also associated with atherosclerosis and is a genetic impairment of vitamins B_6 and B_{12} and folic acid metabolism, which leads to an increase in plasma levels of homocysteine.

Table 12.1   Effects of concurrent conditions on drug choice in hyperlipidaemia

Conditions	Effects on drug choice	Comments
Liver disease	A reason to avoid statins and severe disease would be a reason to avoid fibrates	Anion-exchange resins are contraindicated in complete biliary obstruction because they are ineffective
Gall stones	Fibrates can cause gallstones	Avoid in patients who have gallbladder disease
Hypertension	It is well established that thiazides alter lipid profile, by raising cholesterol and triglycerides. Statins may themselves lower blood pressure, when used with antihypertensive drugs	Whether the increase in cholesterol with thiazides is sustained is unclear, but this adverse reaction may have a bearing on the treatment of borderline cases of hyperlipidaemia
Recent heart attack	The PRISM trial (PRISM Investigators 2002) has indicated that patients who are taking a statin before an MI are at increased risk of further cardiac events for the following week if the statin is abruptly withdrawn at the time of the initial event	This effect appeared to be independent of the effects of the statins on plasma lipids and may be due to the loss of other beneficial effects. This suggests that statin therapy should not be withdrawn abruptly in these patients
Renal impairment	May necessitate dose reductions (consult BNF)	The risk of rhabdomyolysis is increased in those with renal impairment (CHM). Modified-release bezafibrate is not appropriate in renal impairment
Diabetes mellitus	Fibrates improve glucose tolerance with an additive effect in combination with hypoglycaemic agents	A reduction in the dose of hypoglycaemic agent may be necessary, particularly with clofibrate. Nicotinic acid should be used with caution
Gout	Nicotinic acid should be used with caution in gout	
Dementia	A report (Jick et al 2000) has also claimed that statins, in the absence or presence of hyperlipidaemia, reduce the risk of dementia and this may also have a bearing on its selection	
Hypothyroidism	Increased risk of rhabdomyolysis with statins and fibrates (CSM/CHM)	
Pregnancy	Statins, nicotinic acid and fibrates are contraindicated in pregnancy and breast-feeding	With statins, adequate contraception should be used during treatment and for 1 month after stopping
Postmenopausal osteoporosis	Statins may reduce bone turnover (Rejnmark et al 2002)	
Peptic ulcer	Nicotinic acid should be used with caution	

BNF, British National Formulary; MI, myocardial infarction; CHM, Commission on Human Medicines; CSM, Committee on Safety of Medicines; PRISM, Platelet Receptor Inhibition in Ischemic Syndrome Management.

Table 12.2   Summary of interactions within drugs used in hyperlipidaemia

Interaction	Consequences	Comments
Fibrates and statins	This beneficially results in additional lipid lowering but increases the risk of myopathy	The adverse interaction appears rare but the agents should be used with caution. The interaction is substantial with cerivastatin and gemfibrozil; cerivastatin has now been withdrawn
Colestyramine with fluvastatin/pravastatin	Increased lipid-lowering effect but reduced bioavailability of the statins	Colestyramine binds these statins and so giving the statins several hours afterwards improves bioavailability

This induces oxidative stress, which predisposes towards atherosclerosis and thrombogenesis. Folic acid is thought to reduce plasma homocysteine levels and reduce the progression of atherosclerosis.

Concurrent illnesses

Clinically significant hyperlipidaemia that necessitates treatment is likely to occur in the older patient population where a range of other illnesses may coexist. Of specific importance to atherosclerosis are diabetes mellitus and hypertension, both of which should be treated in concert with lipid lowering. Some considerations of drug prescribing in concurrent conditions are summarized in Table 12.1.

Drug interactions

When considering drug choice within the lipid-lowering agents, interactions should be considered (Table 12.2).

In addition to within-group interactions, antihyperlipidaemic drugs show a range of interactions and some important examples are summarized in Table 12.3.

Drug safety

Statins and fibrates are both, to varying degrees, associated with myopathy presenting as muscle pain, which may potentially lead to rhabdomyolysis; this is the breakdown of muscle, which may lead to the release of myoglobin and is associated with renal damage. It is for this reason that cerivastatin was withdrawn in 2001. Despite this, the instances of myopathy with elevated creatine kinase are very rare and occur in less than 1 in every 10 000 patients on standard dose statin. The risk is, however, increased with interacting drugs or concomitant fibrates. Statins are also commonly associated with derangements of hepatic transaminases but not liver damage. Therefore, with appropriate counselling and monitoring, statins are regarded as safe medicines.

General counselling

In a patient with hyperlipidaemia the counselling should first be directed at lifestyle advice to attempt to reduce plasma cholesterol and other risk factors for atherosclerosis. In relation to hyperlipidaemia it may be worth talking in terms of the blood containing too much of a fatty substance which, over time, can lead to the patient having a heart attack or stroke. The good news is that, by altering diet, with or without taking drugs, the risk of having a heart attack or stroke is reduced. The patient would be advised to reduce the intake of fatty foods, especially dairy products, and perhaps to consider a Mediterranean diet with plenty of oily fish, fruit and vegetables. Dietary changes alone may cause a modest reduction in plasma cholesterol but this

Table 12.3   Summary of interactions with drugs used in hyperlipidaemia

Interacting drugs	Consequences	Comments
Warfarin with fibrates or statins	Fibrates and some statins (Chapter 15) may increase the anticoagulant effect of warfarin	INR should be monitored
Warfarin with fish oils	Fish oils may have anticoagulant effects	Additional monitoring of clotting seems appropriate
Simvastatin and macrolides	This can lead to increases in the concentration of simvastatin and the risk of rhabdomyolysis	It may be appropriate to avoid this combination
Simvastatin and grapefruit juice	High consumption of grapefruit juice can increase substantially the plasma concentrations of simvastatin. This is less marked for atorvastatin whereas pravastatin appears unaffected	Patients taking simvastatin should avoid drinking grapefruit juice
Statins or fibrates with ciclosporin	Increased levels of ciclosporin and increased risk of rhabdomyolysis with statins, particularly simvastatin, and fibrates	Pravastatin does not appear to interact adversely with ciclosporin
Statins with itraconazole	Itraconazole increases the levels of simvastatin with an increased risk of rhabdomyolysis	
Pravastatin with orlistat	Possible increase in levels of pravastatin	

INR, international normalized ratio.

is limited, because only 25–30% of cholesterol is derived from the diet. The importance of smoking cessation should be emphasized. Weight reduction, increased physical activity and reduction of excessive alcohol consumption would all be beneficial.

Patients with suspected familial hypercholesterolaemia should be advised that other members of their family should be screened and counselled. Specific counselling is detailed below.

Statins

- Statins should be taken at night (this offsets a nocturnal increase in cholesterol synthesis), except atorvastatin (which has a prolonged half-life).
- They may cause myopathy (rarely leading to rhabdomyolysis) and so patients should immediately report any unexplained muscle pains, tenderness or weakness to their GP.

- Patients may expect to suffer from headaches, nausea and gastrointestinal pain. These side effects should improve as treatment continues.
- Statins exhibit a number of interactions. Some statins may enhance plasma levels of warfarin (see Chapter 16), and so patients should be advised to inform other health-care professionals that they are receiving this drug. The international normalized ratio (INR) should ideally be checked before and 5 days after treatment with an interacting drug.
- Simvastatin may interact with grapefruit juice and patients should be counselled to avoid drinking grapefruit juice.
- It is important to continue with the recommended dietary and lifestyle changes.

Fibrates

- Fibrates may cause myopathy (rarely leading to rhabdomyolysis) and so patients should immediately report any muscle pains to their GP.

- Side effects include rash, urticaria, weight gain, impotence and headache.

Anion-exchange resins

- Take other drugs or supplements 1 h before or 4–6 h after colestyramine.
- The powder may be used in sauces or added to fruit juice.
- The dose should be increased gradually and then taken regularly.
- Constipation is a common side effect. Nausea and vomiting, diarrhoea, flatulence and abdominal discomfort may occur but should improve after the first few months of treatment.

Fish oils

- These are best taken with food.
- They may cause occasional nausea and belching.
- Fish oils contain vitamins A and D. Avoid additional supplements containing these vitamins which are stored by the body.

Ispaghula

See Chapter 9.

Monitoring

Liver function

Liver function tests (LFTs) should be carried out before treatment with statins and within 3 months of initiating treatment. Liver function should then be monitored on a fairly regular (6-monthly to yearly) basis. A sustained rise in transaminase levels of three times the upper limit of the reference range would necessitate discontinuation of treatment.

Monitoring advice for patients prescribed fenofibrate indicates that LFTs should be repeated every 3 months for the first year. LFTs are also recommended before initiating long-term treatment with gemfibrozil.

Creatine kinase

A patient reporting muscle pains should have creatine kinase levels measured. A 10-fold elevation would be consistent with myopathy and treatment would be discontinued.

Over-the-counter considerations

In recent years low-dose (10 mg) simvastatin has been made available as an over-the-counter (OTC) medicine for patients who are at moderate risk of cardiovascular disease and these have been identified as:

- all men >55
- men aged 45–55 and women >55 with one of the following:
  - family history of IHD
  - smokers
  - overweight
  - south Asians from the Indian subcontinent.

However, this presents a number of issues and the pharmacist should be vigilant for patients who may be presenting with evidence of IHD (such as angina) and should be referred to their doctor. Similarly, patients require full counselling with respect to reporting muscle pains, should be vigilant for signs of heptatoxicity (jaundice, itching, dark urine), and should be aware of significant interactions (which include those with HIV protease inhibitors, ciclosporin, azoles, fibrates, anticoagulants and macrolides). It would also be good practice to suggest that patients document their use of statins with their GP.

Although the wider availability of statins is a significant step in health care it does raise some issues. Its OTC use does not, surprisingly, require a cholesterol test or liver function monitoring. Furthermore, the use of simvastatin at 10 mg has not been established by trials as providing protection, e.g. the Heart Protection Study (2002a) established the efficacy at 40 mg. There is also the issue that patients may buy simvastatin to offset an otherwise unhealthy lifestyle or bingeing and so its use should be alongside appropriate lifestyle advice.

In a patient with IHD or at a high risk from it, it would be sensible to consider low-dose aspirin as an antiplatelet drug and/or referral for a cholesterol test. Some pharmacists offer 'healthy heart checks', including blood pressure and cholesterol measurement, medical history taking and body mass index calculations to estimate the patient's risk of heart disease while providing lifestyle advice before coronary artery disease becomes symptomatic. High-risk patients should be advised to wear support hosiery during long flights to reduce the risk of thromboembolism (see Chapter 16). These can be purchased over-the-counter.

Requests for supplements should be considered in relation to prescribed treatment, e.g. patients taking warfarin should be advised to have their INR checked if they wish to take fish oils. Ideally, general diet and lifestyle advice should be given to all patients requesting food supplements (see Chapters 3 and 4).

Self-assessment

Consider whether the following statements are true or false. In the management of dyslipidaemia:

1. Simvastatin is best taken at night to avoid sedation during the day.
2. Simvastatin is available as an OTC medicine for patients >18 years of age.
3. Fibrates are most effective in hypertriglyceridaemia.
4. A substantial elevation in creatine kinase in patient taking a statin is consistent with myopathy.
5. Statins are recommended for patients who have suffered a heart attack, irrespective of their cholesterol levels.

Practice points

- Monitoring of cholesterol should be carried out in those at increased risk of heart disease.
- Lifestyle and dietary measures should be tried first and continued alongside pharmacological intervention if ineffective alone. The maintenance of dietary measures may need emphasizing to the patient.
- Statins have been shown to be effective in both primary and secondary prevention.
- The use of OTC statins requires full counselling and should be documented with the patient's GP.
- Fibrates are effective in mixed hyperlipidaemia and hypertriglyceridaemia.
- The Heart Protection Study Collaborative Group (2002a) suggests that 40 mg simvastatin substantially reduces the risk of MI and stroke. This protection relates to patient's overall risk rather than their lipid profile.
- Statins should be taken at night (except atorvastatin) and LFTs performed.
- Low-dose aspirin should be considered for all patients at risk of IHD.
- Health professionals should be alert to reports of muscle pain, tenderness or weakness by patients taking lipid-lowering drugs.

 CASE STUDY

A 58-year-old woman presents you with a prescription for simvastatin (40 mg daily every night). She is also taking atenolol (50 mg daily) having suffered a heart attack last year:

1. Are you happy to dispense the simvastatin? Justify your decision.
   Yes – there is no interaction with atenolol.

continued

CASE STUDY (continued)

2. How would you counsel this patient?
   Take the simvastatin at night.
   Report any muscle pain or weakness immediately: rhabdomyolysis is a rare but important side effect.
   She may also initially expect headache, nausea and gastrointestinal pain.
   Discuss cardiovascular risks – give up smoking if appropriate; low-fat diet; moderate exercise; weight reduction if appropriate?
   Was she taking low-dose aspirin? If not, might this be appropriate?
   It is important that she continues to take the statin long term.
3. Why is the simvastatin to be taken at night?
   Simvastatin is taken at night, when cholesterol synthesis is greatest.
4. The patient would like to know what this new prescription is for; explain in lay terms why she has this new addition.
   The new medicine is to lower the amount of a fatty substance in her blood called cholesterol which is known to cause heart trouble. Lowering the cholesterol should reduce her chances of another heart attack.
   A year later, while being maintained on simvastatin (40 mg daily every night), she presents with a prescription for erythromycin (250 mg four times daily) for sinusitis (she is allergic to penicillin).
5. How would you respond?
   The *British National Formulary* indicates that there is an increased risk of myopathy when simvastatin is used with erythromycin. For the sake of caution the prescriber should be contacted and it might be suggested that a non-penicillin/non-cephalosporin antibacterial such as doxycycline be used as an alternative.

References

ASTEROID Trial Group (2006). Effect of very high-intensity statin therapy on regression of coronary atherosclerosis. *JAMA* **295**: 1556–65.

BIP Study Group (2000). Secondary prevention by raising HDL cholesterol and reducing triglycerides in patients with coronary artery disease: the bezafibrate infarction prevention (BIP) study. *Circulation* **102**: 21–7.

CLARICOR Trial Group (2006). Randomised placebo controlled multicentre trial to assess short term clarithromycin for patients with stable coronary heart disease: CLARICOR trial. *BMJ* **332**:22–27.

Heart Protection Study Collaborative Group (2002a). MRC/BHF Heart Protection Study of cholesterol lowering with simvastatin in 20 536 high-risk individuals: randomised placebo-controlled trial. *Lancet* **360**: 7–22.

Heart Protection Study Collaborative Group (2002b). MRC/BHF Heart Protection Study of antioxidant vitamin supplementation in 20 536 high-risk individuals: randomised placebo-controlled trial. *Lancet* **360**: 23–33.

INVEST (2005). Periodontal Microbiota and Carotid Intima-Media Thickness. The Oral Infections and Vascular Disease Epidemiology Study (INVEST). *Circulation* **111**: 576–82.

Jick H, Zornberg GL, Jick SS *et al* (2000). Statins and the risk of dementia. *Lancet* **356**: 1627–1631.

Kris-Etherton PM, Harris WS, Appel LJ (2002). Fish consumption, fish oil, omega-3 fatty acids and cardiovascular disease. *Circulation* **106**: 2747–57.

Martin J, ed. *British National Formulary*, latest edition. London: British Medical Association and Royal Pharmaceutical Society of Great Britain.

National Institute for Health and Clinical Excellence (2006). *Statins for the Prevention of Cardiovascular Events*. Technology Appraisal 94. London: NICE. Available at: www.nice.org.uk.

PRISM Investigators (2002). Withdrawal of statins increases event rates in patients with acute coronary syndromes. *Circulation* **105**: 1446–52.

Scandinavian Simvastatin Survival Study Group (1994). Randomised trial of cholesterol lowering in 4444 patients with coronary heart disease: the Scandinavian Simvastatin Survival Study (4S). *Lancet* **344**: 1383–9.

Shepherd J, Cobbe SM, Ford I *et al* (1995). Prevention of coronary-heart disease with pravastatin in men with hypercholesterolaemia. *N Engl J Med* **333**: 1301–7.

Shepherd J, Blauw GJ, Murphy MB *et al* (2002). Pravastatin in elderly individuals at risk of vascular disease (PROSPER): a randomised controlled trial. *Lancet* **360**: 1623–30.

VA-HIT Trial Study Group (1999). Gemfibrozil for the secondary prevention of coronary heart disease in men with low levels of high-density lipoprotein cholesterol. *N Engl J Med* **341**: 410–18.

Further reading

Berger J, Moller DE (2002). The mechanisms of action of PPARs. *Annu Rev Med* **53**: 409–35.

Borghi C, Prandin MG, Costa FV *et al* (2000). Use of statins and blood pressure control in treated hypertensive patients with hypercholesterolemia. *J Cardiovasc Pharmacol* **35**: 549–555.

Rejnmark L, Buus NH, Vestergaard P *et al* (2002). Statins decrease bone turnover in postmenopausal women: a cross-sectional study. *Eur J Clin Invest* **32**: 581–9.

Online resources

www.bhf.org.uk

The website of the British Heart Foundation, providing patient information (accessed April 2008).

www.rpsgb.org.uk

The website of the Royal Pharmaceutical Society and it has produced guidelines for the OTC use of simvastatin (accessed April 2008).

13

Obesity

Disease characteristics

Disease prevention is high on the political agenda as the burden of disease attributed to unhealthy lifestyles reaches epidemic proportions. With the exception of genetic causes (which are uncommon), obesity simply results from the intake of calories in excess of those required to meet energy demands. Indeed, the excess intake of small amounts of energy (e.g. 100 calories/day) over several years will lead to obesity. However, this apparently simple relationship is not easily modified, making obesity a particularly challenging condition. The complex picture of obesity includes genetics, lack of education, derangements of appetite, immobility, emotional problems, co-morbidity, e.g. hypothyroidism, and drug therapy. Drugs that are associated with weight gain include:

- antipsychotics
- corticosteroids
- hormone replacement therapy
- lithium
- oral contraceptives
- pizotifen
- sodium valproate
- sulphonylureas
- insulin
- glitazones
- tricyclic antidepressants.

In the UK more than half of women and approximately two-thirds of men are overweight or obese and the increased incidence of obesity in children is also of special concern (National Audit Office 2001, 2006). The main health consequences are hypertension and other cardiovascular disease, type 2 diabetes, gallstones and osteoarthritis (Ali 2002a). Indeed, alongside hypertension and hypertriglyceridaemia, obesity forms the so-called metabolic syndrome. Obesity has also been shown to increase the risk of various cancers (e.g. Reeves *et al* 2007) and the World Health Organization (WHO) has highlighted that, after smoking, obesity is the second most important modifiable risk factor for cancer-related mortality.

The health risks associated with obesity are in part related to the endocrine activity of adipose tissue, leading to the secretion of a wide range of physiological and pathological mediators. Elevated glucose levels and adipose-derived mediators lead to reduced insulin sensitivity and this ultimately leads to type 2 diabetes.

Clinical features

In 2006 the National institute for Health and Clinical Excellence (NICE) produced detailed guidance for the management of obesity in adults and children according to body mass index (BMI in kg/m^2), waist circumference and co-morbidities. It is important to note that BMI should not be considered alone due to limitations of only considering weight and height, i.e. the BMI does not take into account body composition and does not assess the body's adiposity. Therefore people with significant muscle mass, such as rugby players, have high BMIs without the associated health risks. It is also important to note that obesity should be thought of as a clinical condition rather than associated with appearance. Classification using BMI and waist measurement is shown in Tables 13.1 and 13.2. In addition, the distribution of fat is an issue, with central (abdominal) fat posing a risk

Table 13.1   Classification of weight using body mass index (BMI)

Classification	BMI (kg/m^2)
Healthy weight	18.5–24.9
Overweight	25–29.9
Obesity I	30–34.9
Obesity II	35–39.9
Obesity III	≥40

Table 13.2   Classification of waist circumference

Waist circumference	Men (cm)	Women (cm)
Low	<94	<80
High	94–102	80–88
Very high	>102	>88

factor for cardiovascular disease and diabetes and a more pelvic distribution or 'pear-shape' being seen as relatively protective.

Goals of treatment

Successful treatment will produce gradual weight reduction resulting in improved health and self-esteem. Weekly weight loss should not usually exceed 0.5–1 kg with the aim for an overall weight reduction of 5–10%. The central goal is a reduction in the risk of obesity-related conditions, especially cardiovascular disease and diabetes, and their associated mortality.

Management

General advice on healthy weight, diet and lifestyle

Treatment ranges from support and advice on increasing physical activity and reducing calorie intake to drug treatment and surgery. Clearly any diet regimen needs to involve reducing calorific intake to below the daily expenditure (the NICE recommend a deficit of 600 calories/day) and

ensuring that it is balanced and benefits from low glycaemic foods and five portions of fruit and vegetables, and is low in fat and alcohol.

There is no convincing evidence that supports the efficacy of fashionable diets over simple calorie restriction, and the main dietary approach should be a calorie-reduced, balanced diet. Fashionable diets may also be associated with nutritional deficits. Examples include liquid-only or 'soup' diets and high-protein, high-fat diets such as the Atkins diet (Mason 2002b).

Additional treatment options include behavioural intervention such as cognitive–behavioural therapy (CBT) and, as a last resort, surgery. The limited availability of CBT means that it is not currently an option for all patients. CBT addresses both cognitive and behavioural aspects of overeating and is therefore important for producing long-term change (Ali 2002b). Patients need structured guidance to identify and change what may be life-long thinking patterns, attitudes and behaviour such as comfort or binge eating.

Patients who are overweight but have a relatively low waist circumference may benefit from general lifestyle advice as outlined in Chapter 3, together with verbal and written information about reaching a healthy weight and the benefits of this, in terms of reducing cardiovascular risk and the risk of developing diabetes.

Physical activity

All adults are encouraged to take regular exercise because this reduces the risk of type 2 diabetes and cardiovascular disease regardless of weight loss. Recommendations include the following:

- At least 30 minutes of moderate activity on at least 5 days a week in sessions not less than 10 minutes each.
- To prevent obesity 45–60 minutes of exercise per day may be required.
- To sustain target weight 60–90 minutes of exercise per day may be required.
- Ideally activities should form part of daily life, e.g. walking or cycling to work, leaving the bus at an earlier stop, climbing stairs, walking, vigorous house work or gardening.

- Reducing periods of inactivity such as watching television and playing computer games.
- Consider the patient's fitness level, current lifestyle and ability, aiming for gradual and manageable change.

Pharmacological management

Drugs are initiated after a period of diet and lifestyle changes when patients have not reached their target weight. Pharmacological targets include centrally mediated appetite regulation or fat absorption from the gastrointestinal tract. Amphetamines and fenfluramine were used in the past but are no longer recommended due to problems such as dependence, psychosis, valvular heart disease and pulmonary hypertension. Drugs in current use are orlistat, sibutramine and rimonabant.

Orlistat

Orlistat irreversibly inhibits pancreatic lipases, thereby reducing fat absorption. A proportion of dietary fat is therefore excreted in faeces. Indeed, the malabsorption of fat leads to steatorrhoea, which is the passing of oily stools and sometimes the loss of bowel control. These adverse effects actually contribute to the actions of orlistat because the patient would tend to avoid food with a high fat content. The malabsorption of fat also leads to reduced absorption of fat-soluble vitamins such as vitamin D, with possible consequences for calcium balance and bone mineralization.

Sibutramine

Originally developed as an antidepressant, sibutramine inhibits the reuptake of serotonin and noradrenaline (norepinephrine). This effect in the hypothalamus results in reduced food intake. In addition, sympathetic activity maintains the basal metabolic rate, due to effects on thermogenesis, and this would usually be reduced after weight loss (Ali 2002c). However, increases in blood pressure and heart rate contraindicate the use of sibutramine in patients with cardiovascular disease.

Rimonabant

Rimonabant is a cannabinoid CB_1-receptor antagonist that opposes the central actions of endogenous cannabinoids involved in the control of appetite. Recent interest has focused on its use in patients with concurrent diabetes where, in addition to weight loss, it appears to cause an improvement in some metabolic indices, such as decreased triglycerides and an increase in high-density lipoprotein (HDL) (Scheen *et al* 2006). The antagonism of cannabinoid receptors has been anticipated to block many of their physiological roles and this has led to rimonabant being associated with depression and mood changes, which are more pronounced when used at higher doses than recommended.

Drug choice

The NICE (2006) guidelines indicate that drug treatment should be initiated after a period of lifestyle and dietary change, for patients who have not reached their target weight. It should be stressed that lifestyle and dietary changes should be continued alongside drug treatment. The choice of drugs is essentially governed by their adverse effect profile, with sibutramine being avoided in uncontrolled hypertension or following an increase in blood pressure on starting treatment, and rimonabant being avoided in patients with depression. Dyslipidaemia or type 2 diabetes is a compelling reason to choose rimonabant.

Orlistat

Orlistat is recommended for patients with a BMI $\geq$28.0 kg/m^2 with co-morbidities or BMI $\geq$30 kg/m^2. With the exception of patients with type 2 diabetes, treatment is restricted to 3 months if the patient has lost <5% of their initial weight since starting the drug.

Sibutramine

Sibutramine is used for patients with BMI $\geq$27.0 kg/m^2 with co-morbidities or BMI $\geq$30 kg/m^2. Co-prescribing of drugs for obesity is not recommended. Treatment is licensed only for 12

Table 13.3   Prescribing considerations when concurrent conditions are present

Condition	Effects on drug choice	Comments
Cardiovascular disease	Sibutramine contraindicated	
Cerebrovascular disease or uncontrolled hypertension		
History of major eating disorders or psychiatric illness		
Hyperthyroidism		
Prostatic hypertrophy		
History of drug or alcohol abuse		
Chronic malabsorption syndrome	Orlistat contraindicated	
Cholestasis		
Contraception required	Combined oral contraception used with caution if BMI >30 kg/m² and contraindicated for BMI >39 kg/m²	
Pregnancy	Antiobesity drugs are contraindicated	
Depression	SSRIs may be preferred because these drugs are often associated with weight loss	Consider rimonabant as a cause. This is contraindicated in depression and should be stopped if depression occurs
Diabetes	Metformin is preferred because it is not associated with weight gain	Orlistat is used with caution. Rimonabant may be preferred due to its apparent metabolic benefits
Osteoporosis	Multivitamin may be co-prescribed with orlistat	Consider risk of deficiency of fat-soluble vitamins particularly in patients with additional risk factors for osteoporosis
Schizophrenia	Antipsychotics are associated with weight gain and therefore risk vs benefit should be considered in obesity	Lifestyle advise should be given as appropriate when antipsychotics are prescribed

BMI, body mass index.

months and continued after 3 months only as described for orlistat.

Rimonabant

Use is limited to 2 years for patients with a BMI ≥ 30 kg/m² or ≥ 27 kg/m² when additional risk factors such as type 2 diabetes or dyslipidaemia are present.

Despite the availability of anti-obesity drugs, a recent meta-analysis has concluded that weight loss above placebo for these three agents was relatively modest (2.9–4.7 kg) and that drug choice should be determined by cardiovascular profile and their adverse effect profiles (Rucker *et al* 2007).

Concurrent illnesses

Prescribing for patients with obesity will take into account weight gain as a possible adverse effect, once diseases such as hypothyroidism have been excluded. Additional risks associated with excess weight such as type 2 diabetes, hypertension and hyperlipidaemia will also be explored, necessitating the introduction of treatment such as antihypertensives, or the exclusion of drugs such as sibutramine due to adverse cardiovascular effects (Table 13.3).

Monitoring

Sibutramine

- Blood pressure and pulse should be checked every 2 weeks for the first 3 months, then every month for 3 months and then a minimum of every 3 months.
- Treatment is discontinued if blood pressure >145/90 mmHg or systolic or diastolic pressure is increased by >10 mmHg or pulse is increased by 10 beats/min at two consultations.
- Use with caution in mild-to-moderate renal impairment.

Drug interactions (Table 13.4)

Drug interactions involving drugs used to treat obesity often occur due to reduced absorption, as might be expected with orlistat, and additive pharmacology in the case of rimonabant and sibutramine. Rimonabant is metabolized by the cytochrome P450 isoenzyme CYP3A4 and therefore also exhibits metabolic interactions with drugs that alter the activity of this isoenzyme.

Over-the-counter considerations

It is anticipated that orlistat will soon be available over-the-counter and pharmacists should be vigilant to its use as a substitute to healthy eating or lifestyle. In the meantime, pharmacists should be alert for the misuse of laxatives and herbal preparations, and patients referred to their GP or local slimming club as appropriate. Herbal preparations for weight loss may contain compounds associated with laxative, diuretic or metabolic effects such as increasing thyroid function. St

John's wort has also been used due to increased serotoninergic effects but evidence is lacking for its efficacy (Mason 2002a). Similarly, food supplements such as L-carnitine, chitosan and lecithin are also available but there is no convincing evidence to support their usage (Mason 2002a).

General counselling

The health benefits of losing weight should be emphasized. These include increased mobility and therefore improvement in arthritis, a greater feeling of wellbeing and reduced risk of diseases such as coronary heart disease, type 2 diabetes and some cancers. Advice should be practical and easily incorporated into people's lives, e.g. simple changes can include walking to school or the shops, taking the stairs rather than the lift. Recommended changes should be tailored to individual patients and include the following.

Weight

Ideal weight and waist measurement should be calculated and a realistic target of weight loss given. Weight loss should be no more than 0.5–1 kg/week.

Diet

Modifications to the diet need to be manageable. The recommendations for a healthy, balanced diet are given in Chapter 3.

Exercise

Exercise that is appropriate to the patient's current level of fitness and health should be recommended and preferably something that the person enjoys. The advice of the patient's GP should be sought in the presence of concurrent morbidity such as heart disease, diabetes and arthritis. Patients, including children, should be advised to reduce the time spent watching the television and playing computer games.

Table 13.4   Examples of drug interactions involving drugs used to treat obesity

Interacting drugs	Consequences	Comments
Orlistat with:		
Acarbose	Unknown	Manufacturers recommend avoidance of concurrent use
Other antidiabetics, e.g. glipizide, metformin, insulin	Glycaemic control may improve	Blood glucose levels should be monitored and doses of antidiabetic drugs reduced as appropriate
Ciclosporin	Absorption reduced significantly, possibly >50%	Closer monitoring is required and the dose of ciclosporin adjusted as appropriate
Contraceptives	Possible contraceptive failure has been reported	Additional contraception is recommended during severe diarrhoea
Warfarin	Possible increased INR	INR should be monitored closely for the first 4 weeks
Vitamins	Reduced absorption	Multivitamins should be taken at least 2 hours after orlistat or at bedtime
Sibutramine with:		
Antidepressants (SSRIs, MAOIs)	Risk of serotonin syndrome due to further inhibition of serotonin uptake	Avoid combination
Dextromethorphan Lithium Opioids	Risk of serotonin syndrome	Contraindicated
Rimonabant with:		
Ketoconazole and possibly other CYP3A4 inhibitors, e.g. clarithromycin, itraconazole	Increased plasma levels of rimonabant	Monitor for adverse effects CYP3A4 inducers may reduce effect of rimonabant, e.g. carbamazepine, phenytoin
Antidepressants	See above	Contraindicated

INR, international normalized ratio; MAOI, monoamine oxidase A inhibitor; SSRI, selective serotonin reuptake inhibitor.

Children

The NICE (2006) guidelines recommend that clinical judgement be used do decide when it is necessary to measure the weight and height of children and that BMI charts are referred to. Routine waist measurement is not recommended. Physical activity should include at least 60 min of moderate exercise daily or several shorter sessions of at least 10 min each. It is useful for pharmacists to liaise with health visitors about local guidelines for dealing with excessive weight gain in children. The NICE guidance does not advocate the use of drug treatments unless there are compelling reasons such as co-morbidities.

Action points

NICE (2006) has produced guidelines which include:

- setting healthy target weight, with the aim of loosing approximately 5–10% of initial weight
- a maximum weight loss of 0.5–1 kg/week
- emphasis on long-term lifestyle changes
- using a variety of approaches to improve **both** diet and exercise

- recommending a healthy balanced diet
- the provision of safe and realistic advice on increasing activity
- addressing techniques for changing behaviour such as encouraging patients to keep a diary and developing strategies to deal with regression to old habits
- patients should be given access to continued support.

Specific counselling points

Orlistat

- Should be taken in addition to long-term dietary and lifestyle changes.
- Take immediately before, during or up to one hour after each main meal (max. 360 mg/day).
- Dose should not be taken if a meal is missed or does not contain fat.
- Multivitamins should be taken at least 2 hours after orlistat or at bedtime.
- May cause liquid or oily stools and reducing fat intake should lessen these side effects.
- It should be used regularly, rather than avoided after fatty meals. Some patients might omit a dose after a fatty meal to avoid the unpleasant side effects of fatty stools and this undermines the purpose of the drug treatment (Ali 2002c).
- Other common side effects include respiratory tract infection, headache, gum problems and irregular periods.

Sibutramine

- Dose should be taken in the morning.
- Do not take for longer than 12 months.
- Most side effects occur during the first 4 weeks of treatment and improve as treatment continues. These include dry mouth, nausea, constipation, insomnia and palpitations.
- Blood pressure may increase and this should be checked regularly.
- Avoid OTC decongestants that may also increase blood pressure. Also mention any use of NSAIDs that may also increase blood pressure.

Rimonabant

- Do not take for longer than 2 years.
- Weight is known to increase when treatment is stopped so it is important to continue lifestyle changes.
- Contact GP if suffer changes in mood or other signs of depression.
- Other common side effects include nausea, upper respiratory tract infections, anxiety and dizziness.

Future drug treatment

Drug development is currently targeting neuroendocrine molecules such as cholecystokinin involved in the production of satiety. Central nervous system targets include the neurotransmitters NPY (neuropeptide Y) and melanocortins. Melanocortin MC4 receptor agonists are also being investigated but have problematic side effects such as penile erection (Adan *et al* 2006).

Self-assessment

Consider whether the following statements are true or false:

1. Rimonabant is a cannabinoid receptor agonist used to treat obesity.
2. Antipsychotics should not be given to obese patients because they cause weight gain.
3. The INR may increase in patients taking warfarin when orlistat is introduced.
4. Sibutramine may increase blood pressure.
5. Tricyclics are the preferred option for treating depression in obese patients.

Practice points

- Be alert for weight gain as an adverse drug reaction and counsel patients as appropriate. The balance of risks versus benefits of treatment should be considered carefully.
- Sign posting to local slimming clubs may help patients find the support that they need to lose weight. Check that these clubs meet best-practice standards set out by NICE.
- Consider setting up an obesity clinic, which could possibly target certain groups more likely to gain excess weight such as ante- and postnatal women, people attempting to stop smoking or menopausal women (Ali 2002d).
- Obesity should be thought of as a clinical condition rather than associated with appearance.
- Emphasize that exercise produces health benefits even in the absence of weight loss. This may prevent patients from giving up exercise if they are not losing weight.
- Display leaflets and posters supporting health campaigns. These are available from organizations such as the Food Standards Agency and the British Heart Foundation.

 CASE STUDY

A 60-year old woman who is visibly obese is having concerns about her health since turning 60. Her GP advised her to lose weight and increase physical activity but she has not reached her target weight and is finding it difficult to exercise due to painful knees. She refuses to be weighed or to allow measurement of her waist circumference. She has a family history of cardiovascular disease, has worked in a smoky environment for many years and had an early menopause. She is currently taking:

atenolol 50 mg (every morning)
indapamide 2.5 mg (every morning)
atorvastatin 40 mg (once daily)
glucosamine with chondroitin for painful knees.

What risk factors does this patient have?

- Diabetes due to obesity and combined use of β blocker with thiazide diuretic.
- Osteoporosis due to early menopause.
- Cardiovascular disease due to obesity, hyperlipidaemia, passive smoking, family history and early menopause.

What changes to treatment might her GP consider?

- ACE inhibitor: this would be appropriate, especially in view of her risk of diabetes.
- Stopping the β blocker. Since 2006, β blockers are no longer recommended for the management of hypertension and, if an ACE inhibitor alone is ineffective at controlling blood pressure, the A/CD rules would suggest that a calcium channel blocker be used.
- Orlistat: her history of hypertension might favour the use of orlistat over sibutramine.
- Vitamin D supplement if orlistat is prescribed.

continued

CASE STUDY (continued)

Her treatment is changed to:

enalapril 5 mg (once daily)
amlodipine 10 mg (daily)
simvastatin 40 mg (every night)
orlistat 120 mg (three times daily)
glucosamine with chondroitin.

How would you counsel the patient regarding her new prescription for orlistat?
Drug-specific counselling for orlistat should focus on its role alongside a healthy balanced diet and the avoidance of fat. Indeed, consumption of fat will lead to oily stools. The tablets should be taken during or just after a meal. Provide advice on exercise that the patient could try such as swimming, and reinforce healthy eating information. It may help to motivate the patient to lose weight knowing that weight loss may help her painful knees. The patient is likely to be particularly receptive to advice given her health concerns since turning 60. Local slimming clubs could also be recommended so long as these incorporate NICE 2006 best-practice criteria

References

Adan RAH, Tiesjema B, Hillebrand JJG *et al* (2006). The MC4 receptor and control of appetite. *Br J Pharmacol* **149**, 815–27.

Ali O (2002a). Get to grips with obesity: (1) Incidence and associated risks. *Pharm J* **268**: 616–18.

Ali O (2002b). Get to grips with obesity: (2) Non-drug strategies. *Pharm J* **268**: 652–4.

Ali O (2002c). Get to grips with obesity: (3) Pharmacotherapy. *Pharm J* **268**: 687–9.

Ali O (2002d). Get to grips with obesity: (4) How pharmacists can contribute to obesity management. *Pharm J* **268**: 720–2.

Mason (2002a). Slimming. (1) OTC weight control products. *Pharm J* **269**:103–5.

Mason (2002b). Slimming. (2) Popular slimming diets. *Pharm J* **269**: 135–7.

National Audit Office (2001). *Tackling Obesity in England*. London: NAO.

National Audit Office (2006). *Tackling Child Obesity, First Steps*. London: NAO.

National Institute for Health and Clinical Excellence (2006). *Obesity*. Clinical Guideline 43. London: NICE.

Reeves GK, Pirie K, Beral V *et al* (2007). Cancer incidence and mortality in relation to body mass index in the Million Women Study: cohort study. *BMJ* **335**:1134–8.

Rucker D, Padwal R, Li SK *et al* (2007). Long term pharmacotherapy for obesity and overweight: updated meta-analysis. *BMJ* **335**: 1194–9.

Scheen AJ, Hollander P, Jensen MD *et al* (2006). Efficacy and tolerability of rimonabant in overweight or obese patients with type 2 diabetes: randomised controlled trial. *Lancet* **368**: 1660–72.

Online resources

www.rpsgb.org/pdfs/obesityguid.pdf
The RPSGB provide a document for pharmacists on the management of obesity (accessed 27 January 2008).

www.nationalobesityforum.org.uk
The website of the National Obesity Forum, providing

professional and patient information (accessed 27 January 2008).

www.weightconcern.org.uk
The website of the charity Weight Concern which contains patient, self-help information (accessed 27 January 2008).

14

Ischaemic heart disease

Disease characteristics

Ischaemic heart disease (IHD), which is also referred to as coronary artery disease (CAD) or coronary heart disease (CHD), is the biggest killer in the western world and so represents a crucial area for both prevention and treatment. IHD may manifest as either angina or myocardial infarction (MI) and is an important cause of chronic heart failure (see Chapter 15). In both cases, IHD is generally associated with atherosclerosis within the coronary artery, leading to impaired blood flow or thromboembolic occlusion. In angina the reductions in coronary blood flow mean that perfusion does not match demand, leading to ischaemia, which provokes the symptoms. In MI, there is often thromboembolic occlusion of the coronary artery, which may lead to acute left ventricular failure and/or arrhythmias; these are the leading cause of early mortality.

Risk factors for IHD include:

- male gender
- family history
- smoking*
- diabetes mellitus*
- hypercholesterolaemia*
- hypertension*
- sedentary lifestyle*
- obesity*.

*Modifiable.

Angina pectoris

Angina may be divided into two groups: stable and unstable. Stable angina reflects athero-sclerotic disease, which limits the heart's ability to respond to increased demand and is characterized by symptoms that appear on exertion but are relieved by rest. By contrast, unstable angina is generally due to plaque rupture and the formation of a non-occlusive thromboembolism, or, less commonly, vasospasm (Prinzmetal's angina), both of which give rise to symptoms at rest.

The characteristic feature of angina is a crushing chest pain, which may radiate to the arm and jaw. Of course, chest pain may reflect a number of other causes (see Chapter 1):

- MI
- dyspepsia
- musculoskeletal pain
- pulmonary embolism.

A diagnosis may be made on the basis of history and, in the case of stable angina, its provocation by exercise or eating a meal. The pain should be relieved by glyceryl trinitrate (GTN) and in stable angina is relieved by rest. An electrocardiogram (ECG) during an attack would confirm a diagnosis by showing ST-segment depression. Angina may also be secondary to increased cardiac work in anaemia (see Chapter 17) and hyperthyroidism (see Chapter 36), which should be excluded.

Goals of treatment of angina

Angina is a manifestation of IHD and the principal goal of treatment is the reduction of cardiovascular risk. In relation to the management of angina the specific goals are to:

- reduce symptoms
- improve exercise capacity

- reduce the risk of a heart attack
- stabilize or bring about regression of atherosclerotic lesions.

Management of angina

In the first instance, attention should be paid to reducing cardiovascular risk by smoking cessation, weight loss and dietary changes (see Chapters 3, 11 and 12). Treatment options include percutaneous transluminal coronary angioplasty (PTCA) to open the occlusion and may include placing a stent. This often produces relief but is associated with a high rate of restenosis (reocclusion) because the resulting physical damage promotes proliferation of vascular smooth muscle. Recent advances have included the fitting of stents, which are essentially 'cages' that may be inserted at the diseased area to hold the vessel open and prevent restenosis. In some cases the stents are impregnated with drugs to suppress the growth of blood vessels locally. Alternatively, coronary artery bypass grafting (CABG) is a surgical option in which the diseased artery is bypassed by a saphenous vein or internal mammary artery. CABG has been proved to offer longer-term relief of symptoms but is associated with a degree of operative mortality.

Pharmacological basis of the management of angina

Drug treatment is aimed at reducing cardiac work or improving coronary blood flow. The first group of agents to consider is the nitrates.

Nitrates: GTN, isosorbide mononitrate

Nitrates cause vasodilatation via the release of nitric oxide (NO), which gives rise to an increase in guanosine cyclic 3':5'-monophosphate (cGMP). In the context of angina, their beneficial effect is largely via venodilatation, leading to a decrease in preload and a reduction in cardiac work, although they may also cause coronary vasodilatation to improve coronary flow.

GTN is widely used for rapid symptomatic relief of an attack or may be given before exercise, which may provoke an attack. GTN may be given by a spray under the tongue or as a sublingual tablet. Isosorbide mononitrate tablets may be given orally with the aim of giving longer-term nitrate treatment.

β Blockers

These are dealt with in detail in Chapter 11. In the context of angina they should be considered as first-choice drugs for prevention, with their negative inotropic and chronotropic effects reducing cardiac work and preventing symptoms. As coronary flow occurs only during diastole, then by slowing the heart the diastolic period will be increased, as will the time for coronary blood flow. They also have anti-arrhythmic effects and reduce the risk of MI.

Calcium channel blockers, e.g. amlodipine, diltiazem, felodipine, nifedipine, verapamil

Once again, these are dealt with in detail in Chapter 11. The calcium channel blockers give rise to vasodilatation and improve coronary blood flow, so preventing symptoms. In addition, verapamil, and to a lesser extent diltiazem, also have myocardial-depressant and bradycardic actions, so reducing cardiac work. Verapamil also exerts class IV antiarrhythmic activity.

Angiotensin-converting enzyme inhibitors

Angiotensin-converting enzyme (ACE) inhibitors are dealt with in detail in Chapters 11 and 15. In addition, the Heart Outcome Prevention Evaluation (HOPE) trial (Yusuf et al 2000) indicated that ramipril reduced mortality in patients with IHD and it may therefore be worth considering the addition of ramipril (or presumably any ACE inhibitor) to treatment of a patient with IHD.

Potassium channel activators: nicorandil

Nicorandil is a recent addition and is a combined NO donor and activator of adenosine triphosphate (ATP)-sensitive K^+ channels. The release of

NO leads to an elevation in cGMP levels and the independent activation of ATP-sensitive K+ channels leads to vascular smooth-muscle hyperpolarization with coronary artery vasodilatation and improved coronary flow. The vasodilator actions of nicorandil contribute towards its side effects of flushing and reflex tachycardia.

Ivabradine

This agent was approved for use in 2005 and inhibits pacemaker sodium and potassium currents in the sinoatrial node of the heart. This leads to bradycardia and reduces the work of the heart, which is of benefit in angina. Although its place in therapy has yet to be established, the INITIATIVE trial (INITIATIVE Investigators 2005) indicated that it was equally effective as atenolol but without the side effects associated with β blockers.

Choice of drugs (Figure 14.1)

All patients with angina are at a high risk of having an MI and so all patients should be considered for antiplatelet treatment with low-dose aspirin or, if they are intolerant to aspirin, clopidogrel. Low-dose aspirin is now well established as playing a major role in the primary and secondary prevention of MI. Aspirin inhibits irreversibly both platelet and endothelial cyclooxygenases (COXs). The endothelial cells may regenerate COX but the platelets lack nuclei and cannot, so endothelial production of prostacyclin may be resumed shortly afterwards, although the production of thromboxane is impaired until a new cohort of platelets are produced. This leads to a state that opposes platelet aggregation. Other non-steroidal anti-inflammatory drugs (NSAIDs) may cause reversible inhibition of COX, leading to transient antiplatelet actions, so they are not suitable for primary or secondary prevention. A small-scale study has in fact suggested that ibuprofen administered before aspirin may inhibit the actions of aspirin, presumably by protecting COX against aspirin (Catella-Lawson *et al* 2001).

Clopidogrel is an equally effective alternative antiplatelet drug for patients intolerant of aspirin.

Clopidogrel inhibits adenosine diphosphate (ADP)-induced expression of platelet glycoprotein IIb/IIIa, which is involved in aggregation by cross-linking fibrin.

A significant proportion (around a quarter) of patients are now recognized as being resistant to the protective effects of low-dose aspirin and do not derive benefit from this treatment. This resistance is apparently independent of its action at COX and it appears that patients do not benefit from other antiplatelet drugs. To confound the matter, this cohort of patients is also at a greater risk of cardiovascular events compared with aspirin-sensitive patients (Krasopoulos *et al* 2008).

Attention should be paid to controlling blood pressure (to obtain a target of 140/85 mmHg; see Chapter 11) and managing hypercholesterolaemia (see Chapter 12).

For symptomatic relief or occasional treatment, a GTN spray or sublingual tablets would be appropriate. In terms of continuous, the following are the preventive treatments:

- First choice: β blockers should be used for more pronounced stable and unstable angina (but not Prinzmetal's angina). Oral long-acting nitrates may be added.
- Second choice: if a β blocker is ineffective or contraindicated, then verapamil (or diltiazem) would be used or, failing that, a long-acting dihydropyridine. Calcium channel blockers are particularity effective at reversing vasospasm and are first choice drugs for Prinzmetal's angina.
- In refractory disease: a β blocker may be used with dihydropyridine calcium channel blockers *but not with verapamil* because there is a severe risk of asystole; diltiazem and β blockers may be used with caution. Nicorandil may also be added to therapy. If two agents fail to control the disease then surgical treatment may be required.

Although the role of nicorandil in therapy has been uncertain, the large-scale Impact Of Nicorandil in Angina (IONA) clinical trial (IONA Study Group 2002) has found that in stable angina nicorandil, in addition to standard therapy, reduced the incidence of cardiovascular events. This indicated that nicorandil afforded

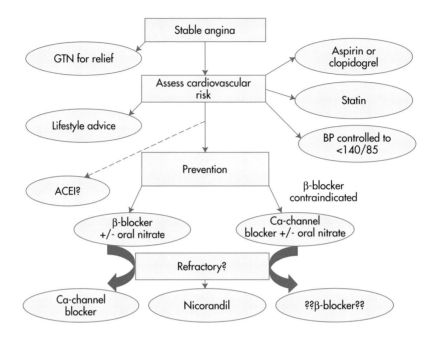

Figure 14.1 A scheme indicating a typical approach to the management of ischaemic heart disease. It should be re-emphasized that, if a β blocker is combined with a calcium channel blocker, this is usually safe with dihydropyridines, but rate-limiting agents such as verapamil and diltiazem pose a serious risk of asystole and should be avoided. ACEI, angiotensin-converting enzyme inhibitor; GTN, glyceryl trinitrate.

cardioprotection and it was proposed that by activating cardiac mitochondrial K_{ATP} channels it was able to mimic ischaemic cardiac preconditioning, the natural phenomenon whereby short periods of ischaemia protect the heart. This points to nicorandil as being of particular benefit in IHD.

Some compelling indications and contraindications are indicated in Table 14.1. In addition, patients with unstable angina are likely to be maintained on a low-molecular-weight heparin.

Drug interactions

Within antianginal drugs, the major within-group interaction is between β blockers and verapamil, because in combination they may cause asystole. All of the agents, by acting as vasodilators, may lead to hypotension, with the possibility of a fall in elderly people.

General counselling

Counselling should be directed towards a reduction in cardiovascular risk, with smoking cessation, weight reduction, increased exercise, reduced alcohol intake and dietary changes, to reduce the intake of saturated fats and increase oily fish in the diet or supplementation with fish oils. When explaining the disease to patients, one approach might be to tell them that their heart muscle is not getting enough blood to do the job that it used to do, and that the pains that they experience are similar to muscle cramp.

Nitrates

- GTN sprays or sublingual tablets should be used before an event likely to provoke an attack.
- The patient should be counselled on how to use a GTN spray and supervised in its use.

Table 14.1   Other considerations in the choice of antianginal agents

Condition	Drug choice	Comments
Heart failure	β Blocker can be used with caution (Chapter 15) Verapamil is contraindicated	
Arrhythmias	May be a reason to use a β blocker or verapamil	Both agents are antiarrhythmic
Chronic obstructive pulmonary disease (COPD) and asthma	Contraindication for β blockers in asthma and caution in COPD	β Blockers may lead to bronchospasm
Migraine	β Blocker	β Blockers are effective in migraine prophylaxis
Diabetes mellitus	May be a reason to avoid β blockers	β Blockers may reduce the warning signs of hypoglycaemia
Hyperthyroidism	An indication for a β blocker	For reduction of cardiac effects in hyperthyroidism
Glaucoma	Closed-angle glaucoma is a contraindication for nitrates Chronic simple glaucoma is an indication for a β blocker	In glaucoma, β-blocker eye drops are absorbed and should not be used in addition to an oral β blocker

- GTN sprays or sublingual tablets may cause pronounced hypotension and are best taken while sitting.
- If a patient feels faint after GTN tablets the tablet should be spat out or swallowed; the patient could also bend over and place the head between the knees.
- GTN tablets have a short shelf-life of 8 weeks once opened and should be discarded after this time.
- When taking isosorbide mononitrate or dinitrate, there is a substantial risk of nitrate tolerance. This may be reduced by having a nitrate-free period, usually at night when symptoms are less. Patients may be advised to take their twice-daily nitrate tablets 8 h apart, at say 8am and 4pm, to give a nitrate-free period. GTN patches should also be removed for several hours each day, perhaps at night.
- If GTN does not relieve an episode of chest pain, medical help should be sought immediately.
- Drugs that cause a dry mouth may reduce the effects of sublingual GTN.

β Blockers

- See Chapter 11.
- Great emphasis should be made to ensure that patients do not stop taking the β blocker suddenly, because this is likely to lead to a worsening of symptoms and may increase their chances of having an MI.

Calcium channel blockers

See Chapter 11.

Nicorandil

- Nicorandil may affect driving or operating machinery.
- Side effects are related to vasodilatation and may include headache.

Myocardial infarction

MI is often due to the formation of a thrombus at the site of rupture of an atherosclerotic plaque, leading to cardiac ischaemia and damage, with early deaths resulting from arrhythmias and late deaths from damage to the myocardium, which may cause heart failure. The necrotic muscle may rupture, leading to rupture of the ventricles (giving rise to tamponade) or pulmonary oedema if papillary muscles rupture and there is severe mitral regurgitation. Rupture of the septum leads to shunting, which requires surgery.

In full-thickness infarctions, the infarct may undergo thinning and stretch, causing ventricular dilatation and hypertrophy, which may lead to the development of heart failure at a later date.

Symptoms of MI

- Prolonged cardiac pain – chest, throat, arms, epigastrum or back.
- Breathlessness.
- Collapse.
- Anxiety.
- Nausea/vomiting.

Signs of MI

- Pallor/sweating/tachycardia (due to sympathetic activation).
- Vomiting/bradycardia (vagal).
- Signs of impaired cardiac function.
- Hypotension, oliguria, cold extremities.
- Weak pulse.
- Lung crepitations.
- Some (especially elderly) patients have a 'silent MI' with no signs or symptoms.

Differential diagnosis

- Dyspepsia.
- Angina (which is relieved by GTN).
- Musculoskeletal pains.
- Panic attacks.
- Pulmonary embolism.

Diagnosis

The diagnosis is based on ECG changes (including ST-segment elevation) and increases in cardiac enzymes released by infarcted tissue. These are creatine kinase (CK), troponin T (TrT), aspartate aminotransferase (AST) and lactate dehydrogenase (LDH).

Management

The initial management of MI is beyond the scope of this book. However, a brief summary is given in Table 14.2.

For patients who survive the initial MI the outlook can be good, with on average 80% being alive after 1 year, although the outlook is influenced by the initial presentation and development of heart failure. Therefore, in primary care the central issues are secondary prevention and prevention of long-term complications such as heart failure. All patients should be counselled with respect to lifestyle changes:

- weight reduction
- dietary advice, including increased intake of oily fish
- smoking cessation
- appropriate exercise.

Secondary prevention

In terms of drug treatment for secondary prevention in patients who have already had an MI there are a number of considerations and the following takes account of the National Institute for Health and Clinical Excellence (NICE) guidelines issued in 2007:

- Antiplatelet therapy with low-dose aspirin (75–150 mg) is established as substantially reducing reinfarction. In patients who are intolerant of aspirin due to asthma, clopidogrel is indicated, and it is equally effective. Low-dose aspirin is associated with gastric damage, and prophylaxis with a proton pump inhibitor may be required (see Chapter 7). The addition of aspirin and clopidogrel can result in additive protective effects and they may be used in combination.
- β Blockade: all patients should be considered for a β blocker to limit cardiac work and reduce the risk of rupture, to manage stable

Table 14.2   Management of a myocardial infarction

Treatment	Comments
Immediate	
Soluble or chewable aspirin (150–300 mg)	This may be given as a first-aid measure as an antiplatelet treatment to reduce further thrombus formation
Oxygen	To reduce hypoxia
Nitrates	To reduce ischaemia, but they have no bearing on mortality
IV morphine or diamorphine with antiemetics (cyclizine (but only if left ventricular function is satisfactory), prochlorperazine or metoclopramide)	• Morphine for relief of dyspnoea; also causes venodilatation to reduce preload and induces a degree of calm • An antiemetic to reduce nausea associated with opioids
Thrombolytic agent (e.g. alteplase, streptokinase, reteplase)	• Should be given to dissolve the clot as soon as possible (ideally within 90 min) and certainly within the first 12 h, unless contraindicated (including recent surgery, peptic ulceration, current menstruation, pregnancy, recent stroke, history of haemorrhagic stroke) • Streptokinase can be given up to 4 days after an initial dose, but thereafter it should not be given for at least 12 months, if at all • Streptokinase may be ineffective in patients who have recently had a streptococcal sore throat, due to the production of antibodies • Streptokinase may cause an allergic reaction • Certain thrombolytic agents are now licensed for use before admission
Subsequent use of acute treatments	
ß Blocker	• IV atenolol or metoprolol given early reduces arrhythmias and improves survival • Improves myocardial perfusion and reduces infarct size • Reduces chance of cardiac rupture • If β blockade is contraindicated and in the absence of heart failure then verapamil might be used
ACE inhibitors	The European Society of Cardiology recommends the use of an ACE inhibitor within the first 24 h if there is evidence of heart failure emerging
Anticoagulants	Heparin given for 7–10 days post-MI after thrombolysis may prevent reinfarction
Nitrates	If systolic blood pressure >100 mmHg they may be given in the first 24 h to reduce cardiac work
Antiarrhythmics	• Despite arrhythmias complicating post-MI, antiarrhythmics may increase mortality • Antiarrhythmics may be proarrhythmic on the ischaemic myocardium • β Blockade is likely to have been initiated • Lidocaine is indicated for ventricular ectopics but is less widely used now
Insulin	Patients with diabetes often receive intensive insulin therapy from admission for 3 months because this reduces mortality

IV, intravenous; ACE, angiotensin-converting enzyme.

angina and hypertension and as an anti-arrhythmic. β Blockers are contraindicated in bradyarrhythmias. Long-term β blockade is well established at reducing reinfarction. If the patient has heart failure, the β blocker may be introduced (after an ACE inhibitor) at a low dose and under expert supervision, and would be contraindicated in severe heart failure.

- ACE inhibitors: all patients with heart failure should receive an ACE inhibitor. NICE guidelines point to an ACE inhibitor also being considered for patients without heart failure after they have been considered for a β blocker.
- Calcium channel blockers: these should be considered only for patients who are intolerant of β blockers or ACE inhibitors and for the relief of angina and/or hypertension, because there is no evidence that they reduce mortality. Diltiazem or verapamil should be used with caution because of their cardiodepressant actions.
- Statins: these should be considered for all patients. Currently plasma cholesterol should be measured within 24 h of the MI because it is believed that cholesterol falls for the first 3 months afterwards. Statins are believed to be equally effective to β blockers and antiplatelet drugs in secondary prevention.

- Diuretics: patients with symptomatic heart failure benefit from loop diuretics or thiazides. Patients in moderate-to-severe failure benefit from the addition of spironolactone.
- Antiarrhythmics: there is no evidence that long-term treatment with these agents confers any benefit in the patient post-MI, but they may be needed in some patients.
- Anticoagulants: these drugs do not appear to have a long-term role in most patients and do not appear to confer any additional benefit to aspirin, except in patients with atrial fibrillation. Fiore et al (2002) have reported that the addition of warfarin to low-dose aspirin does not confer further benefit in the secondary prevention of MI. NICE guidance suggests that moderate intensity warfarin therapy is appropriate for patients who cannot receive antiplatelet drugs.

Additional considerations

There is a high incidence of depression after an MI. In terms of drug treatment this may present a question of drug choice because tricyclic antidepressants have been associated with increased mortality in patients post-MI, especially if class I antiarrhythmics are also used. Currently,

Table 14.3   Examples of conditions that may be affected by a previous myocardial infarction

Condition	Problems	Comments
Migraine	• $5HT_{1D}$-receptor agonists (triptans) are contraindicated in patients with IHD • Ergotamine is contraindicated in IHD	The triptans may cause coronary artery spasm (Chapter 22)
Nicotine addiction	Nicotine replacement products should be avoided immediately post-MI	
Depression	Tricyclic antidepressants are contraindicated after recent MI and used with caution in cardiac disease	SSRIs appear to be more appropriate (Chapter 24)
Hypothyroidism	Levothyroxine	May cause anginal symptoms; monitor and reduce dosage in IHD (Chapter 36)
Impotence	Sildenafil	Risk of severe interactions with nitrates, as sildenafil inhibits phosphodiesterases and prevents the breakdown of cGMP. It is contraindicated after recent MI.

5HT, 5-hydroxytryptamine (serotonin); cGMP, guanosine cyclic 3′:5′-monophosphate; IHD, ischaemic heart disease; MI, myocardial infarction; SSRIS, selective serotonin reuptake inhibitors.

selective serotonin reuptake inhibitors (SSRIs, particularly sertraline) are considered more suitable.

A history of IHD may affect other treatments, which are detailed in Table 14.3.

Specific counselling

All of the counselling for specific drugs or classes is detailed in other sections:

- β blockers (see Chapters 11 and 15)
- ACE inhibitors (see Chapters 11 and 15)
- statins (see Chapter 12)

The only additional consideration is to advise patients who have received streptokinase to carry a card to alert medical staff who may treat them at a subsequent MI that they have previously received this agent.

Self-assessment

Consider whether the following statements are true or false:

1. In ischaemic heart disease stable angina is best managed by atenolol and verapamil.
2. In stable angina glyceryl trinitrate spray should provide rapid relief of symptoms.
3. In stable angina warfarin is the drug of choice to prevent thrombosis.
4. After a heart attack thrombolytic drugs are used to promote reperfusion.
5. After a heart attack, patients are routinely discharged from hospital on an ACE inhibitor, a β blocker, a statin and low-dose aspirin.

Practice points

- NICE guidance should be consulted for secondary prevention.
- For secondary prevention after an MI, patients are often prescribed a β blocker, an ACE inhibitor, a statin and an antiplatelet drug.

 CASE STUDY

Mr PS (56 years) has recently suffered an MI and is on a cardiac ward. He was initially treated with streptokinase (1.5 million units i.v.), diamorphine (5 mg i.v.), cyclizine (50 mg i.v.) and atenolol (10 mg i.v.; then 50 mg twice daily for 2 days). On discharge he is now written up for:

aspirin 75 mg daily
atenolol 50 mg daily.

1. Explain the use of all of the above drugs:
    - streptokinase – to destroy the clot, leading to reperfusion
    - diamorphine – pain relief (pain can be severe in MI), and may induce some euphoria
    - cyclizine – H$_1$-receptor antagonist used as an antiemetic to prevent diamorphine-induced emesis
    - atenolol – an antiarrhythmic: reduces infarct size and cardiac work (risk of cardiac rupture); improves survival
    - aspirin – antiplatelet drug.

continued

CASE STUDY (continued)

2.   What considerations were made before streptokinase was administered?
   – Had the patient had an MI? This would be confirmed by an ECG.
   – Was the MI recent, within the last 12 h? Streptokinase is of real benefit only in the first 12 h.
   – Had the patient had any evidence of recent surgery, recent haemorrhagic stroke, active gastric ulceration or previous treatment with streptokinase? All of these are contraindications.
   His lipid biochemistry has revealed a total cholesterol level of 7.1 mmol/L (ideal <5.2 mmol/L), triglycerides of 1.9 mmol/L (ideal < 1.9 mmol/L) and HDL of 0.9 mmol/L (ideal > 0.9 mmol/L).
3.   What advice would you give concerning the management of this patient?
   – Hypercholesterolaemia: there is a need to reduce total cholesterol and LDL; statins should be given to MI patients, have been proved to reduce cardiovascular risk and may cause regression of coronary artery disease.
   – Simvastatin (40 mg every night) should be prescribed.
   – Statins reduce total cholesterol and LDL.
   – Statins (except atorvastatin) are taken at night to offset the nocturnal increase in cholesterol synthesis.
   – Liver function tests should be carried out before and 1–3 months after starting the statin.
   – All post-MI patients should be discharged on an ACE inhibitor if appropriate.
4.   How would you counsel the patient with regard to treatment with streptokinase and simvastatin?
   – Streptokinase: the patient should carry a streptokinase card. Further treatment with this agent may be ineffective or provoke an anaphylactic reaction due to the antibodies raised.
   – Simvastatin: this should be taken at night; the patient should stick to the recommended diet and report muscle pains straight away because they may indicate rhabdomyolysis. Ten per cent of patients have gastrointestinal disturbances.
   On presentation of a repeat prescription to his community pharmacist, Mr PS complains of indigestion-type discomfort.
5.   What do you advise?
   – Refer to the GP – the discomfort may be due to cardiac symptoms or gastric irritation due to aspirin.
   Several years later Mr PS is experiencing chest pains and is prescribed GTN sublingual tablets (500 micrograms as required).
6.   How would you counsel Mr PS?
   – Take the GTN when symptoms develop or before provoking event.
   – Sit down while taking the GTN.
   – Place the tablet under the tongue.
   – Spit it out or swallow the tablet if feel faint.
   – Keep in the original container and discard after 8 weeks of opening.
   – Any headache may be managed with paracetamol.
   The above treatment is only partially successful and Mr PS is now prescribed verapamil (80 mg three times daily).
7.   Are you happy to dispense the new prescription?
   – No – we do not know whether he is still taking atenolol. There is a risk of a serious interaction of ß blockers and verapamil, and the cardiac depression could cause asystole.

References

Catella-Lawson F, Reilly MP, Kapoor SC *et al* (2001). Cyclooxygenase inhibitors and the antiplatelet effects of aspirin. *N Engl J Med* **345**: 1809–17.

Fiore LD, Ezekowitz MD, Brophy MT *et al* (2002). Department of Veterans Affairs Cooperative Studies Program clinical trial comparing combined warfarin and aspirin with aspirin alone in survivors of acute myocardial infarction – primary results of the CHAMP study. *Circulation* **105**: 557–63.

IONA Study Group (2002). Effect of nicorandil on coronary events in patients with stable angina: the Impact Of Nicorandil in Angina (IONA) randomised trial. *Lancet* **359**: 1269–75.

INITIATIVE Investigators (2005). Efficacy of ivabradine, a new selective I_f inhibitor, compared with atenolol in patients with chronic stable angina. *Eur Heart J* **26**: 2529–36.

Krasopoulos G, Brister SJ, Beattie WS *et al* (2008). Aspirin 'resistance' and risk of cardiovascular morbidity: systematic review and meta-analysis. *BMJ* **33**: 195–8.

National Institute for Health and Clinical Excellence (2007). *MI Secondary Prevention*. Clinical Guideline 48. London: NICE. Available at: www.nice.org.uk.

Yusuf S, Sleight P, Pogue J *et al* (2000). Effects of an angiotensin converting-enzyme inhibitor, ramipril, on cardiovascular events in high-risk patients. The Heart Outcomes Prevention Evaluation Study Investigators. *N Engl J Med* **342**: 145–53.

Cohen H W, Gibson G, Alderman M H (2000). Excess risk of myocardial infarction in patients treated with antidepressant medications: association with use of tricyclic agents. *Am J Med* **108**: 2–8.

de Bono DP, Hopkins A (1994). The management of acute myocardial infarction: guidelines and audit standards. *J R Coll Phys Lond* **28**: 312–17.

ISIS-2 (Second International Study of Infarct Survival) Collaborative Group (1988). Randomised trial of intravenous streptokinase, oral aspirin, both, or neither among 17187 cases of suspected acute myocardial infarction: ISIS-2. *Lancet* **ii**: 349–60.

McGlynn S, Reid F, McAnaw J *et al* (2000). Coronary heart disease. *Pharm J* **265**: 194–205.

Roose SP (2000). Considerations for the use of anti-depressants in patients with cardiovascular disease. *Am Heart J* **140**(suppl S): 584–8.

Saltissi S, Mushahwar S (1995). Myocardial infarction: prophylaxis after infarction. *Prescribers J* **35**: 149–58.

Scandinavian Simvastatin Survival Study Group (1994). Randomised trial of cholesterol lowering in 4444 patients with coronary heart disease: the Scandinavian Simvastatin Survival Study (4S). *Lancet* **344**: 1383–9.

Online resources

www.bhf.org.uk
The website of the British Heart Foundation, providing patient information (accessed April 2008).

Further reading

ACE Inhibitor Myocardial Infarction Collaborative Group (1998). Indications for ACE inhibitors in the early treatment of acute myocardial infarction. *Circulation* **97**: 2202–12.

15

Heart failure

Disease characteristics

In simple terms, heart failure may be viewed as a failure of the heart as a pump to meet circulatory needs and this may be either acute (e.g. following a heart attack or volume loading) or chronic. The underlying cause is failure of the heart muscle, sustained arrhythmias (such as atrial fibrillation) or failure of the heart valves (through infection or ageing-related changes).

The leading causes (70%) of chronic heart failure (CHF) are ischaemic heart disease and hypertension. In the case of hypertension, the increased afterload leads in time to hypertrophy. The cardiac enlargement thus increases the work of the heart and lessens the ejection fraction. Indeed, a compelling reason to treat hypertension is to reduce the likelihood of developing CHF. Heart failure associated with ischaemic heart disease (IHD) results from reduced blood flow, leading to impaired cardiac muscle function, with a reduction in pump performance. Cardiomyopathies due to alcohol abuse, infection and drug treatment (e.g. anthracycline anticancer drugs) may also cause CHF. Other causes of heart failure are pregnancy, anaemia, thyrotoxicosis, excessive infusion of intravenous fluids and fluid-retaining drugs (e.g. non-steroidal anti-inflammatory drugs [NSAIDs], corticosteroids, mineralocorticoids, glitazones) and these should be excluded.

Underlying pathology

The key change, to which therapy is ideally targeted, is inappropriate neurohormonal adaptation. As a pathophysiological adaptation, in an attempt to compensate for circulatory failure, there is activation of the sympathetic nervous system and the renin–angiotensin–aldosterone system (RAAS), with increased release of anti-diuretic hormone (ADH), although there is also a release of atrial natriuretic peptide (ANP) from the dilated heart. Although these activations may seem logical to restore circulatory function, the increased sympathetic and RAAS activities increase arterial vascular resistance (afterload) and venous return (preload), thus increasing the workload of the heart. The increased sympathetic activity will also attempt to increase the force of cardiac contraction but will predispose towards arrhythmias. The attendant increase in circulating volume, evoked principally by the RAAS, will similarly increase preload and afterload on the heart. Consequent on the increased resistance there is impaired renal function, with additional salt and water retention and further activation of RAAS. Hence a vicious cycle develops which further impairs the pump activity of the heart. A consequence of these changes is oedema (congestion) at different sites in the body and the term 'congestive heart failure' is also widely used (Figure 15.1).

The neurohormonal activation also leads to myocyte dysfunction, with increased aldosterone activity leading to fibrosis and stiffening of the cardiac muscle, further impairing pump activity.

Classification

Left-sided failure

- This is the most common form of heart failure, and is often secondary to hypertension.

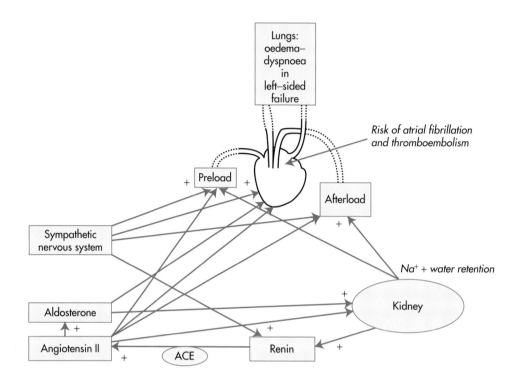

Figure 15.1 Schematic diagram of the principal pathophysiological changes and interactions in chronic heart failure. Activation of the renin–angiotensin systems leads to increased levels of angiotensin II (via angiotensin-converting enzyme [ACE]) which activates the release of aldosterone, promotes sodium retention, and causes arterial and venous vasoconstriction, and cardiac remodelling. The sympathetic nervous system also stimulates renin release and causes both arterial and venous vasoconstriction. Aldosterone promotes sodium retention and is associated with cardiac fibrosis. Sodium and water retention increase the circulating volume, with increases in preload and afterload.

- Left ventricular (systolic) function is impaired, with poor output leading to increased left atrial and pulmonary venous pressures with pulmonary congestion and oedema.

Right-sided failure

- Right-sided failure is often due to chronic lung disease (cor pulmonale).
- Right ventricular output falls, leading to increased venous pressure, with peripheral oedema.

Biventricular failure

- Both main chambers are affected because left and right ventricular failure often coincide. Diseases such as IHD may have affected both ventricles.

- Often, left ventricular failure leads to pulmonary congestion, which in turn impairs right ventricular function, causing failure on the right side as well.

Clinical features

As one might predict from a failure of the heart to meet circulatory needs, cardiovascular-related features are:

- reduced ejection fraction (<45%), as identified on an echocardiogram; this leads to impaired exercise tolerance
- hypotension, leading to tiredness and possibly dizziness
- reduced urine flow
- cold peripheries

- breathlessness
- oedema.

  With associated, non-specific symptoms:

- fatigue, listlessness
- poor exercise tolerance (determines grade)
- weight loss or even gain due to oedema.

Left ventricular failure

The key feature is pulmonary oedema, which leads to dyspnoea with a sensation of drowning. There is often marked orthopnoea, because lying down leads to further venous congestion, which is relieved on sitting up or standing. This is particularly pronounced in bed and patients often describe having to go to the window 'to get air'. Using pillows to prop the patient up may relieve orthopnoea in bed and the number of pillows used may be a guide to the severity of this symptom. The pulmonary congestion may also lead to a cough, with sputum, which may or may not be frothy and contain blood.

Right ventricular failure

The leading feature of right ventricular failure is raised venous pressure, which leads to peripheral oedema (typically in the ankles on standing, and which may shift to the sacral regions while lying down). The raised venous pressure will also manifest as raised jugular venous pressure (JVP, which is raised if >4 cm from the clavicular line). The increased venous pressure may also lead to hepatomegaly (enlarged liver), with abdominal discomfort.

Although a diagnosis may be made on clinical features, it should be established by an echocardiogram. Heart failure may also be suggested by increased plasma levels of B-type natriuretic peptide (BNP), and this is being introduced as a screening test to aid diagnosis.

Atrial fibrillation

A major and common consequence of cardiac failure is a build-up of back-pressure in the heart, as there is impaired ejection. This often leads to dilatation of the left atrium and the physical distension of the muscle causes disturbances in atrial electrical activity, resulting in atrial fibrillation. This does not greatly impair cardiac function; however, the consequent stasis of blood in the left atria increases the likelihood of thrombi forming. These may dislodge and travel to the cerebral circulation, giving rise to thromboembolic occlusion, resulting in transient ischaemic attacks or stroke.

The key feature of a patient with atrial fibrillation is an irregularly irregular pulse. Atrial fibrillation is readily identified on an electrocardiogram (ECG) as the absence of P waves and irregular QRS complexes.

Goals of treatment

The main goal of treatment is to improve the quality of life by relieving symptoms and, if possible, to reverse or modify the disease processes.

The simplest approach is to treat any underlying causes, such as valvular disease, IHD or atrial fibrillation. In these cases this may involve cardiac surgery.

The principles of medical management using drugs are to:

- decrease cardiac work, which may be achieved by using diuretics or vasodilators
- increase cardiac output, which may be achieved by using positive inotropic agents
- counteract maladaptation: the key goal, which involves blocking and reversing the neurohormonal adaptation; if this is achieved then the outcome should be improved.

If atrial fibrillation is present, additional aims are to control ventricular rate and prevent thrombus formation, reducing the likelihood of a transient ischaemic attack.

Pharmacological basis of management (Table 15.1)

ACE inhibitors, e.g. captopril, enalapril, lisinopril, perindopril, ramipril

Angiotensin-converting enzyme (ACE) inhibitors are now recognized as first-line therapy in CHF

Table 15.1 Summary of principal effects of drugs used in heart failure

Drug	Pharmacological targets	Mechanism	Effects
ACE inhibitors	Renin–angiotensin system (RAS)	Inhibition of ACE	• Decreased arterial and venous vasoconstriction • Decreased blood volume • Decreased compensatory effects of RAS
Loop diuretics	Kidney: loop of Henle	Inhibition of $Na^+/K^+/2Cl^-$ transporter in loop of Henle	• Na^+ excretion • Decreased blood volume • Decreased plasma K^+
Thiazide diuretics	Kidney: distal convoluted tubule	Inhibition of Na^+/Cl^- reabsorption	• Na^+ excretion • Decreased blood volume • Decreased plasma K^+
Potassium-sparing diuretics (amiloride)	Kidney: aldosterone-responsive segment of distal tubule	Decreased Na^+ permeability due to blockade of Na^+ channels	• Weak diuretic effect (increased Na^+ excretion) with decreased K^+ excretion
Potassium-sparing diuretics (spironolactone)	Kidney: as above	Aldosterone receptor antagonist	• Weak diuretic effect (increased Na^+ excretion) with decreased K^+ excretion • Reverses adverse effects of aldosterone on the heart
Beta-blockers	Myocardium	Antagonism of cardiac β-adrenoceptors	• Reduce sympathetic drive to the heart • Oppose neurohormonal adaptation • Antiarrhythmic actions
Digoxin	Myocardium, AV node	Inhibition of Na^+ pump	• Positive inotropic effects • Induces a degree of AV block
Nitrates	Vascular smooth muscle	Increased cGMP production	• Vasodilatation
α Blockers (prazosin or mixed α/β blocker carvedilol)	Sympathetic nervous system	α-Adrenoceptor antagonists	• Vasodilatation

ACE, angiotensin-converting enzyme; AV, atrioventricular; cGMP, guanosine cyclic 3':5'-monophosphate.

and may be given to asymptomatic patients. They have been proved to both reduce symptoms and improve prognosis (Cooperative North Scandinavian Enalapril Survival Study [CONSENSUS] trial: Swedeberg, 1987). By inhibiting ACE, they lead to reductions in the neurohormonal adaptation due to angiotensin II and aldosterone, with the following consequences:

• reduction in arterial and venous vasoconstriction (reduced after- and preload)
• reduction in salt and water retention, hence reduced circulating volume
• indirect positive inotropic effect
• prevention and reversal of cardiac remodelling due to RAAS.

Clinical use

By nature of their action, ACE inhibitors may cause severe hypotension (in about 2% of patients) and are best given initially on retiring at night. A low starting dose should be used and titrated up to the maximum tolerated dose. In certain patients at high risk, including those with a systolic blood pressure <90 mmHg, treatment should be initiated in hospital under supervision. There should be close monitoring of creatinine, urea and electrolyte levels before and after each dosage change.

The renin–angiotensin system is activated in renovascular disease in order to maintain renal perfusion and filtration. Hence ACE inhibitors may cause deterioration of renal function in pre-existing renal disease, and these patients should be identified by measurement of plasma creatinine and monitoring of renal function throughout treatment.

Angiotensin II receptor antagonists, e.g. candesartan, irbesartan, losartan, valsartan

This newer class of drugs blocks the action of angiotensin II at the angiotensin AT_1-receptor, which will also reduce the stimulation of aldosterone release. Hence AT_1-receptor antagonists act in a similar manner to ACE inhibitors but do not give rise to a cough. The ELITE II trial (Pitt *et al* 2000) reported that losartan was equally effective at reducing mortality in elderly patients with heart failure to captopril, but it was also better tolerated. Similarly results (Val-HeFt: Cohn and Tognoni 2001) have indicated that valsartan improves the quality of life in patients with heart failure. AT_1-receptor antagonists may also be used together with ACE inhibitors.

Diuretics: thiazides and related agents (e.g. bendroflumethiazide, indapamide, metolazone)and loop diuretics (e.g. furosemide)

Diuretics are the mainstay of drug treatment in heart failure and provide rapid symptomatic relief. Diuretics reduce circulating volume, thus decreasing pre- and afterload, and hence cardiac work. In addition, they may have direct vascular effects leading to venodilatation, which further reduces preload. Diuretics provide relief for the symptoms of congestion but do not affect the progression of the disease.

Thiazides act in the distal convoluted tubule to inhibit Na^+/Cl^- reabsorption. Loop diuretics inhibit the $Na^+/K^+/2Cl^-$ co-transporter in the thick ascending limb of the loop of Henle, inhibiting the establishment of a hyperosmotic interstitium and so reducing the ability of the kidneys to produce concentrated urine, leading to profuse diuresis.

Clinical use

The rational use of diuretics includes situations where there is oedema (peripheral or pulmonary). Thiazides induce modest diuresis and are used in mild failure or in elderly people. Loop diuretics, which are more extensively used, cause very pronounced diuresis and are especially useful in causing rapid relief of pulmonary oedema. Indeed, intravenous furosemide rapidly reduces the dyspnoea associated with pulmonary oedema in acute left ventricular failure. This effect precedes the diuresis and is thought to be due to venodilatation reducing preload on the heart.

Why do thiazides and loop diuretics cause hypokalaemia?

Hypokalaemia is a major side effect of these diuretic agents. By acting on the kidney, largely before the distal tubule, these agents increase the sodium content in the tubular fluid. Under the control of aldosterone, the distal tubule attempts to reabsorb sodium (via amiloride-sensitive sodium channels) but at the cost of excreting potassium. In addition, these agents will also provoke the release of renin and the activation of RAAS, which will further promote the excretion of potassium. By contrast, ACE inhibitors will oppose the aldosterone-sensitive potassium loss and there is a risk of significant hyperkalaemia if the ACE inhibitor is given in addition to potassium supplements or potassium-sparing diuretics (e.g. amiloride, spironolactone).

Spironolactone

This is an aldosterone receptor antagonist, which acts as a weak potassium-sparing diuretic. It is now used at a low dose (25 mg), which does not have pronounced haemodynamic effects but reverses the aldosterone-mediated neurohormonal changes. Even after ACE inhibition, aldosterone levels may still be appreciable, so spironolactone is able to exert substantial beneficial effects. It is thought that spironolactone inhibits aldosterone-induced fibrosis, which otherwise stiffens the heart and is associated with arrhythmias. It may also inhibit the adverse effects of aldosterone on autonomic and baroreceptor function. The RALES trial (Pitt *et al* 1999), in which low-dose spironolactone was added to conventional therapies, indicated that this treatment reduced mortality by 30%.

Digoxin

Digoxin used to be the mainstay of therapy and has been in and out of fashion over many years. Its principal action is as a positive inotrope by inhibiting Na^+/K^+ ATPase (which causes a rise in intracellular sodium, promoting calcium entry, and leading to increased force of contraction). However, digoxin also directly and indirectly (via central vagal activation) impairs atrioventricular conduction. This induction of heart block and bradycardia is beneficial in heart failure with atrial fibrillation because it controls ventricular rate. Indeed, it is now widely believed that digoxin should be reserved for heart failure with atrial fibrillation, or when treatment with an ACE inhibitor and a diuretic is inadequate for patients in sinus rhythm.

Clinical usage

Digoxin improves the patient's symptoms, reduces hospitalization but does not affect all-cause mortality (DIG trial: Digitalis Investigation Group 1997). Digoxin has a very narrow therapeutic window and is largely renally excreted, which means that renal function should be taken into account, with dose reductions to prevent increased plasma concentrations and toxicity.

Digoxin is associated with a range of significant side effects which include:

• anorexia
• nausea
• gastrointestinal disturbances
• visual disturbances
• arrhythmias.

β Blockers: bisoprolol, carvedilol and metoprolol

β-Adrenoceptor antagonists have traditionally been contraindicated in heart failure, because they reduce sympathetic drive to a failing heart or may precipitate failure in compensated failure. However, there is now evidence that they reduce disease progression, symptoms and mortality (CIBIS-II Investigators and Committee 1999; MERIT-HF Study Group 1999). Principally, β blockers:

• reduce sympathetic stimulation, heart rate and oxygen consumption
• reduce sudden death by their antiarrhythmic properties
• oppose the neurohormonal activation which leads to myocyte dysfunction.

In addition, carvedilol causes vasodilatation as it is also an α blocker, and its antioxidant properties may be beneficial.

Clinical usage

Metoprolol, bisoprolol and carvedilol are now being increasingly used in patients with stable, moderate heart failure, and are especially useful in patients with cardiac ischaemia. However, they should be used with caution in patients with chronic obstructive pulmonary disease (COPD), which is relatively common in the patient population with the highest incidence of heart failure. Their use would also be contraindicated in hypotension and marked bradycardia.

β Blockers should be initiated starting with a low dose under the supervision of a cardiologist or general practitioner (GP) experienced in their usage. The β blocker may initially cause a worsening of symptoms but benefit may become apparent after several weeks.

Vasodilators

Nitrates in particular may have a role in CHF because they will cause venodilatation, leading to a reduction in preload. Many patients will also have IHD and so nitrates will be of benefit in these patients. Nitrates may be suitable for people in whom ACE inhibitors are not tolerated but are contraindicated in hypotension and marked anaemia.

Other vasodilators that may be added on to therapy are α blockers such as prazosin, which will reduce peripheral resistance by opposing sympathetic activity. They are of no proven benefit. The arterial vasorelaxant hydralazine is also used as an add-on drug or for those intolerant of ACE inhibitors.

Other positive inotropes

In addition to digoxin, phosphodiesterase inhibitors (PDEIs) such as milrinone have a limited role. These drugs act to potentiate adenosine cyclic 3′:5′-monophosphate (cAMP) in myocytes and so have positive inotropic effects; they are used in end-stage failure on a short-term basis in hospital. It should be noted that their long-term use is associated with increased mortality.

Amines such as dobutamine, which acts as a β agonist, similarly may have a role in the management of acute failure and end-stage failure in the context of specialist hospital care.

Choice of drugs

This is largely stage (New York Heart Association or NYHA) dependent:

* stage I (asymptomatic)
* stage II (slight limitations through breathlessness/fatigue on normal exertion)
* stage III (marked limitations through breathlessness/fatigue on normal exertion)
* stage IV (breathless at rest).

The guidance of the National Institute for Health and Clinical Excellence (NICE 2003) suggests that ACE inhibitors have a central role and should be used in all cases of left ventricular systolic dysfunction. If patients are intolerant of ACE inhibitors due to the associated cough then AT_1-receptor antagonists may be used instead. Diuretics are used for symptomatic relief where there is oedema. Although β blockers are now recognized as having an important role, they should be added cautiously to therapy in patients with moderate but stable heart failure. Despite these recommendations it appears that in practice the use of β blockers is less common than would be expected. Digoxin is recommended for refractory disease or in patients with concurrent atrial fibrillation, and spironolactone is also used in cases of CHF that do not respond to optimal therapy (Figure 15.2).

Concurrent disease

Additional considerations when prescribing in CHF:

* Renal impairment may preclude the use of ACE inhibitors and thiazides and lead to a dose reduction with digoxin. In moderate failure higher doses of loop diuretics are required and in anuria their use would be precluded.
* Liver function: close monitoring with ACE inhibitors is important in liver disease. Warfarin and carvedilol should be avoided and a reduced dose of metoprolol may be required. The use of potassium-sparing diuretics may be necessary. This is due to the risk of precipitating coma if hypokalaemia develops during treatment with loop and thiazide diuretics. There is also an increased risk of hypomagnesaemia in alcoholic cirrhosis. Thiazides should be avoided in severe liver disease.
* Atrial fibrillation would be a compelling reason to use digoxin and an indication for an anticoagulant (see Chapter 16). Amiodarone may also be required.
* Asthma would preclude the use of a β blocker because of the risk of bronchospasm. This is less clear cut in the case of COPD, where the beneficial effects of β blockers in heart failure are significant. The current view is that in

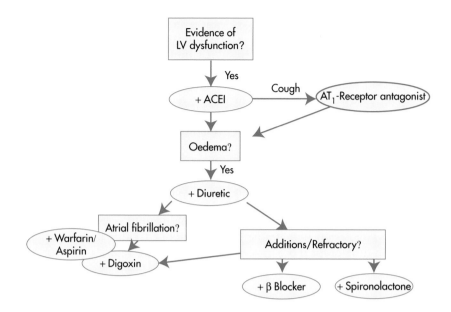

Figure 15.2 A summary of current approaches to the management of chronic heart failure incorporating National Institute for Health and Clinical Excellence (NICE 2003) guidance. Approaches to managing atrial fibrillation in chronic heart failure are also indicated. ACEI, angiotensin-converting enzyme inhibitor; AT, angiotensin; LV, left ventricular.

patients with concurrent COPD the cautious use of cardioselective β blockers is acceptable.

• Diabetes mellitus may be a reason not to use a thiazide (due to risk of hyperglycaemia) but may be a compelling reason to use an ACE inhibitor (see Chapter 35). Blood pressure and plasma glucose concentration should be monitored regularly.

• History of stroke would be an indication for perindopril alone or in combination with indapamide. The PROGRESS Collaborative Group (2001) trial has indicated that perindopril alone or in combination with indapamide reduces the incidence of stroke (both haemorrhagic and thromboembolic) in patients who have previously suffered any type of stroke. It remains to be determined if this is specific to perindopril and indapamide or whether it applies to any ACE inhibitor plus a thiazide. Cerebral haemorrhage would be a contraindication for the use of nitrates.

• Ischaemic heart disease would be a reason to add a β blocker and nitrates. Attention should also be paid to primary or secondary prevention with antiplatelet agents and correction of hyperlipidaemia (see Chapter 12).

• Risk of infection from influenza and pneumonia would be a reason to consider immunization with influenza and pneumococcal polysaccharide vaccines, respectively.

Additional considerations are: Wolff–Parkinson–White syndrome (contraindication for digoxin); closed-angle glaucoma (contraindication for nitrates); Addison's disease (contraindication for thiazides); and gout (contraindication for thiazides).

CHF may itself influence drug choice in unrelated conditions: important examples are summarized in Table 15.2.

Drug interactions

In the context of drug choice, the interactions between drugs used in CHF should be considered (Table 15.3).

Table 15.2   Examples of how chronic heart failure may influence drug choice in other conditions

Condition	Drugs	Comments
Diabetes	Glitazones	These may cause oedema and exacerbate CHF. They should be avoided
Migraine	5HT$_1$-receptor agonists – triptans and ergotamine	Coronary vasoconstriction. CHM warning against use in ischaemic heart disease or Prinzmetal's angina. Also contraindicated with nitrates
Glaucoma	Timolol eye drops	Systemic effects of β blockade
Thyroid disease	Levothyroxine	Risk of rapid increase in metabolism and activation of sympathetic nervous system
Bipolar affective disorder	Lithium	Lithium concentrations increased by ACE inhibitors and diuretics
Depression	Tricyclic antidepressants	Prolongation of Q–T interval. Risk of arrhythmias and sudden death
Pain	NSAIDs	Risk of Na$^+$ and fluid retention, renal failure with ACE inhibitor
	Sodium load from soluble paracetamol	
Indigestion	Antacids	Na$^+$ content should be considered. Absorption of prescribed drugs may be affected
Infection	Erythromycin, clarithromycin	Prolongation of Q–T interval. Risk of arrhythmias and sudden death. Macrolides interact with amiodarone, warfarin, digoxin and antihyperlipidaemic agents
Menopause	HRT (also oral contraception)	Contraindicated in thromboembolic disorders
Angina, hypertension, Raynaud's phenomenon	Verapamil, diltiazem, nifedipine	May cause or worsen CHF (bradycardia)
COPD	High doses and chronic use of β$_2$-adrenoceptor agonists	CHM warning of serious hypokalaemia. Regular monitoring required

ACE, angiotensin-converting enzyme; CHF, chronic heart failure; COPD, chronic obstructive pulmonary disease; CHM, Commission on Human Medicines; HRT, hormone replacement therapy; NSAIDs, non-steroidal anti-inflammatory drugs.

General counselling

One approach to explaining CHF to a patient is that the heart is simply not able to pump the blood as well as it used to, making exercise more difficult. Patients may notice that they have become increasingly breathless and their ankles swell. In some cases it may be appropriate to avoid mentioning failure, and use of terms such as 'congestion' may be helpful. The purpose of the drug treatment is either to reduce the work of the heart or to make it beat more forcefully. Other points to consider:

- General counselling would follow the lifestyle advice outlined in Chapters 3 and 11.
- If the patient is taking diuretics, it would be worth suggesting cutting out excess salt in the diet, because this would undo the beneficial effects of the diuretic.
- Patients are at risk of developing secondary depression as a consequence of reduced quality of life or with the realization of the seriousness of their condition. The GP should be alert to this and may wish to consider anti-depressant therapy.
- In the presence of orthopnoea, patients would be advised to prop themselves up with pillows in bed at night.

Table 15.3 Summary of important interactions within drugs used in chronic heart failure

Interaction	Consequences	Comment
ACE inhibitor with potassium-sparing diuretics or potassium supplements	Hyperkalaemia	ACE inhibitors and potassium-sparing diuretics both oppose aldosterone, leading to potassium retention
Loop diuretics or thiazides with digoxin	Enhanced effects of digoxin	Diuretic-induced hypokalaemia will enhance the actions of digoxin
Digoxin with captopril, telmisartan, amiodarone or spironolactone	Increased plasma concentrations of digoxin	Pharmacokinetic interaction
Digoxin with β blockers	Bradycardia, increased AV block	Addition of actions
Diuretics with vasodilators	Hypotension	Addition of actions

ACE, angiotensin-converting enzyme; AV, atrioventricular.

- Patients taking ACE inhibitors, diuretics, α and β blockers, and nitrates should be alerted to the problems of hypotension and orthostatic hypotension, and the possibility of having a fall. They should be advised to stand up slowly.
- Patients should be advised to report muscle cramps, pain, nausea or vomiting, which may indicate hypokalaemia. Confusion may point to hyponatraemia.
- Patients should be alert for changes in heart rate and palpitations.

Specific counselling

ACE inhibitors

- Patients may experience pronounced first-dose hypotension; it is best to take the first doses of the ACE inhibitor immediately before retiring to bed at night. First-dose hypotension may be worse if the patient is also taking diuretics and the diuretic may be stopped for a few days before the ACE inhibitor is initiated.
- Discuss any cough with the GP. Patients should be encouraged to persist with the ACE inhibitor, because this is the most effective treatment. The ACE inhibitor could be changed or an angiotensin receptor antagonist used.
- Consult a pharmacist before purchasing other medicines or supplements, e.g. avoid use of

potassium salts (salt substitute, effervescent preparations, cystitis treatments), and to use caution with NSAIDs.

Diuretics

- Male patients should be informed of possible impotence as a side effect.
- Diuretics (or 'water tablets') will cause an increase in urine flow, usually after 2 h of taking the dose. This may subside after a couple of weeks. In the case of furosemide, it may be worth pointing out that diuresis may be pronounced.
- It is best to take the diuretic in the morning to limit sleep disturbance. A dose may be taken later in the day to avoid the need for urination interfering with social engagements during the day. If two daily doses are required, they may be taken at 7am and 1pm.
- Omit a dose during periods of diarrhoea and vomiting to prevent dehydration and electrolyte disturbances.
- If appropriate, correction of oedema may be monitored by the patient's weight.
- Sunscreen advice may be appropriate to avoid photosensitivity reactions.

Digoxin

- Patients should be advised to report signs of toxicity, e.g. nausea, vomiting, diarrhoea, disturbances of vision or loss of appetite.

- As digoxin may cause arrhythmias, patients should also report dizziness, an irregular heartbeat or palpitations.
- Ensure the pulse does not fall below 60 beats/min. If this occurs, the patient should omit the next dose.

β Blockers

- Beneficial effects may not be immediate and there may be a worsening of symptoms.
- Male patients may experience impotence.
- Report any additional breathlessness (due to worsening of symptoms or blockade of bronchial β_2-adrenoceptors); cold extremities or peripheral weakness may reflect blockade of vasodilator β_2-adrenoceptors.
- Do not stop taking the tablets suddenly.

Nitrates

Patients may experience a throbbing headache, which should be relieved with paracetamol.

Spironolactone

Male patients may be advised of the small risk of breast enlargement (gynaecomastia), which in itself is harmless.

Hydralazine

Patients should report any weight loss, arthritis or ill health because this may suggest systemic lupus erythematosus.

α Blockers

- Patients should be alert to first-dose hypotension.
- Patients may also experience urinary incontinence.

Monitoring

Renal function (creatinine)

- This should be monitored before treatment to determine glomerular filtration rate, because this may be impaired through age or CHF. This is important, because thiazides (except metolazone, which is rarely used) are ineffective in moderate renal failure. Furthermore, digoxin

is largely, but not entirely, excreted renally and so in renal impairment there should be a dose reduction or digitoxin, which is not renally excreted, should be used instead.
- ACE inhibitors are contraindicated in renovascular disease.
- Creatinine and urea may rise slightly after initiating an ACE inhibitor or diuretic and this may require dose reduction. Creatinine, urea and electrolyte levels should then be checked after 2 weeks and after each dose change.

Electrolytes

Ideally, potassium levels should be monitored a week after starting diuretic treatment or adjusting treatment and then at least annually once the regimen is stabilized. Sodium may also be affected, presenting as hyponatraemia in which the patient may become confused. Thiazides are also associated with hypomagnesaemia and hypercalcaemia.

Hyperkalaemia

ACE inhibitors, by inhibiting the production of angiotensin II and aldosterone, will tend to cause potassium retention, leading to hyperkalaemia. This may become significant if the ACE inhibitor is taken with a potassium-sparing diuretic or potassium supplements, and their concurrent use is contraindicated or they should be used with great care (e.g. regular monitoring).

Hypokalaemia

Thiazides (especially) and loop diuretics cause hypokalaemia, which is associated with increased fatal arrhythmias. Hypokalaemia is less of a problem if ACE inhibitors are also used because they have the opposite effect (as mentioned above). Hypokalaemia is especially problematic in patients taking digoxin, because hypokalaemia potentiates its pharmacological actions and may lead to toxicity. If hypokalaemia occurs in patients not receiving an ACE inhibitor (unlikely nowadays), the patient may benefit from the addition of a potassium-sparing diuretic or, less commonly, potassium supplements. Digoxin should be withheld until the hypokalaemia is corrected.

Table 15.4   Over-the-counter (OTC) medicines to avoid in chronic heart failure

OTC products	Comments
Na+: table salt, high-salt foods (bacon, crisps, etc.), soluble preparations, indigestion remedies (Na+-free alternatives are available), cystitis treatments	Increased Na+ will reduce the effect of treatment or enhance renal impairment with ACE inhibitors
K+: salt substitute, cystitis treatments (low-sodium or potassium citrate mixture), some indigestion remedies	Interaction with ACE inhibitors and K+-sparing diuretics with a risk of hyperkalaemia
Cough and cold remedies containing decongestants (pseudoephedrine, phenylpropanolamine)	Decongestants may increase blood pressure due to sympathomimetic activity
NSAIDs (aspirin, ibuprofen, ketoprofen) in oral and topical analgesics	In addition to drug interactions, the use of NSAIDs may exacerbate heart failure. Gout may be a side effect of thiazides and ibuprofen would be unsuitable
Laxatives (senna, lactulose)	Chronic use of laxatives may cause electrolyte disturbances
Caffeine (analgesic preparations)	Caffeine may cause myocardial ischaemia

ACE, angiotensin-converting enzyme; NSAIDs, non-steroidal anti-inflammatory drugs.

Digoxin

Ideally, plasma levels should be measured on a regular basis, although this does not often happen in practice. Plasma concentrations of digoxin should be measured (6–12 h post-dosing, see Appendix 2) at regular intervals because toxicity is a common occurrence. As commented above, patients or their carers should be told to ensure that their heart rate does not fall below 60 beats/min, and this will also act as a rough therapeutic monitor.

Over-the-counter considerations (Table 15.4)

The main problems with over-the-counter (OTC) products result from sodium or potassium content, sodium retention or sympathomimetic activity. Due to the complex nature of CHF treatment there is also a great potential for drug interactions. The pharmacist is ideally placed to identify concordance problems, side effects of prescribed medicines or worsening symptoms, and can advise the patient accordingly, e.g. a classic side effect of ACE inhibitors is a persistent cough, which may result in failure of treatment due to poor patient concordance. Patients should be encouraged to continue with the ACE inhibitor despite the cough, because alternative treatments may be less effective.

Alternative medicine

In an attempt to avoid polypharmacy and in the absence of reliable clinical trial data, the concurrent use of herbal drugs and conventional medicines should be discouraged. Many herbal drugs exhibit pharmacological activity and therefore have the potential to produce the undesirable side effects outlined with conventional medicines above, e.g. there is some evidence that herbal medicines may exhibit sympathomimetic activity, diuretic or antiplatelet effects. Food supplements may also interact with conventional medicines (see Chapters 3 and 4).

Self-assessment

Consider whether the following statements are true or false. In the management of chronic heart failure:

1. ACE inhibitors should be titrated up to the maximum tolerated dose.

2. ACE inhibitors are initially taken on retiring to bed due to the risk of first-dose hypotension.
3. Loop diuretics are proven to prolong life and reduce mortality.
4. β Blockers are contraindicated.
5. When digoxin is used the patient should ensure that the pulse does not rise to >60 beats/min.

Practice points

- Be observant for symptoms suggestive of heart failure, particularly in high-risk patients such as after a myocardial infarction.
- Treatment should be aimed at relieving symptoms and reducing the risk of death.
- Take steps to prevent readmission to hospital: ensure good symptom control, improve concordance with medicines and diet, reduce alcohol consumption, recognize psychological problems and lack of social support.
- Lower doses of diuretics should be used initially in elderly people due to an increased risk of side effects.
- ACE inhibitors improve both symptoms and prognosis and have a major role in the management of CHF.
- Regular monitoring is essential, particularly for patients taking digoxin. Potassium-sparing diuretics can cause severe hyperkalaemia in patients taking an ACE inhibitor.
- Angiotensin AT_1-receptor antagonists may have an important role in patients intolerant of ACE inhibitors.
- β Blockers are now recognized as having an important role in improving quality of life and reducing mortality.
- When β blockers are used the recommendation is 'to start low and go slow'.
- People with CHF are at high risk of developing arrhythmias and of sudden death. Arrhythmias should be investigated and treated as appropriate.
- Be vigilant of the use of OTC medicines and supplements in patients with CHF.
- Patients should be warned about first-dose hypotension with ACE inhibitors and α blockers (extra caution in combination with diuretics).

 CASE STUDY

Last year Mr AH (65 years) found himself increasingly short of breath while walking to the shops and he was referred by his GP for cardiological investigations. A physical examination did not reveal any abnormalities but a chest X-ray revealed cardiomegaly without evidence of pulmonary oedema. A subsequent echocardiogram revealed a reduction in ejection fraction. A diagnosis of chronic heart failure was made and the cardiologist prescribed lisinopril starting at 2.5 mg daily (every night) and this was increased over several weeks by his GP to 20 mg daily.

1. Comment on the clinical findings.
   – His shortness of breath is a symptom of CHF.
   – Cardiomegaly is an enlarged heart, and is consistent with CHF.
   – Reduced ejection fraction on an echocardiogram is diagnostic of CHF.
2. What is the purpose of the lisinopril?
   – The ACE inhibitor will inhibit angiotensin II production and aldosterone release.
   – It reduces cardiac work.
   – It opposes neurohormonal changes in the heart.

continued

CASE STUDY (continued)

3. How should the patient be counselled with respect to taking the lisinopril for the first time?
   - The patient should be warned of first-dose hypotension and advised to take the first dose before retiring to bed.
   - The patient may develop a cough. This should be reported to the GP but the benefits of the drug outweigh the cough so he should be encouraged to persist with the medicine if possible.
   - He should report any rashes or swellings, which may be due to angio-oedema.

   After his initial treatment, Mr AH felt substantially better. However, after 6 months he was admitted to hospital with breathlessness, which had become worse while taking bed rest. This time a physical examination and chest X-ray revealed pulmonary oedema and the patient rapidly responded to diamorphine 5 mg i.v. stat and was started on furosemide 40 mg every morning.

4. Comment on the use of diamorphine and furosemide.
   - Diamorphine induces a degree of euphoria. It opposes dyspnoea and cough associated with pulmonary oedema.
   - Furosemide will cause venodilatation to reduce preload. It induces diuresis, reducing fluid and relieving pulmonary oedema.

   Mr AH's condition is currently well managed but he is admitted to hospital once again to monitor his progress. This time his GP is concerned with a new addition made by the consultant to the patient's prescription. The addition is for bisoprolol (1.25 mg every morning). The GP remembers from medical school something about β blockers being contraindicated in CHF, and comments: 'Surely the consultant means bisacodyl?'

5. How do you respond to the GP?
   - The consultant is indeed correct. The bisoprolol may be given. Previously it was thought that β blockers were contraindicated due to negative inotropic effects but now evidence points to cardioselective ones being safe in stable CHF. Start with a low dose.

6. What is the rationale for the consultant's new addition?
   - To oppose the neurohormonal maladaptation due to catecholamines. Also it is antiarrhythmic.

References

CIBIS-II Investigators and Committee (1999). The Cardiac Insufficiency Bisoprolol Study II (CIBIS-II): a randomised trial. *Lancet* **353**: 9–13.

Cohn JN, Tognoni G (2001). A randomized trial of the angiotensin receptor blocker valsartan in chronic heart failure. *N Engl J Med* **345**: 1667–75.

Digitalis Investigation Group (1997). The effect of digoxin on mortality and morbidity in patients with heart failure. *N Engl J Med* **336**: 525–33.

MERIT-HF Study Group (1999). Effect of metoprolol CR XL in chronic heart failure: Metoprolol CR XL Randomised Intervention Trial in Congestive Heart Failure (MERIT-HF). *Lancet* **353**: 2001–7.

National Institute for Clinical Excellence (2003). *Chronic Heart Failure: Management of chronic heart failure in adults in primary and secondary care*. Clinical guidance 5. London: NICE.

Pitt B, Zannad F, Remme WJ *et al* (1999). The effect of spironolactone on morbidity and mortality in patients with severe heart failure. *N Eng J Med* **341**: 709–17.

Pitt B, Poole-Wilson PA, Segal R *et al* (2000). Effect of losartan compared with captopril on mortality in patients with symptomatic heart failure: random-ised trial – the Losartan Heart Failure Survival Study ELITE II. *Lancet* **355**: 1582–7.

PROGRESS Collaborative Group (2001). Randomised trial of a perindopril-based blood-pressure-lowering regimen among 6105 individuals with previous stroke or transient ischaemic attack. *Lancet* **358**: 1033–41.

Swedeberg K (1987). Effects of enalapril on mortality in severe congestive-heart failure – results of the Cooperative North Scandinavian Enalapril Survival Study (CONSENSUS). *N Engl J Med* **316**: 1429–35.

Further reading

Cleland JGF, Swedberg K, Poole-Wilson PA (1998). Successes and failures of the current treatment of heart failure. *Lancet* **353**(suppl): 19–28.

Cowie MR, Zaphiriou A (2002). Management of chronic heart failure. *BMJ* **325**: 422–5.

Perry G, Brown E, Thornton R *et al* (1997). The effect of digoxin on mortality and morbidity in patients with heart failure. *N Engl J Med* **336**: 525–33.

Seed A, McMurry J (2001). Current approaches to treating heart failure. *Prescriber* **12**: 75–95.

Online resources

www.bhf.org.uk
The website of the British Heart Foundation, providing patient information (accessed April 2008).

16

Thromboembolic prophylaxis

Thrombosis

Thrombosis is the unwanted formation of blood clots and may be venous or arterial. Venous thrombosis is associated with stasis of blood: the major problem is that the clot may become dislodged and travel to the lungs, leading to a life-threatening pulmonary embolism. By contrast, thrombosis formed at an atherosclerotic site may lead to arterial blockage in the heart (myocardial infarction; see Chapter 14), cerebral vessels or the peripheral circulation, resulting in ischaemia and infarction. In addition, atrial fibrillation is associated with the stasis of blood and the formation of thrombi in the left atria, which may become dislodged and result in embolism of cerebral vessels, leading to a cerebrovascular accident. Other important thrombogenic sites include artificial mechanical heart valves.

Venous thrombosis is largely associated with an inappropriate activation of the clotting cascade; the thrombi formed have a high fibrin but a low platelet content. Once again, arterial thrombosis has different characteristics, with platelet activation playing a central role. This has a bearing on prevention, because venous thrombosis is largely managed by anticoagulants and arterial thrombosis largely by antiplatelet agents (see Chapter 14), although anticoagulants may also have a role in limiting recruitment of the clotting cascade in arterial thrombosis. Thrombosis associated with atrial fibrillation involves activation of both clotting factors and platelets, hence anticoagulants are predominantly used, although aspirin may also be effective as prophylaxis in low-risk patients.

Risk factors for venous thrombosis include oral contraceptives, hormone replacement therapy, a history of thrombosis, recent surgery, immobility, obesity, pregnancy, malignancy and previous myocardial infarction. Risk factors for arterial thrombosis are detailed in Chapter 14.

Goals of treatment

The goals of treatment are prophylaxis against either arterial or venous thrombosis, and the preventive treatment is targeted at those at risk. Specific targets for treatment with anticoagulants are detailed in Table 16.1.

Pharmacological basis of management

Anticoagulants

Injectable anticoagulants: unfractionated heparin and low-molecular-weight heparins (e.g. dalteparin, enoxaparin, tinzaparin)

Heparin is a glycosaminoglycan found naturally in mast cells and the vascular endothelium. Due to the size of this polymer, heparin is poorly absorbed from the gastrointestinal tract and is therefore given by subcutaneous or intravenous injection. Heparin activates antithrombin III, a natural protein, which inactivates some clotting factors and thrombin by complexing with their serine protease component. Accordingly, the effects of heparin are rapid in onset and are given when anticoagulation is required immediately. Heparin is available as either unfractionated heparin (average molecular mass 15 kDa) or low-molecular-weight heparin (LMWH) (average

Table 16.1   Target international normalized ratios (INRs) for various indications for warfarin

Indication	Target INR	Duration of treatment
Pulmonary embolism	2.5	6 months
Proximal deep vein thrombosis	2.5	6 months
Calf vein thrombosis (non-surgical)	2.5	3 months
Postoperative calf vein thrombosis	2.5	6 weeks
Recurrence of deep vein thrombosis or pulmonary embolism in patients not taking warfarin	2.5	Indefinite
Recurrence of deep vein thrombosis or pulmonary embolism in patients already taking warfarin	3.5	Indefinite
Atrial fibrillation	2.5	Long term
Mural thrombosis after an MI	2.5	3 months
Mechanical prosthetic heart valves	2.5–3.5 (depends on valve type)	Lifelong

Information obtained from the oral anticoagulant guidelines of the British Society for Haematology (1998; updated 2005).
MI, myocardial infarction.

molecular mass 4.5 kDa). Compared with unfractionated heparins, LMWHs have greater activity against factor Xa and less against thrombin. Unfractionated heparins may also reduce platelet aggregation, which does not occur with LMWHs.

Oral anticoagulants: warfarin

Warfarin is a vitamin K antagonist, which inhibits the enzyme vitamin K reductase required for vitamin K to act as a cofactor in the production of clotting factors. In this regard, vitamin K is essential for the post-translational modification by carboxylation of glutamic acid residues of prothrombin and factors VII, IX and X. Accordingly, warfarin inhibits the hepatic synthesis of these clotting factors and its action is apparent only after several days, once the existing clotting factors have been replaced by these newly synthesized, defective factors. The inhibition persists for 4–5 days after the withdrawal of warfarin.

Antiplatelet drugs

Aspirin and clopidogrel are dealt with in Chapter 14, in the context of their major role in the primary and secondary prevention of myocardial infarction and cerebrovascular accidents. Dipyri-

damole is also an antiplatelet drug that is thought to act via phosphodiesterase inhibition and so potentiate camp (adenosine cyclic 3':5'-monophosphate, cAMP), leading to an inhibition of platelet activation. This mechanism of action will potentiate endogenous prostacyclin and synergize with low-dose aspirin.

Thrombin inhibitors

The difficulty in using warfarin has meant that drug discovery has aimed to develop safer oral anticoagulants. Dabigatran has recently been introduced to therapy and acts via inhibition of thrombin in the coagulation cascade. Although experience is limited with this group of drugs, there are fewer interactions and their actions appear more predictable. This class of drugs, therefore, has promise as a safer alternative to warfarin.

Clinical use of anticoagulants

Oral anticoagulants have a number of indications to prevent thrombosis, which are listed in Table 16.1. To initiate treatment with warfarin it must be borne in mind that it will take several days for full effects to become apparent, while in the meantime there may be an increased chance of clotting due to lowering of the levels of protein C (a protein generated from a vitamin K-dependent precursor, which destroys certain clotting factors). Therefore, heparin is started at the same time to 'anticoagulate' the patient and this should be continued until the target international normalized ratio (INR) has been achieved and maintained for 2 days.

Use of heparin

Heparin may be used to initiate anticoagulant treatment or is given for a short, defined period for the prevention of postoperative thromboembolism, e.g. after surgery and in particular after orthopaedic surgery. In terms of clinical use, LMWHs have the advantage of once-daily administration by subcutaneous injection.

The anticoagulant effects of unfractionated heparin are monitored daily by the activated partial thromboplastin time (APTT), with a target value of 1.5–2.0, and the dose is altered to maintain this. By contrast, LMWHs do not require monitoring because their effects are predictable (and they do not prolong APTT). In addition, the use of heparin is associated with thrombocytopenia (less so with LMWH) and with sustained use (>5 days) the platelet count should be monitored.

Initiation of warfarin

Before starting warfarin, it is appropriate to monitor liver function and the INR. The INR is the key anticoagulant screen for warfarin and is the prothrombin time (the normalized time for thromboplastin to cause clotting when added to citrated plasma compared to a standard). The INR is measured during initiation to achieve a target, which depends on the indication (Table 16.1), and should be maintained at this level by altering the dose of warfarin. The INR should be determined daily or on alternate days and then at longer intervals, depending on response (unless a change in clinical condition or administration of other drugs dictates otherwise). Once stabilized, the INR should be monitored at least every 12 weeks.

Warfarin is not indicated for ischaemic stroke without atrial fibrillation. After coronary artery thrombosis, coronary artery bypass grafting or coronary angioplasty, low-dose aspirin (see Chapter 14) and/or heparin should be considered. Heparin is also considered for unstable angina.

When initiating treatment, the patient is typically loaded with warfarin doses of 10 mg, 10 mg and then 5 mg on 3 consecutive days and the INR should be reviewed on day 4 to determine the maintenance dose. In patients who initially have a higher INR (>1.2), e.g. through age, liver disease or warfarin-potentiating drugs, the loading doses should be reduced.

For patients whose anticoagulant therapy is poorly controlled and who have an elevated INR, a number of procedures may be carried out. These are given in more detail in the *British National Formulary* (Section 2.8.2) but, depending on the extent of increase, involve dose reduction or withholding doses, oral or intravenous vitamin K and, in the presence of severe bleeding, the administration of clotting factors or, failing that, fresh frozen plasma. Heparin is reversed with protamine, although it is less effective against LMWHs.

Drug choice

Before initiating warfarin treatment, patients must be identified as able to adhere strictly to the regimen and sufficiently motivated and compliant to ensure that their INR is monitored regularly.

Pregnancy

Warfarin is teratogenic if it is given during the first trimester and particularly after 6 weeks of gestation. During the last few weeks of pregnancy and during delivery warfarin may cross the placenta, leading to a risk of placental or fetal haemorrhage. Vitamin K deficiency of neonates may also be an issue. Warfarin should therefore be avoided during pregnancy and in particular during the first and third trimesters. Heparin does not cross the placenta into the fetus and may be used under expert supervision, although prolonged use is associated with osteoporosis.

Non-rheumatic atrial fibrillation

The prevention of stroke in this condition is subject to various views. The Oral Anticoagulant guidelines of the British Society for Haematology (1998, updated 2005) suggest that warfarin is appropriate in moderate- and high-risk patients (those with hypertension, previous thromboembolism, heart failure or left ventricular dysfunction). Guidance from Clinical Knowledge Summaries (formerly called PRODIGY, see www.cks.library.nhs.uk) suggests that warfarin should be prescribed to patients aged >65 years or <65 years with risk factors (hypertension, diabetes mellitus, previous thromboembolism, heart failure or left ventricular dysfunction). With regard to the benefits of using warfarin in atrial fibrillation, some evidence-based guidelines have been produced by Thomson *et al* (2000). In low-risk patients (with no risk factors), low-dose aspirin alone may be sufficient. Aspirin should also be considered for patients who are unsuitable for warfarin. In general, warfarin reduces the incidence of stroke by two-thirds and aspirin by about one-fifth. Patients with permanent atrial fibrillation who are candidates for electrical cardioversion should receive warfarin for 3 weeks before this procedure.

Atrial fibrillation in rheumatic heart disease

This presents a much higher risk for stroke and the current guidelines of the British Society for Haematology recommend warfarin for all patients.

Deep vein thrombosis

Deep vein thrombosis (DVT) is associated with immobility leading to stasis of blood and hypercoagulability: pregnant and postoperative patients are at an increased risk. The major complication is that the thrombus may dislodge and lead to a life-threatening pulmonary embolism. Patients with DVTs should be heparinized and non-pregnant patients should then be initiated on warfarin.

'Economy-class syndrome'

This term describes DVT leading to pulmonary embolism associated with prolonged travel; whether it is exacerbated by air travel has yet to be established. It is associated with immobility, and so exercise and wearing compression stockings may be effective. Recommended exercises include short walks, bending and straightening legs, feet and toes, and pressing feet on the ground. Passengers should also avoid excess alcohol and becoming dehydrated. Passengers with a moderate risk for DVT (e.g. pregnancy, heart disease, family history of DVT, hormonal contraception, hormone replacement therapy) may consider low-dose aspirin and support stockings. Recommending low-dose aspirin to all passengers seems unwise, as the risk of gastric bleeding in the general population is greater than the risk of DVT. The Department of Health (2001) has advised that patients at high risk due to previous DVT, clotting tendency (thrombophilia), a history of cancer, major surgery in the past 3 months (including hip or knee replacement) or stroke should consult their GP. High-risk patients may be prescribed an LMWH and/or advised to wear compression stockings.

Concurrent disease

Warfarin is contraindicated in peptic ulcer disease, severe hypertension and bacterial endocarditis and should not be used in cerebral thrombosis or peripheral arterial occlusion as first-line therapy. It should be used with caution after recent surgery. Warfarin itself is associated with a significant risk of haemorrhagic stroke.

Heparin is also contraindicated in patients with peptic ulcer, severe hypertension in addition to haemophilia and other haemorrhagic disorders, thrombocytopenia, recent cerebral haemorrhage, severe liver disease including oesophageal varices, major trauma or recent surgery.

Hepatic disease

Oral anticoagulants should be avoided in severe liver disease, particularly if the prothrombin time is already prolonged. The dose of heparin should be reduced in severe liver disease.

Renal disease

Oral anticoagulants should be avoided in severe renal impairment. There is an increased risk of bleeding when heparin is given in severe renal impairment.

Monitoring

INR, APTT and platelets

See earlier.

Electrolytes

Heparin inhibits aldosterone secretion and may possibly result in hyperkalaemia. The risk increases with prolonged therapy and in patients with diabetes mellitus, chronic renal failure, acidosis and those taking drugs that increase plasma potassium (such as potassium-sparing diuretics and angiotensin-converting enzyme [ACE] inhibitors; see Table 2.2, and Chapters 11 and 15). Potassium levels should be monitored before starting heparin in patients at risk and regularly throughout treatment, particularly if the treatment period is >7 days.

Drug interactions

Potentiation

Warfarin shows a notoriously wide range of drug interactions, which are of clinical importance because of its narrow therapeutic index. The most common interactions usually result in the enhancement of anticoagulant activity, and this appears largely to result from competition or inhibition of hepatic metabolism, although it is sometimes through displacement from protein-binding sites. The enhancement may lead to increased bleeding. Inhibitors of metabolism are likely to have rapid effects on the levels of warfarin. However, this alteration will take several days to have an effect on the INR and these effects will reverse on stopping the inhibitor, although, in the case of drugs with long half-lives, such as amiodarone, they may persist for some time. The dose of warfarin may then need to be altered.

In choosing drugs for patients who are taking warfarin the ideal is to select drugs that do not interact. When starting drugs known to interact with warfarin the British Society for Haematology (1998) recommends the following:

- For drug changes lasting less than 5 days with a known potentiating drug: no change, minor dose reduction for warfarin or omit one dose of warfarin.
- For longer drug changes: monitor INR after 1 week and alter warfarin dose accordingly.

In addition, when warfarin is initiated in a patient who is already taking a known interacting drug, the loading dose may need to be altered.

Some important drugs that may enhance the actions of warfarin (D indicates that a dose reduction of warfarin is likely) include:

- allopurinol
- amiodarone – may persist after discontinuation of amiodarone due to its long half-life (D)
- azapropazone (contraindicated)
- azoles – fluconazole, ketoconazole, miconazole
- clarithromycin
- co-trimoxazole (D)
- cytotoxic agents (carboplatin, mustine, cyclophosphamide, doxorubicin, etoposide, 5-fluorouracil, ifosfamide/mesna, methotrexate, procarbazine, vincristine and vindesine)
- disulfiram (D)
- erythromycin
- fibrates (D)
- H_2-receptor antagonists, cimetidine (famotidine, nizatidine and ranitidine are less likely to interact)
- hydrocodone (rarely)
- interferon
- isoniazid (rarely)
- lansoprazole (rarely)
- levothyroxine (D)
- metronidazole (D)
- non-steroidal anti-inflammatory drugs (NSAIDs) – diclofenac and flurbiprofen may increase INR
- omeprazole

- paracetamol – monitoring is required if taken regularly, but safer than aspirin
- penicillins (occasionally)
- quinolones
- selective serotonin reuptake inhibitors (SSRIs): fluoxetine (rarely)
- statins
- sulfinpyrazone (D)
- sulphonamides (D)
- tamoxifen (D)
- tetracyclines (rarely)
- tricyclic antidepressants
- zafirlukast (D).

In addition the anticoagulant effects of warfarin may lead to enhanced bleeding with antiplatelet drugs (aspirin, clopidogrel, dipyridamole) or drugs that lead to gastric bleeding. Aspirin may be combined with warfarin but there is an increase in bleeding tendency, although this is less marked with low doses. Warfarin may also lead to gastric bleeding with aspirin and other NSAIDs. Patients should be advised to use paracetamol for pain relief.

Reduced activity

Less frequently agents will reduce the activity of warfarin and this appears to be due to induction of its metabolism. In dealing with inducers, they take several days to alter the concentrations of warfarin and longer to alter the INR, and these effects are likely to persist for some time after an inducer is stopped. The dose of warfarin may then need to be altered.

Some important drugs that may reduce the actions of warfarin include:

- barbiturates
- carbamazepine – oxacarbazepine appears safe
- colestyramine – separate doses
- cytotoxic agents (azathioprine, cyclophosphamide, mercaptopurine and mitotane)
- disopyramide
- griseofulvin
- phenytoin – monitoring of both warfarin and phenytoin is required (see Chapter 23)
- rifampicin – the dose of warfarin may need to be increased (two- to threefold) several days after rifampicin is started
- St John's wort (avoid)

- vitamin K supplements and diet (including spinach, Brussels sprouts, broccoli, liver, lettuce)
- oral contraceptives – contraindicated in thromboembolic disorders.

The above lists have largely been compiled from *Stockley's Drug Interactions* by Baxter (2008). The list gives some important examples but more complete information should be sought from more detailed sources, including *Stockley's Drug Interactions*.

Over-the-counter considerations

Health professionals should be aware of products containing vitamin K, which may antagonize the effect of warfarin, e.g. multivitamin supplements and liquid dietary supplements. Herbal drugs also have the potential to interact with warfarin (see Chapter 4), e.g. close monitoring is required with garlic supplements. The dose of warfarin may need to be adjusted.

General counselling

In talking to patients, warfarin ('rat poison') is usually referred to as 'thinning the blood'. It should be made absolutely clear to patients that they must stick to their dosage regimen and take it at the same time of day, conventionally at 6pm. If they miss a dose they should not take two doses together and they should inform their doctor at the next blood test.

- Patients should be informed that they must tell any doctor, dentist or pharmacist who treats them that they are receiving warfarin. The need to mention their treatment is essential when purchasing over-the-counter (OTC) medicines (including creams and gels, e.g. antifungal imidazoles) and supplements. Preparations containing vitamin K should be avoided.
- Females of child-bearing age should be advised not to become pregnant while taking warfarin.

- Alcohol may be consumed in moderation but not in excess.
- Patients should avoid excessive consumption of green vegetables (particularly spinach, Brussels sprouts, lettuce, broccoli) and beetroot and liver. Changes to diets rich in vitamin K should be discussed with a health-care professional, because a dose change of warfarin may be required. Warfarin therapy may also be altered after the consumption of regular or large quantities of foods such as avocado, ice cream, soybean protein and the sweetener aspartame.

Patients should report:

- haemoptysis
- blood in faeces
- blood in urine
- nose bleeds
- easy bruising
- skin changes (necrosis)

and consult their doctor if they have diarrhoea or vomiting for 2 days or more.

Self-assessment

Consider whether the following statements are true or false. In terms of anticoagulants:

1. Heparin acts immediately.
2. The actions of heparin are monitored by the INR.
3. Warfarin inhibits blood coagulation in a test tube.
4. The actions of warfarin are opposed by vitamin B_{12}.
5. The activity of warfarin is often enhanced by concomitant erythromycin.

Practice points

- Patients require extensive counselling to ensure compliance.
- Guidelines on oral anticoagulation of the British Society for Haematology (1998) should be consulted.
- Warfarin interacts with many drugs and the pharmacist should be vigilant of this and look for signs of enhanced actions of warfarin.
- Consider all requests for OTC medicines (especially NSAIDs) as a potential for drug interactions.

   CASE STUDY

A 70-year-old man who has chronic atrial fibrillation associated with left ventricular failure is currently receiving:

lisinopril 10 mg once daily
furosemide 40 mg every morning
digoxin 62.5 micrograms once daily
amiodarone 200 mg once daily.

continued

CASE STUDY (continued)

Make a recommendation for thromboembolic prophylaxis.

- The patient is over 65 years old, and has heart failure, which means that he is at moderate risk of thromboembolic complications. Given his moderate risk, he is likely to receive warfarin (if anticoagulation is required immediately then he might also receive heparin). However, it should be noted that amiodarone will enhance the actions of warfarin so, unless an alternative anti-arrhythmic (sotalol) or digoxin alone is considered sufficient, his loading dose may need to be reduced and his INR (target 2.5) will need to be closely monitored with a view to dose reductions. Note the low maintenance dose of digoxin, which has been used as amiodarone increases the plasma concentrations of digoxin.

He is stabilized on warfarin but develops a bacterial chest infection. Comment on antibiotic treatment.

- Amoxicillin is first choice and, according to *Stockley's Drug Interactions* (Baxter 2008), only rarely interacts with warfarin. Monitoring is, however, advisable, at least before the antibiotic is added. Second-line agents include erythromycin, which may enhance the actions of warfarin.

References

Baxter K, ed. (2008). *Stockley's Drug Interaction*, 8th edn. London: Pharmaceutical Press.

Department of Health (2001). *Advice on Travel-related Deep Vein Thrombosis*. London: Department of Health.

British Society for Haematology (1998). Guidelines on oral anticoagulation. *Br J Haematol* **101**: 374–87. Updated in 2005, *Br J Haematol* **132**: 277–85.

Martin J, ed. *British National Formulary*, latest edition. London: British Medical Association and Royal Pharmaceutical Society of Great Britain.

Thomson R, Parkin D, Eccles M *et al* (2000). Decision analysis and guidelines for anticoagulant therapy to prevent stroke in patients with atrial fibrillation. *Lancet* **355**: 956–62.

Further reading

Heck AM, DeWitt BA, Lukes AL (2000). Potential interactions between alternative therapies and warfarin. *Am J Health Syst Pharm* **13**: 1221–7.

Hoffbrand AV, Pettit JE, Moss PAH (2001). *Essential Haematology*, 4th edn. Oxford: Blackwell Science.

Lip GYH, Lowe GDO (1996). ABC of atrial fibrillation: antithrombotic treatment of atrial fibrillation. *BMJ* **312**: 45–9.

17

Anaemias

As with several medical specialities, haematology encompasses both minor and serious conditions. Of relevance to the pharmacist are the anaemias, because these are important conditions that are encountered on a regular basis: simple iron-deficiency anaemia is of particular importance.

Anaemias are characterized by reduced levels of haemoglobin and occur when the haemoglobin is <13.5 g/dL in males and <11.5 g/dL in females. The signs and symptoms depend on the severity but are related to impaired oxygen transport and delivery due to reduced levels of haemoglobin. Key symptoms include:

- weakness
- lethargy
- impaired exercise tolerance
- shortness of breath.

although cardiovascular adaptations, coupled to reduced blood viscosity, may result in tachycardia. In severe anaemia, particularly in more elderly people, there may be angina due to impaired delivery of oxygen to the cardiac muscle, and anaemia may also lead to heart failure. Skin colour is not a reliable sign, because this is determined by blood flow, but pale nail beds and conjunctiva may be present. In haemolytic anaemias, jaundice may be present.

Iron-deficiency anaemia

As the name implies, it is due to impaired iron balance and for this to occur the bone marrow's iron stores must be depleted. The deficiency in iron leads to impaired synthesis of haemoglobin and the production of smaller red cells, which have a reduced mean corpuscular volume (MCV <75 fL; see Appendix 2), and this is referred to as microcytic anaemia. In addition to the above features, the patient may also have:

- spoon nails (koilonychia)
- sores on the corner of the mouth (angular stomatitis)
- painful, red tongue (glossitis)
- unusual food cravings.

As commented above, for iron-deficiency anaemia to develop the iron stores must be depleted. As the diet normally provides the body's requirement for iron, coupled with the fact that iron is efficiently recycled from destroyed red cells, iron-deficiency anaemia is a chronic condition that occurs when input is impaired, output is increased or there are increased demands.

Input is reduced with:

- poor diet (in infants)
- surgical removal of stomach
- malabsorption (coeliac disease, Crohn's disease).

Clinically the main cause is when there is chronic and excessive blood loss through:

- gastrointestinal bleeding (often from ulcers and chronic non-steroidal anti-inflammatory drug [NSAID]-induced damage, but also from colitis, carcinoma, haemorrhoids)
- chronic heavy menstruation (menorrhagia); hence iron-deficiency anaemia is more common in women due to a more precarious iron balance

Demand is increased in pregnancy due to the fetal requirements and the expansion in the maternal circulating volume, and anaemia, to varying degrees, is very common. Pregnancy tends to increase corpuscular volume and any iron deficiency tends to reduce the volume; these opposing factors may cancel out, leading to normocytic anaemia.

Goals of treatment

These are twofold: to identify and treat the underlying cause and to restore both the iron stores and the level of haemoglobin.

Pharmacological management

The most straightforward approach to restoring iron stores is to give ferrous iron. This is generally in the simple and inexpensive form of oral ferrous sulphate, although this may be poorly tolerated due to gastric irritation and other forms may be used, such as ferrous fumarate. Slow-release preparations have lower bioavailability, as the iron is released in the lower small intestine, where it is not absorbed. The ferrous sulphate is given as 200 mg up to three times daily (once or twice daily in less severe anaemia) with a view to building up the iron stores and increasing the haemoglobin at a rate of approximately 1 g/dL per week. The first response that may be measured is an increase in the reticulocyte count, due to newly formed maturing red blood cells. Once the haemoglobin has returned to normal, iron therapy should be continued for 3 months to build up the iron stores. In prophylaxis of anaemia in pregnancy, the iron may be combined with low doses of folic acid, to ensure an adequate supply of folate.

Interactions with iron therapy

Iron preparations exhibit a range of interactions, largely related to the reduced absorption of the iron or the interacting drug from the gastrointestinal tract. Some important examples are detailed in Table 17.1.

Counselling

The patient should be counselled that the anaemia is likely to be a symptom of another

Table 17.1   Clinically significant interactions of iron preparations with other drugs

Interacting drugs	Consequences	Comments
Ferrous salts with antacids	Antacids reduce the absorption of ferrous salts	Their administration should be separated. H_2-receptor antagonists do not significantly affect the absorption of ferrous salts
Ferrous salts with colestyramine	Colestyramine binds ferrous salts and may reduce their absorption	Their administration should be separated
Ferrous salts with neomycin	Neomycin may increase or decrease the absorption of ferrous salts	
Ferrous salts with quinolones	Ferrous salts decrease the absorption of quinolones	The quinolone should be taken at least 2 h before the ferrous salt
Ferrous salts with tetracyclines	Concomitant administration of these agents reduces the plasma concentrations of both iron and tetracyclines	Their doses should be separated
Ferrous salts with levodopa or carbidopa	Ferrous sulphate reduces the bioavailability of these antiparkinsonian drugs	Their doses should be separated and the control of Parkinson's disease monitored
Ferrous sulphate with levothyroxine	Ferrous sulphate reduces the effects of levothyroxine	Their doses should be separated

condition, which should be identified and treated. If patients request iron tablets without a diagnosis, they should be referred to their GP for a blood test and, if appropriate, identification of the underlying cause.

Iron

Clearly, counselling should be directed towards ensuring compliance and completing the course of iron until stores are replenished. The doses should be evenly spaced or at least 6 h apart because absorption may be reduced by the previous dose. Patients should also be alerted to any important interactions and advised not to take over-the-counter antacids at the same time as the iron salt. The patient should also be made aware of the side effects of iron; these largely affect the gastrointestinal tract and include:

• gastric irritation, which may be reduced by taking the iron with food; however, this may reduce its absorption (although foods rich in vitamin C may actually enhance absorption)
• nausea
• altered bowel habits with constipation or diarrhoea
• the stools will be darkly coloured
• excessive iron is toxic in children.

Foods rich in iron include (Webster-Gandy *et al* 2006):

• Meat (especially liver)
• Eggs
• Fish
• Dark-green leafy vegetables and pulses
• Bread and flour
• Yeast extract
• Breakfast cereals (especially bran flakes).

Megaloblastic anaemia

This is a rarer form of anaemia due to abnormal red blood cell maturation as a result of defective DNA synthesis, and the bone marrow contains megaloblasts, abnormal precursor cells in which nuclear maturation is impaired in relation to that of the cytoplasm. The abnormal production of red cells results in increased cell volume and is referred to as macrocytic anaemia (MCV >95 fL); there is also a reduced level of haemoglobin. An increased MCV without anaemia may be due to alcohol misuse – a common cause of macrocytosis, which is unrelated to megaloblastic anaemia. However, in severe alcoholism, the toxic effects of alcohol on the bone marrow may lead to megaloblastic anaemia.

In megaloblastic anaemia the symptoms are those of mild anaemia and may also include jaundice, because the enlarged red cells are more likely to undergo haemolysis, raising the level of bilirubin. Megaloblastic anaemia is due to a deficiency of either vitamin B_{12} or folate, and this may be associated with a painful red tongue (glossitis), sores at the corner of the mouth (angular stomatitis) and neuropathy (in vitamin B_{12} deficiency).

Vitamin B_{12} (as a cofactor) and folate (as component) are essential for DNA synthesis, and a deficiency of either impairs synthesis. As there is a substantial rate of red blood cell production with a high requirement for DNA synthesis, impaired DNA synthesis results in the formation of megaloblasts in the bone marrow. In severe forms impaired DNA synthesis may lead to reduced production of white blood cells and/or platelets.

Deficiencies of vitamin B_{12} can be due to:

• vegan diet
• Crohn's disease, which leads to impaired absorption of vitamin B_{12}
• gastrectomy, which leads to the loss of the intrinsic factor for the absorption of vitamin B_{12}
• metformin, which may reduce the absorption of vitamin B_{12}.

In addition, pernicious anaemia is a special subset and is due to an autoimmune destruction of the intrinsic factor, which is released by the stomach to facilitate the absorption of vitamin B_{12}.

Folate deficiency may be due to:

• dietary deficiency in people with alcohol problems
• pregnancy due to increased demand
• malabsorption in coeliac disease

- chronic inflammatory conditions such as Crohn's disease, rheumatoid arthritis, tuberculosis
- drug induced: methotrexate and trimethoprim are folate antagonists by inhibition of dihydrofolate reductase; phenytoin and phenobarbital may also cause deficiency, possibly due to enzyme induction increasing the requirement for folate.

Pharmacological management

This clearly depends on the cause. If a deficiency of vitamin B_{12} is identified as the cause then hydroxocobalamin is given intramuscularly, which avoids the need for absorption from the gastrointestinal tract, because this may be impaired. Oral vitamin B_{12} may of course be used in otherwise healthy vegans. Once the stores have been replaced, maintenance treatment may need to be continued for life. Intramuscular hydroxocobalamin is also appropriate as prophylaxis in patients who have had gastrectomy or ileal resection.

Folate deficiency is simply treated by oral folic acid (5–15 mg daily) and this, depending on the cause, may need to be life long.

Drug interactions

The drugs used to treat megaloblastic anaemia have a limited number of interactions (Table 17.2).

Other anaemias

There is a range of other anaemias that are beyond the scope of this book. However, a brief description of some of them may be appropriate.

Renal anaemia

The kidney is the source of the hormone erythropoietin, which is released in hypoxia (secondary to anaemia, climbing to altitude and chronic obstructive pulmonary disease, for example) and acts on the bone marrow to increase the production of red blood cells. Renal failure is associated with reduced levels of erythropoietin, which leads to normocytic anaemia. Patients with renal failure and those on dialysis accordingly receive erythropoietin. They may also receive prophylactic iron and folic acid (see Chapter 18).

Table 17.2   Clinically significant interactions of folic acid or vitamin B_{12} with other drugs

Interacting drugs	Consequences	Comments
Folic acid with phenytoin, phenobarbital	As commented above, these anticonvulsants may lead to folate deficiency	In patients treated with folate, the concentrations of the anticonvulsants may fall, leading to impaired seizure control. Monitoring and dose adjustment may be required
Folic acid with trimethoprim, co-trimoxazole	The weak antifolate actions of trimethoprim may substantially reduce the effectiveness of folic acid	They should not be used together
Folic acid with magnesium trisilicate	The absorption of folic acid is reduced	
Folic acid with sulfasalazine	The absorption of folic acid is reduced	
Vitamin B_{12} with H_2-receptor antagonists	H_2-receptor antagonists reduce the absorption of oral vitamin B_{12}	Analogues given by injection are not affected

Haemolytic anaemias

This is a class of anaemia and is due to excessive destruction of red cells, which leads to reduced haemoglobin levels. The increased breakdown of red blood cells leads to raised bilirubin levels and this results in jaundice. This may occur in megaloblastic anaemia. The increased erythropoiesis required to replace the cells may actually lead to folate deficiency. Examples of this include:

- spherocytosis: a genetic and abnormal reduction in the red blood cell membrane protein, spectrin, which leads to fragile cells
- sickle cell anaemia: due to the haemolysis of the sickle-shaped cells
- in glucose-6-phosphate dehydrogenase (G6PD) deficiency, where certain drugs may cause red cell damage (see Chapter 5)
- infections such as malaria.

Aplastic anaemia

This is a serious condition in which there is insufficient production of red blood cells, white blood cells and platelets (pancytopenia). The patient has decreased resistance to infections, increased bleeding and the symptoms of anaemia. Most cases are acquired due to viral infection, radiation or drugs (including cytotoxic agents, chloramphenicol, sulphonamides and insecticides). Treatment is via antilymphocyte globulin to prevent suppressor killer T cells from damaging the stem cells, ciclosporin and sometimes bone marrow transplantation for cure.

Drug-induced haematological changes

See Chapter 5.

Self-assessment

Consider whether the following statements with regard to anaemias are true or false:

1. Iron deficiency anaemia is macrocytic.
2. Iron deficiency anaemia is most commonly caused by a poor diet.
3. Haemolytic anaemias may lead to jaundice.
4. Megaloblastic anaemia is best managed by vitamin K injections.
5. Pregnancy is a contraindication to iron sulphate therapy.

Practice points

- Iron-deficiency anaemia is a common occurrence and its underlying cause should be identified and treated.
- Iron-deficiency anaemia may be a presenting feature of NSAID-induced gastric damage.
- Iron preparations have a range of drug interactions.

Reference

Webster-Gandy J, Madden A, Holdsworth M, eds (2006). *Oxford Handbook of Nutrition and Dietetics*. Oxford: Oxford University Press.

Further reading

Hoffbrand AV, Pettit JE, Moss PAH (2001). *Essential Haematology*, 4th edn. Oxford: Blackwell Science.

18

The renal patient

This chapter deals specifically with the management issues surrounding patients with renal impairment, which may be associated with other conditions such as diabetes mellitus, hypertension or chronic heart failure. Renal failure has important implications for drug treatment but is a condition in its own right, which must be managed with a view to preserving renal function and dealing with its complications such as anaemia, bone disease, hypertension and uraemia. The focus of this chapter is on renal impairment and chronic renal failure, which are likely to be encountered in primary care, whereas acute renal failure is largely beyond the scope of this book.

Renal function is reflected by the glomerular filtration rate (GFR), which may be estimated from plasma creatinine levels (see Chapter 2) or estimated GFR (eGFR). In terms of renal function, the following classes are used to classify chronic kidney disease (CKD):

GFR: >90 mL/min per 1.73 m^2 with signs of kidney damage (CKD stage 1)
GFR: 89–60 mL/min per 1.73 m^2 – mild renal impairment (CKD stage 2)
GFR: 59–30 mL/min per 1.73 m^2 – moderate renal impairment (CKD stage 3)
GFR: 29–15 mL/min per 1.73 m^2 – severe renal impairment (CKD stage 4)
GFR: <15 mL/min per 1.73 m^2 or dialysis – renal failure (CKD stage 5).

Renal failure may be acute or chronic and is classified according to cause:

- Prerenal: this involves reduced renal perfusion, as occurs acutely in hypovolaemia, and secondary to heart failure or renal artery stenosis.

- Intrinsic: this represents pathological damage to the tubular, interstitial or glomerular regions that occurs in the kidney itself and may be due to diabetic nephropathy, hypertension, glomerulonephritis (which is largely an immunological disease), pyelonephritis (associated with infection) or nephrotoxic damage, e.g. caused by drugs (see Chapter 5).
- Postrenal: this is secondary to impaired renal outflow as occurs with renal stones, tumours and prostatism.

Acute renal failure

Management of acute renal failure

This topic is beyond the scope of this book but the mainstays of therapy are diuretics and the use of dopamine as a renal vasodilator, coupled with the correction of potassium levels.

Chronic renal failure

Chronic failure represents a long-term deterioration in renal function with the progressive loss of nephrons and impaired renal function over many years. The most common causes are glomerulonephritis, diabetic nephropathy and hypertension. The consequences of chronic renal failure are related to the extent of impairment. Characteristically there is protein loss in the urine (proteinuria), which leads to less protein in the plasma (hypoalbuminaemia). This resulting reduction in colloidal osmotic pressure in the plasma, coupled with reduced water excretion, leads to tissue oedema. Impaired excretion of toxins leads to uraemia which represents the build-up of urea, phosphate, guanidines, phenols and organic acids in the blood, and leads to the following clinical features:

- skin coloration (lemon tinge)
- itching
- nausea and vomiting
- constipation
- pericarditis
- neurological changes, which may include personality changes and cognitive impairment
- fatigue, which is an important presenting complaint.

The impaired renal function leads to significant changes in blood biochemistry which may include:

- increased creatinine and urea
- hyperkalaemia
- hyponatraemia or normal sodium levels
- hypocalcaemia
- hyperphosphataemia
- acidosis.

In addition, chronic renal failure is associated with the following complications.

Complications

Anaemia

Normocytic anaemia occurs secondary to chronic renal failure, as the kidneys produce erythropoietin (EPO) which regulates red cell production (see Chapter 17) and its absence will reduce red cell synthesis. In addition, the uraemic toxins may cause bone marrow suppression and further depress red cell synthesis.

Renal bone disease (renal osteodystrophy)

The kidneys play a major role in calcium balance and renal failure also has consequences for bone mineralization. In this respect the kidney is involved in the activation of vitamin D_3 (colecalciferol). Specifically, dietary and endogenously synthesized colecalciferol is converted by the liver to 25-hydroxycolecalciferol, which is then converted by renal 1α-hydroxylase to 1,25-hydroxycholecalciferol. This more active derivative is involved in promoting calcium uptake from the gastrointestinal tract, and is consequently impaired in renal failure. This reduction in calcium absorption leads to less calcium for bone mineralization. Furthermore, the reduced levels of 1,25-hydroxycholecalciferol lead to an increase in the release of parathyroid hormone (PTH) from the parathyroid gland as a negative feedback in response to reduced levels of 1,25-hydroxycholecalciferol. In addition, low calcium also stimulates the release of PTH and this results in hyperparathyroidism, which is associated with increased osteoclastic resorption of bone and calcium release. The calcium may be deposited at sites other than skeletal muscle such as blood vessels. In addition, phosphate excretion is impaired in renal failure, leading to increased phosphate in the plasma, which also promotes calcium loss from the bones. Consequently, renal failure is associated with impaired bone mineralization, which carries the risk of fractures.

Hypertension

Hypertension is associated with renal failure because renal ischaemia leads to activation of the renin–angiotensin–aldosterone system, resulting in salt and fluid retention together with vasoconstriction. These in turn lead to hypertension and an ensuing vicious circle, which causes further renal damage. Both the hypertension and fluid overload may precipitate heart failure.

Renal failure and impaired drug excretion

Many drugs and/or their metabolites are excreted by the kidneys, especially via the weak acid and base transporters in the proximal tubule.

Consequently, in renal impairment and chronic renal failure, drugs may accumulate and reach toxic levels. Therefore, for renally excreted drugs, impairment should be determined by measuring plasma creatinine levels and estimating the GFR. The *British National Formulary* contains an extensive section dealing with the use of drugs in renal impairment. More specialist and detailed literature includes *Renal Drug Handbook* (Ashley and Currie 2004) which details how specific regimens should be altered. Generally, the approaches to renal impairment are dose reduction of the maintenance dose, increasing the dosing interval or choosing an alternative drug that is not extensively cleared by the kidneys, e.g. digoxin is largely renally excreted and plasma levels will rise in renal impairment. This is dealt with by either reducing the maintenance dose of digoxin or using digitoxin as an alternative that largely undergoes hepatic elimination. When a loading dose is required, and the patient has a 'normal' extracellular volume, then the initial dose is unaffected (see Chapter 6), but it may need to be increased if the volume is increased due to oedema or ascites.

Patients with impaired renal function may be more sensitive to the pharmacological actions and side effects of certain drugs, e.g. in the volume-depleted state, α blockers such as prazosin have enhanced hypotensive effects.

Although impaired renal function may lead to drug toxicity through impaired excretion, this may reduce the effectiveness of drugs that require renal excretion for their actions. Examples of these include thiazide diuretics, drugs used in urinary tract infections that require excretion into the bladder to act (e.g. nalidixic acid, nitrofurantoin) and uricosuric agents that promote excretion of uric acid (e.g. probenecid).

Goals of treatment

These are to reduce the progressive loss of renal function, to limit or reverse complications such as anaemia, hypertension and renal bone disease, to reduce uraemia and provide symptomatic relief, and to normalize the electrolytic balance of the body.

Management of chronic renal failure

The degree of intervention required is governed by the degree of renal impairment. Detailed guidance produced by the Renal Association (www.renal.org) and should be consulted.

Management of early chronic renal failure

Early chronic renal failure may be managed with diuretics (see Chapters 11 and 15) and a diet that is low in sodium, potassium and protein. In choosing a diuretic, attention must be paid to renal function, as thiazides and thiazide-like agents (except metolazone) are ineffective in moderate renal failure because they are themselves renally excreted to enable them to act at their site of action, the distal tubule. Loop diuretics may be used in moderate and severe renal impairment but high doses may be required. The object of the low-protein diet is to slow down the accumulation of nitrogenous end-products of protein metabolism. A low-protein diet is, however, associated with malnutrition and the loss of muscle mass and reduced immune responses that are adverse to health.

Management of itching due to uraemia

Chlorphenamine may be used to relieve itching associated with uraemia.

Management of nausea

See Chapter 8.

Management of hypertension

As commented above, hypertension may lead to renal damage and may also be induced in renal damage as a consequence of activation of the renin–angiotensin–aldosterone system. What is clear is that reducing blood pressure with antihypertensive drugs will reduce the rate of loss of renal function, as assessed by a reduction in the rate of decline of GFR and protein excretion. A target blood pressure of 130/80 mmHg or less is aimed for in patients with stable renal failure and a target of 125/75 mmHg in patients with progressive disease with proteinuria.

The Ramipril Efficacy In Nephropathy (REIN) trial by the GISEN Group (1997) reported that ramipril was more effective than blood pressure lowering alone at reducing proteinuria and the rate of decline in GFR in non-diabetic nephropathy. The implication from this is that ramipril, and other angiotensin-converting enzyme (ACE) inhibitors, may be renally protective in renal failure and that ACE inhibitors should therefore be used to treat the hypertension associated with renal failure. Although it should be noted that ACE inhibitors may themselves lead to renal impairment (especially in renovascular disease) and renal function should be monitored, ACE inhibitors may increase potassium and this may enhance hyperkalaemia associated with renal failure. ACE inhibitors may also reduce the release of EPO which may compound the associated anaemia. Angiotensin receptor antagonists can substitute for ACE inhibitors in type 2 diabetes for renal protection (see Chapter 35), but whether this is the case for patients who are not diabetic remains to be determined.

Generally speaking, ACE inhibitors have a significant role in the management of hypertension in renal disease, especially when there is proteinuria. Calcium channel blockers are also widely used.

Hyperlipidaemia

There is an association of hypercholesterolaemia and hypertriglyceridaemia with renal failure and statins are often prescribed (see Chapter 12) to lower plasma cholesterol and reduce the cardiovascular risk. The dose of statin should take account of the level of renal impairment with appropriate reductions, and fluvastatin should be avoided in severe renal impairment.

Management of renal anaemia

Oral iron is often given initially to build up iron levels before treatment with EPO. EPO may then be given subcutaneously or intravenously, with the dose adjusted to restore haemoglobin levels to a target of >10 g/dL. The treatment of anaemia should improve exercise tolerance and reduce the risk of precipitating heart failure. EPO is, however, associated with an increase in blood pressure in a number of patients. There are also rare reports of pure red cell aplasia (failure of red cell production) in patients receiving EPO-α by the subcutaneous route. This is believed to be due to the production of antibodies to EPO and treatment with EPO should be stopped.

Management of renal bone disease

1α-Hydroxycholecalciferol (alfacalcidol) and calcitriol are hydroxylated derivatives of vitamin D and are given in renal failure to compensate for impaired endogenous production. Patients taking these agents should have their calcium levels measured to avoid hypercalcaemia and the dose is chosen to correct the increased PTH levels.

The additional problem contributing to renal bone disease is phosphate, because its elimination is impaired in renal failure. To reduce this problem, phosphate binders are taken with meals to bind phosphate in the gastrointestinal tract and prevent its absorption. Foods rich in phosphate include protein-rich foods, dairy products, cereals, nuts, chocolate and cola drinks. Phosphate binders used are aluminium hydroxide and calcium salts (carbonate or acetate). Calcium carbonate is the preferred agent, because, although it is less effective, it is safer than aluminium and may also provide a calcium supplement. Aluminium hydroxide has the problem that aluminium may build up in the plasma, with the risk of toxicity, including dementia and aluminium bone disease. Sevelamer is a phosphate binder that is available for patients on haemodialysis.

Aluminium- and calcium-based phosphate binders show a range of interactions by increasing gastric pH and altering the absorption of certain drugs (see Chapters 5 and 7 dealing with antacid interactions). For agents affected in this way, the dose should be separated in time from the phosphate binder. A particularly important interaction is between citrate (in vitamin supplements and effervescent drug formulations) and aluminium hydroxide, which leads to an increase in aluminium levels in the blood and the possibility of encephalopathy. Accordingly, the combination of citrate and aluminium should be avoided.

Management of constipation

Constipation may occur as a result of fluid restriction and the use of aluminium as a phosphate binder, and this may be managed by lactulose and/or senna.

Hyperkalaemia

Increased plasma levels of potassium occur in renal failure and are potentially life threatening if they rise too high. Hyperkalaemia may be prevented by polystyrene sulphonate ion exchange resins such as calcium polystyrene sulphonate, which is given orally or rectally. Sodium polystyrene sulphonate exchanges sodium for potassium in the gastrointestinal tract and is excreted rectally. Sodium polystyrene sulphonate may lead to sodium overload, which should be avoided. These resins are also constipating and a laxative should be given.

Severe hyperkalaemia is treated with insulin (given with glucose to prevent hypoglycaemia), which promotes cellular uptake of potassium.

Dialysis

Once renal function is substantially impaired and pharmacological and dietary means alone do not control the condition, renal function must be replaced by artificial means, involving either peritoneal dialysis or haemodialysis, before transplantation.

Continuous ambulatory peritoneal dialysis

A permanent indwelling catheter is implanted through the abdominal wall. Sterile salt solution (2–3 L), similar to plasma but with no protein or potassium, is repeatedly run into the peritoneal cavity where it lies next to the mesenteric blood vessels. Uraemic substances accumulating in the blood enter the fluid and approach equilibrium. The solution is then discarded and replaced, and this crudely performs the main functions of the kidney. As the dialysate has zero potassium, it equilibrates with plasma and so draws potassium off down its diffusion gradient, e.g. if the plasma potassium concentration is 4 mmol/L then 10 L of dialysate fluid per day transfers 40 mmol of potassium per day. Therefore, dietary potassium must not exceed this or hyperkalaemia will occur. Adding osmotic solute (glucose) to the peritoneal dialysate can produce 1–1.5 L/day of peritoneal water loss by osmosis and the intake must be controlled to match this. This method of dialysis carries a significant risk of peritoneal infection.

Haemodialysis

This involves the exchange of substances from the blood with dialysate across an artificial semipermeable membrane outside the body using a machine. Once again, substances diffuse into the dialysate and altering potassium and glucose concentrations may enable regulation of potassium and circulating volume. Patients receiving haemodialysis are usually anticoagulated with heparin to prevent activation of clotting triggered by the foreign surfaces of the machine.

Drug choice and dialysis

Both continuous ambulatory peritoneal dialysis (CAPD) and haemodialysis provide routes for drug elimination and certain drugs may be efficiently removed from the body via these routes. The elimination will be determined by their permeability across the natural or artificial membranes, protein binding (drugs with high binding are less likely to be eliminated), the degree of hepatic elimination and water solubility. Hence in choosing drugs for patients on dialysis it is important to establish how the particular form of dialysis (as they may handle drugs differently) will affect drug elimination. In addition, antihypertensive drugs may be omitted or delayed on the day of haemodialysis to prevent hypotension. Accordingly, specialist advice and literature should be consulted when prescribing for patients on dialysis. Specialist books that detail how regimens for an extensive range of drugs should be altered in dialysis include *Renal Drug Handbook* (Ashley and Currie 2004).

Renal transplantation

Renal transplantation of kidneys from a living donor or cadaveric donor represents the best chance of a cure in end-stage renal failure. Replacement of the kidney will restore renal function, including vitamin D_3 activation and the production of EPO, and their replacement will no longer be required. However, to prevent an immunological rejection of the transplanted kidney, lifelong immunosuppression will be required (except in donations from an identical twin).

Table 18.1   Summary of actions and adverse effects of some immunosuppressant agents

Immunosuppressant	Mechanism of action	Comments
Azathioprine	Inhibits nucleic acid synthesis and prevents lymphocyte production	May lead to bone marrow suppression with reductions in red cell, platelet and white blood cell production
Ciclosporin	Prevents activation of T lymphocytes	Ciclosporin has many drug interactions; its metabolism may be inhibited by cytochrome P450 inhibitors such as macrolides, imidazoles, diltiazem, verapamil and cimetidine. Its metabolism may be induced by antiepileptic drugs, rifampicin and St John's wort. It is nephrotoxic and may cause hypertension
Corticosteroids	A range of immunosuppressant actions	Widespread steroid side effects
Tacrolimus	Prevents the activation of T lymphocytes	
Mycophenolate mofetil	Is converted to mycophenolic acid which has a more selective action than azathioprine and inhibits DNA synthesis	May cause gastrointestinal side effects such as diarrhoea and vomiting. It is less likely than azathioprine to cause leukopenia

Immunosuppression

A range of immunosuppressants is used in various combinations: triple therapy of ciclosporin, prednisolone and azathioprine is commonly used. The immunosuppressants are summarized in Table 18.1.

Over-the-counter considerations

Renal impairment and failure represent an important consideration for providing over-the-counter (OTC) medicines as certain products may not be suitable. An important example of this are the non-steroidal anti-inflammatory drugs (NSAIDs) which are available over-the-counter (aspirin and ibuprofen as either tablets or topical preparations) because they may cause sodium retention and also a deterioration in renal function, and should be avoided. Paracetamol is considered a safe alternative. Similarly, effervescent products should not be used due to their appreciable content of sodium, which may lead to fluid overload in renal impairment.

Other considerations include avoiding oral rehydration therapy for diarrhoea, which will also increase the salt load; antidiarrhoeal agents such as loperamide would be a better alternative. The load of electrolytes should also be considered when using antacids, and OTC H_2-receptor antagonists are suitable alternatives for dyspepsia. Also aluminium and calcium salts used as phosphate binders will provide relief.

Herbal medicines

It is especially important that renal patients report their usage of herbal medicines, because some herbal preparations such as cat's claw and juniper berries may cause renal damage. Furthermore, herbal remedies may interact with prescribed medicines, e.g. St John's wort induces the metabolism of ciclosporin, and could of course render the immunosuppressant less effective and potentially lead to rejection of a transplanted kidney.

Counselling

Phosphate binders

- These should be taken 10–15 min before meals.
- They should also be taken with snacks containing protein.
- Alu-Cap, Renagel and Phosex should be swallowed whole; Calcichew and Titralac may be chewed.
- They should not be taken with antacids which contain aluminium or calcium.
- Aluminium salts may cause constipation.
- Phosphate binders should not be taken at the same time as iron tablets.

Immunosuppressants

- These must be taken continuously or the transplanted kidney may be rejected; patients should stop taking them only if advised by their doctor.
- Patients should ensure that they have adequate supplies.
- Patients taking immunosuppressants should not receive live immunizations.
- Patients taking steroids should consult their GP if they come into contact with chicken-pox.
- Patients taking immunosuppressants are more susceptible to infections and are regarded as a 'special group', who should have a lower threshold for referral.
- Patients taking tacrolimus, sirolimus or ciclosporin should avoid grapefruit and grapefruit juice for 1 h before taking the drug.
- Patients taking tacrolimus may develop headaches, nausea and trembling, and should consult their GP.
- Patients taking azathioprine or mycophenolate mofetil should consult their GP if there is easy bruising or signs of infection that may be due to bone marrow suppression.
- Patients should always take the same brand of ciclosporin.
- The administration of ciclosporin and sirolimus requires counselling (see *British National Formulary*).

- Tacrolimus has been associated with cardiomyopathy, which should be monitored.
- Immunosuppressants (except corticosteroids) are associated with an increased risk of skin cancer and patients taking them should wear sunblock in sunny weather.
- Tacrolimus has been reported to interact with ibuprofen (and this may also occur with other NSAIDs), leading to renal impairment.

Practice points

- Many patients with chronic renal failure also have diabetes mellitus and the treatment of these conditions should occur in tandem. *Metformin should be avoided.*
- Blood pressure should be at or below the target levels.
- ACE inhibitors play a major role in the management of hypertension in patients with chronic renal disease.
- Renal patients are likely to be taking many different drugs, which should be reviewed regularly.
- Patient compliance may be improved by producing a list of drugs to take and when.
- Patients with chronic renal failure should be considered for the management of anaemia, renal bone disease (involving phosphate binders and vitamin D) and hypertension.
- Renal impairment and failure and also dialysis have implications for the use of many prescription and OTC drugs.
- *Renal Drug Handbook* (Ashley and Currie 2004) is an essential resource.

Self-assessment

Consider whether the following statements are true or false. In a patient with chronic renal disease:

1. Creatinine levels will be lower.
2. There is a risk of normocytic anaemia.
3. Renal bone disease may be prevented by adding phosphate to the diet.

4. Tight management of blood pressure is essential.

5. ACE inhibitors are effective at preventing diabetic nephropathy.

References

Ashley C, Currie A, eds (2004). *Renal Drug Handbook.* 2nd edn. Oxford: Radcliffe.

GISEN Group (1997). Randomised placebo-controlled trial of the effect of ramipril on decline of glomerular filtration rate and risk of terminal renal failure in proteinuric, non-diabetic nephropathy. *Lancet* **349**: 1857–1863.

Martin J, ed. *British National Formulary*, latest edition. London: British Medical Association and Royal Pharmaceutical Society of Great Britain.

Further reading

Ashley C, Morlidge C, eds (2008). *Introduction to Renal Therapeutics.* London: Pharmaceutical Press.

Online resources

www.renal.org
The website of the Renal Association, which produces clinical guidelines on the management of renal disease (accessed April 2008).

www.kidney.org.uk
The website of UK National Kidney Foundation, which provides patient information (accessed April 2008).

www.renalpharmacy.org.uk
The website of the UK Renal Pharmacy Group (accessed April 2008).

Part E
Respiratory diseases

19

Coughs and colds

This is clearly a key topic in community practice, with many patients having consultations for a range of related illnesses. Nevertheless, this can be a controversial area as some commonly used remedies are of questionable value.

Colds or acute coryza

This is a very common occurrence, usually resulting from either rhino- or adenovirus infections, which produce symptoms of a runny nose (rhinorrhoea), sneezing and pyrexia. The common cold is often referred to as a 'flu-like' illness but it should be noted that influenza is an entirely different and more serious infection. Infants may have around 12 colds per year and adults can expect to have 1–2 per year. Colds are self-limiting with a typical course of 1 week. However, there are a number of complications, including sinusitis, otitis media and secondary chest infections.

Treatment of a cold

Treatment of the cold is generally directed at symptomatic relief. The mainstay of treatment should be regular ibuprofen and/or paracetamol to reduce the increased temperature. Additional simple measures include steam inhalation, which appears to hydrate the airways and promote the removal of mucus. Zinc lozenges have been advocated for reducing the length of colds but there is no evidence to support this.

Nasal decongestants

Topical nasal decongestants are also effective at reducing the symptoms of excessive mucus production. Topical decongestants, such as xylometazoline and oxymetazoline, are α-adrenoceptor agonists which cause nasal vasoconstriction and so reduce the flow of mucus. The only major problem is that prolonged use (5–7 days) may lead to rebound congestion (rhinitis medicamentosa).

Systemic decongestants are also widely used but are probably less effective than topical agents and their systemic administration may be associated with side effects. Systemic agents include phenylephrine, which has direct sympathomimetic activity, whereas pseudoephedrine and phenylpropanolamine both have direct and indirect sympathomimetic vasoconstrictor actions, leading to nasal vasoconstriction. Their sympathomimetic activity also means that they are unsuitable for patients with:

- severe ischaemic heart disease
- uncontrolled hypertension
- hyperthyroidism
- diabetes.

Indeed, phenylpropanolamine, when used at higher doses than those in the UK, has been implicated in causing stroke in patients in the USA. The former Committee on Safety of Medicines (CSM; now known as the Commission on Human Medicines, CHM) has now indicated that the daily dose of phenylpropanolamine should not exceed 100 mg. In theory, pseudoephedrine should cause bronchodilatation via activation of β_2-adrenoceptors on the bronchial smooth muscle, which may be of benefit in infections that involve the airways. Sympathomimetics

Table 19.1   Some interactions of drugs with oral sympathomimetic agents

Drugs	Consequences	Comments
Phenylephrine with MAOIs	The pressor activity of phenylephrine is substantially enhanced by MAOIs	This is largely because phenylephrine is normally metabolized by MAO and only small amounts enter the circulation. In the presence of an MAOI, this may lead to a fatal hypertensive crisis. Their concurrent use should be avoided
Indirectly acting sympathomimetic agents (e.g. phenylpropanolamine, pseudoephedrine) with MAOIs	This combination may lead to a fatal hypertensive crisis	Their concurrent use should be avoided
Indirectly acting sympathomimetic agents (e.g. phenylpropanolamine, pseudoephedrine) with tricyclic antidepressants	The actions of indirectly acting sympathomimetic agents would be expected to be reduced by tricyclic antidepressants	This is not believed to be significant
Phenylephrine with tricyclic antidepressants	The pressor actions of phenylephrine would be expected to be increased by tricyclic antidepressants	This is not believed to be significant
Phenylephrine/ phenylpropanolamine with β blockers	No significant interaction between OTC phenylephrine and β blockers occurs	Phenylpropanolamine has been shown to cause a pressor effect in patients taking β blockers but this is not regarded as clinically significant. The CSM (2001) has advised that phenylpropanolamine should not be taken by patients with hypertension, heart disease or hyperthyroidism
Phenylpropanolamine with caffeine	The pressor effects of phenylpropanolamine are enhanced by caffeine and this may result in hypertension in susceptible patients	

CSM, Committee on Safety of Medicines; MAOIs, monoamine oxidase inhibitors; OTC, over-the-counter.

show a range of interactions and in particular will be potentiated by monoamine oxidase inhibitors (MAOIs), which precludes their concurrent use. Some important interactions are detailed in Table 19.1.

Cough mixtures

Antitussives, e.g. codeine, dextromethorphan, pholcodine; expectorants, e.g. guaifenesin, ipecacuanha, ammonium chloride

Although a cough is a symptom and not an illness, it is appropriate to consider cough mixtures here because they are widely used in colds. Cough mixtures are divided into antitussives (cough suppressants) and expectorants. In general, cough mixtures are of doubtful medicinal value but do provide an appreciable placebo effect, from which patients may derive benefit. Antitussives contain opioids that act on the cough centres in the brain to suppress the cough. Codeine in particular has the potential for dependence and pronounced opioid side effects such as constipation. These agents will suppress the cough and remove the symptoms. However, the cough serves the purpose of clearing the lungs and cough suppression may be inappropriate. Indeed, retention of sputum means that they are harmful in chronic obstructive pulmonary disease (COPD) and asthma, and may also mask worsening symptoms. Expectorants are intended to facilitate mucus removal but there is no convincing evidence to support this occurring at the doses used.

Given the apparent lack of efficacy of cough mixtures, a simple linctus may be beneficial by a soothing action and a placebo effect.

Compound preparations

Many proprietary compound preparations are available and typically contain some of the following: an antitussive, an antipyretic (paracetamol or ibuprofen), a systemic decongestant and an antihistamine. The effectiveness of each agent has been considered above, except antihistamines. Sedating (or old) antihistamines such as promethazine will promote sleep (which could be disturbed by the cough) and their antimuscarinic side effects will help dry up the secretions.

Over-the-counter medicines and young children with colds

Many cold preparations contain powerful opioids, sympathomimetics and antihistamines and there is a significant risk of overdose, particularly in young children. It is for this reason that they should not be sold for children under the age of 2 years. Once again, ibuprofen or paracetamol should be the mainstay of therapy.

Echinacea

Echinacea is widely used to shorten the duration and reduce the severity of cold symptoms. To date, there have been trials that both confirm and question its efficacy. A systematic review has indicated that echinacea can reduce the duration, but not prevent a cold, and that the beneficial effects may vary between actual preparations (Linde *et al* 2001).

Influenza

As commented above, this must be distinguished from flu-like illnesses. Influenza is an upper respiratory tract infection that has a more severe course and is associated with more complications and significant mortality. Indeed, more people died in the epidemic of Spanish flu (1918–19) than were killed in the First World War. It is caused by influenza viruses A, B and C. The associated symptoms include pyrexia, chills, headache, muscle aches, backache, sore throat, cough and runny nose, and it is followed by postviral debilitation which may persist for several weeks after the infection.

Treatment of uncomplicated influenza is directed towards symptomatic relief, including ibuprofen and/or paracetamol for pain relief and reduction of pyrexia. A recent development has been the introduction of viral neuramidase inhibitors, such as zanamivir and oseltamivir, which prevent the entry and release of viral particles from host cells. These drugs are effective against influenza A and B. Zanamivir is given by inhalation and this has occasionally been associated with bronchospasm and so should be used with caution in asthma (a bronchodilator should be available) and avoided in severe asthma. In 2002, the National Institute for Health and Clinical Excellence (NICE) released guidance recommending that zanamivir was not for use in normally healthy patients but was appropriate for:

- patients >65 years of age
- patients with chronic respiratory diseases
- patients with cardiovascular disease (but not hypertension)
- immunocompromised patients
- patients with diabetes mellitus.

It is now extended to chronic renal disease and must be started within 48 h of the start of symptoms.

Amantadine (an anti-parkinsonian drug) also has a limited role in the prevention of influenza A and acts by inhibiting viral DNA replication. It is best used as prophylaxis in patients who are at risk but who cannot be immunized or while immunization takes effect (2 weeks).

Immunization now plays an important role in the prevention of influenza in vulnerable patients and annual immunization is recommended for:

* patients >65 years of age
* people in residential care homes
* patients with:
    – chronic respiratory conditions
    – chronic heart disease
    – chronic renal failure
    – diabetes mellitus
    – immunosuppression due to drugs, disease or following a splenectomy.

Acute bronchitis

A potential complication of an upper respiratory infection is acute bronchitis, which may be viral or bacterial. A viral infection may give rise to a dry cough, whereas a secondary bacterial infection is more often associated with the production of thick green sputum. Additional symptoms may include a wheeze and breathlessness.

In healthy patients acute bronchitis usually resolves spontaneously in 1–2 weeks but may exacerbate asthma and COPD (see Chapter 21) and there is a risk of bronchopneumonia. As mentioned in Chapter 21, patients with COPD may be given prophylactic antibiotics to take at the start of an exacerbation, and if appropriate may receive a steroid. In normally healthy patients symptomatic relief may be all that is required. Elderly patients or those with concurrent illnesses such as heart disease or diabetes may be treated with amoxicillin; in patients who are penicillin allergic, tetracycline or erythromycin may be prescribed. Failure of initial treatment with amoxicillin may be followed by the use of co-amoxiclav, tetracycline or a macrolide.

Pneumonia

Pneumonia involves infection of the alveoli as opposed to the bronchi. This may lead to sputum (which may be blood stained, and is often rusty in appearance), breathlessness, pleuritic chest pains and fever. In pneumonia acquired in the community (as opposed to hospital) the principal causative agents are *Streptococcus pneumoniae* (most), *Haemophilus influenzae* and *Chlamydia pneumoniae*, while *C. psittaci* is associated with contact with birds. Given the potential seriousness of pneumonia, antibacterial treatment is appropriate with amoxicillin (or erythromycin if penicillin allergic) being used first line for mild, community-acquired infections. Depending on response and the strain of bacteria, other agents that may be used include: tetracycline, flucloxacillin, erythromycin, clarithromycin, cefuroxime, cefotaxime and gentamicin, alone or in various combinations, *C. psittaci* and *C. pneumoniae* are treated with a macrolide or tetracycline, and *H. influenzae* with cefaclor (see Chapter 32). As a preventive measure immunization against *Streptococcus pneumoniae* is recommended for patients aged >65 years and patients at risk (including those with chronic respiratory, cardiac, renal and hepatic diseases), and patients with diabetes mellitus.

Acute sinusitis

This is infection of the facial sinuses, and is usually bacterial, with *S. pneumoniae*, *H. influenzae* and *Staphylococcus aureus* being the common causative organisms. Sinusitis is associated with discomfort and purulent discharge. Treatment may include nasal decongestants and analgesics to provide symptomatic relief. Sinusitis should normally resolve spontaneously but, in severe or poorly resolving cases, systemic antibiotics (amoxicillin, co-amoxiclav, erythromycin or doxycycline) are appropriate. There is no evidence that topical antibacterial agents are effective.

Otitis media

This is earache due to middle-ear infection and is very common in children, often after a cold or sore throat. On examination the eardrum is bulging and inflamed. The cause is often viral but may also be bacterial (mostly due to *S. pneumoniae, H. influenzae, Moraxella catarrhalis* and, less commonly, *S. pyogenes*) and there is no way of identifying the causative agent unless the eardrum is perforated and a swab taken for culture.

The initial management is for pain relief with either paracetamol and/or ibuprofen, and this is certainly appropriate for the first day or so because most cases will resolve spontaneously. Further treatment with antibiotics is controversial as many cases are viral. Some practitioners prescribe antibiotics blind and amoxicillin is used, but 15% of *H. influenzae* are resistant due to β-lactamase production and so co-amoxiclav or cephalosporins may be more appropriate; macrolides may also be considered. However, evidence indicates that antibiotics shorten the course of the infection by only a couple of days, and then only in about 15% of patients, so their empirical use is often unnecessary (Damoiseaux *et al* 2000). Furthermore, the use of antibiotics is associated with side effects (such as diarrhoea and nausea) and overuse has been implicated in secretory otitis media ('glue ear').

Sore throats – pharyngitis and tonsillitis

Pharyngitis, other than that due to irritation (e.g. smoke), is mostly viral in origin and thus requires symptomatic relief. This typically involves paracetamol or ibuprofen. Interestingly, antibacterial lozenges are of no value and may in fact irritate the inflamed mucosa, whereas local anaesthetic lozenges may sensitize the mucosa. Indeed, simple sugar-free boiled sweets may provide relief.

Some sore throats are caused by bacteria, generally due to infection with group A β-haemolytic streptococci. It is particularly difficult to distinguish a bacterial sore throat from a viral infection. Some features that may point to a bacterial infection are an inflamed pharynx with yellow/white exudates on the tonsils, enlarged, tender cervical lymph nodes, and a sore throat in isolation not accompanied by upper respiratory tract infection. Bacterial sore throats may be treated with antibiotics when there is proven streptococcal infection, they fail to resolve spontaneously, the symptoms are severe and may involve systemic symptoms such as scarlet fever, or in children with diabetes mellitus. Currently phenoxymethylpenicillin for 10 days is the standard first-line drug treatment for infections by β-haemolytic streptococci but cephalosporins and macrolides are also effective. Amoxicillin and ampicillin should not be used blind, because in glandular fever they frequently lead to a maculopapular rash.

Previously rheumatic fever and glomerulonephritis were occasional complications of streptococcal throat infections. This is because *S. pyogenes* antigens cross-react with human connective tissue. Group A streptococci share antigenic properties with heart valve glycoprotein leading to damage, nephritis and also arthritis. This complication is very rare nowadays but patients who have previously had endocarditis, a history of nephritis or artificial heart valves should receive antibiotics during throat infections.

Sore throats are a common occurrence in patients with drug-induced neutropenia and patients who are taking:

- carbamazepine
- phenytoin
- clozapine
- mianserin
- gold salts
- carbimazole
- 5-aminosalicylates
- azathioprine

should be counselled to report sore throats because this may indicate neutropenia and a white blood cell count is required. Inhaled steroids may also promote candidal infections of the throat (see Chapter 21).

Cough

A cough is not an illness but a symptom of a range of other conditions, from trivial to serious (see Chapter 1).

Self-assessment

Consider whether the following statements are true or false. With regard to coughs and colds:

1. Uncomplicated otitis media in a child is usually managed by using simple analgesia.
2. Prolonged use of nasal decongestants can lead to long-term inhibition of mucus production.
3. A sore throat can indicate neutropenia.
4. Coughing up blood (or haemoptysis) is a serious alerting symptom.
5. Amoxicillin is commonly prescribed for simple chest infections.

Counselling and practice points

It is impossible to provide generic counselling for the infections described above; however, there are several important points that should be borne in mind:

- Simple analgesia and antipyretic treatment with paracetamol and/or ibuprofen has a major role in many of these conditions. Paracetamol tends to be used first line in pyrexia and is favoured because it has limited adverse drug reactions (ADRs) and interactions; ibuprofen may be added in resistance.
- Symptomatic relief has a major role in colds, sore throats, otitis media and sinusitis. Reassurance of parents plays an important role with children.
- Cough mixtures generally lack efficacy but have an appreciable placebo effect.
- Antitussive agents may cause sputum retention that is potentially harmful in COPD and asthma.
- Sympathomimetic agents are best via the topical route; with the oral route there is the potential for systemic effects and life-threatening interactions with concurrent MAOIs.
- Over-the-counter (OTC) cold remedies containing opioids, sympathomimetics and antihistamines should not be used in children aged <2 years.
- In pharyngitis and otitis media, most cases are viral and it is difficult to identify bacterial infections. Antibiotic treatment is appropriate on the suspicion of a bacterial infection, in a poorly resolving infection or in patients who are at risk.
- Be alert for pharyngitis as a symptom of neutropenia as an adverse drug reaction (ADR).
- Be alert for cough as a symptom of a range of diseases (see Chapter 1).
- When a course of antibiotics is prescribed, the importance of completing the course should be emphasized and instructions given about when to take the agent in relation to food.
- In influenza, zanamivir has been recommended for use in vulnerable patients, but must be started within 48 h of the appearance of symptoms. It carries the risk of bronchospasm and patients with asthma should have a bronchodilator available.
- Given the need for prompt initiation of zanamivir, systems should be in place to ensure that it is available for immediate dispensing.
- Immunization against influenza and *Streptococcus pneumoniae* are recommended for patients at a high risk of complications.

CASE STUDIES

Case 1
Mr NC (35 years old), who has previously been in good health, visits his GP complaining of a 'nasty, painful and irritating cough'. On questioning, the GP establishes that the patient has retrosternal pain on coughing and that the cough is non-productive. The GP recommends paracetamol if there is any fever.

The GP's next patient is Mr CC (65 years), who has previously been in good health and is complaining of a 'nasty cough', is slightly breathless and has been coughing up thick green sputum for 5 days. On auscultation the GP hears wheezing in a previously healthy chest. The GP prescribes amoxicillin 250 mg three times daily to be taken for 1 week and recommends paracetamol if required.

Why has the GP treated these patients differently?
Mr NC probably has a viral infection leading to a non-productive painful cough, whereas Mr CC appears to have acute bronchitis, which may well be secondary to a recent bout of viral tracheitis – the bacterial infection is indicated by a cough productive of green sputum. Antibiotics may be appropriate, although less so in a previously healthy chest.

How would you counsel Mr CC?
- He should complete the course, even if the cough clears up, because there may still be bacteria present (especially the more resistant strains), so the complete course is required for full eradication.
- He should take the antibiotic three times a day: breakfast, lunch and bedtime is a traditional and convenient spacing.
- As a common side effect of antibiotic treatment, he might get diarrhoea.

Case 2
Mrs PT visits the above GP complaining of a sore throat and a raised temperature. Following an examination, the GP recommends that she take either paracetamol or ibuprofen, rest and take plenty of fluids.

Mrs SP is the next patient and complains of the same symptoms. Following a throat examination the GP observes pus exudates and enlarged cervical lymph nodes. Phenoxymethylpenicillin 500 mg four times daily was prescribed for 10 days.

Why has the GP treated these patients differently?
Most cases of pharyngitis are viral and thus require symptomatic relief. Some infections are bacterial (streptococcal) and present with similar symptoms. On examination, the bacterial infection may be suggested by an inflamed pharynx with yellow/white exudates visible on the tonsils. The patient may have enlarged, tender cervical lymph nodes. Mrs PT has a viral infection and Mrs SP a presumed bacterial infection.

continued

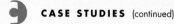
CASE STUDIES (continued)

Comment on the choice of antibiotic.
Phenoxymethylpenicillin is recommended first line. Amoxicillin and ampicillin should not be used blind in a sore throat because in glandular fever they generally lead to a maculopapular rash.

Case 3
An 18-year-old female student visits her GP complaining of a sore throat and general tiredness. Following a limited consultation the GP gives her a prescription for amoxicillin 250 mg three times daily. The following day, the student develops a maculopapular rash and seeks your advice.

How might you respond to the rash?
She should stop taking the amoxicillin. She should take an antihistamine (loratadine 10 mg daily or chlorphenamine 4 mg four times daily, but sedation may be a problem) for relief of the rash.

What are the likely causes of the rash?

- Penicillin allergy.
- Glandular fever; amoxicillin should not be given blind for a sore throat as 90% of patients with glandular fever develop a rash. This does not mean a lifelong allergy to penicillins.

What further tests and treatment may be appropriate for this patient?

- A blood test (Monospot or Paul–Bunnell test) for glandular fever. If she has glandular fever then symptomatic relief is required and she should avoid alcohol.
- If she has a penicillin allergy, she should be prescribed a non-penicillin, non-cephalosporin such as erythromycin (250 mg four times daily) and the allergy documented on her medical records.

References

Committee on Safety of Medicines (2001). Current problems: Phenylpropanolamine and haemorrhagic stroke. *Curr Prob Pharmacovigilance* 27: 1–8.

Damoiseaux RAMJ, van Balen FAM, Hoes AW *et al* (2000). Primary care based randomised, double blind trial of amoxicillin versus placebo for acute otitis media in children aged under 2 years. *BMJ* 320: 350–4.

Linde K, Barrett B, Bauer R *et al* (2007). Echinacea for preventing and treating the common cold. *Cochrane Database Systemat Rev* Issue 3: CD000530.

National Institute for Clinical Excellence (2002). *Guidance of the use of zanamivir (Relenza) in the treatment of influenza.* Technology Appraisal Guidance no. 15. London: NICE. Available at: www.nice.org.uk).

Further reading

Brooks A, Ryan R (2001). Diagnosis and treatment of otitis media in children. *Prescriber* 12: 84–91.

Jewes L (2000). When and how to treat URTI with antibiotics. *Prescriber* 11: 97–109.

Rice P (2002). Influenza – recommended treatment and prevention. *Prescriber* 13: 48–57.

Schroeder K, Fahey T (2002). Systematic review of randomised controlled trials of over the counter cough medicines for acute cough in adults. *BMJ* 324: 329–31.

Wilkinson M (2001). Chest infections: causes and when to treat. *Prescriber* 12: 25–32.

20

Allergy

Allergy may be viewed as an inappropriate immune response provoked by a foreign agent, the allergen, which leads to a troublesome pathophysiological response; in the extreme there may be life-threatening anaphylaxis.

In an allergic response an antigen (allergen) leads to increased immunoglobulin E (IgE) synthesis. The IgE becomes attached to mast cell surfaces and the cross-linking of IgE by the allergen leads to calcium entry. This is followed by mast cell degranulation and the release of inflammatory mediators (including histamine and leukotrienes) leading to increased vascular permeability, chemotaxis, and increased production of mucus and oedema (due to increased vascular permeability and vasodilatation in response to histamine).

There are a number of conditions associated with allergic responses and these include allergic rhinitis, allergic asthma, contact dermatitis (see Chapter 34), drug-induced skin reactions (see Chapter 5) and anaphylaxis.

Allergic rhinitis

Disease characteristics

Allergic rhinitis may be perennial (throughout the year), seasonal (as in hayfever) or occupational, resulting from exposure to chemicals, dusts, and animal dander and urine. The clinical features include:

- nasal itching
- rhinorrhoea
- sneezing
- itchy throat

- wheezing
- conjunctival symptoms, which involve itchiness and bilateral red eye, worsened by irritants such as smoke.

The precise balance of symptoms may vary between the causes, with the perennial disease having less prominent eye symptoms.

In response to allergen exposure, mast cells and T lymphocytes are activated with tissue recruitment of basophils and eosinophils. Histamine is the primary mediator from mast cells and basophils and acts largely on H_1-receptors to evoke the characteristic symptoms, whereas actions at H_2- and H_3-receptors also occur, leading to nasal obstruction. In addition, leukotrienes, prostaglandins and kinins also contribute to the inflammatory response.

Goals of treatment

These are to provide symptomatic relief with the minimum of side effects.

Management

The first approach is to minimize exposure to allergens such as grass pollen in the spring, tree pollen at other times and house-dust mites; simple measures such as vacuuming the house, washing bed clothes at 60°C and freezing pillows may help.

Antihistamines

Initial pharmacological treatment is directed against histamine and involves H_1-receptor antagonists or antihistamines. These agents remove the symptoms of rhinorrhoea, itching, conjunctivitis and sneezing but not nasal obstruction. Older sedating agents include:

- chlorphenamine (Piriton)
- promethazine (Phenergan)
- alimemazine (Vallergan).

Some antihistamines (especially promethazine) have prominent antimuscarinic effects, which may limit their use. More recently, non-sedating agents have been introduced that have a better side-effect profile, which favours their use. Examples of non-sedating antihistamines include:

- acrivastine (Benadryl)
- cetirizine (Zirtek)
- fexofenadine (Telfast)
- loratadine (Clarityn)
- desloratadine (Neoclarityn), which is a metabolite of loratadine

and all, except acrivastine, can be used once daily.

Topical antihistamines

Antihistamines such as azelastine are available as topical nasal and eye drops for the rapid relief of nasal and eye symptoms. Patients are probably better maintained on oral antihistamines but topical antihistamines may have a limited role as 'on demand' treatment against a background of continuous oral drug treatment. In addition, ocular antihistamines may be of use for the relief of occasional symptoms. Some ocular preparations may also contain sympathomimetic vasoconstrictors such as xylometazoline to reduce red eye.

Topical intranasal corticosteroids, e.g. beclometasone, budesonide, fluticasone and triamcinolone

Corticosteroids reduce the production of cytokines and chemokines, and the infiltration of antigen-presenting cells, T cells, eosinophils in the tissue and mast cells in epithelial mucosa. Clinical trials have shown that they are superior to oral or topical antihistamines for nasal symptoms but take several days for an effect, during which time an oral antihistamine is appropriate.

Administration via the nasal route reduces the side effects associated with corticosteroids, such as the risk of hypothalamic–pituitary–adrenal axis suppression, but in children their height should be monitored for height suppression. Patients with allergic rhinitis may also be asthmatic and, although the topical nasal steroids may be used in addition to inhaled steroids, there is an increased risk of side effects. Intranasal steroids should be avoided during nasal infection.

Oral steroids are not recommended as first-line treatment but can be used for short periods (<2 weeks) in severe disease or when control of symptoms is essential, e.g. during examination times. Indeed, by reducing mucus production in severe disease, they may enable topical agents to penetrate more easily.

Topical cromones: sodium cromoglicate and nedocromil sodium

The action of cromones is poorly defined but they may inhibit cytokine release from mast cells, possibly by blocking calcium channels. They may also inhibit sensory nerve activity and suppress local reflexes. Their effects are weak but they are devoid of side effects and are largely for seasonal disease. Eye drops containing cromones may also be effective for conjunctival symptoms. In both cases it may take several days for cromones to exert an effect.

Muscarinic antagonists: ipratropium

The muscarinic antagonist ipratropium is available as a nasal spray and will reduce the rhinorrhoea but will not affect other nasal symptoms such as itchiness. The older antihistamines also have appreciable antimuscarinic activity, which will contribute to their actions.

Decongestants, e.g. oxymetazoline, xylometazoline

These sympathomimetic agents are dealt with in Chapter 19. In the context of allergic rhinitis,

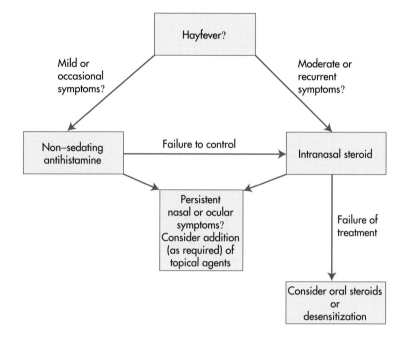

Figure 20.1 A flow diagram showing the typical management of allergic rhinitis. The scheme indicates the central role of either oral antihistamines or intranasal corticosteroids with 'add ons' of topical agents.

these are applied topically and provide relief from nasal obstruction but once again their use should be limited to a week due to rebound congestion.

Hyposensitization

This involves desensitization of a patient towards an allergen but is very rarely carried out these days. To achieve this the patient is challenged with increasing subcutaneous doses of the allergen over time, starting with a very low dose, and this is believed to reduce the IgE response. This may be effective for severe allergic rhinitis when the allergen is identified and conventional treatment has failed, and may also be appropriate for wasp and bee venom stings. However, the process carries a significant risk of anaphylaxis and so hyposensitization for allergic rhinitis is contraindicated in people with asthma, although, in the case of bee and wasp stings, the allergic response may be fatal and so asthma is not an absolute contraindication.

A recent introduction has been Grazax, which is a sublingual tablet containing an extract of Timothy grass to cause desensitization. It is appropriate for patients with a proven grass allergy and who fail to respond to standard treatment. For it to be effective it should also be given for 16 weeks before and during the grass pollen hayfever season. At the moment its place in therapy remains to be established.

Choice of drugs (Figure 20.1)

Oral antihistamines and/or intranasal steroids seem to be the mainstay of therapy, with other agents being added to treatment in response to symptoms. Oral antihistamines tend to be used for mild or intermittent disease, whereas intranasal steroids are perhaps best used for persistent, moderate and severe disease, especially with nasal symptoms. Combining oral antihistamines and regular intranasal steroids would probably be the best approach in more severe disease. Other considerations are detailed in Table 20.1.

Table 20.1   The effects of concurrent conditions on drug choice in allergy

Condition	Effect on drug choice	Comments
Symptoms affecting sleep	This would favour the use of a sedating antihistamine	
Patient must be alert (e.g. driving, exams)	This would preclude the use of a sedating antihistamine	The sedating effects are enhanced by alcohol
	Non-sedating antihistamines would be appropriate or nasal or, rarely, oral steroids	There is no evidence that alcohol enhances the effects of the newer, non-sedating antihistamines but patients should exercise caution
Glaucoma, prostatic hypertrophy, urinary retention	Ipratropium is best avoided	Newer, non-sedating antihistamines are generally devoid of antimuscarinic actions and would be appropriate
	Antimuscarinic side effects of certain older antihistamines mean that they should be used with caution in these conditions. Nasal steroids may rarely affect glaucoma. Vasoconstrictors, such as xylometazoline, should be avoided in angle-closure glaucoma	The use of other drugs with antimuscarinic effects should be taken into account
Q–T prolongation	Avoid mizolastine	Mizolastine is associated with Q–T prolongation, leading to arrhythmias
Epilepsy	Antihistamines may occasionally lead to convulsions	Caution should be exercised
Porphyria	Avoid certain antihistamines	Cetirizine, chlorphenamine, cyclizine, doxylamine, loratadine and alimemazine are considered safe. Refer to the *British National Formulary*
Asthma	Steroids and leukotriene receptor antagonists are also used for asthma	Intranasal steroids may be used concurrently with inhaled steroids taken for asthma, but this may increase the chances of an ADR
	Antihistamines are of no clear benefit in asthma	Leukotriene receptor antagonists reduce the symptoms of allergic rhinitis and this may be a reason to choose them in concurrent asthma
Risk of anaphylaxis	This may be a reason to avoid continuous use of antihistamines	Antihistamines may mask the early warning symptoms
Renal impairment	Avoid acrivastine in moderate impairment. Chlorphenamine is used for pruritus associated with renal failure	

ADR, adverse drug reaction.

Drug interactions

The most significant interactions in the past have resulted from the increase in plasma concentrations of terfenadine due to various inhibitors of cytochrome P450, including macrolides. Inhibition of cytochrome P450-dependent metabolism prevents the breakdown of terfenadine to its active metabolite (fexofenadine), and the augmentation of terfenadine levels is associated with Q–T prolongation and fatal arrhythmias. In 1997 this resulted in terfenadine being changed from an over-the-counter (OTC) medicine to a prescription-only medicine (POM) and, since the

Table 20.2 Examples of interactions with antihistamines

Drugs	Consequences	Comments
Alcohol with sedating antihistamines	The sedating effects are enhanced by alcohol	There is no evidence that alcohol enhances the effects of the newer non-sedating antihistamines but patients should exercise caution
Mizolastine with erythromycin, ketoconazole or antiarrhythmics (class I and III) which prolong Q–T interval	Concomitant use should be avoided due to the risk of potentially fatal torsade de pointes arrhythmias	Caution with cimetidine, ciclosporin and nifedipine
Older antihistamines with antimuscarinic agents (e.g. tricyclic antidepressants, certain antipsychotics)	Potentiation of antimuscarinic side effects	These will also oppose the actions of acetylcholinesterase inhibitors used in dementia

introduction of fexofenadine, it has been discontinued. Other specific interactions are detailed in Table 20.2.

Counselling

General counselling may be directed at avoiding contact with allergens and limiting them in the home. Patients with hayfever may benefit from wearing sunglasses and should avoid going outdoors and keep the windows closed when the pollen count is high. For occupation-related allergies the patient should be advised to wear suitable protective clothing.

Antihistamines

- Patients taking sedating antihistamines should be advised that their ability to drive or operate machinery may be impaired. The sedation will be enhanced by alcohol.
- Non-sedating antihistamines rarely affect skilled tasks in this way but patients should be advised to exercise caution.

Topical antihistamines

Nasal antihistamines would be best used as an add-on to oral treatment with worsening symptoms.

Decongestants

These should only be used for 5–7 days due to the risk of rebound congestion.

Ocular agents

- Ocular antihistamines are best used for occasional eye symptoms.
- Long-term use of eye drops containing xylometazoline should be avoided due to vasoconstrictor effects on the eye.
- Contact lenses should not be worn during conjunctival symptoms or after the application of drugs.

Topical corticosteroids

- In seasonal rhinitis treatment should be started a week or two before the appearance of pollen.
- These drugs will take several days to act and in the meantime an oral antihistamine may be used for relief.
- They should be used continuously, even if the patient feels better.

Cromones

- They will take a few days for an effect to occur.
- They should be used continuously, even if symptoms resolve.

Intranasal agents

Correct application is important. The patient should shake the container, close the other nostril with a finger, bend forward, spray and inhale, but avoid sniffing.

Allergy and anaphylaxis

Many foreign substances can elicit an allergic response, affecting many systems, including the skin and airways. Examples of important allergens include:

- drugs (especially penicillins, streptokinase, non-steroidal anti-inflammatory drugs [NSAIDs] including aspirin, monoclonal antibodies, vaccines, radiological contrast media)
- food (particularly nuts and seafood) but should be distinguished from food intolerance
- insect bites
- snake venom
- latex
- household chemicals or pollutants.

Drug-induced allergy

This is a serious type B adverse drug reaction and affects a minority of patients on second exposure to the drug, even to minute doses, and manifests as an allergic response. Allergic drug reactions are dealt with in more detail in Chapter 5.

Management of allergic reaction

Regardless of the cause, the first measure is to remove the patient from exposure to the allergen or prevent exposure. In an allergic reaction leading to a maculopapular rash or urticaria, an oral antihistamine should be considered the mainstay of treatment. In local allergic responses to insect stings, an oral antihistamine should be given and topical hydrocortisone may be applied. In both cases, topical antihistamines such as mepyramine should be avoided because they may irritate the tissue. As a secondary measure for more severe reactions, an oral steroid may be appropriate.

Prophylaxis

When it is anticipated that medical treatment, such as the use of radiological contrast media or monoclonal antibodies, may lead to an allergic response, patients may receive a prophylactic oral antihistamine and possibly a corticosteroid.

Anaphylaxis

Anaphylactic shock is a serious life–threatening allergic reaction due to production of IgE and involves high yields of mediators, especially histamine. Anaphylactoid shock is related to anaphylaxis but does not involve IgE. Anaphylaxis may manifest within 30 min of exposure and symptoms include:

- angio-oedema (including swollen lips, eyelids and tongue)
- shortness of breath
- wheezing
- generalized itch
- hypotension.

Oedema is an important feature, with extravasation of fluid from the circulation leading to hypotension and airway obstruction. Antihistamines may mask the early symptoms of anaphylaxis and so they should be avoided as continuous treatment in patients at risk.

Treatment of anaphylaxis

Basic life support measures are essential and involve maintaining airways and laying the patient flat. Treatment is aimed at bronchodilatation, supporting the circulation and suppressing the immune response. To this end 'shock boxes' containing adrenaline (epinephrine), chlorphenamine and hydrocortisone are available.

Initially adrenaline is given intramuscularly and this may be repeated at 10-min intervals according to blood pressure and respiration. The purpose of administering adrenaline is to restore blood pressure by increasing cardiac output, via activation of cardiac β_1-adrenoceptors, and vasoconstriction via α-adrenoceptors. The adrenaline will also act on bronchial β_2-adrenoceptors to oppose the bronchospasm. In patients who are receiving non-selective β blockers, the effects of adrenaline will be reduced and so intravenous salbutamol should also be considered. Further measures include oxygen, an inhaled β_2 agonist if there is a wheeze, a saline infusion to restore circulating volume in hypotension and intravenous antihistamine (e.g. chlorphenamine) to oppose the effects of histamine.

As a secondary measure to suppress the immune response, hydrocortisone may be given intravenously.

Adrenaline for self-administration

Patients at risk of anaphylaxis may be given adrenaline for self-administration via intramuscular injection as required, e.g. after a bee sting. These patients require instructions in the use of the adrenaline administration devices and should be advised to wear a MedicAlert bracelet.

Drug interactions with adrenaline

As commented above, adrenaline may be less effective in patients taking β blockers and higher doses of adrenaline or intravenous salbutamol should be used. The interaction between non-selective β blockers (such as propranolol) and adrenaline in normotensive patients is discussed in Chapter 5. Topical β blockers such as timolol eye drops for glaucoma may also interact with adrenaline. In patients who are at risk of anaphylaxis it may be sensible, if possible, to swap from β blockers to alternative drugs.

The effects of adrenaline are enhanced by tricyclic antidepressants which prevent the uptake of adrenaline and so increase its concentration. Accordingly, lower doses of adrenaline should be used in patients who are taking tricyclic antidepressants. Alternatively, the antidepressant may be changed to a selective serotonin reuptake inhibitor, which should not interact with adrenaline.

Practice points

- Oral antihistamines and/or nasal steroids should be regarded as the mainstay of therapy for allergic rhinitis.
- Prompt recognition of the symptoms of anaphylaxis is essential.
- Patients at risk of anaphylaxis should be counselled on how to use an adrenaline autoinjector.

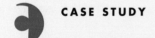

CASE STUDY

A 40-year-old lorry driver visits his community pharmacy complaining of hayfever, which he had as a child but remembers the drugs that he took as being 'awful' as they made him feel worse than the hayfever.

Past medical history: asthma

Drugs:

salbutamol 200 micrograms as required
beclometasone 200 micrograms twice daily

1. What symptoms is the patient likely to have?
   – nasal itching, rhinorrhoea, sneezing and conjunctival symptoms, which are worsened by irritants

continued

CASE STUDY (continued)

2. He would like something that will clear up his hayfever; what do you suggest?
   – A non-sedating H_1-receptor antagonist such as loratadine or acrivastine may be recommended. These are available over-the-counter and should not interfere with his ability to drive.

   Several weeks later he complains that, although he is much better, his nose is still blocked and his eyes are still watery.
3. What OTC medication might you prescribe?
   Possibilities include:
   – a topical nasal steroid such as beclometasone for prophylaxis and treatment; it may be added to the inhaled steroid
   – sodium cromoglicate nasal spray or eye drops, but these will take several days to act; he should not drive immediately after the drops if his vision is blurred
   – antihistamine eye drops for fast relief.

Reference

Martin J, ed. *British National Formulary*, latest edition. London: British Medical Association and Royal Pharmaceutical Society of Great Britain.

Further reading

Croom A (2002). Anaphylaxis: prevention and acute treatment. *Prescriber* **13**: 18–28.

Rusznak D, Davies RJ (1998). ABC of allergies. Diagnosing allergy. *BMJ* **316**: 686–98.

21

Respiratory diseases: asthma and chronic obstructive pulmonary disease

Asthma

Disease characteristics

Asthma is a common clinical condition affecting 5–10% of the population and appears to be on the increase. It is especially prevalent in children but also has a high incidence in more elderly patients. Asthma is defined as reversible increases in airway resistance, involving both bronchoconstriction and inflammation.

Underlying pathology

In order to appreciate the causes and treatment of asthma, it is important to understand the control of bronchial calibre, and hence airway resistance. Parasympathetic innervation results in acetylcholine acting on bronchial muscarinic M_3-receptors, which cause bronchoconstriction and increased mucus secretion. The bronchial smooth-muscle cells also contain β_2-adrenoceptors, which are linked via adenosine cyclic 3':5'-monophosphate (cAMP) to bronchodilatation. The β_2-adrenoceptors have no direct innervation but are responsive to circulating adrenaline (epinephrine), which stimulates bronchodilatation (Figure 21.1). In addition, the mucous glands contain β_2-adrenoceptors, which inhibit mucus secretion. There are also a limited number of sympathetic fibres that release noradrenaline (norepinephrine), acting on β_2-adrenoceptors at parasympathetic ganglia to inhibit transmission. Non-adrenergic non-cholinergic (NANC) fibres also play a role in which nitric oxide and vasoactive intestinal polypeptide are inhibitory transmitters and substance P is an excitatory transmitter. These sensory nerve fibres are thought to play a role in local reflex responses to irritant stimuli.

An asthma attack may comprise an early (immediate) phase with bronchospasm which may be followed by a late phase (Figure 21.2), characterized by both increased airway resistance and inflammation. Other variations include an immediate phase alone, a late phase without an immediate phase and recurrent late phases.

An asthma attack is often provoked by allergens, cold air, viral infections, smoking, certain foods or exercise. It should also be noted that asthma has a genetic component and is associated with atopy. The immediate phase of the

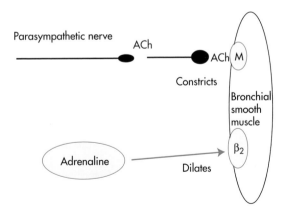

Figure 21.1 Schematic diagram showing the autonomic control of bronchial smooth muscle with direct parasympathetic innervation (leading to bronchoconstriction) and circulating adrenaline (leading to bronchodilatation). ACh, acetylcholine; M, muscarinic.

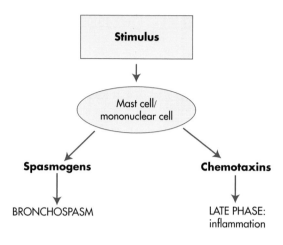

Figure 21.2   A summary of phases of asthmatic attack with early bronchospasm and the late inflammatory phase.

attack is associated with the release of spasmogens (histamine, prostaglandin D_2, leukotrienes LTC_4 and LTD_4, and platelet-activating factor [PAF]) from mast cells and mononuclear cells, which lead to rapid bronchospasm (Figure 21.3). Chemotaxins (including LTB_4 and PAF) then attract leukocytes (especially eosinophils and mononuclear cells), which lead to inflammation and airway hyperactivity, associated with the late phase. This second phase occurs some 3–6 h after the initial release of the mediators.

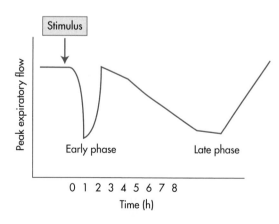

Figure 21.3   An idealized asthma attack with stimulus leading to the early phase with this being followed several hours later by a late phase. The attack is shown by the decreases in peak expiratory flow, indicating an increase in airway resistance.

Long-term growth changes in the bronchial smooth muscle in asthma lead to hyperplasia, with associated increases in airway responsiveness. This is referred to as remodelling.

Drug-induced asthma

Non-steroidal anti-inflammatory drugs (NSAIDs) may provoke asthma in a number of sensitive individuals (about 15% of people with asthma). This is achieved by inhibition of cyclo-oxygenase, and is thought to lead to more arachidonic acid being available as a substrate, resulting in increased leukotriene production.

β Blockers may also induce bronchospasm, by blocking the β_2-adrenoceptors on the bronchial smooth muscle. It is for this reason that β blockers (even in eye drops for glaucoma) are contraindicated in asthma (and often, but not always, avoided in chronic obstructive pulmonary disease [COPD]). β_1-Adrenoceptor antagonists should be used only in *extreme* circumstances in patients with asthma and under supervision.

Clinical features

The leading clinical features are wheezing, breathlessness, a tight chest and cough, which are intermittent and may be worse at night or on exercise.

Asthma is due to reversible increases in airway resistance, characterized by reversible decreases in the ratio of forced expiratory volume in the first second (FEV_1) to the forced vital capacity (FVC). A value of less than 70% suggests increased airway resistance and in asthma the change should be reversed by a β_2-adrenoceptor agonist. In diagnosis, the following point to asthma (British Thoracic Society [BTS] and Scottish Intercollegiate Guidelines Network [SIGN] joint British guidelines 2003):

- a variation of peak expiratory flow (PEF) of >20% on 3 days or more in a week over 2 weeks or
- an FEV_1 that improves by more than 15% with an inhaled β_2-adrenoceptor agonist or

- an FEV_1 that improves by more than 15% after a 14-day trial of oral steroids (30 mg prednisolone per day) or
- an FEV_1 that decreases by more than 15% after 6 min of exercise (running)

In people with asthma the airway resistance may also show variations throughout the day and typically increases in the morning; this is termed 'morning dipping'. In children, the diagnosis is often based on a history that may include wheezing, cough (a persistent dry nocturnal cough may be the only feature), exacerbations on infection and a family association. Asthma is associated with atopy and individuals are likely to have a history of eczema and/or hayfever.

Asthma is divided further into episodic asthma and chronic asthma. Episodic asthma tends to occur in atopic individuals who have periods of attacks associated with provoking factors such as viral infection, allergens or exercise. The attacks include wheezing and breathlessness but the patient shows no symptoms between attacks. Chronic asthma runs a course of prolonged periods of breathlessness and wheezing, with a cough and wheezing at night. The cough is often productive of mucoid sputum. Severe acute asthma (status asthmaticus) is a serious and potentially life-threatening occurrence that involves severe bronchospasm: its management is considered later.

Goals of treatment

Given the two key phases of an asthmatic attack, treatment is divided into relief of symptoms, which is achieved by bronchodilators (relievers) and may reverse the early phase, and prevention using anti-inflammatory agents (preventers).

Pharmacological basis of management

β-Adrenoceptor agonists, e.g. salbutamol, terbutaline

These are the agents of first choice and act on β_2-adrenoceptors on the bronchial smooth muscle to increase cAMP, leading to rapid bronchodilatation and reversal of the bronchospasm

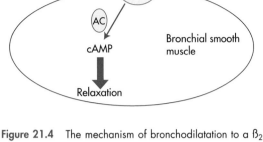

SALBUTAMOL

Figure 21.4 The mechanism of bronchodilatation to a β_2 agonist. This leads to activation of AC (adenylyl cyclase) and increase in intracellular cAMP (adenosine cyclic 3':5'-monophosphate).

associated with the early phase (Figure 21.4). Prolonged use is associated with receptor down-regulation, making them less effective. However, there is some evidence that concomitant treatment with corticosteroids may reduce receptor down-regulation.

Long-acting β-adrenoceptor agonists: e.g. formoterol (eformoterol), salmeterol

Although these are also β_2-adrenoceptor agonists, which cause bronchodilatation, their rate of onset is slow and, more importantly, through its lipophilic properties the molecule is retained near the receptor for a prolonged period, which means that its action persists. Accordingly, they are not used to reverse an attack but cause prolonged bronchodilatation, which is preventive. They are more effective than xanthines or cromones.

Xanthines: aminophylline, theophylline

These are also bronchodilators, but are not as effective as β_2-adrenoceptor agonists and are given orally (theophylline or aminophylline, which is theophylline with ethylenediamine) or occasionally intravenously (aminophylline with improved solubility). Pharmacologically, their actions are less clear; they are phosphodiesterase III and IV inhibitors and so will potentiate cAMP by preventing its breakdown, which leads to bronchodilatation. Additional therapeutic actions may include blockade of adenosine receptors, which leads to bronchial smooth-muscle relaxation, and anti-inflammatory actions through a reduction in mediator release. Xanthines show a narrow therapeutic window (see Chapter 6), with toxic concentrations leading to nausea and central nervous system (CNS) stimulation as side effects.

Muscarinic M-receptor antagonists: ipratropium

Ipratropium is given by inhalation and blocks parasympathetically mediated bronchoconstriction with only limited systemic side effects. Tiotropium bromide is a new long-acting member and may be given once a day. The bronchodilator effects of muscarinic antagonists are less than those of β_2-adrenoceptor agonists. Indeed, BTS/SIGN guidelines (2003) indicate that they are of little or no value in the treatment of asthma.

Corticosteroids: inhalation (beclometasone, budesonide, fluticasone) and oral (prednisolone)

These agents have an anti-inflammatory action via activation of intracellular receptors, leading to altered gene transcription. This results in decreased cytokine production and the synthesis of lipocortin, which inhibits phospholipase A_2, and the production of prostaglandins and leukotrienes.

Fungal oral infections occur as a common side effect with inhalation, due to local immuno-suppression. Laryngeal myopathy may also lead to hoarseness. Systemic steroid effects, including adrenal suppression and bone resorption, occur with high-dose inhalation or oral dosing.

Cromones: nedocromil sodium, sodium cromoglicate

Sodium cromoglicate prevents both the early and late phases of an attack. Its action is uncertain but may include a reduction in sensory nerve reflexes, stabilization of mast cells, and a reduction in the release of PAF and cytokines. Cromones are effective only in a few patients:

prevention of bronchoconstriction is an early effect and prevention of the late phase may require up to a month of treatment to occur. The BTS/SIGN guidelines do not support the use of cromoglicate in children. Nedocromil sodium is of benefit only in children aged 5–12 years, although cromones may be affective in exercise-induced asthma.

Leukotriene receptor antagonists: montelukast, zafirlukast

This is a newer class of orally active drugs that block leukotriene receptors and so will oppose the bronchoconstrictor and inflammatory actions of leukotrienes. However, the Commission on Human Medicine (CHM, formerly the Committee on Safety of Medicines or CSM) has warned that they should not be used to reverse an attack but should be used as a 'preventer'.

IgE antibodies: omalizumab

This novel agent has a role in treatment-resistant asthma. It is a monoclonal antibody that is directed against free immunoglobulin E (IgE), but not bound IgE, and prevents IgE from binding to immune cells that would otherwise lead to allergen-induced mediator release in allergic asthma.

Choice of drugs

The initial approach is to educate the patient to recognize and avoid trigger factors such as dust, animals, smoke and cold air. Lifestyle advice regarding weight reduction may be beneficial in overweight patients. Breast-feeding of infants is also recommended because it protects against the development of asthma.

Drugs have a major role in the management of asthma but two major problems limit their effectiveness: undertreatment and poor patient compliance, largely due to poor inhaler technique. The pharmacological basis of the treatment of asthma is well established and described in the BTS and SIGN joint British guidelines (2003) and has a stepped-care approach (Figure 21.5). These guidelines differ from previous

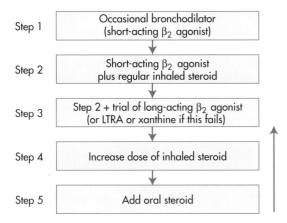

Step 1 — Occasional bronchodilator (short-acting β₂ agonist)

Step 2 — Short-acting β₂ agonist plus regular inhaled steroid

Step 3 — Step 2 + trial of long-acting β₂ agonist (or LTRA or xanthine if this fails)

Step 4 — Increase dose of inhaled steroid

Step 5 — Add oral steroid

Figure 21.5 A flow diagram summarizing the stepped-care approach to the management of asthma in adults according to British Thoracic Society (BTS) and Scottish Intercollegiate Guidelines Network (SIGN) (2003) guidelines. LTRA is a leukotriene receptor antagonist.

recommendations by favouring the use of alternative drugs before increasing the dose of inhaled steroids. Another important feature is the emphasis that inhaled steroid dosages should be the minimum required for control.

The treatment should be reviewed regularly (3 months) and a step-down considered in patients who are stabilized. If a reduction in the dose of the inhaled drug is appropriate then it should be reduced by 25–50%, with further reductions considered thereafter at 3-monthly intervals.

The role of leukotriene receptor antagonists has now been established in the BTS/SIGN guidelines. In addition, their pharmacological action suggests that they would oppose NSAID-induced asthma, by blocking the actions of leukotrienes, which are implicated in this adverse drug reaction.

Long-acting β₂-adrenoceptor agonists have a valuable role in addition to, and not in place of, inhaled steroids. Their prolonged action means that they are of particular benefit in nocturnal asthma but it is important that their effectiveness does not lead to reduced compliance with inhaled steroids. Indeed, combined preparations of long-acting β₂-adrenoceptor agonists and corticosteroids may help improve compliance and these are recommended by the National

Institute for Health and Clinical Excellence (NICE 2008) for suitable patients aged 12 years and over.

There has been some concern in the USA that long-acting β₂-adrenoceptor agonists have been associated with increased mortality but it is believed that this may be due to their use in the absence of inhaled steroids, which is not what is recommended in the BTS/SIGN guidelines.

Intercurrent infections: the previous BTS guidelines (1997) suggested that the dose of inhaled steroid should be doubled in patients with asthma during an acute exacerbation in infections. Evidence for the effectiveness is unproven and the current BTS/SIGN guidelines (2003) comment that this increased dose is of benefit only at low doses of steroids. Immunizations against pneumococcal infection and influenza are appropriate for patients with asthma.

In severe disease, and to reduce the need for steroids ('steroid sparing'), immunosuppression with ciclosporin or methotrexate is used in some patients. In asthma that proves to be mediated by IgE and not controlled by full optimum therapy (stage 5 of BTS guidelines), omalizumab may be added (NICE 2007).

Children

In children there is also a stepped-care approach with different BTS/SIGN guidelines for those aged <5 years. Essentially steps 1 and 2 are similar to those in adults, except at step 2 a leukotriene receptor antagonist can be used if an inhaled steroid is inappropriate while at step 3 a leukotriene receptor antagonist can be added to a steroid. However, if this fails to control the child's asthma, referral should be made to a respiratory physician.

During treatment, the BTS/SIGN guidelines (2003) recommend that the child's height should be monitored in relation to the adverse effects of uncontrolled asthma on height and steroid-induced growth retardation.

In very young children under 18 months, it is unclear whether the β₂-adrenoceptors are fully functional. β₂-Adrenoceptor agonists have been viewed as being less effective and ipratropium has been used in their place. However, the recent BTS/SIGN guidance (2003) supports the use of β_2-adrenoceptor agonists whereas muscarinic receptor antagonists are not recommended.

Exercise-induced asthma

The BTS/SIGN guidelines indicate that β_2-adrenoceptor agonists (long and short acting), inhaled steroids, xanthines, leukotriene receptor antagonists and cromones protect against exercise-induced asthma whereas antimuscarinic agents do not. The guidelines also suggest that exercise-induced asthma may indicate poor management of asthma and that treatment should be reviewed.

Pregnancy

During pregnancy control of asthma is important. The BTS/SIGN guidelines (2003) recommend that β_2-adrenoceptor agonists and inhaled steroids are used as normal and that oral steroids may be used as normal in severe asthma. Leukotriene receptor antagonists may be continued if they were essential for control before pregnancy but should not be introduced.

Choice of inhaler

The choice of an inhaler device is crucial for effective delivery of the drugs. Metered dose inhalers (MDIs) are the most commonly used; however, it should be recognized that many patients have a poor inhaler technique and require counselling in their use. To overcome problems of coordination of breathing with administration, a spacer may be used in which the drug is distributed for inhalation. This may also reduce steroid-induced oral candidiasis.

In addition, in the selection of an inhaler the following should be taken into account:

- The age of the patient: for children under 5 years of age, the NICE (2000) recommends that inhaled therapy should be via a pressurized MDI and spacer, with a mask if required. When this is not possible or effective, then nebulized therapy is appropriate; a dry powder inhaler may also be considered for 3 to 5 year olds. NICE guidelines (2002) recommend that, for children aged 5–15 years, a pressurised MDI and spacer be used for regular corticosteroid therapy, unless adherence is problematic. For other inhaled therapy, especially bronchodilators, the device that best allows spontaneous use should be chosen. The inhaler requirements should be reviewed at least annually.
- Impaired respiratory function: this may make a breath-activated device impossible to use.
- The lifestyle of the patient: can the inhaler be used at school or work?
- The physical ability of the patient, e.g. patients with arthritis may not be able to activate the pressurized inhalers or refill devices. Patients with poor eyesight may be unable to read the dose counters.

When patients are changed to newer inhalers with chlorofluorocarbon (CFC)-free propellant, the dose of steroid (but not β_2-adrenoceptor agonists) may need to be reduced in well-managed asthma; the *British National Formulary* should be consulted.

Adverse drug reactions and interactions

Asthma therapy largely involves inhalation, which limits systemic effects. Having said that, over-administration or absorption may of course lead to side effects. Systemic effects of β_2-adrenoceptor agonists include tremor and tachycardia, due to activation of peripheral β_2-adrenoceptors and cardiac β-adrenoceptors respectively. The sympathomimetic actions of β_2-adrenoceptor agonists mean that they should be used with caution in conditions where increased sympathetic activity would be undesirable, such as in hyperthyroidism, arrhythmias, hypertension and diabetes mellitus. Prolonged overuse of β_2-adrenoceptor agonists is also associated with hypokalaemia, caused by activation of the sodium pump, leading to cellular uptake of potassium.

Systemic side effects of ipratropium are antimuscarinic in nature but are limited. When using nebulized ipratropium, the drug should not come into contact with the eyes because this may lead to glaucoma.

Table 21.1   Some drugs that may influence plasma levels of theophylline

Drugs that may increase plasma levels of theophylline	Drugs that may decrease plasma levels of theophylline
Aciclovir	Barbiturates
Amiodarone (rare)	Carbamazepine
Oral contraceptives (but not thought to lead to toxicity)	Rifampicin
Disulfiram	Ritonavir
Erythromycin: this is much less of a problem with clarithromycin	Tobacco smoke
Fluvoxamine	Levothyroxine
Cimetidine	Ketoconazole (isolated reports)
Phenylpropanolamine	
Ciprofloxacin	
Carbimazole	
Nifedipine, verapamil and fluconazole (isolated reports)	

Xanthines are given either orally or intravenously and will of course have systemic effects. This is important because xanthines have a narrow therapeutic window and toxicity may lead to gastrointestinal and CNS side effects. Accordingly, monitoring of plasma levels and side effects is important.

Side effects of inhaled corticosteroids are dose related and are more pronounced at the higher doses (>800 micrograms of beclometasone dipropionate equivalent in adults and 400 micrograms of beclometasone dipropionate equivalent in children). These include height suppression in children (which should be monitored), adrenal suppression, osteoporosis, skin thinning, cataracts and anti-insulin effects leading to diabetes. Inhalation of the steroid may lead to impaction on the throat, which may promote local candidiasis. In 2002, the CSM brought to the attention of practitioners the need to be vigilant of adrenal suppression in children. They pointed out that adrenal suppression was a recognized adverse effect of inhaled steroids and may present as non-specific symptoms such as weight loss, nausea, hypoglycaemia and reduced consciousness. To avoid these problems, the maximum licensed doses should not be exceeded and the lowest effective dose should be used. Oral corticosteroids are more likely to lead to systemic effects and are associated with gastric damage (see Chapter 7).

Leukotriene receptor antagonists have been associated with Churg–Strauss syndrome (lung vasculitis), which may be accompanied by a rash. This may be more likely to occur when oral steroid therapy is reduced or stopped.

In terms of drug interactions, there are no obvious intergroup interactions that would have a significant bearing on therapy. However, xanthines, by preventing the breakdown of cAMP, will potentiate the actions of β_2-adrenoceptor agonists. This is generally considered desirable but the side effects of β_2-adrenoceptor agonists (including risk of hypokalaemia) may also be enhanced. The hypokalaemic effect of β_2-adrenoceptor agonists and xanthines will also be potentiated by concomitant corticosteroids and potassium-losing diuretics (loop diuretics and thiazides). The CHM has advised that plasma potassium levels should be monitored in patients with severe asthma.

Theophylline, in particular, has a number of significant interactions. These interactions are largely at the level of cytochrome P450, with some inducers of cytochrome P450 reducing the concentrations of theophylline, whereas some inhibitors may augment the plasma levels. In view of its narrow therapeutic window, theophylline should be used with caution and monitored appropriately and the dosage altered if necessary. Some drugs that may influence plasma levels of theophylline are summarized in Table 21.1.

In addition, theophylline may enhance renal excretion of concomitant lithium therapy, leading to reductions in its plasma concentrations, which should be monitored and the dosage increased if necessary.

β_2-Adrenoceptor agonists and corticosteroids used in combination are particularly effective in the control of asthma. A laboratory-based study by Roth *et al* (2002) demonstrated that β_2-adrenoceptor agonists and corticosteroids interact at the cellular level to enhance gene transcription. It was proposed that this might contribute to their antiproliferative effects on the bronchial smooth muscle.

Over-the-counter considerations

Respiratory complaints form a large proportion of requests for over-the-counter (OTC) medicines such as cough mixtures and sympathomimetics (see Chapter 19). This raises issues for patients with asthma or COPD. In both conditions a cough may suggest poor control or an exacerbation and review of inhaler technique or a referral is appropriate. Furthermore, as commented above, a nocturnal cough in a child may arouse the suspicion of asthma. Of particular importance, antitussive agents are contraindicated in COPD because they may lead to sputum retention.

Despite many people's perceptions, asthma alone is not a sound reason to avoid sympathomimetics. However, on theoretical grounds they would be expected to enhance the sympathetic actions and side effects in patients taking β_2-adrenoceptor agonists and should be used with caution. Topical agents are less likely to have systemic effects and are preferred to oral ones (see Chapter 19), although, once again, the request for a sympathomimetic may indicate an intercurrent infection.

Counselling

Counselling has a major role in ensuring patient compliance and correct inhaler technique. General counselling should include advice to avoid precipitating factors, including caution with NSAIDs and avoidance in patients with a known sensitivity to them. Smoking and smoky atmospheres must be avoided. Patients should always have a short-acting β_2-adrenoceptor agonist inhaler available and should ensure that they do not run out of supplies. Attention should be paid to inhaler technique because a significant number of patients are incapable of using a pressurized inhaler or have a poor technique leading to failure of treatment. Patients should monitor their own PEF and may require counselling in the use of peak flow meters. Specific advice is as follows.

Spacers

- The device should be washed out monthly and left to air dry after use to prevent static electricity from causing the drug particles to stick to it.
- They should be replaced every 6–12 months.

Short-acting β_2-adrenoceptor agonists

- They should be used as required to relieve an attack.
- They may be used before an event that may trigger asthma such as exercise.
- If they are required more than once a day, patients should consult their GP with a view to moving up the ladder of care.
- Patients should not exceed the maximum dose or frequency in 24 h.
- CFC-free inhalers may taste and feel different to CFC-containing preparations.

Long-acting β_2-adrenoceptor agonists

These will not relieve an attack but are used to prevent an attack.

Inhaled corticosteroids

- The judicious use of steroids outweighs any adverse effects, even in children.
- Inhalation limits their systemic effects.
- These will take several days to have an effect.
- If taking with a β_2-adrenoceptor agonist, the β_2 agonist should be taken first to dilate the airways, which will aid deposition of the steroid.

- They may cause a sore throat: to reduce the chances of this occurring, patients should rinse their mouth or gargle after use.
- High-dose steroids from an MDI should be administered with a spacer device, to prevent impaction on the throat.
- These are preventive and should be taken even when the patient is stabilized with few or no attacks.
- Patients may have previously been advised by their GP to double the dose in acute exacerbations of asthma. However, BTS/SIGN guidelines (2003) indicate that the benefit of this has yet to be established.
- Steroid cards should be issued to those with high-dose inhalers.
- With doses exceeding 800 micrograms beclometasone (or equivalent) per day, there is a risk of osteoporosis. Measures to avoid this should be encouraged, such as exercise, adequate calcium and vitamin D intake, smoking cessation and hormone replacement therapy, if appropriate.

Oral steroids

- These may have an important role in poorly controlled asthma.
- They should be taken in the morning.
- Any indigestion should be reported.
- The patient should not stop taking the steroid suddenly if the course is longer than 3 weeks.
- If patients have never had chickenpox, they should avoid contact with the virus and consult their GP if they are exposed to it.

Xanthines

- Patients should be vigilant for signs of toxicity such as tremor, palpitations, nausea and CNS stimulation.
- Patients should avoid excess caffeine.
- Patients should not change from brands on which they are stabilized.

Cromones

They may themselves cause wheezing due to the irritant effects of the powder on the airways.

Leukotriene receptor antagonists

- These should not be used for an acute attack.
- They may cause a headache.
- Any rash while taking them should be reported.
- Patients taking zafirlukast should report nausea, jaundice or other signs of liver damage.

Acute severe asthma

Although acute asthma attacks are largely beyond the scope of this book, a brief description of their features and management is appropriate. It should be recognized that asthma may be life threatening and prompt recognition of clinical features is important. In a severe attack the following may be present:

- The patient is unable to complete a sentence.
- There may be tachycardia (>110 beats/min; greater in children).
- There may be tachypnoea (>25 breaths/min; greater in children).
- Peak flow >35 to <50% of predicted.

Signs and symptoms of life-threatening attacks include:

- a silent chest
- cyanosis
- bradycardia
- exhaustion
- peak flow <35% of predicted.

In a severe acute attack the treatment is:

- oxygen (40–60%)
- nebulized β_2-adrenoceptor agonist (e.g. salbutamol or terbutaline) as soon as possible
- oral prednisolone or intravenous hydrocortisone; prednisolone 40–50 mg daily should be continued for at least 5 days.

In a life-threatening attack the following may be added:

- nebulized ipratropium
- intravenous magnesium sulphate
- intravenous aminophylline, provided that the patient is not already receiving a xanthine.

Chronic obstructive pulmonary disease

Disease characteristics

COPD encompasses both chronic bronchitis and emphysema, and is typically a disease of late onset with a very close association with a history of smoking. Some smokers are more susceptible to developing COPD than others, while a smoker's cough may be an early manifestation of the disease. COPD may also appear in former smokers decades after they have stopped smoking. In most patients, COPD is generally a combination, to varying degrees, of both chronic bronchitis and emphysema.

In the past chronic bronchitis was defined as sputum production for 3 months of the year for 2 consecutive years. A more helpful definition of COPD is a chronic reduction in the predicted FEV_1 (<80%), with the following grades:

- Mild COPD: FEV_1 is 80–50% of predicted.
- Moderate COPD: FEV_1 is 49–30% of predicted.
- Severe COPD: FEV_1 is <30% of predicted.

The FEV_1/FVC ratio is likely to be <0.7 and, unlike asthma, there is little variation in PEF. Absolute PEF measurements tend to underestimate the extent of COPD, and FEV_1 is the measurement recommended by the BTS for diagnosis and monitoring.

Chronic bronchitis is an inflammatory response (usually following many years of smoking), leading to proliferation of goblet cells with excess mucus production, which leads to airway obstruction. The chronic inflammation, oedema and fibrosis also lead to increases in airway tissue thickness. These changes lead to the symptoms of a productive cough, wheeze, dyspnoea and acute exacerbations with infections. In more severe disease, the dyspnoea is disabling, there may be secondary polycythaemia and pulmonary hypertension may lead to right-sided heart failure (cor pulmonale). Emphysema is similarly linked to smoking, although in a very small proportion of patients it is due to a genetic deficiency of α_1-antitrypsin. There is marked destruction of the alveoli, leading to dilatation, with reduced elastic recoil of the airways, so the airways are held open during expiration.

Goals of treatment

The prognosis of COPD depends on severity but is generally poor with progressive deterioration. The key goal of treatment is to improve respiratory function.

Management (Figure 21.6)

The treatment of COPD was reviewed by the BTS in 1997 and NICE in 2004 and their guidelines should be consulted. In the first instance, smoking cessation must be emphasized, because this may lead to a slowing of the disease process and a reduction of carboxyhaemoglobin. The pharmacological management is based on the drugs used in asthma, described above.

Bronchodilators

In general, patients with COPD are less responsive to bronchodilators because bronchospasm is not a feature of COPD. However, some patients do benefit from β_2-adrenoceptor agonists and they are widely prescribed for the relief of symptoms and for use before exercise. Traditionally, muscarinic antagonists such as ipratropium have also been used to oppose vagally mediated bronchoconstriction and appear to be as effective as β_2-adrenoceptor agonists, but have a slower rate of onset and so are less effective as relievers. More recently the longer-acting muscarinic antagonist, tiotropium, has been introduced. The combination of a β_2-adrenoceptor agonist and muscarinic antagonist may give an even better response.

The BTS guidelines suggest that all patients with COPD should receive a bronchodilator reversibility test. Here a positive response is defined as >200 mL increase in FEV_1 and >15% increase of the baseline value in response to inhaled bronchodilators. This should identify patients who would benefit most from bronchodilator therapy. Responses with >500 mL increase in FEV_1 may, in fact, reveal asthma.

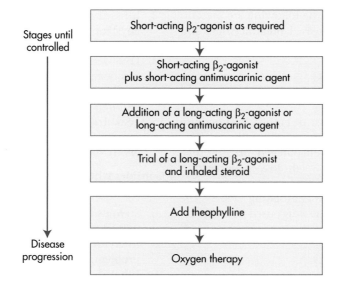

Stages until controlled

Disease progression

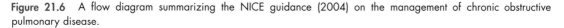

Figure 21.6 A flow diagram summarizing the NICE guidance (2004) on the management of chronic obstructive pulmonary disease.

The role of long acting β_2-adrenoceptor agonists in COPD has now been established and they are of benefit in addition to short-acting β_2-adrenoceptor agonists and muscarinic antagonists.

Xanthines have less of a role in COPD due to their narrow therapeutic window and offer no advantages over β_2-adrenoceptor agonists or muscarinic antagonists. However, some patients may empirically show an improvement with xanthines.

The role of corticosteroids

Despite the inflammatory nature of COPD, corticosteroids are relatively ineffective in most patients; indeed the disease process may make the patients less responsive to steroids. However, approximately 15% of patients respond to corticosteroids and this is often due to undiagnosed asthma as opposed to COPD. NICE (2004) recommends that, in moderate disease, an inhaled steroid in combination with a long-acting β_2-adrenoceptor agonist should be tried for a month. In addition, all patients with FEV_1 that is 50% or less than predicted and who have had two exacerbations in a year should receive an inhaled steroid.

Other considerations

The BTS and NICE recommend that patients with COPD should be immunized against influenza and pneumococcal infection, although evidence for the effectiveness of the latter is yet to be fully established. Depression should be identified and treated.

Long-term oxygen therapy is the only treatment known to improve the outlook in patients with severe COPD. By providing 24–28% oxygen for at least 15 h a day the consequences of hypoxia (e.g. pulmonary hypertension, cor pulmonale and polycythaemia) are reduced. The oxygen concentration should not exceed 28%, because higher concentrations will lead to carbon dioxide trapping.

In the presence of cor pulmonale, leading to peripheral oedema, the administration of diuretics is appropriate. Venesection (bleeding the patient) should be considered for polycythaemia.

In an acute exacerbation, the use of bronchodilators may be increased. Oral steroids may also be added for 7–14 days. Antibiotics may be of benefit in acute exacerbations and may be given to motivated patients who would be able to initiate treatment at the start of an exacerbation. The BTS recommends that antibiotics are of value only if at least two of the following are present: purulent sputum, increased breathlessness and increased volume of sputum.

Counselling

Smoking cessation must be emphasized because this will slow the progression of the disease. Exercise should be encouraged to improve exercise tolerance and weight loss encouraged in overweight patients.

For drug-specific counselling, see the comments above for the drugs used in asthma.

Self-assessment

Consider whether the following statements re the management of asthma are true or false:

1. If a patient is using their short acting β_2-agonist (such as salbutamol) on a daily basis the asthma is not being fully controlled.

2. Inhaled steroids should be used for several days for their beneficial effects to become apparent.
3. Long-acting β_2-agonists (such as salmeterol) can be used to relieve an attack.
4. Cromones are the agents of choice in children.
5. Leukotriene receptor antagonists (such as montelukast) would be a logical choice for NSAID-induced asthma.

Consider whether the following statements re a patient with COPD are true or false:

6. Steroids form the mainstay of therapy.
7. β Blockers should never be used.
8. Intercurrent infections pose an important problem.
9. Inhaled muscarinic antagonists (such as ipratropium) are rarely effective.
10. In severe disease, pure (100%) oxygen is required.

Practice points

- Asthma can kill.
- Many patients with asthma may be undertreated.
- Be alert for the overuse of bronchodilators. In asthma, if a short-acting β_2-agonist is required for relief more than three times a week, the patient should be reviewed with a view to stepping up treatment.
- Poor inhaler technique is a major cause of undertreatment.
- In both cases, smoking cessation is essential.
- The BTS provides detailed guidelines for the treatment of both asthma (in conjunction with SIGN) and COPD.
- In asthma a written action plan improves health outcome.
- Some patients with COPD demonstrate a positive response to steroids and these patients should be identified and treated.
- Patients with COPD are often maintained on a number of drugs and it may be difficult to deduce rationally which agents confer the most benefit.

CASE STUDY

Mr SM (aged 65) has COPD with an FEV_1 of 55% predicted. He is a current smoker with a 50 pack-year history (i.e. he has smoked the equivalent of one packet of cigarettes per day for 50 years). He has been prescribed:

salbutamol MDI 200 micrograms as needed
ipratropium MDI 80 micrograms three times daily.

How should you counsel this patient?

- He should be advised that giving up smoking will slow down the progression of COPD.
- He should take salbutamol as required, and before activities that may provoke shortness of breath. Taking salbutamol before ipratropium may help more ipratropium get into the lungs.

Several months later Mr SM is still taking salbutamol and ipratropium but now with beclometasone 500 micrograms twice daily. However, he is short of breath and has thick green sputum, which is occasionally streaked with blood. What is the likely cause of this exacerbation?

- The symptoms may point to acute bronchitis.

What treatment may be appropriate?

An antibacterial such as amoxicillin 250–500 mg three times daily or erythromycin or tetracycline. He should also be advised to increase his use of the bronchodilators and may be prescribed a short course of oral steroids.

Several weeks later the patient's condition has not improved. What tests may be appropriate?

- Further investigations are appropriate. As he is a smoker this may point to other serious pathologies (e.g. lung cancer, tuberculosis) and a chest X-ray is appropriate.

References

British Thoracic Society (1997). BTS guidelines for the management of chronic obstructive pulmonary disease. *Thorax* 52(suppl 5): S1–S28.

British Thoracic Society (BTS) and Scottish Intercollegiate Guidelines Network (SIGN) (2003). British guidelines on the management of asthma. *Thorax* 58: suppl I.

Martin J, ed. *British National Formulary*, latest edition. London: British Medical Association and Royal Pharmaceutical Society of Great Britain.

National Institute for Clinical Excellence (2000). *Guidance of the use of inhaler systems (devices) in children under the age of 5 years with chronic asthma.* Technology Appraisal Guidance no. 10. London: NICE.

National Institute for Clinical Excellence (2002). *Inhaler devices for routine treatment of chronic asthma in older children (aged 5–15 years).* Technology Appraisal Guidance no. 38. London: NICE.

National Institute for Clinical Excellence (2004). *Chronic obstructive pulmonary disease: Management of chronic obstructive pulmonary disease in adults in primary and secondary care.* Clinical Guideline no 12. London: NICE.

National Institute for Health and Clinical Excellence (2007). *Omalizumab for severe persistent allergic asthma.* Technology Appraisal Guidance no. 133. London: NICE.

National Institute for Health and Clinical Excellence (2008). *Inhaled corticosteroids for the treatment of chronic asthma in adults and children aged 12 years and over.* Technology Appraisal Guidance no. 138. London: NICE.

Roth M, Johnson PRA, Rudiger JJ *et al* (2002). Interaction between glucocorticoids and β_2 agonists on bronchial airway smooth muscle cells through synchronised cellular signalling. *Lancet* **360**: 1293–9.

Online resources

www.asthma.org.uk
The website of the UK National Asthma Campaign (accessed April 2008).

www.brit-thoracic.org.uk
The website of the British Thoracic Society and provides professional information, including clinical guidance (accessed April 2008).

Further reading

Tattersfield AE, Knox AJ, Britton JR *et al* (2002). Asthma. *Lancet* **360**: 1313–22.

Part F
Central nervous system disorders

22

Migraine

This is a common and often debilitating condition, which is frequently under-treated. It is characterized by a severe headache, which may be unilateral and throbbing, and lasts for 4–72 h. There may also be vomiting, photophobia, phonophobia and sensitivity to movement. Migraine is more common in women. In 10–25% of patients with migraine (migraineurs) the headache is preceded, by approximately 1 h, by an aura with visual (flashing and zigzag lines) and other sensory disturbances, and this is referred to as 'classic migraine'. Most cases of migraine are, however, without an aura and termed 'common migraine'. In terms of diagnosis, migraine must be differentiated from cluster and tension headaches and other causes of headache.

Pathophysiology

Migraine is a neurovascular disease and is thought to be due to an abnormal neuronal discharge, which initiates a train of further neurological activations (Ferrari 1998; Goadsby *et al* 2002). The precise mechanisms underlying an attack are not fully understood and this is an area of much controversy. There is thought to be 'cortical spreading depression', a wave of depolarization across the cortex, which depresses neuronal activity, and this may lead to an aura. There is also activation of serotoninergic (5-hydroxytryptamine/serotonin or 5HT) neurons, leading to perivascular inflammation and the release of vasodilator and pain mediators, namely prostanoids, calcitonin gene-related peptide (CGRP) and kinins, resulting in vasodilatation and pain. In summary, there is a humoral response, which leads to a vascular response with disturbed brain function and pain.

Although the precise causes are unclear, migraine may be triggered by a range of influences including emotions (e.g. anxiety, depression and fatigue), hormonal influences (e.g. menstrual cycle, puberty, oral contraceptives, pregnancy and menopause), vision, sound, smoking, smell, unaccustomed exercise, and too much or too little sleep. The role of foods such as cheese, red wine, chocolate, citrus fruits and coffee is unclear.

Goals of treatment

These are twofold: prevention and relief of attacks. In the first instance therapy is directed at relief but, in recurrent attacks, prophylaxis is introduced.

Pharmacological basis of management

Analgesics, e.g. aspirin, diclofenac, ibuprofen, paracetamol, tolfenamic acid

These may be used in an acute attack to inhibit the production of the noxious and vasodilator prostanoids. As discussed in Chapter 29, preference for paracetamol or a non-steroidal anti-inflammatory drug (NSAID) will be determined by side effects and concurrent illness. In addition to the analgesics, antiemetics such as metoclopramide, domperidone, cyclizine or prochlorperazine may be given, because these will reduce any associated nausea. In the case of metoclopramide and domperidone, the prokinetic actions of these drugs will also increase gastric emptying and accelerate the uptake of the analgesics given at the same time. This is particularly important, because migraine is associated with gastrointestinal disturbances, which may reduce transit. Diclofenac may be given as suppositories or intramuscularly when there is vomiting, because absorption via the oral route will be limited.

The use of low doses of codeine in over-the-counter (OTC) preparations may be inappropriate because the doses present have only weak analgesic effects but have marked opioid side effects (e.g. constipation), and may lead to analgesic or overuse headache with persistent use (see Chapter 29).

Triptans, e.g. almotriptan, eletriptan, naratriptan, rizatriptan, sumatriptan, zolmitriptan

Sumatriptan, the prototypical member of this group, was developed to revolutionize the management of migraine. Triptans are $5HT_{1D}$ full agonists but they also activate $5HT_{1B}$- and $5HT_{1F}$-receptors; these actions cause cerebral vasoconstriction to abort an attack. Triptans may also act presynaptically to inhibit neuronal CGRP release, which is associated with inflammation and vasodilatation. In addition, they may act directly on neuronal cells to reduce excitability. The use of 5HT-receptor agonists to manage migraine may seem counterintuitive, given the role of 5HT in migraine, but it should be noted that these agonists are selective for subtypes of $5HT_1$-receptor and are used to abort an attack after its initiation (which is thought to involve 5HT acting at $5HT_2$-receptors). They should be taken when there is mild pain and not during any aura.

The vasoconstrictor action of triptans means that they may cause chest pain and are therefore contraindicated in patients with ischaemic heart disease, peripheral vascular disease or a history of cerebrovascular accident. Sumatriptan tablets have poor bioavailability but may also be given by a nasal spray or subcutaneously by an auto-injector. The newer agents may be given as tablets or in some cases (rizatriptan and

zolmitriptan) as wafers that dissolve on the tongue. If a patient fails to respond to the first triptan used, switching to an alternative triptan may be effective.

Ergotamine

This is an ergot alkaloid with $5HT_{1D}$ partial agonist activity, so it acts in a similar manner to the triptans but its use is limited by widespread side effects including nausea, vomiting and gastrointestinal disturbances.

Prophylactic drugs

This class includes pizotifen, an antagonist of both $5HT_2$- and histamine H_1-receptors. By blocking $5HT_2$-receptors, pizotifen will oppose the 5HT neuronal activation associated with the initiation of migraine attacks, and is therefore used as a preventive measure. Methysergide is also a $5HT_2$-receptor antagonist but is toxic and its use is limited to prescription by hospital consultants.

Certain β blockers (propranolol, metoprolol, atenolol and bisoprolol) are also widely used for prophylaxis. In addition, tricyclic antidepressants (amitriptyline), sodium valproate, calcium channel blockers (verapamil) and the α_2-adrenoceptor agonist, clonidine, are also used for prophylaxis. The therapeutic action of these diverse agents in preventing migraine is unclear.

Drug choice

Migraine management should be reviewed regularly with a stepped-care approach (Figure 22.1), moving up the scale when the measures taken are inadequate on several (usually three) occasions. The guidelines produced by the British Association of the Study of Headache in 2007 (available at www.bash.org.uk) should be consulted. Some key points are summarized here:

• Step 1: for mild and occasional attacks simple analgesia (aspirin or ibuprofen) with or

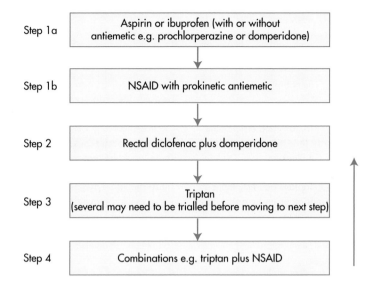

Step 1a	Aspirin or ibuprofen (with or without antiemetic e.g. prochlorperazine or domperidone)
Step 1b	NSAID with prokinetic antiemetic
Step 2	Rectal diclofenac plus domperidone
Step 3	Triptan (several may need to be trialled before moving to next step)
Step 4	Combinations e.g. triptan plus NSAID

Figure 22.1 A flow diagram summarizing the stepped-care approach to the management of migraine as advocated by the British Association of the Study of Headache. NSAID, non-steroidal anti-inflammatory drug.

without an antiemetic, taken as soon as possible. The inclusion of domperidone or metoclopramide as antiemetics will enhance absorption.
- Step 2: when step 1 is inadequate, diclofenac suppositories plus domperidone suppositories should be used. This step is not popular with patients and is often avoided and step 3 used.
- Step 3: when step 2 is insufficient then a triptan should be used, with choice being governed by cost. Some patients may not respond to a particular triptan but this should be tried on three occasions before swapping to another triptan.
- Step 4: combinations, e.g. triptan plus an NSAID.

For severe or frequent attacks (more than two per month) prophylaxis may be added. Prophylaxis should be used for 4–6 months and then reviewed. Ergotamine may be used in place of a triptan but should be given at least 12 h after the triptan. Despite the addition of prophylaxis, many patients are resistant to this and also find the associated side effects unacceptable.

Drug choice will be influenced by concurrent illness and conditions; migraine may also influence other drug choices such as oral contraceptives and some considerations are summarized in Table 22.1.

Drug interactions

The interactions of triptans and other anti-migraine drugs are complex. Although certain drugs are predicted to interact with triptans, evidence for these adverse effects is often lacking or incomplete. The reader is therefore referred to specialized literature such as *Stockley's Drug Interactions* (Baxter 2008). Some important interactions are summarized in Table 22.2.

Over-the-counter medicines and dietary supplements

Sumatriptan has recently been re-classified as an OTC medicine for the acute treatment of migraine attacks with or without aura in adults aged 18–65 years. Practice guidance for pharmacists may be downloaded from the Royal Pharmaceutical Society of Great Britain's (RPSGB's) website (see Online resources at end of chapter).

Table 22.1   Some considerations for the choice of drugs in migraine

Condition	Drugs affected	Comments
Vomiting	Sumatriptan	If vomiting occurs then the subcutaneous route should be used. The nasal spray is not appropriate because ingestion is also involved
Ischaemic heart disease	Triptans and ergotamine	Contraindicated in ischaemic heart disease because these agents may cause coronary vasoconstriction
Ischaemic heart disease or hypertension	β Blockers	These would be reasons to choose β blockers for prophylaxis
Peripheral vascular disease	Triptans and ergotamine	These should be avoided due to vasoconstriction
Cerebrovascular accidents	Triptans and ergotamine	These should be avoided due to vasoconstriction
Age	Triptans	Triptans are not recommended in patients aged >65 years
Wolff–Parkinson–White syndrome	Zolmitriptan	This is contraindicated
Asthma or peptic ulceration	NSAIDs should be used with caution or avoided	See Chapters 7 and 21
Contraception	Combined oral contraceptives	• Migraine is associated with an increased risk of ischaemic stroke. As combined oral contraceptives may compound this risk they should be avoided in patients with migraine with aura, in severe migraine and in migraine without aura but with at least one other risk factor (aged >35 years, smoking, diabetes mellitus, hypertension, hyperlipidaemia, obesity, family history). They should be used with caution in patients with migraine without aura, who do not have any of these risk factors • Patients who develop migraine or who have increased incidences or severity after starting combined oral contraceptives should stop taking them • Progesterone-only contraceptive pills may be used with caution • A current focal migraine attack is a contraindication to emergency hormonal contraception • Migraine is not a contraindication to hormone replacement therapy
Menstrual migraine		This is migraine without aura around the time of menstruation. It may be managed by mefenamic acid or transdermal oestrogen for 3 days before menstruation and for 7 days afterwards
Depression	Amitriptyline	This would be a reason to choose amitriptyline as a prophylactic agent. Similarly, amitriptyline would be appropriate if there are sleep problems
Depression	Clonidine, β blockers	This would be a reason to avoid β blockers and clonidine because they may aggravate depression

NSAIDs, non-steroidal anti-inflammatory drugs.

Table 22.2   Some important interactions of antimigraine drugs

Interacting drugs	Consequences	Comments
Triptans with nitrates or β blockers	Triptans should not be taken with either nitrates or β blockers in ischaemic heart disease due to the risk of coronary vasoconstriction	
Triptans with antidepressants	The combination of an SSRI and sumatriptan is contraindicated by the manufacturers due to the possible potentiation of 5HT	This only occasionally leads to adverse effects
Ergotamine with triptans	These combinations are contraindicated due to enhanced vasoconstrictor effects	Concurrent ergot derivatives and rizatriptan are contraindicated by the manufacturers, who recommend that ergot derivatives should be taken at least 6 h after rizatriptan and that rizatriptan should be taken 24 h after ergots. The manufacturers advise that zolmitriptan and ergotamine should be taken at least 6 h apart
Sumatriptan with lithium	This combination is contraindicated	
Sumatriptan, rizatriptan with MAOIs	MAOs metabolize sumatriptan and rizatriptan and so MAOIs may increase their concentrations	These combinations are contraindicated
Sumatriptan with sibutramine	Possible potentiation of 5HT effects	This combination is contraindicated but there is no evidence of adverse reactions
Rizatriptan with propranolol	Propranolol doubles the plasma levels of rizatriptan	The dose of rizatriptan should be halved to 5 mg and the doses separated by 2 h
Tolfenamic acid with magnesium hydroxide or aluminium hydroxide	Magnesium hydroxide accelerates the rate of absorption of tolfenamic acid (this will enhance the onset of action) whereas aluminium hydroxide may slow the rate of absorption	Aluminium hydroxide should be given separately
Ergotamine with erythromycin	Erythromycin may inhibit the metabolism of ergotamine, leading to severe side effects such as peripheral vasoconstriction	Their concurrent use should be avoided
Ergotamine with tetracycline	Risk of ergotism	Concurrent use should be monitored
Ergotamine with methysergide	Risk of severe vasoconstriction	This combination should be avoided
Pizotifen with triptans	There is no evidence that pizotifen interacts with sumatriptan and zolmitriptan	
Methysergide with tolbutamide	Methysergide has been shown to enhance the actions of tolbutamide	

5HT, 5-hydroxytryptamine or serotonin; MAOIs, monoamine oxidase inhibitors; SSRI, selective serotonin reuptake inhibitor.

As outlined above, sumatriptan is recommended when appropriate use of analgesics with or without antiemetics has been ineffective. Important considerations for OTC supply:

- It is not suitable for a first attack or for patients who have had fewer than five previous attacks.
- The first attack should have occurred more than 12 months previously.
- The occurrence of four or more attacks per month or requests for four or more packs per month warrant referral.
- Pharmacists should be alert for the increased risk of stroke with sumatriptan in women taking combined oral contraceptives. Worsening symptoms and migraine with aura should be referred.

In addition, patients with three or more risk factors for cardiovascular disease should not be supplied with OTC sumatriptan. These include:

- obesity (body mass index or BMI >30 kg/m^2)
- diabetes
- men >40 years and postmenopausal women
- hypercholesterolaemia
- smoker (10 or more a day)
- family history of heart disease <55 years for men and <65 for women.

Alternative therapies

Supplements requested in the pharmacy for the treatment of migraine include feverfew, riboflavin (vitamin B$_2$) and magnesium. Feverfew is a herbal preparation, riboflavin a water-soluble vitamin and magnesium an essential mineral. In the case of feverfew a systematic Cochrane review (Pittler *et al* 2002) concluded that there was a lack of evidence to support the effectiveness of feverfew in the treatment of migraine.

Counselling

The first general advice, which may be effective in some patients, is the identification and avoidance of trigger factors as mentioned above (certain foods, emotional stress, changes in sleep patterns and hormonal changes, including oral contraceptives). Indeed, a trigger diary may be helpful in identifying and avoiding stimuli. Rest and sleep may provide some relief from an attack. Specific counselling points are described below.

NSAIDs and paracetamol

See Chapter 29.

- These should be taken at the start of an attack, even before the headache develops.
- The use of diclofenac suppositories does not avoid side effects, including gastrointestinal toxicity or hypersensitivity.

Triptans

- Triptans should be taken at the onset of a headache and not during the aura because they will not stop the aura and not all auras lead to a headache.
- Side effects of triptans include nausea, dizziness, dry mouth, warm sensations and tingling, and transient increases in blood pressure.
- Some patients experience chest symptoms of tightness, shortness of breath and occasionally pain. If there is chest pain, patients should consult their GP.
- Wafers should be placed on the tongue and allowed to dissolve.
- Triptans may cause drowsiness.
- In a high proportion of patients taking a triptan, the migraine may recur within 12 h.
- Frequent use may lead to chronic daily headache or exacerbation of migraine.

Ergotamine

- If patients develop numbness and tingling of extremities they should stop taking ergotamine and report this to their GP.
- Important side effects may include nausea, vomiting, headache and chest pains.

Prophylactic agents

Some of these are covered in Chapters 11 (β blockers, clonidine, calcium channel blockers), 23 (sodium valproate) and 24 (tricyclic anti-depressants).

Pizotifen

- Pizotifen may cause drowsiness and weight gain.
- Pizotifen is best taken at night due to its sedating actions.

Methysergide

- This may cause drowsiness and affect the ability to operate machinery or drive.

- It may cause a range of other side effects, including nausea, vomiting and rashes.

Self-assessment

Consider whether the following statements are true or false. In the management of migraine:

1. Gastrointestinal stasis may delay the onset of simple analgesics and prokinetic drugs may be helpful.
2. Triptans are 5HT antagonists.
3. Triptans are best taken during an aura.
4. If a triptan fails to control migraine then the other triptans are likely to be ineffective.
5. Certain β blockers may be used for prophyl-axis.

Practice points

- Pharmacological treatment is via a stepped-care approach, with simple analgesia providing the first effective step.
- Soluble preparations are preferred due to delayed gastric emptying during migraine.
- Triptans are recommended when treatment with simple analgesia with or without antiemetics has failed.
- Nausea and vomiting may make the oral route ineffective.

 CASE STUDY

A 35-year-old woman who has a history of migraine since the age of 15 years now requires further medication, as ibuprofen is ineffective at managing her condition.

Her current medication is:

sertraline 50 mg once daily
Microgynon.

1. Comment on her current medication: first, it should be noted that combined oral contraceptives may lead to increases in migraine. Instead, progesterone-only contraceptives pills may be used. Her age and obesity (revealed later on) would also favour the use of progesterone-only contra-ceptives pills (with caution) or alternative contraceptive measures.
   Sertraline is a selective serotonin reuptake inhibitor (SSRI) that may lead to headaches and nausea, and so one needs to be certain that her symptoms are not related to the SSRI.

continued

CASE STUDY (continued)

2. What antimigraine treatment would be appropriate in her case?
   – The next likely step would be simple analgesic with an antiemetic plus a triptan (sumatriptan, zolmitriptan or rizatriptan as first-line). Step 2 of diclofenac suppositories plus domperidone suppositories is often unacceptable to patients. If she is maintained on the sertraline then the use of a triptan is contraindicated by manufacturers of sumatriptan due to the possibility of CNS toxicity through potentiation of the effects of 5HT. However, *Stockley's Drug Interactions* (Baxter 2008) points out that the combination of sumatriptan and an SSRI only occasionally leads to adverse effects and suggests that they may be used together with caution.

   Her depression is compounded by her obesity (BMI = 35) but she has shown motivation in losing weight and her GP is prepared to prescribe an antiobesity drug.
3. What advice would you give her GP in drug choice?
   – The choice of antiobesity drugs is between sibutramine and orlistat. If she is taking a triptan and/or sertraline then sibutramine would be contraindicated, because there is a risk of CNS toxicity through potentiation of the effects of 5HT. Therefore, orlistat, which acts on pancreatic lipases, would be a safer choice. In terms of future antimigraine treatment, pizotifen should be avoided because this may cause weight gain. She should be encouraged to take regular exercise and maintain a healthy diet.

References

Baxter K, ed. (2008). *Stockley's Drug Interaction*, 8th edn. London: Pharmaceutical Press.

Ferrari MD (1998). Migraine. *Lancet* **351**: 1043–51.

Goadsby PJ, Lipton RB, Ferrari MD (2002). Migraine – current understanding and treatment. *N Engl J Med* **346**: 257–70.

Pittler MH, Vogler BK, Ernst E (2002). Feverfew for preventing migraine (Cochrane review). In: *The Cochrane Library* issue 2. Oxford: Update Software.

Further reading

Goadsby PJ, Olesen J (1996). Fortnightly review: diagnosis and management of migraine. *BMJ* **312**: 1279–83.

Online resources

www.bash.org.uk
The website of the British Association for the Study of Headache, providing guidelines for all healthcare professionals in the diagnosis and management of migraine, tension-type, cluster and medication-overuse headache (accessed January 2008).

www.rpsgb.org/pdfs/otcsumatriptanguid.pdf
The RPSGB guidance document for OTC sumatriptan (accessed February 2008).

www.migrainetrust.org
The website of the Migraine Trust, with professional and patient information on migraine (accessed April 2008).

23

Epilepsy

Disease characteristics

This is the most common serious neurological condition, with 3–5% of the population experiencing some form during their lifetime. There are several forms, ranging from temporary loss of concentration (absences) to full-blown seizures with convulsions and loss of consciousness. The seizures are divided into partial and generalized seizures and the major forms are described below.

Generalized seizures

In generalized seizures, abnormal electrical activity spreads simultaneously throughout the cerebral cortex and there are several forms:

- Tonic–clonic convulsions (or grand mal seizures) involve sudden loss of consciousness; the limbs may stiffen (tonic) and then jerk (clonic). There is often tongue biting and incontinence. On regaining consciousness, the patient is often drowsy and confused.
- Tonic seizures involve going stiff but without loss of consciousness.
- Atonic seizures involve loss of tone and becoming limp.
- Absences (or petit mal epilepsy) often occur in children who go blank and stare for approximately 10–30 s: this may be mistaken for daydreaming.
- Myoclonic epilepsy is characterized by abrupt jerks, which may affect the whole body, arms or legs.

Partial seizures

These are focal seizures that are localized to a brain region and produce simple symptoms such as muscle contractions and abnormal sensory changes without collapsing. Simple partial seizures involve changes in activity whereas complex partial seizures involve changes in awareness. In secondary generalized seizures activity starts in one area and then spreads, which may lead to a full seizure.

Causes

In general, epilepsy is due to abnormal neuronal discharges, which may or may not spread across the brain. The cause may be the result of a structural lesion, secondary to trauma or caused by some unidentified change. Biochemical changes such as hypoglycaemia, hyperglycaemia, hyponatraemia or alcohol abuse may also lead to seizures, and infections such as meningitis may cause seizures. In some cases, particularly those appearing later in life, they may be due to lesions such as brain tumours, which should be excluded. Therapeutic drugs, particularly when used in combination, may induce seizures in patients with or without a history of epilepsy and important examples are:

- quinolones
- tricyclic antidepressants
- selective serotonin reuptake inhibitors (SSRIs)
- antihistamines
- bupropion (amfebutamone)
- donepezil
- baclofen
- lithium

Table 23.1   Summary of the pharmacological actions and adverse effects of antiepileptic drugs

Antiepileptic drug	Mechanism of action	Adverse effects and comments
Sodium valproate	Acts weakly by potentiating GABA and causing use-dependent blockade of Na+ channels	• Sedation, ataxia, diplopia, nystagmus, weight gain, nausea, hair loss and tremor • May rarely cause thrombocytopenia and agranulocytosis • Liver dysfunction and failure have occurred • Pancreatitis may also occur • Associated with high incidence of birth defects
Carbamazepine	Use-dependent blockade of Na+ channels	• Induces its own metabolism and so the dosage is increased gradually • It is associated with sedation, erythematous rashes, dizziness, and diplopia (double vision) • It is also associated with hyponatraemia, which itself may reduce seizure threshold • May cause agranulocytosis and thrombocytopenia • It is an important enzyme inducer
Oxcarbazepine	Derivative of carbamazepine	As for carbamazepine but causes less enzyme induction and skin rashes. Hyponatraemia is more problematic than with carbamazepine
Phenytoin	Use-dependent blockade of Na+ channels	• It shows zero-order pharmacokinetics (Chapter 6), so achieving therapeutic concentrations is difficult and side effects such as nystagmus are indicative of toxic effects • It frequently causes adverse effects, including gingival hypertrophy, hair growth, coarsening of facial features, diplopia, sedation and ataxia. It may cause agranulocytosis • Risk of folate deficiency leading to megaloblastic anaemia • It is an important enzyme inducer
Lamotrigine	Use-dependent blockade of Na+ channels and decreased release of the excitatory transmitter, glutamate	• Less sedating than the older agents but there may be dizziness and ataxia • It is associated with skin reactions, including toxic epidermal necrolysis and Stevens–Johnson syndrome
Gabapentin	Uncertain	Associated with dizziness, ataxia, somnolence, diplopia, nystagmus and nausea
Vigabatrin	Potentiates GABA by inhibiting its metabolism via the GABA transaminase enzyme	Associated with drowsiness and fatigue. It may cause irreversible visual field defects
Topiramate	Uncertain, but it may act via blockade of sodium channels and/or enhancing the actions of GABA by binding to a modulatory site	CNS side effects such as confusion, dizziness, fatigue and memory impairment

Continued

Table 23.1 (Continued)

Antiepileptic drug	Mechanism of action	Adverse effects and comments
Ethosuximide	Inhibition of T-type calcium channels	Associated with gastrointestinal side effects, drowsiness and dizziness
Phenobarbital	Enhances the effects of GABA at opening the GABA receptor-associated chloride channel	• Sedation is a major problem and it is rarely used • It is an important enzyme inducer • Tolerance is a problem • Rebound seizures on withdrawal are common
Primidone	Metabolized to phenobarbital	As for phenobarbital
Benzodiazepines, e.g. clonazepam, clobazam diazepam	Enhance the actions of GABA via the benzodiazepine receptor	Sedation and dependence
Levetiracetam	Uncertain	Dizziness, somnolence, diplopia, tremor, depression and headaches
Tiagabine	Inhibitor of GABA reuptake	Dizziness, somnolence, nervousness and tremor

CNS, central nervous system; GABA, γ-aminobutyric acid.

- mefloquine
- theophylline
- tramadol.

In addition, withdrawal from alcohol, benzodiazepines and barbiturates is associated with seizures.

Goals of treatment

These are to control seizures with the lowest possible dose, and with fewest side effects.

Pharmacological management

For a first seizure it is important to exclude other pathologies that may have caused the seizure, important examples of which are detailed above. In the absence of any obvious cause, a first or isolated seizure may go untreated, because in a high proportion of patients (up to 50%) they may not recur. However, once a patient has a subsequent seizure, epilepsy may be diagnosed and antiepileptic drugs (AEDs) are prescribed to prevent further seizures. In general, AEDs either reduce neuronal excitability, and so prevent the spread of neuronal discharges or potentiate inhibitory transmitters such as α-aminobutyric acid (GABA). Given these depressant actions on the brain, AEDs are associated with a wide range of central side effects, which are summarized together with their modes of action in Table 23.1.

Vagal nerve stimulation

This involves insertion of a generator into the chest, with electrodes connected to the vagus nerve. The stimulator provides electrical impulses every 3–5 min and, during an aura or the early stages of a seizure, the patient or an observer can activate the stimulator to stimulate the vagus, which is thought to disrupt attacks. The mechanism by which this occurs is unclear.

Drug choice

The aim of pharmacological therapy is to control seizures and this is ideally achieved by using one drug at an effective dose. If the first drug fails to control epilepsy at its maximum dose, a second drug is often tried as the first drug is withdrawn slowly. Only after failure of monotherapy is

Table 23.2   Summary of drug choices in the different forms of epilepsy

Form of epilepsy	First-line	Second-line	Antiepileptic drugs to avoid
Absence	Sodium valproate Lamotrigine	Ethosuximide	Carbamazepine
Generalized tonic–clonic	Sodium valproate Lamotrigine Carbamazepine	Levetiracetam	Vigabatrin
Myoclonic	Sodium valproate	Clonazepa Ethosuximide Lamotrigine	Carbamazepine
Partial seizures	Sodium valproate Carbamazepine Lamotrigine	Phenytoin Gabapentin Vigabatrin Clonazepam	

combined therapy used. Currently, sodium valproate and carbamazepine are widely used, with lamotrigine having a much increased role, and phenytoin and phenobarbital being less widely used. Some choices of AEDs are summarized in Table 23.2.

Currently gabapentin, levetiracetam, tiagabine, topiramate and vigabatrin (except as monotherapy for infantile spasms) are licensed only as add-on drugs where control is not attained with monotherapy.

In some cases, seizures increase around menstruation and this is termed 'catamenial epilepsy'. In these patients the benzodiazepine clobazam may be used around that time.

In status epilepticus, a prolonged seizure lasting more than 30 min, benzodiazepines such as diazepam, lorazepam or clonazepam may be given to stop the attack. The rectal route may be more practical during a seizure. If this fails to control the seizure, intravenous phenytoin or phenobarbital may be used or even general anaesthetics.

Other considerations include concurrent diseases or conditions and some important examples are depression and pregnancy.

Affective disorders

Depression is an important consideration, and this may well occur secondary to patients developing epilepsy. The use of antidepressants is associated with decreasing the seizure threshold, which may lead to episodes of epilepsy, and so antidepressants should be used with caution in epilepsy. In concurrent bipolar affective disorder carbamazepine may be considered as a compelling choice because it is effective in this condition. It should be noted that carbamazepine may be used effectively with lithium, but there have been instances of increased neurotoxicity with this combination.

Pregnancy

Pregnancy is a major issue in patients with epilepsy because the associated physiological changes may increase the incidence of seizures. Furthermore, AEDs are associated with a range of birth defects, e.g. carbamazepine and sodium valproate are associated with increased risks of neural tube defects and phenytoin and phenobarbital are associated with cleft palates. Other adverse effects may include impaired psychomotor development in the child, cardiac defects and facial abnormalities. Some patients who are seizure free for some time may have their AED withdrawn before conception. However, if this is not the case, continuing AEDs during pregnancy is considered important because seizures during pregnancy may have serious consequences for both the mother and the fetus. Pharmacokinetic changes in pregnancy may also reduce the effectiveness of some AEDs.

The management of epilepsy during pregnancy is usually under specialist care. There has been much debate around the safety of AEDs in pregnancy, with lamotrigine and carbamazepine being favoured in females of child-bearing age and sodium valproate being associated with a high incidence of birth defects. Sodium valproate and older agents such as phenobarbital and phenytoin should be avoided in women of child-bearing age if possible, due to the increased risk of birth defects. To reduce the chances of neural tube defect, patients often receive 5 mg folic acid daily before conception and for at least the first 12 weeks of pregnancy. Carbamazepine, phenytoin and phenobarbital are also associated with increased neonatal bleeding (including intracranial bleeds) and vitamin K is given to the mother from week 36 of pregnancy before delivery and to the baby at birth.

Breast-feeding

Breast-feeding is considered safe for mothers taking carbamazepine, phenytoin and sodium valproate. Breast-feeding while taking phenobarbital, primidone, vigabatrin (risk of visual defects) and ethosuximide should be avoided. Breast-feeding is considered safe with newer agents such as lamotrigine, and gabapentin if taken during pregnancy. Non-hormonal methods of contraception may be required during breast-feeding by patients prescribed enzyme-inducing drugs because progestogen-only contraceptives may be less effective.

Contraception

Compounding the issue of pregnancy is the established interaction of the enzyme-inducing AEDs (carbamazepine, oxcarbazepine, phenytoin, phenobarbital and topiramate) with oral contraceptives; they accelerate their metabolism, which may lead to contraceptive failure. To overcome this problem alternative contraception such as barrier methods or intrauterine devices should be used. Alternatively a high-dose oestrogen (50 microgram ethinylestradiol)-containing pill might be prescribed. The guidance of the National Institute for Health and Clinical Effectiveness (NICE 2004) recommends that progestogen-only pills should be avoided but depot injections of progesterone might be used although at shorter intervals than normal. As lamotrigine does not interact with oral contraceptives, this may be a reason to choose this agent in favour of enzyme-inducing agents.

Young children

It should be noted that young children may require higher doses per kilogram of body weight of antiepileptics, with more frequent doses due to more rapid metabolism of these drugs.

Drug interactions

AEDs show a wide range of interactions and the reader is referred to specialized literature such as *Stockley's Drug Interactions* (Baxter 2008). However, a few important points to note are that carbamazepine (oxcarbazepine to a lesser extent), phenytoin and phenobarbital induce cytochrome P450, and accelerate the metabolism of other drugs. Indeed, one reason to favour monotherapy is that many of the AEDs interact with each other, often increasing each other's metabolism. By contrast, sodium valproate inhibits the metabolism of lamotrigine, thus increasing its plasma half-life. Some important examples of other interactions due to induction of metabolism are as follows.

Carbamazepine, phenytoin and phenobarbital may significantly accelerate the metabolism of:

- doxycycline but not other tetracyclines
- warfarin (phenytoin may also potentiate the actions of warfarin)
- indinavir, nelfinavir, saquinavir
- dihydropyridines
- corticosteroids
- oestrogens and progestogens
- theophylline
- levothyroxine
- certain other AEDs.

In addition, given the hepatic route of metabolism of some AEDs, there is scope for inhibitors of these pathways to interact with AEDs, resulting in increased concentrations and promoting toxicity. Important examples of this are the interactions of carbamazepine with erythromycin, clarithromycin, diltiazem, verapamil, certain selective serotonin reuptake inhibitors (SSRIs, e.g. fluoxetine and fluvoxamine) and cimetidine (transiently). St John's wort may induce the metabolism of carbamazepine, making it less effective. Having commented on the extensive range of drug interactions with AEDs, it should also be noted that gabapentin is not known to have any significant interactions.

Monitoring

AEDs are associated with a range of serious adverse drug reactions (ADRs) affecting the liver (see Chapter 5) and haematological system (see Chapter 5), so monitoring is appropriate. Baseline monitoring of haematology and biochemistry is often carried out before starting treatment. Liver function tests (LFTs) are essential with sodium valproate before treatment and during the first 6 months, including a determination of the international normalized ratio (INR). Some of the inducing AEDs may alter LFTs (see Chapter 2) via enzyme induction (e.g. increased levels of γ-glutamyl transferase [GGT]), and may also promote damage due to the enhancement of drug metabolism, which may give rise to toxic metabolites.

Blood counts should be determined if there are signs of reduced white cell counts (leukopenia due to agranulocytosis) such as increased infections (e.g. sore throats, fevers, mouth ulcers) or thrombocytopenia (increased bruising), which may occur with carbamazepine, ethosuximide, lamotrigine, phenytoin (the manufacturer recommends monitoring of blood counts) and sodium valproate (principally thrombocytopenia). If serious blood disorders such as leukopenia or thrombocytopenia are identified then the AED should be withdrawn under the cover of another agent.

Visual fields should also be measured every 6 months with vigabatrin.

Withdrawing antiepileptic drugs

In many patients it is undesirable that they are maintained indefinitely on AEDs; indeed, the condition that may have led to their seizures may have resolved. Therefore, after a suitable seizure-free period, the patient and doctor may consider withdrawal of therapy. Typically, patients who are seizure free for 2–4 years are considered, because a substantial proportion will remain seizure free on withdrawal. Withdrawal of AEDs may itself decrease the seizure threshold, so this should be gradual with a dose reduction over time. Typical reducing regimens are dose reductions (e.g. carbamazepine by 100 mg, sodium valproate by 200 mg) every 4 weeks. Benzodiazepines and phenobarbital should be withdrawn over several months. During the withdrawal period, and for 6 months afterwards, patients should not drive, because the withdrawal may precipitate seizures or the patient's epilepsy may return. When changing medication, the original drug should be withdrawn only once the new drug is established.

Over-the-counter medication and supplements

Over-the-counter (OTC) issues in epilepsy involve screening for ADRs and drug interactions and providing support to patients to aid compliance. Drugs such as cimetidine, a cytochrome P450 inhibitor, should be avoided (see earlier). Female patients should be advised to consult their doctor before planning a pregnancy, for counselling and prescription of folic acid together with a medication review. Patients with epilepsy should not take evening primrose oil or ginkgo biloba due to a risk of seizures with these agents.

Counselling

To achieve adequate control of epilepsy, patients should be informed of the importance of compliance, because omitting doses or abrupt withdrawal may cause a rebound increase in the occurrence of seizures.

Informing family and colleagues about their condition and what to do in the event of a seizure may help as seizures can appear frightening.

Haematological and hepatic adverse effects

Patients taking carbamazepine, oxcarbazepine, ethosuximide, gabapentin, lamotrigine, phenytoin and sodium valproate should be counselled to report promptly signs of blood disorders such as sore throats, mouth ulcers, fevers or easy bruising. In the case of lamotrigine, patients should also report rashes or flu-like illnesses. Patients taking carbamazepine, oxcarbazepine and sodium valproate should report symptoms that may indicate liver damage such as jaundice, itching, nausea and vomiting.

Skin reactions

Many of the AEDs may cause skin reactions (see Chapter 5). Although many of these are harmless, some may be serious, so patients should consult their doctor.

Sedation

Many of the AEDs may cause sedation, so patients should be warned of this possibility. When taking carbamazepine, gabapentin, vigabatrin, topiramate, barbiturates and benzodiazepines, patients should be specifically advised that sedation may affect their ability to operate machinery.

Driving

This is subject to clear regulations of the driving licensing authorities (see the *British National Formulary*) and the onus is on patients to report their condition. Patients should also stop driving for 6 months on withdrawal of AEDs. In addition, all of the AEDs may impair driving and so patients should be alerted to this.

Alcohol

Alcohol may enhance central nervous system (CNS) side effects such as sedation in some AEDs such as carbamazepine. Excessive fluid intake may also predispose patients taking carbamazepine and oxcarbazepine to hyponatraemia, which itself may lead to seizure. Hence patients should be cautioned against excessive alcohol intake.

Drug interactions

Patients should inform all healthcare professionals that they are taking AEDs.

Pregnancy

Female patients should be advised to discuss with their GP the issues surrounding pregnancy and epilepsy (see above) before stopping contraception. Advice should be given on the interaction of antiepileptics and oral contraceptives, the risks associated with unplanned pregnancy and the risks/benefits of AED use during pregnancy.

Bone

The enzyme-inducing AEDs (carbamazepine, phenytoin and phenobarbital) have been associated with accelerated metabolism of vitamin D, leading to impaired calcium levels. These effects have been associated with rickets and osteomalacia, so the importance of a balanced diet should be stressed. This may be particularly important in the presence of additional risk factors such as early menopause and use of corticosteroids.

Side effects

In addition to the extensive range of side effects reported above, some other drug-specific counselling points are as follows.

Phenytoin
This may cause increased growth of the gums.

Vigabatrin
This may cause irreversible changes in vision, which should be reported.

Practice points

- Epilepsy is a common condition, which is usually managed by drugs.
- Monotherapy is preferred.
- Pharmacists have an important role in ensuring adherence to AEDs.
- AEDs have a wide range of interactions and the enzyme inducers may cause a failure of oral contraception.
- AEDs are associated with a range of side effects and may cause birth defects.
- In treatment failure, check that the dose has been increased to an appropriate maintenance dose, and/or check blood levels before a new prescription, e.g. carbamazepine induces its own metabolism, requiring a gradual dose increase.

Self-assessment

Consider whether the following statements are true or false. In the management of epilepsy:

1. Antiepileptic drugs are usually used in combination.
2. Oral contraceptive may make antiepileptic drugs less effective.
3. Sodium valproate is often avoided in females of child-bearing age.
4. Carbamazepine is associated with causing neutropenia.
5. Antiepileptic drug therapy is usually life long.

 CASE STUDY

A 25-year-old man has been diagnosed with tonic–clonic epilepsy. Antiepileptic treatment was initiated with carbamazepine (100 mg once daily) and subsequently maintained at a total daily dose of 800 mg.

1. How would you counsel this patient with respect to treatment with carbamazepine?
   He should:
   – not discontinue his medicine without advice
   – report any unexplained sore throats, mouth ulcers, rashes, bleeding or bruising to his GP.
   After several weeks he complains to you, as his community pharmacist, of a persistent sore throat.
2. What action should you take?
   – He should be referred to his GP.
3. What tests are appropriate? Why?
   – He should have a full blood count, because carbamazepine is associated with agranulocytosis which results in reduced white blood cell counts (leukopenia).
4. Considering the different potential outcomes of the test(s), what actions might be taken?
   – If there is neutropenia, the carbamazepine should be stopped under the cover of another antiepileptic. Neutropenia is not a class effect and another antiepileptic might be tried. If the white blood count is normal, the sore throat should be treated. If this is bacterial, phenoxymethylpenicillin or cephalosporins might be used or, if it is viral, simple linctus or soothing sugar-free sweets could be recommended.

References

Baxter K, ed. (2008). *Stockley's Drug Interactions*, 8th edn. London: Pharmaceutical Press.

Martin J, ed. *British National Formulary*, latest edition. London: British Medical Association and Royal Pharmaceutical Society of Great Britain.

National Institute for Health and Clinical Excellence (2004). *The epilepsies: diagnosis and the management of the epilepsies in adults in primary and secondary care.* Clinical Guideline 20. London: NICE. Available at: www.nice.org.uk.

Further reading

Brodie MJ, French JA (2000). Management of epilepsy in adolescents and adults. *Lancet* **356**: 323–9.

Craig J, Sisodiya S (2001). Guide to the management of epilepsy in pregnancy. *Prescriber* **12**: 30–6.

Feely M (1999). Drug treatment of epilepsy. *BMJ* **318**: 106–9.

Online resources

www.epilepsy.org.uk
The website of Epilepsy Action (British Epilepsy Association), a very useful resource for information on epilepsy, with excellent patient information (accessed 1 February 2008).

www.epilepsynse.org.uk
The website of National Society for Epilepsy, a very useful resource for information on epilepsy with excellent patient information (accessed 1 February 2008).

24

Affective disorders

Disease characteristics

Affective (emotional) disorders consist of changes in mood, with the most common manifestation being depressed mood. Typically this is a long-standing condition that may be associated with feelings of low self-esteem, a lack of motivation and an inability to derive pleasure, and sleep may be disturbed, often with early waking. The cause is often difficult to identify and may be multifactorial with risk factors including creative, perfectionist and neurotic personality types, stressful life events, history of abuse in childhood, the later stages of pregnancy, after childbirth and with a hereditary link, particularly in bipolar disorder. There is also a close association with chronic illnesses (such as multiple sclerosis, myocardial infarction, stroke, Parkinson's disease, cancer, human immunodeficiency virus [HIV]), and may be precipitated by major events such as bereavement. Depression may complicate or worsen pre-existing diseases. In addition certain drugs may lead to or exacerbate depression, e.g. isotretinoin, corticosteroids, mefloquine, rimonabant, varenicline, benzodiazepines and alcohol. Substance misuse is also a significant cause. For detailed guidance on the management of depression the reader is referred to guidance of the National Institute for Health and Clinical Excellence (NICE 2004, 2007).

Underlying pathology

The underlying pathology of affective disorders is poorly understood. The classic explanation comes from the monoamine theory, which is now over 50 years old, but does not, however, satisfactorily account for all of the pathology. This theory links reduction in the monoamine neurotransmitters noradrenaline (norepinephrine) and 5-hydroxytryptamine (5HT, serotonin) as the main biochemical changes linked to clinical symptoms of depression. The theory was developed after the observation that drug-induced changes in monoamine neurotransmitters either caused or improved symptoms of depression, e.g. the antihypertensive reserpine was withdrawn due to side effects of depression, which were thought to be caused by a reduction in noradrenaline and 5HT-mediated transmission in the brain. By contrast the antituberculosis drug isoniazid, which increased levels of catecholamines, enhanced mood. Antidepressant drugs were, therefore, designed to increase the availability of noradrenaline and 5HT in the brain, leading to a clinical response.

Anomalies exist in the theory in that some drugs affect noradrenaline and/or 5HT activity without evoking changes in mood, e.g. methysergide, a 5HT antagonist, does not produce a depressed mood, as might be predicted. A further discrepancy in the monoamine theory is the delayed onset of antidepressant action despite a rapid change in monoamine levels detectable by analysis of noradrenaline and 5HT metabolite concentrations in cerebrospinal fluid or urine. A change in receptor numbers has therefore been proposed as an important mechanism because a common and delayed down-regulation of β-adrenoceptors and $5HT_2$-receptors is observed after prolonged antidepressant treatment.

More recent theories focus on long-term changes in the neuronal development and plasticity of neuronal circuits. Interest has focused on the changes in the cAMP response element-binding protein (CREB), which is a transcription factor that has been shown to be up-regulated by chronic antidepressant treatment and could influence neuronal development (Thome *et al* 2000).

Despite the anomalies in the monoamine theory, increased availability of monoamines in the brain remains the most effective bio-chemical manipulation used in the treatment of depression, being common to all antidepressant drugs.

Classification and clinical features

Depressive illness is classified according to the criteria of the *Diagnostic and Statistical Manual of Mental Disorders*, 4th edition (DSM-IV: American Psychiatric Association 1995) and the *International Statistical Classification of Diseases and Related Health Problems* 10th revision (ICD-10: World Health Organization 1992). These classifications are intended to differentiate between normal and pathological states through assessment of behavioural, psychological and biological dysfunction, with the aim of classifying disorders, not people. There is considerable overlap and mutual working between the two classifications. The following section therefore considers the DSM-IV criteria to prevent repetition.

The previous terminology used in the classification of affective disorders comprised reactive, endogenous, manic, psychotic and neurotic. The terms 'reactive' and 'endogenous' differentiated between depression occurring in response to life events or depression tending to have a hereditary component without associated life events, respectively. The types of depressive illness are currently classified as postnatal depression, seasonal affective disorder (SAD), dysthymia, unipolar depression (in response to stressful life events) and bipolar depression (previously manic depression). Psychotic symptoms may be present but do not constitute a distinct disorder.

Postnatal depression

The diagnosis of postnatal depression is made if any of the criteria below are met and symptoms occur within 4 weeks of childbirth.

Seasonal affective disorder

It is increasingly recognized that affective disorders may follow a seasonal pattern, with onset during the winter months. Accordingly, the DSM-IV criteria recognize SAD, when a regular and recurrent temporal relationship is observed and seasonal psychosocial stressors are excluded (e.g. unemployment every winter). In addition, two major depressive episodes will have been present in 2 years. Full remission or a switch from depression to mania or hypomania also follows a temporal relationship, such as occurs in spring-time. Major depressive episodes should also be absent outside the seasonal episodes. Finally, major depressive episodes with a seasonal onset should outnumber those without seasonal onset during the patient's life.

Dysthymic disorder

The DSM-IV criteria for dysthymic disorder include depressed mood for most of the day for most days for at least 2 years. The symptoms cause significant distress or reduced social or occupational functioning. At least two or more of the following symptoms are present with no more than 2 months without symptoms:

- poor appetite or overeating
- altered sleep requirements
- reduced energy or fatigue
- low self-esteem
- poor concentration or indecisiveness
- feelings of hopelessness.

In addition, the criteria require that no major depressive episodes have been diagnosed within the first 2 years. This excludes the possibility of partial remission after a major depressive episode. Full remission would include being symptom free for 2 months. Diagnosis is made after the exclusion of other mental disorders, drug abuse, medication (see Chapter 5) or underlying disease such as hypothyroidism.

Children

Dysthymic disorder may present as irritable mood in children and adolescents, with duration of at least 1 year.

Unipolar affective disorder (major depression)

Unipolar depression is the most common disorder, affecting one in six people. As many as one in three is likely to suffer an episode of unipolar depression in his or her lifetime. Diagnosis of a major depressive episode according to the DSM-IV criteria is currently considered when five or more of the following symptoms have been present on most days or nearly every day for 2 weeks and are causing clinically significant distress or impaired functioning. In addition, one of the symptoms must be one of the first two symptoms listed below. Major depressive disorder is diagnosed following one or more major depressive episodes, including:

- depressed mood
- loss of interest or pleasure in all or most activities
- increased or decreased appetite, particularly associated with significant weight change (more than 5% in a month and not dieting)
- altered sleep
- psychomotor agitation or retardation
- fatigue
- worthlessness or excessive or inappropriate guilt
- reduced ability to think or concentrate or indecisiveness
- recurrent thoughts of death or suicide.

The diagnosis is made only after the exclusion of substance abuse, bereavement (see below) or general medical conditions such as hypothyroidism.

Children

In children and adolescents, the symptom of depressed mood (first point above) may present as irritable mood. In addition, weight changes may present as a failure to make expected weight gains (see below).

Psychotic depression

A depressive episode may also present with additional psychotic symptoms. The term 'psychosis' is used to describe severe mental illness with loss of contact with reality. Thought processes are often altered and patients suffer hallucinations and delusions (see Chapter 27). Psychosis is a component of severe schizophrenia, depression and bipolar affective disorder. For a discussion of the psychotic symptoms associated with antimuscarinic drugs, see Chapter 27.

Severity

The severity of a depressive episode may be mild, moderate or severe. An episode is described as mild if the number of symptoms required for a positive diagnosis is exceeded only marginally. The impact of a minor episode produces only limited effects on social and occupational functioning. By contrast, a severe episode will present with numerous additional symptoms to those required to make a diagnosis, and a marked disruption to normal functioning occurs. Moderate illness falls between the two extremes.

Elderly patients and bereavement

The recognition and treatment of depression in elderly people are important but bereavement and/or dementia may complicate diagnosis. Bereavement is differentiated from depression if symptoms develop within 2–3 weeks of the death of a close friend or relative and resolve spontaneously. Dementia may be excluded depending on the magnitude of decline in memory.

Children

Depression in children and adolescents is now increasingly recognized, often presenting as self-criticism, pessimism about the future, lack of energy, sleep disturbance, stomachache, headache, indecision and difficulty concentrating (see also DSM-IV criteria listed above). Children may lack interest in activities that they previously enjoyed. Risk factors include a family history of affective disorders, stress, viral infections and a history of abuse. There is sparse information relating to the treatment of childhood depression but this may involve cognitive–behavioural therapy (CBT) and possibly the selective serotonin reuptake inhibitor (SSRI) fluoxetine, according to clinical trial data. The Commission on Human Medicines (CHM) has warned that the risks of other SSRIs such as citalopram, paroxetine and sertraline generally outweigh the benefits in children aged <18 years. There is no good evidence for the use of tricyclic antidepressants (TCAs) for depression in children. Recent NICE guidance has reminded practitioners that, in prescribing antidepressants for patients <18, the advantages must outweigh the disadvantages and, when treatment is indicated, fluoxetine should be used and paroxetine avoided. Monitoring for behavioural changes and suicidal thoughts is essential, particularly during the early stages of treatment.

Goals of treatment

Treatment aims are to improve the quality of life, including the ability to work and function socially, together with the prevention of suicide. This should of course be achieved with the minimum of side effects. Drug treatment should ideally be used with appropriate CBT or psychotherapy, which may hasten recovery and prevent recurrence. Detailed guidance for the provision of psychological interventions is given by NICE (2004, 2007).

Pharmacological basis of management

SSRIs, e.g. citalopram, escitalopram (active isomer of citalopram), fluoxetine, fluvoxamine, paroxetine, sertraline

As the name implies, SSRIs selectively inhibit the neuronal reuptake of 5HT, thus enhancing synaptic concentrations of 5HT and downregulating presynaptic 5HT-receptors. SSRIs have a different side-effect profile to TCAs, including nausea, diarrhoea, constipation, dizziness, headache, altered platelet function, anorexia, insomnia, loss of libido, and delay or failure of orgasm. Some SSRIs are also licensed for the treatment of anxiety, panic and obsessive–compulsive disorders (see Chapter 25).

TCAs, e.g. amitriptyline, dosulepin (dothiepin), imipramine, lofepramine, nortriptyline

TCAs are similar in structure to phenothiazines (prochlorperazine, thioridazine) and inhibit the neuronal uptake of noradrenaline and 5HT, leading to augmented concentrations in the synaptic cleft. The increase in catecholamines may lead to down-regulation of presynaptic α_2-adrenoceptors and 5HT receptors and postsynaptic β-adrenoceptors. In addition, TCAs exhibit binding at a range of receptors, including muscarinic receptors, histamine, α_1-adrenoceptors and 5HT-receptors. The inhibition of muscarinic receptors results in side effects such as dry mouth, blurred vision, constipation and urinary retention. TCAs vary in the degree of sedation that they cause (with amitriptyline and dosulepin having significant effects and lofepramine being less sedating) and this may have a bearing on their use where sedation may be an advantage or unwanted. TCAs may cause cardiac effects such as Q–T interval prolongation and the potentiation of catecholamines also predisposes to heart block and arrhythmias. The cardiac effects of TCAs (except lofepramine), together with increased effects of alcohol, including respiratory depression, mean that these agents are dangerous in overdose. They are not suitable for patients with ischaemic heart disease, aged >70 years or those patients who are thought to be at high risk of attempting suicide.

Monoamine oxidase inhibitors: isocarboxazid, moclobemide, phenelzine, tranylcypromine

Monoamine oxidase inhibitors (MAOIs) are rarely used because of their widespread side effects and drug interactions, including those with tyramine-containing foods. They were the first antidepressants used after the observation that treatment with isoniazid for tuberculosis improved mood. MAOIs inhibit the MAOs, which metabolize catecholamines. Once again, their action is to increase the concentration of these neurotransmitters. As a result of this effect, MAOIs also prevent the breakdown of tyramine, the indirectly acting sympathomimetic amine, which is present in the diet. By preventing the breakdown of tyramine, this amine causes the release of catecholamines and leads to a hypertensive response. Tyramine is present in certain foods such as yeast extracts (including Bovril and Marmite), some wines and beers, avocado, banana, pickled herring and cheese, and this response is known as the 'cheese reaction'. As most MAOIs inhibit MAO irreversibly, these reactions may persist for 2–3 weeks after the cessation of treatment until a new MAO is synthesized.

MAO exists as either MAO-A, which metabolizes predominantly noradrenaline and 5HT, or MAO-B, for which phenylethylamine is a substrate. Tyramine and dopamine are metabolized by both subtypes. In an attempt to reduce side effects and interactions, selective inhibitors of MAO have been developed, e.g. moclobemide, a selective reversible inhibitor of MAO-A (RIMA), reduces interactions with food because tyramine is metabolized by MAO-B. The MAO-B inhibitor selegeline is used to treat Parkinson's disease.

Noradrenaline reuptake inhibitors: reboxetine

Reboxetine is one of the newer noradrenaline reuptake inhibitors (NARIs). It selectively inhibits noradrenaline reuptake, providing an option for patients who cannot take TCAs (Table 24.1) but who are resistant to the effects of SSRIs.

Serotonin–noradrenaline reuptake inhibitors: venlafaxine

A relatively new reuptake inhibitor is venlafaxine. The mechanism of action involves the inhibition of both serotonin and noradrenaline reuptake, as with TCAs. Serotonin–noradrenaline reuptake inhibitors (SNRIs), however, fail to bind to additional receptors and therefore demonstrate fewer side effects compared with TCAs, including a lack of sedative and antimuscarinic side effects, but do cause gastrointestinal side effects. In addition, an analysis of fatal toxicity of antidepressants in the UK reported that venlafaxine toxicity is greater than for other serotoninergic agents and similar to some TCAs (Buckley and McManus 2002). In May 2006, the MHRA (Medicines and Healthcare products Regulatory Agency) highlighted problems of serious cardiac arrhythmias and cardiotoxicity in overdose with venlafaxine.

Noradrenergic and specific serotoninergic antidepressants: mirtazapine

Observations of the pharmacological activity of mianserin have been exploited in the development of mirtazapine. This agent exhibits α_2-adrenocepter antagonist activity, inhibiting negative feedback by these presynaptic receptors and thus producing an increase in noradrenaline and 5HT transmission. Mirtazapine also inhibits $5HT_2$- and $5HT_3$-receptors, preventing sexual dysfunction and nausea, respectively. Sedation predominates in early treatment but antimuscarinic side effects are limited.

Serotonin receptor modulators: nefazodone and trazodone

Nefazodone and trazodone are similar in structure and exhibit mixed serotoninergic activity, including both inhibition of serotonin reuptake and the selective inhibition of postsynaptic 5HT-receptors. Trazodone also acts at noradrenaline receptors, with nefazodone exhibiting less activity at these receptors.

TCA-related antidepressants: bupropion, maprotiline, mianserin

In the ongoing search for antidepressants with fewer side effects, reduced toxicity in overdose and no delayed onset of action, a number of agents have been developed that do not fit the above classes of MAOI, SSRI or TCA, e.g. some agents possess a non-TCA structure but exhibit similar modes of action. The mechanisms thought to be involved in the antidepressant effects of these TCA-related agents include:

- the inhibition of noradrenaline uptake (nomifensine and maprotiline)
- a small reduction of 5HT uptake and possibly inhibition of dopamine uptake (nomifensine)
- agents that do not affect amine uptake (mianserin, bupropion)
- inhibition of 5HT- and α_2-adrenoceptors, thereby inhibiting negative feedback and increasing release of noradrenaline without the conventional effects on the reuptake of noradrenaline and serotonin (mianserin)
- unknown mechanisms – bupropion is efficacious but fails to demonstrate biochemistry in common with conventional antidepressant activity.

Benzodiazepines (e.g. clonazepam, lorazepam) and β blockers

These are used on a temporary basis in depression with a component of severe anxiety or hyperactivity (see Chapter 25), e.g. a short-acting benzodiazepine such as lorazepam may be used when antidepressants are initiated, before the onset of efficacy. Long-term use may worsen depression and lead to addiction to benzodiazepines and apparent worsening anxiety (withdrawal reactions, see Chapter 5).

Flupentixol

Lower doses of flupentixol compared with those used in schizophrenia are indicated for the treatment of depressive illness.

L-Tryptophan

L-Tryptophan, a precursor for 5HT, is an amino acid found in food. It has a mild antidepressant effect but use is limited to prescribing by hospital specialists for patients with chronic severe depression who are already taking other antidepressants. This is mainly due to the risk of eosinophilia–myalgia syndrome (increased eosinophils in blood, with muscle pain) and close monitoring of the eosinophil count and muscle symptoms is required.

Electroconvulsive therapy

Electroconvulsive therapy (ECT) is reserved for severe and suicidal depression, with greatest efficacy in depression with psychomotor retardation (literally, a slowing of muscular and mental activity), such as depressive stupor. This is a condition of near unconsciousness, apparent mental inactivity and a reduced response to stimulation. The procedure is carried out under general anaesthesia and a convulsion is induced by passing an electric current through the brain. The main side effects are temporary confusion and memory loss. This treatment should therefore be used with caution in elderly patients with cognitive impairment. Other risks to be considered are those associated with general anaesthesia and the use of ECT during pregnancy. These risks are considered alongside the benefits and potential risks of withholding treatment. The mechanism involved remains unclear but ECT is an effective treatment with rapid onset.

Lithium

Lithium is a useful adjunct in the treatment of resistant depression. It may be added to TCA or SSRI treatment under specialist supervision. The use of TCAs and SSRIs is associated with a risk of switching patients into mania, a particular problem when treating the depressive phase of bipolar disorder. The highest risk is associated with the use of TCAs.

Non-pharmacological therapy

Structured counselling based on theoretical models includes psychotherapy or CBT. Psychotherapy may be of particular benefit to patients with a history of abuse or social history such as stressful life events. CBT has been shown to be effective in mild depression and in combination with antidepressants in moderate depression (Scott *et al* 1997). This would seem logical because neurotic, perfectionist, obsessional or anxious personality types may be linked to depression. The negative thought patterns associated with these personality types are

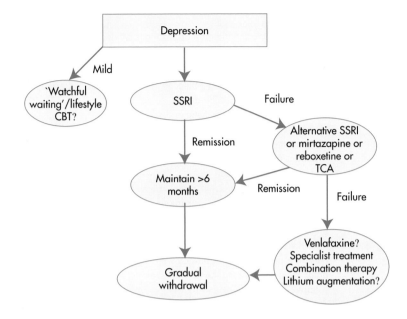

Figure 24.1   A flow diagram summarizing the management of unipolar depression, which incorporates NICE (2004) guidance. CBT, cognitive–behavioural therapy; SSRI, serotonin selective reuptake inhibitor; TCA, tricyclic antidepressant.

identified and addressed during CBT. In addition, increased insight and the avoidance of overly stressful situations contribute to successful treatment. The reader is referred to *Mind over Mood* (Greenberger and Padesky 1995) for an excellent CBT-based workbook for motivated patients. Computerised CBT is also recommended for the treatment of mild depression (NICE 2004, 2007). In addition, a meditation-based approach to CBT known as mindfulness-based CBT has been developed and is recommended by NICE for patients with recurrent depression. This is not widely available at the moment but workbooks such as *The Mindful Way through Depression* (Williams *et al* 2007) and *Mindfulness-Based Cognitive Therapy for Depression: A new approach to preventing relapse* (Segal *et al* 2002) are available for patients and therapists, respectively. Patients with SAD may benefit from light therapy (Levitt *et al* 2002).

Choice of drugs in unipolar affective disorder

NICE guidance recommends that, before drug treatment in mild depression, a 2-week period of 'watchful waiting' is appropriate with advice on exercise, sleep and anxiety management. CBT is also recommended. When drug treatment is appropriate the choice is between an SSRI and a TCA, with the most appropriate drug class being selected, according to:

- sedative properties
- side-effect profile
- previous response
- potential for toxicity in overdose
- concurrent disease (Table 24.1).

Although SSRIs and TCAs are generally regarded as equally effective, NICE guidance (2004) indicates that SSRIs have a superior side-effect profile and are safer in overdose and so should be regarded as first-line agents. Current guidance indicates that antidepressants should not be used in mild depression and that they are really effective only in moderate-to-severe cases. The NICE indicates that either fluoxetine or citalopram is appropriate for first-line usage. TCAs should be used only if SSRIs fail to control the condition or are contraindicated. In cases where sedation is required TCAs such as amitriptyline might be chosen in preference to SSRIs.

Table 24.1   Some considerations when choosing the most appropriate antidepressant

Condition	Cautions and contraindications	Compelling drug choices
Cardiovascular disease	All antidepressants, including lithium, should be used with caution due to increased effects of sympathetic and serotoninergic systems. Venlafaxine has been associated with dose-related hypertension	SSRIs are preferred
Recent MI	TCAs are contraindicated	SSRIs considered safe, particularly sertraline (Glassman *et al* 2002)
Arrhythmias	TCAs are contraindicated. Venlafaxine and antipsychotics may cause Q–T prolongation. Atypical antipsychotics have not been associated with this but caution is needed if co-prescribed with drugs known to prolong the Q–T interval (Chapter 5)	SSRIs (not fluoxetine) Avoid fluoxetine and trazodone, which can cause atrial fibrillation
Stroke	Avoid MAOIs due to the risk of a hypertensive episode. Use venlafaxine with caution due to dose-related hypertension (see above)	
Insomnia	SSRIs may occasionally cause insomnia. Lofepramine is a less-sedating TCA	Sedating TCAs (e.g. amitriptyline, dosulepin), maprotiline, mianserin or trazodone
Risk of deliberate self-harm or suicide attempt	See text	
Epilepsy	All antidepressants have the potential to lower the convulsive threshold and should be used with caution and avoided in poorly controlled epilepsy	• Carbamazepine and lamotrigine (unlicensed indication) may be considered in bipolar affective disorder • Additional risk factors include diabetes mellitus or concurrent treatment with drugs known to lower the convulsive threshold (Chapter 23)
Bipolar affective disorder – manic phase	TCAs, MAOIs and SSRIs are contraindicated. Antidepressants may trigger bipolar disorder, particularly in patients with hypomania and/or a family history	Mood stabilizers (lithium, neuroleptics, carbamazepine and valproate – see text). Combining SSRI treatment (avoiding long-acting preparations, e.g. fluoxetine) with a mood stabilizer may reduce the risk of switching to mania (Grunze *et al* 2002)
Anxiety disorders	Long-term use of propranolol and/or benzodiazepines should be avoided because these drugs may aggravate depression	For depression with associated anxiety symptoms, refer to Chapter 25
Migraine	SSRIs may cause headache (Chapter 5)	TCAs may be appropriate (Chapter 22)
Neuropathic pain		TCAs or carbamazepine

Continued

Table 24.1 (Continued)

Condition	Cautions and contraindications	Compelling drug choices
Alcoholism	Sedative effects of TCAs enhanced	
Eating disorders		High-dose fluoxetine is indicated for bulimia nervosa
Parkinson's disease treated with co-beneldopa, co-careldopa, levodopa	Irreversible MAOIs should be avoided with drugs used to increase dopamine	
Peptic ulcer disease	Increased risk of GI bleeds, so caution with SSRIs. Consider high-risk patients such as those with a history of previous GI bleed and/or aged over 80 years (Chapter 7)	
Urinary problems (prostatism), glaucoma and constipation	Caution with TCAs and maprotiline and mirtazapine due to antimuscarinic side effects	
Hyperthyroidism	Caution with TCAs due to augmentation of sympathetic nervous system. Lithium should be used with caution and initiated when patients are euthyroid. Regular monitoring of thyroid function is essential (Chapter 2)	

GI, gastrointestinal; MAOIs, monoamine oxidase inhibitors; MI, myocardial infarction; SSRIs, selective serotonin reuptake inhibitors; TCAs, tricyclic antidepressants.

Treatment should be continued for at least 6 months after symptoms resolve to prevent relapse and recurrence. The recommended length of treatment varies according to the severity of symptoms and the number of episodes suffered. The duration of treatment of a second episode should be at least 12 months. For recurrent depression the NICE (2004) recommends the continuation of antidepressants for 2 years after two or more depressive episodes in the recent past and associated with significant functional impairment. The need for ongoing maintenance treatment is assessed according to age, concurrent conditions and other risk factors.

Risk of suicide

TCAs are avoided in patients considered to be at risk of committing suicide, such as those with a history of contemplating or attempting suicide. This is due to the toxic effects of TCAs (except lofepramine) in overdose. SSRIs are preferred due to relative safety in overdose, although patients should be monitored closely during early treatment with all antidepressants and particularly SSRIs, due to a possible increased risk of suicide attempts. Alternative treatment includes the use of mirtazapine, nefazodone and reboxetine, which are considered to be relatively safe in overdose. For a discussion of the use of venlafaxine, see SNRIs above.

Treatment failure

Failure of treatment (typically after 4 weeks) may lead to a different class being used. It should be noted that a failure of TCAs may reflect too low a dosage being prescribed, because it has been found that older TCAs are more effective in the 125–150 mg dose range than at lower doses. A subsequent failure with TCAs or SSRIs may be a reason to consider using venlafaxine, or in some specialist settings combination therapy may be used. Specialists may also use lithium augmentation.

Effectiveness of antidepressants

The effectiveness of antidepressants has been established over many years by numerous clinical trials, analyses and clinical experience. However, one meta-analysis has indicated that certain agents (fluoxetine, venlafaxine, nefazodone and paroxetine) lack or have limited efficacy beyond a placebo effect (Kirsch *et al* 2008). This analysis is clearly controversial but current opinion and guidance certainly support their use in moderate-to-severe depression.

Bipolar affective disorder

Bipolar depression is characterized by cycling between depression and mania and has a strong hereditary link, although no specific gene(s) has been identified to date. It is less common than unipolar depression, affecting 1 in 100 of the population.

Manic episode

By contrast to the symptoms of depression outlined above, the manic phase of bipolar affective disorder presents as abnormally and persistently elevated expansive or irritable mood. The DSM-IV criteria classify a manic episode when three or more of the following symptoms are significant and present for at least 1 week and/or require hospital admission:

* inflated self-esteem or grandiosity
* reduced requirement for sleep
* rapid speech with pressure to keep talking
* flight of ideas
* distractibility
* increased goal-directed activity or psychomotor agitation (compare psychomotor retardation in depressive symptoms)
* reduced inhibitions such as sexual indiscretion and uncontrolled spending.

In addition, the criteria state that a diagnosis is made when the above symptoms are sufficient to impair normal occupational and social activities and relationships with others, require hospital treatment to prevent self-harm or harm to others, or psychotic features are present. Again, additional causes such as medication, ECT, light therapy, drug abuse or hyperthyroidism should be excluded.

Hypomania

Hypomania is diagnosed when mood becomes persistently elevated, expansive or irritable compared with normal mood and persistent throughout the day for at least 4 days. The significant presence of three or more of the symptoms listed for a manic episode or four if the mood is irritable may result in a diagnosis of hypomania. Additional requirements are that others observe an uncharacteristic change in mood and functioning. A hypomanic episode differs from mania in that there is minimal effect on social or occupational function, hospital admission is not required and psychotic symptoms are absent. Additional causes such as medication should be excluded, as stated previously.

Rapid cycling

The diagnosis of rapid cycling is made when four episodes of mood disturbance occur, according to the above criteria, during a 12-month period. Partial or full remission occurs for at least 2 months between episodes. Alternatively a switch between a depressive and manic episode may occur.

Treatment

Lithium remains the first-line agent for both acute treatment and prophylaxis of bipolar disorder, although a delay in the onset of action necessitates the concurrent use of neuroleptics (see Chapter 27) in acute mania. Lithium is a monovalent cation that mimics the role of sodium ions by permeating fast voltage-sensitive channels responsible for generating action potentials in excitable tissue.

Lithium exerts many effects on neurotransmission and its relatively selective action on the brain and kidney has not been elucidated fully (Williams and Harwood 2000). The main site of action is the inhibition of recycling by hydrolysis of the intracellular second messenger inositol triphosphate (IP_3) to phosphatidyl inositol (PI) in cell membranes. This reduces the effects of substances that activate receptors (e.g. α_1-adrenoceptors) linked to IP_3 generation and subsequent Ca^{2+} release from intracellular stores. The extensive distribution of such receptor systems throughout the body suggests many potential effects of lithium. The apparent selectivity has been suggested to result from selective uptake of lithium dependent on sodium channel activity.

Toxic effects of lithium may result from reduced hormone responses involving the second messenger, adenosine cyclic 3':5'-monophosphate (cAMP), e.g. the inhibition of cAMP-mediated antidiuretic hormone (ADH) activity in the kidney results in polyuria and polydipsia. Sodium ions are retained, leading to increased ADH secretion and possible damage of renal tubules. The failure of the thyroid gland to respond to thyroid-stimulating hormone (TSH) may result in an enlarged thyroid gland and hypothyroidism.

Anticonvulsants, e.g. carbamazepine and valproate

Carbamazepine and valproate are used second line as prophylactic mood stabilizers in bipolar disorder and lack the extrapyramidal effects of the antipsychotic drugs. The mechanism of action has not yet been elucidated fully but is thought to involve effects on ion channels, increasing the release of the inhibitory and excitatory neurotransmitters, γ-aminobutyric acid (GABA) and glutamate, respectively. The anticonvulsants lamotrigine and gabapentin have an unlicensed role in bipolar affective disorder when other treatments have failed.

Antipsychotics, e.g. haloperidol and chlorpromazine

Antipsychotics such as haloperidol and chlorpromazine may be used to control psychotic symptoms, which may be associated with depression and particularly during the manic phase of bipolar disorder. They have a rapid rate of onset and so may be initiated together with lithium, controlling the manic phase until the lithium begins to exert its effects in patients with bipolar disorder. The blockade of dopamine D_2-receptors is thought to be the predominant mode of action. Haloperidol is often preferred due to reduced sedative and cardiovascular effects compared with chlorpromazine. The atypical antipsychotic olanzapine has been licensed for use in bipolar disorder and is less likely to cause extrapyramidal effects compared with the older agents (see Chapter 27).

Thyroid hormones and calcium blockers (verapamil, nimodipine)

There is weak or limited evidence for the use of calcium channel antagonists and thyroid hormones in the treatment of bipolar disorder. High doses of levothyroxine have been used, however, in refractory cases of bipolar disorder, particularly with rapid cycling, but are not licensed for this purpose. Particular caution is required due to cardiovascular side effects.

Drug choice in bipolar affective disorder

The acute (manic) phase of bipolar affective disorder is often associated with psychosis and therefore treated with antipsychotics such as haloperidol and/or benzodiazepines such as lorazepam for severe cases. These drugs are used for a few days until the effects of lithium are achieved. The atypical antipsychotic olanzapine is also used to treat moderate-to-severe manic episodes. However, lithium remains the treatment of choice for both acute and long-term prophylaxis; olanzapine may be added to lithium for patients with residual symptoms. Maintenance treatment is given under specialist supervision according to the risk of withdrawing the drug compared with its benefit. The need for continued treatment is assessed regularly and maintenance is recommended beyond 3–5 years only when the benefit of continuing the drug is apparent, e.g. the presence of symptoms during a trial of gradual dose reduction.

Other agents such as the anticonvulsants valproate and carbamazepine may be considered when treatment with lithium has failed. Carbamazepine is indicated for the prophylaxis of manic–depressive psychoses for patients unresponsive to lithium therapy. Valproic acid in the form semisodium valproate is licensed for acute mania whereas sodium valproate remains unlicensed for this use. Carbamazepine may particularly benefit patients with rapid cycling between mania and depression (four or more episodes per year). Both carbamazepine and valproate are currently considered to be second choice for prophylaxis due to an inferior efficacy compared with lithium. The anticonvulsants lamotrigine and gabapentin are unlicensed for bipolar disorder and should be initiated only by specialists. Lamotrigine may be considered for the treatment of the depressive phase of bipolar depression when TCA- or SSRI-induced 'switching' to the manic phase is problematic (Calabrese *et al* 1999). Guidelines published by the World Federation of Societies of Biological Psychiatry suggest that combining SSRIs (or bupropion) with a mood stabilizer (lithium or lamotrigine) reduces the risk of switching, to a level observed when mood stabilizers are used alone (Grunze *et al* 2002). It was noted that lithium might also possess anti-suicide properties.

Concurrent conditions: additional considerations when prescribing in affective disorders

Some considerations for choosing a suitable antidepressant are summarized in Table 24.1.

Diabetes mellitus

MAOIs should be used with caution due to an increased risk of hypoglycaemia. Lithium ions may impair glucose tolerance and may cause diabetes mellitus. There is no evidence, however, for loss of glycaemic control of existing diabetes but careful monitoring is recommended. Olanzapine has been associated with hyperglycaemia or exacerbation of pre-existing diabetes mellitus and should be used with caution in these patients. Monitoring of patients with risk factors for type 2 diabetes, particularly obesity, is important when prescribing olanzapine, which may also cause weight gain.

Renal impairment

- Lithium should be avoided in renal impairment. For patients with mild renal impairment, a dose reduction and close monitoring are advised.
- SSRIs should be generally avoided in severe renal impairment. In moderate impairment, dose reduction may be needed.
- The dose of venlafaxine also requires reduction in moderate renal impairment.
- Small doses of antipsychotics are used in severe renal impairment. Lower doses of risperidone or olanzapine may be required.

Liver function

TCAs and MAOIs are contraindicated in severe liver disease. TCAs are preferable to MAOIs but sedative effects are increased. Lofepramine is associated with hepatic toxicity. MAOIs are implicated in the development of idiosyncratic hepatotoxicity. Reduced doses of SSRIs are advised with avoidance in severe liver disease. Antipsychotics can precipitate coma and phenothiazines are hepatotoxic. Atypical antipsychotics such as risperidone and olanzapine may be used at reduced doses (*British National Formulary*, Appendix 2).

Pregnancy and breast-feeding

TCAs are preferred if necessary for the treatment of unipolar depression during pregnancy and breast-feeding. This is due to greater experience of their use in pregnancy compared with SSRIs, and lower known risks, with the exception of toxicity in overdose. Fluoxetine is the SSRI of choice in pregnancy if the benefit is judged to exceed risk (NICE 2007). All antidepressants may be associated with withdrawal effects in the infant if prescribed close to the delivery date but these tend to be mild and self-limiting. Concerns over the risk of toxicity with venlafaxine in overdose, together with the risk of increased blood pressure, make it a less suitable choice in pregnancy.

Sertraline may be preferred during breast-feeding because lower levels are found in breast milk compared with fluoxetine. The TCAs imipramine and nortiptyline are suitable choices with low levels found in breast milk (NICE 2007).

Drugs used for bipolar disorders are often associated with abnormalities of the fetus and therefore preconception counselling is important. In view of the teratogenic risk associated with lithium in the first trimester, it is recommended that pregnancy be excluded before the initiation of lithium therapy. Ideally, all treatment is withdrawn for at least the first trimester. Alternatively, reducing the dose, particularly of lithium, is considered. For patients taking carbamazepine, folic acid 5 mg supplements are recommended before conception and up to week 12 of pregnancy (see Chapters 3 and 23).

Miscellaneous

Lithium is not recommended for patients with Addison's disease, because disturbances in sodium homeostasis may result. Blood pressure monitoring is recommended if doses of venlafaxine exceed 200 mg/day.

Drug interactions

Drug interactions involving antidepressants may result from: altered drug levels due to effects on drug absorption, metabolism or excretion; over-stimulation of monoamine neurotransmission; an increased risk of cardiac arrhythmias due to prolongation of the Q–T interval and the risk of convulsions due to a lowering of the convulsive

Table 24.2 Problems associated with the co-prescribing of antidepressants

Interacting antidepressants	Consequences	Comments
Fluoxetine with TCAs (amitriptyline, clomipramine, imipramine and nortriptyline) or trazodone	• Increased levels of TCAs • Increased risk of sedation due to trazodone	• Dose adjustment is required during concurrent use • Trazodone and fluoxetine are effective when co-prescribed but patients may develop increased side effects such as sedation • The long half-life of fluoxetine means that this interaction may persist after the drug is stopped
Fluvoxamine with TCAs (amitriptyline, clomipramine, imipramine and trimipramine) or maprotiline	Increased serum levels of the TCA or maprotiline	• Dose adjustment is required to prevent toxicity • There is no evidence for the same interaction with desipramine
Lithium with TCAs or SSRIs	An unpredictable risk of serious effects such as serotonin or neuroleptic malignant syndromes (see text)	Lithium is occasionally used successfully with TCAs or SSRIs but monitoring for ADRs is important
Paroxetine with TCAs (desipramine, imipramine and trimipramine)	Increased serum levels of the TCA	Patients should therefore be monitored closely for ADRs and the dose reduced if necessary

ADRs, adverse drug reactions; SSRIs, selective serotonin reuptake inhibitors; TCAs, tricyclic antidepressants.

threshold. The following section highlights some examples.

Antidepressant combinations

Co-prescribing two or more antidepressants is not recommended due to the risk of toxicity, e.g. co-prescribing MAOIs, particularly irreversible MAOIs, increases the risk of hypertensive crises and stroke (see above). Despite this, the combinations of some antidepressants such as MAOIs or SSRIs with TCAs or atypical agents may be beneficial but only under expert supervision. Monitoring for adverse drug reactions is advised with all combinations. Examples of problems requiring particular awareness are given in Table 24.2.

Serotoninergic syndrome

The Sternbach diagnostic criteria indicate that three or more of the following symptoms should be present before differentiating serotonin syndrome from neuroleptic malignant syndrome (see Chapter 5): confusion, hypomania, incoordination, tremor, agitation, diaphoresis (sweating), shivering, fever, myoclonus (muscle spasms) and hyperreflexia (Sternbach 1991).

Lithium and olanzapine

It should be noted that there is no evidence for an interaction between lithium and olanzapine. Table 24.3 provides examples of drug interactions involving antidepressants.

Monitoring

Renal function and electrolytes (creatinine and sodium)

Hyponatraemia may occur with high doses of TCAs or SSRIs or in elderly patients, and particularly with either co-prescribed diuretics, laxatives or concurrent illness leading to dehydration. The CHM warns that hyponatraemia should be considered in patients developing confusion, drowsiness or convulsions while taking antidepressants.

Lithium (see Appendix 2)

Urea and electrolytes and full blood count

Baseline measurements of blood urea and electrolytes (U&Es), serum creatinine, thyroid function, a full blood count (FBC) and the exclusion of pregnancy are required before the initiation of lithium therapy. Concurrent diseases such as cardiac disease are also considered (see Table 24.1).

During maintenance therapy, the following monitoring is recommended:

- serum creatinine every 6 months
- thyroid function tests every 6–12 months with counselling to report warning symptoms (4–6 weeks if TSH is elevated)
- an FBC annually
- serum lithium levels at least 3-monthly (see Chapter 6)
- U&Es every 6 months.

Ischaemic heart disease

An electrocardiogram is recommended before the initiation of lithium treatment for patients with a history of cardiac problems.

Liver function

Liver function should be assessed before and during the first 6 months of treatment with sodium valproate or valproic acid (see Chapter 23). Raised liver enzymes may be transient and a clinical assessment of clinical features and liver function tests (see Chapter 2), including pro-thrombin time, should be continued until the levels return to normal. Risk factors include children <3 years of age, metabolic or degenerative disease, organic brain disease or severe seizures with learning disability.

Blood counts

Patients taking mianserin should have blood counts checked every 4 weeks for the first 3 months of treatment. Blood monitoring should be performed for patients taking mianserin or carbamazepine who develop fever, sore throat, stomatitis or other signs of infection. Mirtazapine treatment warrants blood counts and immediate cessation of treatment if blood dyscrasias are suspected.

Table 24.3 Examples of drug interactions involving antidepressants

Drug	Consequences	Comments
Antidepressants with alcohol	• Increased side effects such as drowsiness and reduced alertness • Increased risk of accidents when driving or operating machinery	• Possible antagonism of antidepressant effect with chronic alcohol intake • Temporary mood-enhancing effect may contribute to a vicious cycle of alcohol abuse
Induction of hepatic enzymes		
Carbamazepine with haloperidol, oral contraceptives or phenytoin	Reduced effects of the latter	• Increased doses may be required
SSRI-mediated inhibition of hepatic enzymes		
Fluvoxamine with theophylline	Risk of a rapid and potentially toxic increase in theophylline levels	• The CSM warns that this should be avoided (CSM/MCA 1994) • Alternatively, the theophylline dose should be reduced to about half • Limited evidence suggests that a similar interaction does not occur between fluoxetine and theophylline
Fluoxetine, fluvoxamine, sertraline and paroxetine with anticoagulants, MAOIs, alcohol, selegiline, antipsychotics, lithium, phenytoin, carbamazepine and omeprazole	• Increased effects	• Evidence suggests that the SSRI citalopram does not interact with warfarin • Note that SSRIs differ in their profile of cytochrome P450 inhibition
Lithium levels increased		
ACE inhibitors, diuretics (particularly thiazides) and analgesics	Reduced excretion of lithium	• Consider impairment of renal function as a risk factor • Monitoring is required with a possible reduction in lithium dose • Aspirin and paracetamol are considered safe to use with lithium
Lithium with theophylline or metronidazole	Increased plasma concentrations of lithium	Close monitoring is required
Lithium levels reduced		
Lithium with ispaghula husk	Serum levels of lithium may be reduced	• Monitoring with appropriate dose adjustment is recommended • The mechanism involved may be due in part to the sodium content of effervescent granules
Lithium with methyldopa or clonazepam	Enhanced neurotoxicity	Avoid concurrent use

Continued

Table 24.3   (Continued)

Drug	Consequences	Comments
Lithium with haloperidol	Risk of rare but serious neurotoxic reaction, particularly in patients with a history of extrapyramidal effects with antipsychotics or if high doses of haloperidol are used	• Symptoms include fever, tremor, confusion and extrapyramidal effects • Patients should be monitored closely for ADRs, with prompt withdrawal due to a risk of brain damage • The co-prescribing of haloperidol with lithium in acute mania is extremely beneficial
Lithium with baclofen	Increased risk of baclofen-induced hyperkinetic activity	Patients should be monitored closely
MAOIs with pethidine	Risk of a potentially life-threatening reaction	Pethidine should not be given with MAOIs unless a lack of sensitivity is confirmed
Paroxetine or sertraline with tramadol	The combination of two or more serotoninergic drugs may lead to a potentially fatal condition resulting from overstimulation of 5HT receptors	Monitoring for symptoms of serotonin syndrome is advised (see text)
SSRIs or MAOIs with 5HT agonists (sumatriptan)	Risk of serotonin syndrome (see text)	Avoid concurrent use
SSRIs with NSAIDs	Increased risk of GI bleed	Consider additional risk factors and possible GI protection, e.g. using a proton pump inhibitor (Chapter 7)
TCAs and some atypical antidepressants (venlafaxine) **with** other drugs known to prolong the QT interval	Q–T interval prolongation and risk of potentially fatal arrhythmias	• The CHM warns against the use of more than one drug known to prolong the Q–T interval • If concurrent use is unavoidable, patients should report irregular heart beat, palpitations and dizziness immediately
TCAs or SSRIs with other drugs which lower the convulsive threshold	Increased risk of convulsions	

5HT, 5-hydroxytryptamine or serotonin; ACE, angiotensin-converting enzyme; ADRs, adverse drug reactions; CHM, Commission on Human Medicines; CSM, Committee on Safety of Medicines; GI, gastrointestinal; MAOIs, monoamine oxidase inhibitors; MCA, Medicines Control Agency; NSAIDs, non-steroidal anti-inflammatory drugs; SSRIs, selective serotonin reuptake inhibitors; TCAs, tricyclic antidepressants.

Withdrawal

Once a patient has been in remission, withdrawal of the antidepressant should be considered after a sufficient period of sustained remission. Withdrawal may precipitate a reaction (e.g. depression, sensory and balance problems, mood changes and gastrointestinal disturbances) in any patient (particularly with paroxetine and venlafaxine) and should involve a dose reduction over at least 4 weeks or up to 6 months in patients who have been on long-term maintenance therapy. Abrupt withdrawal of lithium should be avoided because this may increase the frequency of manic episodes and shorten the time to relapse.

Table 24.4 Antidepressants and over-the-counter (OTC) prescribing

OTC medicines	Comments
Sedative antihistamines such as diphenhydramine, promethazine are licensed for the treatment of insomnia	• Use is limited to 2 weeks. Repeated requests may point to depression • They should not be used together with TCAs due to enhanced antimuscarinic effects and sedation
Indirectly acting sympathomimetic decongestants (phenylpropanolamine, pseudoephedrine, ephedrine)	• The action of indirectly acting sympathomimetics is likely to be blocked by TCAs • There is, however, limited evidence for this interaction (Chapter 19) • Avoid with MAOIs (Chapter 19)
Directly acting sympathomimetic decongestants (phenylephrine)	These should not be taken by patients prescribed MAOIs or within 14 days of cessation of MAOIs because there is a substantial risk of enhanced pressor activity (i.e. increased blood pressure) (Chapter 19)
Antacids and sodium-containing preparations (cystitis and effervescent products)	These should be avoided with lithium
Cough preparations containing dextromethorphan	A rare but serious interaction (serotonin syndrome) with paroxetine contraindicates concurrent use
Fybogel	May reduce lithium levels
Cimetidine	This inhibits the metabolism of amitriptyline, doxepin, imipramine, moclobemide, nortriptyline, sertraline Use ranitidine as an alternative
NSAIDs	Ibuprofen increases plasma concentrations of lithium. Aspirin or paracetamol are appropriate alternatives

MAOIs, monoamine oxidase inhibitors; NSAIDs, non-steroidal anti-inflammatory drugs; TCAs, tricyclic antidepressants.

Over-the-counter considerations

An important role of the pharmacist is to recognize and refer patients with symptoms of depression, advise patients about drug inter-actions associated with antidepressant medi-cation, and provide advice and reassurance relating to side effects and the need for prolonged treatment. Table 24.4 highlights important issues and drug interactions associated with anti-depressants and over-the-counter (OTC) pre-scribing.

Alcohol

TCAs, fluvoxamine, isoniazid, maprotiline, mianserin and trazodone may enhance the effects of alcohol. In patients who are taking MAOIs, the hypotensive effects may be enhanced by alcohol and the tyramine content of certain beers and red wines should also be considered. It should also be noted that alcohol misuse may be related to depression. The central nervous system (CNS)-depressant effect of alcohol may cause or exacerbate depression, with the temporary mood-enhancing properties contributing to a 'vicious circle'.

Caffeine

Lithium levels may be reduced by excess caffeine intake. Levels may increase following abrupt withdrawal of caffeine intake (e.g. Pro Plus and some analgesic preparations). The effects of caffeine may also be deleterious in depression associated with anxiety (see Chapter 25).

Dietary supplements

Requests for advice regarding dietary supplements should as always be used as an opportunity to recommend a healthy diet (see Chapter 3), particularly including oily fish and foods rich in folic acid. Patients may request supplements such as dehydroepiandrosterone (DHEA), fish oils (particularly rich in the omega-3 fatty acids eicosapentaenoic acid [EPA] and docosahexanoic acid [DHA]), folic acid, phosphatidylserine or *S*-adenosylmethionine. Preliminary observations are interesting, e.g. patients with depression have been shown to have low levels of fish oils and folic acid but it is not clear if this is a cause or effect of depression.

Preliminary finding of pharmacological activity associated with the supplements phosphatidylserine and *S*-adenosylmethionine may also warrant further investigation, e.g. phosphatidylserine, the most abundant phospholipid in the brain, may interfere with the hypothalamic–pituitary–adrenal (HPA) axis, a potential target for the development of new treatments (see below). *S*-Adenosylmethionine may increase dopamine in the brain and preliminary evidence demonstrates antidepressant activity. The supplement choline has been suggested to improve symptoms of mania by increasing the production of acetylcholine, for which it is a precursor, in the brain. There is insufficient evidence to recommend these products to patients, particularly in combination with conventional antidepressants, but healthcare professionals should be aware that patients may be taking them.

Herbal medicines

Herbal medicines should be used with caution due to the lack of safety data available about combinations with conventional medicines. St John's wort has been shown to be better than placebo as an antidepressant for the short-term treatment of mild-to-moderate depression but is associated with significant side effects and interactions (see Chapters 4 and 5). It has been shown to be ineffective in major depression (Shelton *et al* 2001). In the context of depression, it inhibits the reuptake of 5HT, and may potentiate the action of SSRIs, and so should not be used with conventional antidepressants. A Cochrane systematic review concluded that there is evidence that some preparations of St John's wort demonstrate similar efficacy compared with conventional antidepressants for mild-to-moderate depression (Linde *et al* 2005). However, results cannot be extrapolated to all preparations because content varies. They also warn of the risk of adverse reactions when used in combination with other drugs.

Herbal drugs with sympathomimetic activity (see Chapter 4) should not be used with MAOIs and possibly TCAs. Many herbs possess sedative properties (see Chapter 4) and may therefore increase side effects, particularly with TCAs and benzodiazepines. The CNS-depressant effect of these herbs may also oppose the effect of antidepressants. Herbs containing tryptophan (alfalfa, chaparral, fenugreek, ginkgo and plantain) should also be avoided.

General counselling

General counselling points might include:

- To ensure continued treatment, according to the advice of the prescriber, for 6–24 months after recovery to prevent relapse. The analogy between a broken bone healing while in plaster is a useful explanation for the need to continue treatment even when well.
- Not to stop taking medication suddenly or without the advice of the prescriber, but reassure that antidepressants are not addictive.
- Be prepared for a delayed effect of 2–4 weeks and a possible worsening of symptoms in the first week. Sleep improvement may be an early beneficial effect in those receiving sedative TCAs for this purpose.
- The side effects of antidepressants, particularly nausea, should subside after the first week.
- Patients taking any antidepressant should be cautious when driving due to the risk of drowsiness and impaired reaction times.
- The return of insomnia may provide the first signs of relapse, particularly in bipolar

disorder. Patients should be taught to recognize and report early warning symptoms. Short-term treatment with hypnotics may be appropriate. The maximum benefit of antidepressants is obtained when symptoms are recognized early.

- Women should be advised about adequate contraception and to discuss the issues of antidepressant treatment before planning a pregnancy. This enables the prescriber and patient to discuss the risk versus benefit of antidepressant treatment during pregnancy, the possibility of a trial without treatment or changing to an alternative drug associated with lower risk. This is particularly important for women taking lithium salts and SSRIs.

- In view of the stigma still associated with depression, it may help to reassure patients that depression is common.

- Lifestyle changes such as increasing exercise and reducing alcohol and/or caffeine intake may be beneficial. NICE guidelines (2004) recommend a structured approach to exercise comprising up to three sessions per week of moderate duration (45–60 minutes) for 10–12 weeks.

- Diet is important for mental health (see Chapter 3) and the Mental Health Foundation has provided a useful booklet for patients with depression (see Online resources at end of chapter).

- Counselling may help the patient to make appropriate lifestyle changes when possible to prevent recurrence. It may also be useful to explain the importance of the duration of symptoms, comparing depression with normal 'low mood'. It may help to eliminate fear of relapse if the patient is reminded that experiencing occasional low mood is normal.

SSRIs

- Side effects include gastrointestinal disturbances (nausea, abdominal pain, diarrhoea, constipation, indigestion), postural hypotension, palpitations, increased sweating and sexual dysfunction (impotence, delay or failure of orgasm). There is an increased risk of extrapyramidal effects with paroxetine.

- Sexual dysfunction is a common cause of non-compliance with SSRIs, affecting up to 60% of patients. Sensitive counselling is therefore important when treatment is initiated.

- Reaction times may be impaired and patients should therefore be cautious, particularly when driving.

- Report any rash, particularly with fluoxetine, as treatment may need to be stopped.

- Treatment should not usually be stopped abruptly, particularly paroxetine, because withdrawal symptoms may occur. Patients should be advised to continue their treatment according to the advice of the prescriber, even when feeling better. This prevents the risk of relapse on cessation of treatment, which is withdrawn gradually over at least 4 weeks, or slower if withdrawal symptoms occur.

TCAs

- TCAs may cause drowsiness, so advise caution if driving (less with imipramine and lofepramine). Drowsiness may be enhanced by alcohol.

- The dose should be taken at night if sedation is required and also to limit daytime sedation.

- Side effects of TCAs include dry mouth, blurred vision and constipation. Initial sedation, confusion and motor incoordination should improve after 1–2 weeks of treatment.

- Patients presenting with signs of infection, such as a sore throat, while taking imipramine should be referred for an FBC.

Newer antidepressants

- Trazodone, nefazodone, reboxetine and venlafaxine may cause drowsiness and therefore patients should be advised to exercise caution if driving. Drowsiness may be increased by alcohol.

- Patients taking venlafaxine should report any palpitations or rashes, urticaria or related allergic reactions.

MAOIs

- These may cause drowsiness, so advise caution if driving. Drowsiness may be increased by alcohol.
- Patients should avoid tyramine-containing food such as cheese, red wine, yeast extracts (e.g. Marmite), chicken and beef liver, salami, soy sauce and avocado. Only fresh food should be eaten and stale food avoided.
- A warning card should be given.
- Side effects of MAOIs include overexcitement, insomnia, weight gain, dry mouth, blurred vision, constipation and postural hypotension (increased by alcohol). An early warning of food interactions may be a throbbing headache indicating a rapid increase in blood pressure.

Others (mianserin, mirtazapine, flupentixol)

- Patients taking mianserin or mirtazapine should report signs of infection such as fever or sore throat.
- Flupentixol may cause drowsiness but can also be alerting and therefore should not be taken in the evening.

Lithium

- Patients should maintain adequate fluid intake and avoid dietary changes leading to a change in sodium intake (including use of salt substitute) or the sudden introduction or discontinuation of caffeine (see Table 24.3).
- Alcohol intake should not exceed the recommended limits (see Chapter 3 and Table 24.3).
- A treatment card is available for patients from the National Pharmaceutical Association (www.npa.co.uk).
- Preparations may vary widely in bioavailability. Monitoring may be required if patients change brand.
- Symptoms of drowsiness are usually transient.
- Signs of toxicity, including nausea, vomiting, tremor, lack of coordination, extreme thirst, diarrhoea and excessive urination, should be reported urgently.

- Symptoms of hypothyroidism should prompt referral. These include lethargy, feeling cold and weight gain.
- Fluid loss due to diarrhoea, vomiting and intercurrent infection (particularly with profuse sweating) may necessitate discontinuation of treatment. The prescriber should be contacted.
- Patients should not take ibuprofen.
- Inform patients of the importance of regular blood tests and the need to leave 12 h after the last dose (see Chapter 6).
- Patients should inform health professionals that they take lithium.

Antipsychotics

See Chapter 27.

Anticonvulsants

See Chapter 23.

Benzodiazepines

For short-term use only (see also Chapter 26).

Self-assessment

Consider whether the following statements are true or false. In the management of unipolar depression:

1. SSRIs are more effective than TCAs.
2. Paroxetine is the antidepressant of choice in children under 18.
3. A therapeutic response should occur within 2–3 days.
4. TCAs are associated with causing constipation.
5. SSRIs are best used in combination with St John's wort.

Practice points

- Be alert for signs of depression in patients because stigma may still prevent patients from volunteering symptoms. Depression remains underdiagnosed (particularly in men) in primary care, and undiagnosed or undertreated depression is a significant cause of suicide. Pharmacists may identify patients requesting OTC hypnotics or herbal preparations for stress.
- Mild depression does not warrant the use of antidepressants.
- NICE guidance recommends that an SSRI should be considered as first-line treatment in moderate-to-severe depression.
- Close monitoring for signs of suicide is important during early treatment with all antidepressants. Consider also the danger of TCAs when taken in overdose.
- In patients who are at risk of suicide, only small quantities of drugs should be supplied.
- Compliance with treatment may be improved by warning patients of side effects and worsening of symptoms in the first week of treatment, together with the delayed onset of action.
- In treatment failure, consider compliance and encourage the patient to report troublesome side effects.
- Avoid abrupt withdrawal of antidepressant treatment.
- Most MAOIs inhibit MAO irreversibly, so the potential for drug interactions may persist for 2–3 weeks after the cessation of treatment. The SSRI fluoxetine also has a long half-life.
- Adequate doses, particularly of older TCAs, should be used to obtain a therapeutic effect.
- The National Service Framework currently advises that TCAs should not be prescribed to people aged >70 years because of the increased risk of adverse drug reactions in this age group.
- CBT has been shown to be as effective as antidepressants in mild depression and in combination with antidepressants for moderate depression. Beneficial effects include improved compliance, reduction of negative thought patterns and reduced exposure to stress.
- Regular use of propranolol for anxiety associated with depression may worsen depression. SSRIs should be considered (see Chapter 25).
- Be alert for the use of alcohol for temporary mood elevation, leading to a worsening of symptoms and risk of alcohol misuse.
- The CHM warns that hyponatraemia should be considered in patients developing confusion, drowsiness or convulsions while taking antidepressants.
- Prescriptions for lithium should be written using the brand name.
- It may be useful to repeat patient counselling at least annually during long-term treatment, particularly with lithium, and check that the patient retains the appropriate warning card.

 CASE STUDIES

Case 1
A female patient complains to her pharmacist of anxiety, dizziness, tremor and headache and asks to sit down. She asks if it could be due to stopping her antidepressant treatment. She has been prescribed paroxetine 20 mg daily. How do you reply?

- Patients taking all antidepressants, but particularly paroxetine, may experience a withdrawal syndrome if treatment is stopped suddenly. The patient should be advised to take a paroxetine tablet as soon as possible and return to her GP for a discussion about her treatment. You could enquire about the duration of treatment and, if appropriate, reinforce the importance of continuing to take the tablets after remission. Antidepressants should be withdrawn gradually over at least 4 weeks and up to 6 months after long-term maintenance therapy.

continued

◗ CASE STUDIES (continued)

Case 2
A female patient requests Nytol tablets for insomnia. Her patient medication record (PMR) reveals that she takes diazepam 2 mg as needed. She admits to feeling awful due to a hangover and has been feeling depressed for the last few weeks. Do you sell the Nytol?

- No! She may be suffering from depression and should be referred to her GP for assessment because she may require an antidepressant. Depression may be exacerbated by benzodiazepine treatment. If appropriate, you could educate her regarding the risk of dependence with benzodiazepines.
- You could advise her that alcohol causes insomnia and depression and recommend that she should discuss this with her GP.
- She may have depression associated with anxiety, for which an SSRI may be appropriate (see earlier).
- An additive effect of Nytol with benzodiazepines (and alcohol) may cause increased drowsiness.

Case 3
A 24-year-old male patient presents a prescription for fluoxetine 20 mg daily and trazodone capsules 100 mg per day. Are you happy to dispense this prescription?

- Yes. An interaction between the two drugs may result in elevated plasma concentrations of the trazodone, but concurrent use may be beneficial.
- Co-prescribing antidepressants is not recommended, but in this case a specialist had prescribed the combination. Advise the patient to report side effects and particularly excessive sedation.

Case 4
A National Health Service FP10 prescription is presented for 20 mL/day of fluoxetine liquid 20 mg/5 mL for postnatal depression. The drug was originally prescribed by the hospital. Are you happy to dispense the prescription?

- No. The dose is greater than the maximum daily dose for fluoxetine. This prescription should have been for paroxetine 10 mg/5 mL.

Case 5
A patient presents with a prescription for EpiPen (adrenaline injection). You see from his PMR that he is also prescribed lofepramine. Do you dispense the prescription?

- Interaction between adrenaline and lofepramine may lead to a life-threatening hypertensive crisis.
- If adrenaline is required, an SSRI would be a more appropriate antidepressant.

continued

> **CASE STUDIES** (continued)

Case 6
A 55-year-old man known to you for poor compliance with lithium for his bipolar affective disorder complains of tremor. He has difficulty signing his name. He is also taking amitriptyline and tells you that he only needs this. He's going to stop his lithium because of the tremor. What advice should this patient receive?

- Poor compliance is common in patients with bipolar affective disorder because they may fail to recognize their symptoms as abnormal. It is imperative that the patient be encouraged to continue with his lithium.

What is the most likely cause of his tremor?
Lithium and amitriptyline may interact, causing tremor. The patient should be referred to his GP. The combination of lithium and TCAs can be beneficial but also produces serious and unpredictable problems such as convulsions, serotonin syndrome and neuroleptic malignant syndrome. Patients should be monitored closely. Tremor is a side effect of lithium and severe tremor may also be a sign of lithium toxicity.

References

American Psychiatric Association (1995). *Diagnostic and Statistical Manual of Mental Disorders*, 4th edn (DSM-IV). Washington, DC: American Psychiatric Press.

Buckley NA, McManus PR (2002). Fatal toxicity of serotoninergic and other antidepressant drugs: analysis of United Kingdom mortality data. *BMJ* **325**: 1332–3.

Calabrese JR, Bowden CL, Sachs GS *et al* (1999) A double-blind placebo-controlled study of lamotrigine monotherapy in outpatients with bipolar I depression. Lamitcal 602 Study Group. *J Clin Psychiatry* **60**: 79–88.

Committee on Safety of Medicines/Medicines Control Agency (1994). Fluvoxamine increases plasma theophylline levels. *Curr Probl Pharmacovigilance* **20**: 12.

Glassman AH, O'Connor CM, Califf RM *et al* (2002). Sertraline treatment of major depression in patients with acute MI or unstable angina. *JAMA* **288**: 701–9.

Greenberger D, Padesky CA (1995). *Mind Over Mood.* New York: Guilford Press.

Grunze H, Kasper S, Goodwin G *et al* (2002). World Federation of Societies of Biological Psychiatry (WFSBP) guidelines for biological treatment of bipolar disorders, part 1: Treatment of bipolar depression. *World J Biol Psychiatry* **3**: 115–24.

Kirsch I, Deacon B J, Huedo-Medina TB *et al* (2008). Initial severity and antidepressant benefits: a meta-analysis of the data submitted to the food and drug administration. *Pub Lib Science Medicine* **5**: 260–8 (accessed online at www.plosmedicine.org).

Levitt AJ, Lam RW, Levitan R (2002). A comparison of open treatment of seasonal major and minor depression with light therapy. *J Affective Disord* **71**: 243–8.

Linde K, Mulrow CD, Berner *et al* (2005). St. John's wort for depression. *Cochrane Database System Rev* issue 1: CD000448.

Martin J, ed. *British National Formulary*, latest edition. London: British Medical Association and Royal Pharmaceutical Society of Great Britain.

National Institute for Health and Clinical Excellence (2004, 2007). *Depression: Management of depression in primary and secondary care.* Clinical Guideline 23 (amended 2007). London: NICE.

National Institute for Health and Clinical Excellence (2007). *Antenatal and Postnatal Mental Health: Clinical management and service guidance*. Clinical Guideline 45. London: NICE National Institute for Clinical Excellence.

Scott C, Tacchi M, Jones R *et al* (1997). Acute and one-year outcome of a randomised controlled trial of brief cognitive therapy for major depressive disorder in primary care. *Br J Psychiatry* **171**: 289–92.

Segal Z, Williams M, Teasdale J (2002). *Mindfulness-Based Cognitive Therapy: A new approach to preventing relapse*. New York: Guildford Press.

Shelton RC, Keller MB, Gelenberg A *et al* (2001). Effectiveness of St John's wort in major depression. *JAMA* **285**: 1978–86.

Sternbach H (1991). The serotonin syndrome. *Am J Psychiatry* **148**: 705–13.

Thome J, Sakai N, Shin K-H *et al* (2000). cAMP response element-mediated gene transcription is upregulated by chronic antidepressant treatment. *J Neurosci* **20**: 4030–6.

Williams RSB, Harwood A J (2000). Lithium therapy and signal transduction. *Trends Pharmacol Sci* **21**: 61–4.

Williams M, Teasdale J, Segal Z *et al* (2007). *The Mindful Way through Depression: Freeing yourself from chronic unhappiness*. New York: Guilford Press.

World Health Organization (1992). *The International Statistical Classification of Diseases and Related Health Problems*, 10th revision (ICD-10). Geneva: WHO.

Fraser K, Martin M, Hunter R, Hudson S (2001). Mood disorders: drug treatment of depression. *Pharm J* **266**: 433–42.

Fraser K, Martin M, Hunter R, Hudson S (2001). Mood disorders: implications for primary care. *Pharm J* **266**: 259–62.

Fraser K, Martin M, Hunter R, Hudson S (2001). Mood disorders: bipolar conditions. *Pharm J* **266**: 824–32.

Gaster B, Holroyd J (2000). St John's wort for depression. A systematic review. *Arch Intern Med* **160**: 152–6.

Hazell P (2002). Depression in children. *BMJ* **325**: 229–30.

Hirschfield RM, Keller MB, Panico S *et al* (1997). The National Depressive and Manic-Depressive Association consensus statement on the undertreatment of depression. *JAMA* **277**: 333–40.

Lawlor DA, Hopker SW (2001). The effectiveness of exercise as an intervention in the management of depression: systematic review and meta-regression analysis of randomised controlled trials. *BMJ* **322**: 763.

Macritchie KAN, Geddes JR, Scott J *et al* (2001). Valproic acid, valproate and divalproex in the maintenance treatment of bipolar disorder. *Cochrane Database System Rev* issue 3: CD003196.

Müller-Oerlinghausen B, Berghöfer A, Bauer M (2002). Bipolar disorder. *Lancet* **359**: 241–7.

Perry A, Tarrier N, Morriss R *et al* (1999). Randomised controlled trial of efficacy of teaching patients with bipolar disorder to identify early symptoms of relapse and obtain treatment. *BMJ* **318**: 149–53.

Van Walraven C, Mamdani MM, Wells PS *et al* (2001). Inhibition of serotonin re-uptake by antidepressants and upper gastrointestinal bleeding in elderly patients: retrospective cohort study. *BMJ* **323**: 655–61.

Further reading

Anderson IM (2000). Selective serotonin reuptake inhibitors versus tricyclic antidepressants: a meta-analysis of efficacy and tolerability. *J Affect Disord* **58**: 19–36.

Anon (2000). The drug treatment of depression in primary care. *MeReC Bull* **11**: 33–6.

Anon (2002). Specific issues in depression. *MeReC Briefing* **17**: 1–5.

Barbui C, Hotopf M (2001). Amitriptyline v. the rest: still the leading antidepressant after 40 years of randomised controlled trials. *Br J Psychiatry* **178**: 129–44.

Online resources

www.apni.org
The website for the Association for Post Natal Illness (accessed May 2008).

www.mentalhealth.org.uk
For information about mental health including useful

booklets such as *Healthy eating and depression,* for patients. (accessed 14 April 2008)

www.mind.org.uk
The website for the mental health charity, MIND (accessed May 2008).

www.rcpsych.ac.uk
The website of The Royal College of Psychiatrists (accessed May 2008)

www.sada.org.uk
The website for the Seasonal Affective Disorders Association (accessed May 2008).

www.sane.org.uk
The website of the mental health charity, SANE (accessed May 2008).

25

Anxiety disorders

Anxiety is a disabling condition, often associated with depression. It is more common in women and displays a peak onset in the early 20s. The term 'anxiety' is applied to a disproportionate response to fearful triggers such as flying and many social situations, and encompasses panic, phobic, obsessive–compulsive and general anxiety disorders. There is a significant impact on quality of life and personal achievement and, in extreme cases, patients are unable to leave their home. There is a hereditary component of vulnerability to anxiety, which may be triggered by adverse life events. There is also a link to certain personality traits and anxiety experienced in childhood. Drug-induced causes include:

- caffeine
- initial treatment with selective serotonin reuptake inhibitors (SSRIs)
- sympathomimetics
- nicotine
- overuse of β-adrenoceptor agonists, alcohol, amphetamines, cocaine
- withdrawal from alcohol, amphetamines, cocaine, benzodiazepines or antidepressants.

Disease characteristics

Before considering the characteristics of anxiety, terms in common use are defined:

- Fear: an emotional reaction to danger accompanied by physiological (mainly autonomic) and behavioural changes such as avoidance of fear-producing situations. Short-term fear such as fear of flying may be managed by single doses of benzodiazepines such as diazepam.

- Anxiety: generalized and often pathological fear, which may be unpredictable and often uncontrollable. It differs from fear in that there is not always an identifiable trigger.
- Phobia: a disabling or pathological fear of an object or situation such as social phobia or arachnophobia (a fear of spiders or arachnids).

Underlying pathology

Anxiety is considered to be pathological when a persistent or distressing response is triggered by non-threatening events and causes significant impairment of normal social or occupational functioning. The underlying pathology remains to be elucidated fully but is thought to involve disrupted serotoninergic, glutamatergic, GABA-ergic (GABA is γ-aminobutyric acid) and noradrenergic systems together with the involvement of corticotrophin-releasing factor, particularly in the complex interactions of the limbic system, a group of brain regions involved in the physiology of emotion.

Clinical features

Patients present with heightened autonomic symptoms including palpitations, tachycardia, difficulty breathing, dizziness, sweating, tremor, facial flushing and general feelings of panic. Patients may occasionally appear pale. There may also be profound fear of experiencing a heart attack or severe asthma attack. These symptoms may be caused or exacerbated by a number of other medical conditions. The diagnosis may therefore involve ruling out conditions such as asthma, heart disease, hyperthyroidism, vestibular disorders, menopause, hypoglycaemia, epilepsy and phaeochromocytoma (vascular tumour of the adrenal gland). Questioning patients about the frequency and nature of attacks, together with the presence of any fear or phobias, may point to a diagnosis of anxiety. Symptoms of depression may also be present and may form the primary diagnosis (see Chapter 24).

Classification

The classification of anxiety disorders is defined in the *Diagnostic and Statistical Manual of Mental Disorders*, 4th edition (DSM-IV: American Psychiatric Association, 1995) and the *International Statistical Classification of Diseases and Related Health Problems*, 10th revision (ICD-10: World Health Organization 1992). The following section considers the DSM-IV criteria of more common disorders presented to health professionals. These include panic attacks, phobias, obsessive–compulsive disorder (OCD) and general anxiety disorder (GAD). When considering the symptoms suggestive of these disorders, additional causes such as drug abuse, medication or medical conditions including hyperthyroidism are investigated and first excluded. In addition, as the symptoms of mental disorders often overlap, the criteria for similar disorders are considered before confirming a diagnosis, e.g. patients presenting with anxiety may fulfil the criteria for major depression, with the latter being diagnosed and treated. For further detail and discussion, the reader is referred to the DSM-IV manual (APA 1995).

General anxiety disorder

GAD differs from panic disorder, phobias and OCD in that it is persistent rather than short-lived and tends not to demonstrate situation-specific triggers. It may occasionally remain after unsuccessful treatment of panic or depressive disorders. Symptoms include a more general description of feeling 'on edge', irritable and tense most of the time. Diagnosis of GAD is made in the presence of the following symptoms:

- excessive anxiety and worry for more than 6 months and occurring on most days
- the patient cannot easily control the worry
- three or more of the following are present for more than 6 months and occur most days:
  - restless or 'on edge'
  - easily fatigued
  - difficult concentrating
  - irritability
  - muscle tension
  - sleep disturbance.

Panic disorder: panic attacks

Panic attacks commonly develop from phobic or hypochondriac symptoms and may progress to agoraphobia. A panic attack is defined by an intense period of fear with four or more of the following symptoms present, having developed abruptly and reaching a peak within 10 min:

- palpitations and/or increased heart rate
- sweating
- tremor
- shortness of breath or sensation of smothering
- choking feeling
- chest pain or discomfort
- nausea or abdominal symptoms
- dizzy or faint feeling
- feeling of depersonalization or unreality
- fear of losing control
- fear of dying
- paraesthesia ('pins and needles')
- chills or hot flushes.

A diagnosis of panic disorder is made when patients suffer recurrent panic attacks according to the following DSM-IV classification:

1. Recurrent panic attacks, some of which may occur spontaneously. These may be unpredictable and often unrelated to specific situations
2. At least one of the attacks has been followed 1 month or more later by at least one of the following:
   - worry about future attacks
   - worry about the consequences of an attack such as losing control, suffering an asthma or heart attack
   - a significant change in behaviour due to the attack such as avoidance behaviour.

Agoraphobia

Agoraphobia is indicated by anxiety associated with places or situations and a fear of embarrassment or that it is difficult to escape or that help is not available. These include being alone outside the home, in a crowd, standing in a line, on a bridge, and travelling by bus, train or car. Avoidance behaviour or severe distress occurs in relation to these triggers. Social or specific phobias are considered if avoidance behaviour relates to a limited number of situations such as social situations.

Specific phobias

The sufferer describes excessive fear occurring in response to an object or situation such as flying, animals, heights or the sight of blood. Exposure to the trigger often produces anxiety symptoms and may fulfil the criteria for a panic attack. Avoidance behaviour may be present. Normal social and occupational functioning is adversely affected as a result of the phobia. Again, diagnosis is made after the exclusion of other mental disorders, or disease- or drug-related causes.

Children
Symptoms in children may present as tantrums, crying, freezing or clinging, particularly described as a variant of normal behaviour.

Social phobia

Social phobia is diagnosed in the presence of symptoms described for specific phobias. However, the trigger relates to social situations or performance, during which sufferers worry that they will be humiliated or embarrassed.

Children
Social phobia is identified after an assessment of age-related social relationships with familiar people and the anxiety must occur during interaction with peers and not just with adults. Symptoms are the same as for specific phobias but with a social trigger.

Obsessive–compulsive disorder

OCD comprises a continuous and difficult-to-control preoccupation with an object, activity or recurrent thoughts. With the exception of children, the patient tends to be aware that the behaviour is unnecessary or unreasonable. Again, a diagnosis is also dependent on the duration (e.g. more than 1 hour a day) and/or the impact on the patient's quality of life. The diagnosis of OCD is made in the presence of obsessions or compulsions as follows.

Obsessions

- The presence of inappropriate recurrent and persistent thoughts, impulses or images causing distress or anxiety.
- The above cannot be explained as excessive worries triggered by adverse life events.
- Patients attempt to ignore or substitute the thoughts, impulses or images and recognize them as produced by their own mind.

Compulsions

- The patient feels driven to repetitive behaviour such as hand washing, checking that a door is locked, counting or praying. This occurs in response to an obsession or strict rules, e.g. not stepping on the cracks in the pavement.
- The behaviour is intended to prevent the occurrence of an adverse situation such as injury but is not a realistic method of avoiding such occurrences, e.g. believing that avoiding the cracks in the pavement will prevent a serious illness.

Post-traumatic stress disorder

This involves a reaction to a traumatic event that carries the threat of death or serious injury to the patient or other. There is also a significant level of continued experience in dreams, because 'flashbacks' or feelings associated with the incident are triggered by stimuli reminiscent of the scene, e.g. getting into a car may trigger the distress of a previous car accident. Avoidance behaviour may also be present. Additional symptoms not present before the event and with a duration of at least 1 month include two or more of:

- insomnia
- irritability or outbursts of anger
- poor concentration
- increased vigilance
- exaggerated response to non-threatening stimuli.

Children

The effect of post-traumatic stress in children may present as agitated or disorganized behaviour. The event may be revisited through play or in dreams.

Acute stress disorder

The presentation of acute stress disorder is similar to that for post-traumatic stress disorder but with the exception that the duration is at least 2 days but not more than 4 weeks. Acute stress disorder occurs within 4 weeks of the traumatic event and three or more symptoms of dissociation are present in a positive diagnosis:

- numbness, detachment or lack of an emotional response
- reduced awareness of surroundings or being 'in a daze'
- the situation does not feel real to the patient (derealization)
- the patient feels 'unreal', as in depersonalization
- the patient has incomplete recollection of important aspects of the event (dissociative amnesia).

Goals of treatment

Treatment is initiated when symptoms meet the criteria detailed above together with a significant impairment of social and/or occupational functioning and relationships with others. The goals of treatment are to alleviate the symptoms of panic and anxiety, improve the quality of life, and prevent relapse and recurrence. Initially, this may include identifying and dealing with causes such as associated depression and substance abuse.

Pharmacological management

Drugs such as benzodiazepines or β blockers may offer symptomatic relief though the use of the former is limited due to the risk of tolerance and dependence (see Chapter 26). The use of antidepressants with behavioural therapy combined with lifestyle advice, including the importance of regular exercise and the avoidance of drugs causing anxiety such as caffeine, may improve the long-term outcome.

It should be noted that anxiolytics and particularly benzodiazepines were previously described as 'minor tranquillizers', in an attempt to differentiate these drugs from antipsychotics or 'major tranquillizers'. These terms are inaccurate and therefore no longer used.

β-Adrenoceptor antagonists (propranolol)

Propranolol is the most commonly used β blocker for treating the physical symptoms of anxiety associated with the affects of adrenaline (epinephrine)-mediated activation of β-adrenoceptors. These include palpitations, tremor and tachycardia.

Benzodiazepines

See Chapter 26.

Antidepressants

Many antidepressants have been shown to be effective anxiolytics and, unlike buspirone, are also effective for panic attacks. See also Chapter 24.

Buspirone

Buspirone is rarely used, because antidepressants or occasional use of benzodiazepines is preferred. Buspirone activates serotonin $5HT_{1A}$-receptors, binds to dopamine receptors, and may also target noradrenergic and dopaminergic transmission in the brain. The effects on 5HT are thought to be the main mechanism by which buspirone exerts its anxiolytic effects. Side effects include dizziness, nausea and headache, as occur with selective serotonin reuptake inhibitor (SSRI) antidepressants. There is also a delay of 2–3 weeks before an anxiolytic effect. Buspirone differs from the benzodiazepines in that it does not cause sedation.

Drug choice in anxiety

The treatment of anxiety involves a combination of short-term symptomatic relief and long-term use of drugs such as SSRI antidepressants with or without behavioural therapy.

Symptomatic treatment

For rapid resolution of symptoms, a short course of a benzodiazepine may be indicated if symptoms are severe and disabling. Low doses of the longer-acting benzodiazepines diazepam, alprazolam or chlordiazepoxide are used. Short-acting alternatives such as lorazepam or oxazepam are administered to patients with hepatic impairment but these are more likely to produce withdrawal symptoms.

For patients with significant autonomic symptoms, β-adrenoceptor antagonists such as propranolol are effective and often prescribed for intermittent use. These drugs exhibit a rapid onset of action. Buspirone is also used but a response may be delayed for 2–3 weeks. Symptomatic treatment may help to break the cycle of conditioned anxiety, as occurs when anxiety is experienced in a situation that may have evoked an attack in the past. This short-term treatment, combined with counselling and lifestyle advice, may be sufficient to control anxiety.

Long-term pharmacological intervention

According to severity, SSRIs may be used, particularly if the anxiety is associated with underlying depression (see Chapter 24) or chronic symptoms of more than 4 weeks, or when benzodiazepine treatment has failed (Table 25.1). A delay of 2–4 weeks may precede the onset of efficacy of antidepressants in anxiety disorders. However, symptoms may persist for 4–8 weeks in panic disorder and up to 10 weeks in OCD. Treatment is continued for at least 6 months on cessation of symptoms, as for depression, and maintenance treatment may be indicated for recurrent episodes. The treatment of OCD may be continued for a year or more.

It is important to note that antidepressants and particularly paroxetine are associated with an initial worsening of panic symptoms when used to treat panic disorder. Starting with low doses and co-prescribing a benzodiazepine in the short term prevents this. The most common adverse effects reported by patients taking SSRIs long term include tiredness, weight gain and sexual dysfunction.

Table 25.1   The use of antidepressants in anxiety disorders

Anxiety disorder	Drugs indicated
General anxiety disorder	SSRIs (particularly paroxetine, escitalopram), imipramine (unlicensed), venlafaxine or trazodone
Obsessive–compulsive disorder	Fluoxetine, fluvoxamine, paroxetine, sertraline, clomipramine or escitalopram
Panic disorder	Antidepressants, particularly citalopram or escitalopram, paroxetine, imipramine (unlicensed) or clomipramine (unlicensed)
Panic disorder resistant to antidepressants	Lorazepam or clonazepam (unlicensed indications)
Phobias	Antidepressants generally, particularly clomipramine
Social phobia	Paroxetine, escitalopram or moclobemide
Post-traumatic stress disorder	Paroxetine

SSRIs, selective serotonin reuptake inhibitors.

Non-pharmacological intervention

Counselling such as cognitive–behavioural therapy (CBT) may be used to help the patient overcome fear and phobias, thereby aiding recovery and reducing the risk of relapse as many anxiety disorders follow a chronic course. Patients may also benefit from relaxation techniques such as progressive muscle relaxation. Behavioural therapy may include a gradual exposure to feared situations.

General anxiety disorder

The use of benzodiazepines should be particularly restricted when treating GAD because this tends to be lifelong and therefore represents a high risk for long-term dependence of these agents. The risk of depression resulting from regular use of benzodiazepines and β blockers should also be considered (see Chapter 5).

Buspirone may be effective in GAD, although it exhibits a slower onset of action compared with benzodiazepines. β Blockers do not appear to be effective in GAD. CBT may particularly benefit GAD due to the chronic nature of this disorder. This may be combined with drug treatment, which may produce a more rapid reduction in symptoms. Patients are assisted in identifying and changing negative, worrying and anxious thoughts. Relaxation techniques are also important.

Table 25.1 summarizes the use of antidepressants for anxiety disorders.

Concurrent disease

Prescribing decisions in treating anxiety in the presence of concurrent diseases include the following.

β Blockers (propranolol)

β Blockers are a compelling choice for anxious patients with ischaemic heart disease, hypertension or migraine, but should be avoided in asthma and used with caution in chronic obstructive pulmonary disease (COPD). It should be noted that long-term use may cause or exacerbate depression (see also Chapter 5).

Benzodiazepines

See Chapter 26.

Antidepressants

See Chapter 24.

Buspirone

Buspirone is contraindicated in epilepsy, severe hepatic or renal impairment, pregnancy and breast-feeding.

Drug interactions

These are largely dealt with elsewhere (β-adrenoceptor antagonists, see Chapter 11; benzodiazepines, see Chapter 26; antidepressants, SSRIs, see Chapter 24).

Buspirone

- Contraindicated with monoamine oxidase inhibitors (MAOIs).
- Increased drowsiness and weakness when combined with alcohol.
- Risk of serotonin syndrome with citalopram and possibly fluoxetine and other SSRIs. Fluvoxamine may reduce the effects of buspirone.
- Cytochrome P450 enzyme inhibitors such as erythromycin and itraconazole increase buspirone levels, requiring a dose reduction. Diltiazem, verapamil and possibly ketoconazole may interact by the same mechanism.
- Rifampicin induces cytochrome P450 and may therefore reduce levels of buspirone and necessitate an increased dose.

Herbal medicines

Patients may request or take damiana, cowslip, hops, lady's slipper and St John's wort for anxiety (see Chapter 4). These products cannot be recommended by healthcare professionals on the basis of a lack of clinical evidence for safe and efficacious use, and should be avoided with conventional treatment for anxiety. Of particular note is kava, a herbal preparation for anxiety that has been withdrawn after reports of hepatotoxicity. There was also a case reported in which a patient developed a semi-comatose state after concurrent ingestion of kava and alprazolam.

Patients with anxiety should particularly avoid herbs with sympathomimetic activity (see Chapter 4) and stimulants such as ginseng. Herbs with sedative properties include valerian, St John's wort and possibly ginseng, and should not be taken with benzodiazepines (see Chapters 4 and 26). Other herbs associated with causing anxiety include cola and maté.

Counselling

Patients benefit from an empathic approach together with education to increase their understanding of their symptoms. General counselling may include lifestyle advice, as outlined in Chapter 3. Particular emphasis should be placed on smoking cessation and the avoidance of excessive caffeine intake. Motivation for regular exercise may be gained by an explanation of the 'fright or flight' response as occurs when faced with threatening situations. Anxiety is a magnified reaction to situations that may not actually be threatening but invoke a 'fright or flight' response in the patient. A summary of counselling about non-pharmacological interventions includes the following:

- Avoid excess intake of caffeine, alcohol, nicotine and decongestants. It should be noted that caffeine is present in many over-the-counter (OTC) products, including analgesics, tonics and some products marketed to increase energy.
- Patients may be at risk of abusing alcohol due to a temporary relief of symptoms. A vicious circle may result, as described in Chapter 24, and therefore it is useful to highlight this to patients considered at risk.
- Relaxation tapes may help to alleviate anxiety symptoms.
- Practise relaxation techniques, including:
  - progressive muscle relaxation, involving progressive tensing and relaxing of major muscle groups

  - yoga: a Hindu tradition consisting of a series of exercises encompassing stretching, balance and muscle toning, with a focus on controlled breathing throughout
  - meditation: a method of relaxation of the mind involving repetitive methods such as internal or vocal chanting of a word, phrase or sound.
- A diary of symptoms together with situations that provoke or alleviate symptoms may help the patient to feel in control and serves to highlight progress. It also helps health professionals to determine the severity of the disorder.

Specific counselling

Specific counselling for SSRIs, tricyclic antidepressants, β-adrenoceptor antagonists and benzodiazepines is given in Chapters 11, 24 and 26. Points particularly relevant in the treatment of anxiety include the following.

Antidepressants

Patients may be confused by the use of antidepressants for anxiety. It may therefore be helpful to inform patients that antidepressants are used to treat anxiety disorders even in the absence of depression.

SSRIs

- In the treatment of panic disorder with paroxetine, panic symptoms may worsen during initial treatment. Patients should be reassured that this is normal and not a reason to stop treatment.
- Treatment should not be stopped abruptly and should be continued for at least 6 months or up to 12 months or longer.

Benzodiazepines
These are only recommended for short-term (2–4 weeks) symptomatic relief, e.g. when SSRIs are initiated. Use is restricted due to the risk of tolerance and dependence.

β Blockers (propranolol)
β Blockers treat the symptoms of anxiety and tend to be used on a 'when required' basis. If they

are taken regularly, they should not be stopped suddenly because rebound anxiety will occur, with the risk of developing a 'vicious circle' and subsequent psychological dependence on β blockers.

Buspirone

- A response may not be observed for up to 2 weeks.
- This is indicated for short-term use, although the risk of dependence and abuse is low.
- Side effects include dizziness, headache, nervousness, light-headedness, excitement and nausea. These tend to be transient, occurring at the start of treatment.
- Buspirone rarely causes sedation but patients should be advised not to drive until they have established that they do not suffer any sedative effects with buspirone.

Self-assessment

Consider whether the following statements are true or false. In the management of anxiety:

1. Benzodiazepines reduce the activity of GABA.
2. The effects of benzodiazepines take several weeks to become apparent.
3. The use of β blockers is associated with anxiety.
4. Certain SSRIs are licensed for panic disorder.
5. Buspirone is a $5HT_{1A}$ agonist.

Practice points

- Benzodiazepines are reserved for the short-term treatment of severe anxiety.
- Lifestyle advice is important to prevent long-term psychological dependence on drugs.
- Underlying depression should be identified and treated.
- Some antidepressants are indicated for anxiety disorders.
- β Blockers are associated with a rare but unpredictable life-threatening bronchospasm and should therefore be avoided by patients with asthma and used with caution in COPD. This includes low doses.
- Patients often present with physical symptoms, thereby delaying a diagnosis.

 CASE STUDY

A 26-year-old man reports sporadic difficulty with breathing, which usually occurs when he is sitting in an office full of people at work. He is concerned that he may have asthma but has no history of asthma, although he does suffer from hayfever. He is not taking any medication at the moment. Should this patient receive a salbutamol inhaler?

- This is an interesting case, with vague symptoms that may point to asthma, particularly as he has a history of hayfever. On further questioning, however, the patient also reported an increase in heart rate, sweating, facial flushing and feelings of panic about his breathing. Salbutamol was therefore not appropriate and could have exacerbated his symptoms. He admitted to regular consumption of alcohol and caffeine, although he regularly visited a gym. A diagnosis of panic attacks was made; the patient was advised to cut down on alcohol and particularly caffeine, and continue with his exercise. He was given a prescription for 60 propranolol 10 mg tablets three times daily when required.

continued

CASE STUDY (continued)

What are possible alternative causes of these symptoms?

- Underlying conditions such as hyperthyroidism and asthma may produce the above symptoms and these should be excluded. The exclusion of asthma is particularly important when prescribing propranolol, which would otherwise be contraindicated. The measurement of lung function may be considered (see Chapter 21). Cardiac causes are perhaps unlikely in view of his age. Substance abuse should also be excluded.

What advice should be given about propranolol?

- Propranolol may help with the symptoms of anxiety but regular use may lead to rebound anxiety on withdrawal, and without appropriate advice this may progress to chronic use of propranolol. The patient should be advised to use the propranolol occasionally for the temporary relief of symptoms, e.g. propranolol may be taken before difficult situations known to trigger an attack with a view to breaking the association between the situation and an attack (conditioned anxiety). The importance of lifestyle changes with or without CBT should be stressed.
- The patient should be advised to report symptoms of wheeze and return if his symptoms do not improve. He could also be warned that propranolol will decrease exercise tolerance. Anxiety may be associated with depression, so chronic use of propranolol may not be appropriate because it may cause or exacerbate depression. An SSRI and/or CBT may be indicated. This case was resolved with lifestyle changes and intermittent use of propranolol. The patient identified an association with drinking caffeine and excess alcohol.

References

American Psychiatric Association (1995). *Diagnostic and Statistical Manual of Mental Disorders*, 4th edn (DSM-IV). Washington DC: American Psychiatric Association.

World Health Organization (1992). *The International Statistical Classification of Diseases and Related Health Problems*, 10th revision (ICD-10). Geneva: WHO.

Nash J, Nutt D (2002). Primary-care treatment of panic disorder. *Prescriber* 13: 29–41.

National Institute for Health and Clinical Excellence (2004). *Anxiety: Management of anxiety (panic disorder, with or without agoraphobia, and generalized anxiety disorder) in adults in primary, secondary and community care*. Clinical Guideline 22. London: NICE.

Further reading

Kapczinski F, Schmitt R, Lima MS (2003). The use of antidepressants for generalised anxiety disorder. *Cochrane Database System Rev* issue 1: CD003592.

Livingston M, Jarvie S (2002). Treatment of generalised anxiety disorder. *Prescriber* **13**: 17–28.

Online resources

www.adaa.org

The Anxiety Disorders Association of America, a comprehensive educational site, provides up-to-date information for patients and healthcare professionals on the nature and treatment of anxiety disorders (accessed May 2008).

www.alcoholics-anonymous.org.uk
Alcoholics Anonymous (AA) services, including nation-wide support groups (accessed May 2008).

www.crusebereavementcare.org.uk
Cruse Bereavement Care is a charity providing information about bereavement (accessed May 2008).

www.phobics-society.org.uk
The Anxiety Disorders Charity providing help and advice for patients and carers of phobics, including access to literature, counselling and support groups (accessed May 2008).

www.rcpsych.ac.uk
The website for The Royal College of Psychiatrists (accessed May 2008).

26

Insomnia

Characteristics

Insomnia is an extremely common complaint, affecting 1 in 10 people, particularly elderly patients, and may have multiple causes such as stress, chronic illness, pain and depression. The effects on quality of life are extensive, and insomnia and its treatment are also risk factors for accidents.

Causes of insomnia

There are numerous causes of insomnia, which if addressed may resolve the problem without the requirement for treatment with hypnotic drugs. Causes of insomnia include:

- environmental factors: noise, extremes of temperature, poor ventilation
- lifestyle factors: stress, shift work, jet lag
- disease: poorly controlled asthma or chronic obstructive pulmonary disease, heart failure, chronic pain, hyperthyroidism, dementia, schizophrenia, anxiety and depression, or menopausal symptoms

- drugs, including sympathomimetics, selective serotonin reuptake inhibitors, β blockers, thyroid hormones, corticosteroids, caffeine, statins, theophylline and alcohol
- indirect drug causes: diuretics if taken at night, hypoglycaemia after insulin administration or a persistent cough due to angiotensin-converting enzyme inhibitors
- withdrawal from drugs including nicotine, alcohol, antidepressants, hypnotics, opioids, cannabis, amphetamines, and MDMA (3,4-methylenedioxymethamfetamine) or ecstasy.

Clinical features

Symptoms of insomnia include a delay in falling asleep, failure to maintain sleep or early morning wakening. The result is often permanent tiredness. The most common presentation is a delay in falling asleep, which is particularly associated with stress, shift work, noise or drugs. Insomnia is classified according to the duration of the problem, as shown in Table 26.1.

Table 26.1 Classification of insomnia according to the duration of symptoms

Description of insomnia	Duration	Common causes
Transient	2–3 days	Noise, shift work, jet lag
Short term	3–4 weeks	Stress, depression, drugs such as caffeine or decongestants
Chronic	Most nights for 3 weeks or longer	Severe disease, drug abuse, including alcohol and mild hypnotic dependence

Goals of treatment

Initially, potential causes of insomnia should be identified and any underlying problems such as pain or depression treated. There is an important role for patient education and non-pharmacological methods such as counselling and relaxation techniques. The aim is to establish a normal sleep pattern without the use of long-term hypnotics. Patients dependent on hypnotics, including over-the-counter (OTC) preparations, should be supported during gradual withdrawal from these drugs. Referral for cognitive–behavioural therapy (CBT) or specific abuse counselling may be required for chronic insomnia. Sleep clinic referrals are reserved for sleep apnoea, epilepsy during sleep, long-standing insomnia resistant to treatment or after suspicion of exaggeration by the patient.

Pharmacological basis of management

Benzodiazepines, e.g. flurazepam, loprazolam, lormetazepam, nitrazepam, temazepam

Benzodiazepines reduce anxiety and aggression, induce sleep, reduce muscle tone and coordination, and produce an anticonvulsant effect. The main mechanism of action involves increased activity of the inhibitory neurotransmitter, γ-aminobutyric acid (GABA), in the brain. This occurs after binding of the drug to a regulatory site, the benzodiazepine receptor, on $GABA_A$-receptor complexes. Differences in the sensitivity of numerous subtypes of $GABA_A$-receptors to benzodiazepines account for some of their different clinical uses, e.g. clonazepam and diazepam exhibit greater anticonvulsant activity. Short-acting benzodiazepines such as temazepam, lormetazepam or loprazolam are reserved for the treatment of insomnia to reduce the risk of a hangover effect persisting the following day. Tolerance and dependence are also problematic with benzodiazepines.

Related hypnotics: 'Z-drugs': zaleplon, zolpidem, zopiclone

These newer agents, which have a non-benzodiazepine structure, have been developed with the aim of reducing adverse effects such as hangover and dependence. These drugs exhibit a shorter duration of action and are thought to be selective for subtypes of benzodiazepine receptor and/or selectively target individual subunits of these receptors. In practice, however, the adverse effects appear to be similar to conventional benzodiazepines.

Sedating antihistamines, e.g diphenhydramine, promethazine

Sedating antihistamines are histamine H_1-receptor antagonists (see Chapter 20). They also exhibit antimuscarinic effects, resulting in side effects, including dry mouth, blurred vision, constipation and urinary retention. They are available in OTC preparations for the short-term relief of insomnia.

Barbiturates, e.g. amobarbital, butobarbital, secobarbital

Traditionally, barbiturates were used as hypnotics and tranquillizers. These are non-selective central nervous system (CNS) depressants acting to increase GABA transmission in a less selective manner compared with benzodiazepines. Side effects are therefore even more troublesome than those associated with benzodiazepines, and barbiturates are seldom used, with the exception of anaesthesia and occasionally epilepsy. They exhibit numerous drug interactions due to the induction of hepatic cytochrome P450 enzymes, produce tolerance and dependence, and are toxic in overdose.

Drug choice

Treatment may often require non-pharmacological intervention such as lifestyle changes, or reviewing drug-related causes or treating under-lying illness. Occasionally, pharmacological intervention with benzodiazepines is required but this should be short term due to the follow-ing problems:

- an increased risk of falls in elderly people
- a hangover effect the next morning
- confusion, amnesia, cognitive impairment and impaired coordination
- a risk of road traffic accidents associated with benzodiazepines with long half-lives and the short-acting hypnotic zopiclone
- the disruption of normal sleep patterns
- chronic use associated with anxiety and depression
- tolerance and therefore the requirement for higher doses
- the risk of dependence and abuse
- withdrawal effects, including rebound insomnia
- a risk of life-threatening respiratory de-pression if an overdose of benzodiazepines is taken with alcohol, although they are rela-tively safe if taken without alcohol or other substances of abuse.

Summary

Hypnotics are licensed for the short-term treat-ment of insomnia for no more than 3 weeks and ideally for only 1 week and using intermittent doses such as every third night. Agents with a short half-life should be given. These include temazepam, loprazolam and lormetazepam. Diazepam may be given as a single dose at night if the patient also has anxiety during the day.

Short-acting benzodiazepines (temazepam, loprazolam, lormetazepam)

These agents are preferred due to a reduced risk of hangover effect in the short-term treatment of insomnia. Loprazolam exhibits erratic absorp-tion, which may increase its duration of action.

Long-acting benzodiazepines (diazepam, flurazepam, nitrazepam)

The longer-acting benzodiazepines are rarely used to treat insomnia due to residual side effects, particularly affecting elderly patients. The

exception is diazepam used for insomnia associ-ated with anxiety. It is also the preferred agent for withdrawal from chronic use of benzodiazepines because withdrawal effects are less pronounced.

Other hypnotics

'Z-drugs' are associated with withdrawal symptoms, tolerance and dependence. Current evidence suggests that they offer little advantage over benzodiazepines. Chloral hydrate is no longer recommended because there is no evidence of real benefit for elderly patients and the treatment of children is rarely justified. Clomethiazole is occasionally used for elderly patients due to reduced confusion and hangover effects. Short-term use is again indicated due to the risk of dependence.

Concurrent disease

Table 26.2 indicates disease states that may preclude the use of certain hypnotics.

Hepatic impairment

Hypnotics should be avoided in severe liver disease because they may precipitate coma. Reduced doses of some hypnotics may be used in milder hepatic disease and the *British National Formulary* and/or summary of product character-istics should be consulted.

Renal impairment

Small doses of hypnotics are recommended due to increased cerebral sensitivity associated with severe renal impairment.

Special groups

Pregnancy and breast-feeding

Non-pharmacological treatment is preferred during pregnancy and breast-feeding.

Elderly people

The requirement for sleep is reduced in elderly people and this group is likely to expect to sleep for longer than is actually required. Hypnotic use in this group should be avoided due to an

Table 26.2   Concurrent disease states to be considered when prescribing hypnotics

Disease	Comments
Cardiac disease	Chloral hydrate is contraindicated.
COPD	Hypnotics should be used with caution, particularly in patients with hypoxia, due to reduced respiratory drive
Dementia	• Benzodiazepines may cause or worsen dementia. Avoid if possible, or use low doses of short-acting agents
	• Zolpidem has also been associated with memory impairment and vigilance is required for these effects with all 'Z-drugs'
	• Antimuscarinic effects of OTC older antihistamines oppose effects of acetylcholinesterase inhibitors used in dementia
Depression	• Hypnotics should not be used alone as long-term use may exacerbate depression
	• Sedating TCAs (e.g. amitriptyline, dosulepin), maprotiline, mianserin or trazodone may be appropriate
	• SSRIs may cause insomnia
Gastritis	Chloral hydrate is contraindicated
Glaucoma, prostatic hypertrophy and urinary retention	Antimuscarinic side effects of sedative antihistamines mean that they should be used with caution in these conditions
Muscle weakness	Benzodiazepines should be used with caution.
Osteoporosis	The risk of fractures may be increased in elderly patients due to falls associated with hypnotics
Porphyria	Some antihistamines, benzodiazepines and chloral hydrate may be unsuitable (see *British National Formulary*, Section 9.8.2)
Respiratory depression	All hypnotics should be avoided
Sleep apnoea	Benzodiazepines, zaleplon, zolpidem and zopiclone should be avoided

COPD, chronic obstructive pulmonary disease; SSRIs, selective serotonin reuptake inhibitors; TCAs, tricyclic antidepressants.

increased risk of side effects, particularly drowsiness and confusion, which may increase the risk of falls. The enhanced effects are mainly due to an age-related reduction in hepatic metabolism. Reduced doses are indicated if treatment is necessary.

Children

Hypnotics should not be used in children, with the possible exception of night terrors and somnambulism (sleep walking). Alternatives for treating night terrors include waking the child 15 min before the time that a night terror usually occurs and then allowing him or her to go back to sleep. A bedtime routine is particularly important for children.

Drug interactions

Drug interactions with hypnotics generally result from an additive effect with other drugs with sedative properties such as alcohol, antihistamines, antidepressants and opioids. Barbiturates are rarely used because they exhibit numerous interactions due to activation of hepatic cytochrome P450 enzymes.

Plasma levels of benzodiazepines may be elevated in patients taking cimetidine, due to cytochrome P450 inhibition. However this interaction appears not to be very important clinically. Possible increases in side effects may occur.

Over-the-counter considerations

Sedating antihistamines are available for the short-term relief of insomnia but patients should be advised to consult their general practitioner (GP) if symptoms persist after 2 weeks. However these drugs are associated with a hangover effect and may also lead to tolerance, headaches, psychomotor impairment (including impaired reaction times) and antimuscarinic effects.

Herbal medicines

Patients with insomnia may commonly take or request products containing valerian, camomile, hops, gentian, passionflower (*Passiflora*), wild lettuce and pulsatilla, e.g. combinations of these herbs are present in Kalms, HRI night and Nytol herbal. Until more information about the pharmacological activity, efficacy and safety of these products is available, the same precautions observed with conventional hypnotics may be appropriate, e.g. the potential for drug inter-actions and concurrent disease as outlined above should be considered. Advice about non-pharmacological intervention is also relevant. For a discussion on the recommendation of herbal preparations, the reader is referred to Chapter 4.

Patients who take herbal preparations for insomnia should avoid herbs with sympatho-mimetic activity (see Chapter 4) and stimulants such as ginseng. Herbs with sedative properties (see Chapter 4) should not be taken with hyp-notics. Camomile and pulsatilla have been associated with hypersensitivity reactions and should be avoided by susceptible individuals such as people with asthma.

Dietary supplements

Melatonin is a hormone involved in the sleep–wake cycle, being secreted during the night. This is taken as a dietary supplement for jet lag and by shift workers, but reliable evidence for efficacy and long-term safety is lacking. People with depression, prescribed CNS depress-ants or women trying to conceive should avoid it.

Withdrawal from chronic benzodiazepine treatment

See Chapter 5.

Counselling

General counselling should focus on non-phar-macological options:

- Try to establish a routine of retiring to bed and rising at the same time each day.
- Avoid lying in bed worrying about being awake, because this may also contribute to conditioned insomnia and is more tiring than being awake and not worrying.
- Regular exercise may benefit insomnia but should be avoided a few hours before going to bed. A short walk in the evening may help.
- Alcohol should not be used to aid sleep because it is a diuretic, disturbing sleep in the latter part of the night, and also produces 'unrestful' sleep. Chronic use may itself cause insomnia.
- Avoid caffeine, nicotine (including 24-h patches), thyroid hormones and deconges-tants, particularly after 4pm.
- Do not work, eat or watch television in the bedroom because conditioned insomnia may result whereby the bedroom is associated with being awake.
- Avoid napping during the day.
- Avoid intellectual activity before going to bed.
- Establish a routine each night such as reading, drinking warm milk or having a warm bath with lavender oil before retiring to bed.
- Eliminate environmental causes such as noise, light, extremes of temperature or poor air quality.
- Listen to relaxation tapes.
- Relaxation techniques are particularly useful for patients with stress-related insomnia who have difficulty in falling asleep. These include:
  - progressive muscle relaxation, involving progressive tensing and relaxing of major muscle groups
  - yoga, a Hindu tradition consisting of a series of exercises encompassing stretching, balance and muscle toning, with a focus on controlled breathing throughout

– meditation, a method of relaxation of the mind involving methods such as repetitive internal or vocal chanting of a word, phrase or sound.
• A sleep diary may be useful for identifying the cause, pattern and severity of insomnia. Patients may benefit from feeling more in control of the problem and from observing their progress. This method may also reveal patients with an unrealistic expectation of the duration and depth of sleep required. The following points may be recorded:
  – the time of retiring to bed and approximate time taken to fall asleep
  – the duration of sleep
  – the number of times of waking during the night and the duration
  – a score out of 10 of the feeling of tiredness each day
  – a score out of 10 of the feeling of tension and irritability
  – general comments such as alcohol or caffeine intake and other potential causes.

Counselling and the use of hypnotics

Generally, patients should be warned that hypnotics help only the symptoms and not the causes of insomnia. They are recommended only for short-term intermittent use. Informing patients that withdrawal from regular use of hypnotics causes rebound insomnia leading to the desire to continue taking the treatment may help prevent this road to dependence:

• Intermittent use, preferably every third night, is recommended to avoid tolerance. It may be useful to explain that this means that the sedative effect is lost if hypnotics are taken every night.
• Treatment is ideally restricted to no more than 1 week to prevent the development of dependence.

• Hypnotics may cause drowsiness, which may persist to the next day. Patients should therefore be cautious if driving or performing other skilled tasks. Alcohol adds to these effects and should be avoided.
• Following withdrawal from hypnotics, sleep may be disturbed for a few days and may feature vivid dreams due to increased rapid eye movement (REM) sleep for many weeks.

Practice points

• Reinforce non-pharmacological options for treating insomnia.
• Patients should be asked about the use of OTC hypnotics and frequent requests should lead to a referral to the GP.
• Long-term users of benzodiazepines should be changed to the equivalent dose of diazepam before gradual withdrawal, with regular review and encouragement.
• Patient education relating to the risks and benefits of withdrawing from hypnotics may improve the outcome.

Self-assessment

Consider whether the following statements are true or false. In the management of insomnia:

1. Diuretics may be a cause.
2. Temazepam is a long-acting benzodiazepine.
3. Diet is often an important cause of insomnia.
4. Promethazine is a safe drug for regular treatment of insomnia.
5. Early morning wakening is often associated with depression.

CASE STUDIES

Case 1
A 45-year-old man with a history of bipolar affective disorder requests a sedative antihistamine from his pharmacist. He currently takes lithium and is away from home for a business meeting.

Should a supply be made?

- Insomnia may be an early sign of relapse in patients with bipolar affective disorder and therefore referral to the GP is warranted. This patient was away from home and therefore could not see his GP until the following week and did not want to see a GP not familiar with his case. He was driving and therefore a sedating antihistamine was not the best choice due to the possibility of hangover effect the next morning. However, due to the risk of relapse of bipolar disorder, the problem of driving when tired and the absence of other symptoms, a supply was made with the recommendation that the patient take a tablet only every third night until he returned home. He was advised not to take them too late at night to prevent the residual effects next morning and to consult his GP if his symptoms did not improve within a week. He was also given advice and an information leaflet about non-pharmacological treatment of sleep problems, particularly the importance of avoiding alcohol and caffeine. He telephoned to thank the pharmacist on his return, saying that the advice and treatment helped him through a difficult week and he was now feeling much better.

Case 2
A 25-year-old woman with Crohn's disease presented to her GP complaining of insomnia mainly due to her painful condition. She was taking venlafaxine 75 mg twice daily in addition to her immunosuppressant therapy. She felt that her prednisolone treatment was aggravating her low mood and her Crohn's disease symptoms were still not controlled.

What course of action could the GP take?

- The patient should be referred back to her specialist to review her Crohn's disease medication, because this is likely to be the main cause of her insomnia. However, the GP may consider changing the antidepressant to a more sedating agent such as trazodone and reviewing her medication for pain. General counselling about sleep may also be beneficial, as outlined above.

Case 3
A 20-year-old female student presents with insomnia before her exams and asks for a prescription for sleeping tablets. She says that she 'has a few drinks' every night to help her unwind but wakes up in the night and cannot get back to sleep.

Would a short-term hypnotic help this patient?

- A short-term hypnotic may help depending on the amount of distress to the patient and the nature and duration of the exams. However, non-pharmacological intervention could be considered first, e.g. advising that alcohol is not an effective sedative due to disturbed sleep later in the night. She should be advised not to revise late in the evening and to try to revise somewhere other than where she sleeps. Further questioning of this patient revealed that she was taking Pro Plus, a caffeine-containing product, during the day. She was advised to reduce this gradually and was given a leaflet outlining general counselling for people with insomnia and to return if her problem did not improve.

Reference

Martin J, ed. *British National Formulary*, latest edition. London: British Medical Association and Royal Pharmaceutical Society of Great Britain.

Further reading

Anon (2002). An update on benzodiazepines and non-benzodiazepine hypnotics. *MeReC Briefing* **17**: 6–8.

Hallström C (2002). A primary-care guide to insomnia management. *Prescriber* **13**: 65–74.

Online resource

www.rcpsych.ac.uk
The Royal College of Psychiatrists provides up-to-date information and informative patient information leaflets (accessed May 2008).

27

Schizophrenia

Characteristics

Schizophrenia presents with psychotic symptoms similar to the manic phase of bipolar affective disorder but differs in that deterioration of cognitive function is often observed over time. Many patients suffering from schizophrenia are unable to continue with their normal daily life. Approximately 1% of the population is affected: onset tends to be in the early 20s and has both genetic and environmental components. Patients may be reassured that one in five patients may suffer only a single acute episode, although 7 in 10 suffer at least two acute episodes. Drugs such as amphetamines may induce psychotic symptoms or worsen schizophrenia, mainly as a result of dopamine release.

Clinical presentation

The symptoms of schizophrenia are grouped as positive or negative. Patients may describe positive symptoms as 'dreaming while awake'.

Positive symptoms

* Hallucinations: false perceptions of sounds, images, taste, smells or other sensory images that do not have a real stimulus.
* Delusions: these are irrational beliefs, which cannot be altered by logical reasoning, e.g. being controlled by others.
* Thought disorder and disorganized communication, e.g.:
  - thought broadcasting – thoughts are 'expressed freely' to others
  - thought insertion – thoughts are inserted by another person

  - thought withdrawal – thoughts are stolen by another person.

Negative symptoms

* Reduced activity with emotional flattening (psychomotor retardation, see Chapter 24).
* Withdrawal from society.
* Cognitive deficit and therefore unemployment.

Other: catatonic

A catatonic state encompasses motor (movement) abnormalities, including overactivity and violence or standing in strange positions.

Classification

The term 'schizophrenia' literally translates as 'split mind' and is often misinterpreted as a split personality. According to the *Diagnostic and Statistical Manual of Mental Disorders*, 4th edition (DSM-IV: American Psychiatric Association 1995), a diagnosis of schizophrenia is made if two or more of the following symptoms are present for most of the time over a period of 1 month. The required time period is shorter if the symptoms are treated successfully with medication. Symptoms include:

* delusions
* hallucinations
* disorganized speech
* disorganized or catatonic behaviour
* negative symptoms: affective (emotional) flattening.

Schizophrenia results in considerable impairment of social and occupational functioning, including interpersonal relationships and self-care. A diagnosis may also be made on the basis of the presence of hallucinations alone if these comprise a voice giving a running commentary on the patient's behaviour or thoughts, or two or more voices communicating with each other. A longer period, 6 months or more, of milder symptoms may also result in a diagnosis of schizophrenia and may include milder manifestations of at least two of the above symptoms (such as strange beliefs) or only negative symptoms. Finally, substance abuse and concurrent disease are excluded as the cause before a positive diagnosis of schizophrenia can be made.

Pathophysiology

Schizophrenia is considered a neurodevelopmental rather than a neurodegenerative disease, mainly affecting the cerebral cortex, as predicted from the cognitive symptoms. The pathophysiology of schizophrenia remains elusive, although new and interesting theories are beginning to emerge. Historically, schizophrenia has been associated with overactivity of dopaminergic neurotransmission and conventional treatment has been with dopamine receptor antagonists such as chlorpromazine. This theory, however, does not provide a complete explanation, e.g. the efficacy of antipsychotics (chlorpromazine, clozapine, sulpiride, trifluoperazine) is delayed for 7–10 days or more, suggesting an additional mechanism to simple antagonism of receptors. Alternative mechanisms may include a change in the number of receptors expressed in cells or perhaps an effect on signal transduction within cells.

The modulation of dopaminergic neurotransmission remains important in newer, atypical antipsychotics but the role of serotonin or 5-hydroxytryptamine (5HT) is also recognized and effective treatment such as with clozapine is thought to be due to a greater effect on serotoninergic transmission compared with dopaminergic systems. This may partly explain the beneficial effect of clozapine on negative symptoms. Other systems targeted include glutamatergic, GABAergic (GABA is γ-aminobutyric acid) and noradrenergic, which are involved in the modulation of dopaminergic neurotransmission, e.g. antagonism of the glutamate N-methyl-D-aspartate receptor by drugs such as phencyclidine and ketamine produces symptoms similar to those observed in schizophrenia.

Pharmacological basis of management

All antipsychotics are dopamine D_2-receptor antagonists, thereby inhibiting dopaminergic neurotransmission, and this remains an important target for effective antipsychotic activity. Extrapyramidal and endocrine symptoms are often troublesome, particularly at higher doses, e.g. hyperprolactinaemia may also follow the inhibition of dopamine transmission, resulting in increased prolactin secretion. The reverse occurs when the dopamine receptor agonist bromocriptine is used to suppress lactation. Most antipsychotics also act as antagonists at receptors for other monoamines, including α-adrenoceptors, muscarinic and 5HT-receptors (mainly $5HT_2$). The affinity for these receptors determines the side-effect profile. Histamine receptors may also be modulated by antipsychotics, but this is not thought to result in antipsychotic activity.

Conventional antipsychotics

The conventional antipsychotics were previously termed 'major tranquillizers' but this term is no longer used because this is not the main effect exploited in the treatment of schizophrenia. The term 'antischizophrenic' is also inaccurate because these drugs are 'antipsychotic' and are also used to treat psychotic symptoms associated with major depression and bipolar disorder (see Chapter 24) and delusional disorders. The main groups of these typical antipsychotics include:

- phenothiazines comprising three further groups (see *British National Formulary*):
  - group 1 (aliphatic), e.g. chlorpromazine

– group 2 (piperidine), e.g. pipotiazine
– group 3 (piperazine), e.g. prochlorperazine and trifluoperazine.

The following groups resemble the structure of the group 3 phenothiazines:

- butyrophenones, e.g. haloperidol, droperidol
- diphenylbutylpiperidines, e.g. pimozide
- thioxanthenes, e.g. flupentixol
- substituted benzamides: sulpiride (often grouped with 'atypical' antipsychotics due to its reduced extrapyramidal effects).

Atypical antipsychotics, e.g. clozapine, olanzapine, risperidone, sertindole

Atypical antipsychotics have vastly improved the treatment of schizophrenia, mainly as a result of reduced extrapyramidal effects. In addition, clozapine is one of the only antipsychotics to benefit negative symptoms and has a central role in treatment-resistant schizophrenia. These drugs are now considered for first-line treatment and are also used in the treatment of bipolar affective disorder (see Chapter 24). They are not, however, devoid of adverse effects, e.g. weight gain and metabolic effects (hyperglycaemia and dyslipidaemia with a risk of diabetes mellitus) are significant adverse effects particularly associated with olanzapine and clozapine (Newcomer 2007), and sexual dysfunction is a major factor in reduced compliance. Clozapine is associated with agranulocytosis and is therefore restricted to patients who have failed to respond to at least two antipsychotics (see below). Sertindole is currently restricted to named patients due to its association with arrhythmias and sudden death.

Adverse effects of antipsychotics

With the introduction of atypical antipsychotics, frightening extrapyramidal effects are less common, being associated with conventional antipsychotics and particularly the group 3 phenothiazines, the butyrophenones and especially depot preparations of these groups. Common adverse effects with atypical antipsychotics include weight gain, sexual dysfunction and the risk of diabetes mellitus.

Weight gain

Weight gain is common with antipsychotics and may be a factor in the cause or exacerbation of type 2 diabetes mellitus.

Sexual dysfunction

Sexual dysfunction often has a significant effect on personal relationships and quality of life but is not discussed due to embarrassment. Symptoms range from altered libido to impotence in men or reduced lubrication in women and failure of orgasm. Fertility may therefore be an important issue. Sexual dysfunction is an important cause of non-compliance with both conventional and atypical antipsychotics.

Galactorrhoea and amenorrhoea

Endocrine effects such as galactorrhoea occur due to increased prolactin secretion. This includes an enlargement of the breasts and milk production. Other effects include missed periods (amenorrhoea), reduced libido and therefore reduced fertility.

Movement disorders

As described above, many of the adverse effects of antipsychotics result from the blockade of dopamine receptors and therefore include disorders of movement or endocrine disorders. These include parkinsonian symptoms such as tremor and rigidity. This is not surprising considering the use of levodopa to replenish dopamine levels, thereby improving the symptoms of Parkinson's disease. Antimuscarinic drugs such as procyclidine are prescribed 'when required' to counteract these effects but should be used with caution due to the risk of irreversible tardive dyskinesia. The following terms are used to describe movement disorders.

Extrapyramidal effects
Extrapyramidal neurons comprise a system of nerves connecting the cerebral cortex, basal

ganglia, thalamus, cerebellum, reticular formation and spinal neurons in complex systems not included in the pyramidal system. Extrapyramidal motor disorders are those affecting movement, which is regulated by dopamine in the extrapyramidal system. These include the following:

- Akinesia: literally 'lacking movement', a loss of normal muscular tone or responsiveness.
- Parkinsonism: symptoms associated with Parkinson's disease, including tremor, rigidity, salivation (drooling) and akinesia of the face. These effects are reversible when they are drug induced.
- Acute dystonia: abnormal or impaired posture or muscle spasms due to altered muscle tone. This often involves sustained contractions of neck and facial muscles and is reversible.
- Akathisia: an unwanted effect of antipsychotics (phenothiazines) involving involuntary movements or restless overactivity of the legs and/or body, e.g. pacing up and down, constantly changing leg position or foot tapping. This may easily be confused with the agitation for which the drug was prescribed. There is currently no trial-based evidence for the use of antimuscarinic agents to treat acute akathisia induced by antipsychotics (Rathbone and Soares-Weiser 2006).
- Tardive dyskinesia: a chronic condition characterized by repetitive involuntary movements, usually of the tongue, face, fingers, hands, legs and trunk, and resulting in drooling and lip smacking. The concurrent use of drugs with antimuscarinic activity may aggravate the condition, which may be irreversible, and therefore careful monitoring is important.

Cardiovascular effects

Cardiac arrhythmias are a particular problem with sertindole but may also occur with phenothiazines and particularly chlorpromazine. Sertindole was withdrawn in 1998 but has recently been reintroduced for named patients, only for those stabilized on sertindole and when other antipsychotics are not appropriate.

Both olanzapine and risperidone are associated with an increased incidence of stroke in elderly patients and the former Committee on Safety of Medicines (CSM; now known as the Commission on Human Medicines or CHM) has advised that they should not be used for the management of behavioural symptoms associated with dementia. The increased incidence of stroke in elderly patients would be a reason to avoid these agents but if they are used then patient's cardiovascular risk should be assessed.

Severe postural hypotension may occur with chlorpromazine and other phenothiazines due to the antagonism of α-adrenoceptors (see Chapter 11).

Antimuscarinic effects

The antimuscarinic affects of drugs may be peripheral or central. Peripheral effects such as dry mouth, blurred vision, urinary retention and constipation are summarized in Chapter 5. This pharmacological activity also accounts in part for the use of phenothiazines as antiemetics (see Chapter 8). The following central effects may occur with antipsychotics as a result of antimuscarinic activity:

- confusion
- disorientation
- visual hallucinations
- agitation
- irritability
- delirium
- memory impairment
- aggression and possibly violent behaviour
- sedation.

Caution is required in identifying drug-related central antimuscarinic effects to prevent the co-prescribing of antipsychotics with additional antimuscarinic effects. The subsequent occurrence of extrapyramidal effects such as dystonia, akathisia, tremor or rigidity then becomes apparent, with a risk of further antimuscarinic drugs such as procyclidine being added to control these effects. The iatrogenic problem is then worsened, with the risk of causing serious adverse drug reactions such as irreversible tardive dyskinesia, heat stroke or paralytic ileus (see Chapter 5).

Table 27.1 A comparison of severity of common side effects of phenothiazines

Adverse effect	Phenothiazines		
	Group 1	Group 2	Group 3
Extrapyramidal effects	++	+	+++
Antimuscarinic effects	++	+++	+
Drowsiness	+++	++	+

+++ severe, ++ moderate and + fewer in comparison to the other phenothiazines.
Information derived from *British National Formulary*, vol. 55.

Idiosyncratic and hypersensitivity reactions

Type B adverse drug reactions are less predictable from the pharmacological activity of antipsychotics and include photosensitivity, particularly with chlorpromazine (and also contact sensitivity), agranulocytosis, jaundice and neuroleptic malignant syndrome (see Chapter 5).

Tables 27.1 and 27.2 include a comparison of side effects between different groups of phenothiazines and a consideration of the most prominent side effects, considering both conventional and atypical agents.

Drug choice

The aims of treatment are to manage the initial psychotic symptoms, improve the quality of life and reduce the risk of relapse but with minimum adverse effects (particularly frightening extrapyramidal effects). The most difficult symptoms to treat are negative symptoms, for which clozapine may be required. Atypical antipsychotics have been associated with fewer extrapyramidal side effects and have been recommended by the National Institute for Health and Clinical Excellence (NICE 2002) as first-line treatment for newly diagnosed schizophrenia. Specified agents include amisulpiride, olanzapine, quetiapine, risperidone and zotepine, and low doses should be used for the first episode. This recommendation excludes clozapine due to the risk of agranulocytosis. At the time of writing, olanzapine appears to be associated with a greater risk of metabolic adverse effects including weight gain (Newcomer 2007) and this may make it less suitable as a first-line agent. Additional recommendations by the NICE for the appropriate use of atypical antipsychotics include the following:

- Patients taking conventional antipsychotics and experiencing intolerable side effects (usually extrapyramidal) may be switched to an atypical antipsychotic.
- Patients suffering relapse and symptoms who were previously poorly controlled by conventional agents may benefit from an atypical antipsychotic.
- Symptoms of schizophrenia poorly controlled following trials with two or more antipsychotics (including at least one atypical) for 6–8 weeks may benefit from clozapine but initiated only in a hospital inpatient setting. Patients are required to register with a centralized monitoring service for early detection of agranulocytosis. A second antipsychotic may be added if there is a poor response with clozapine.
- There is convincing evidence that clozapine is more effective than conventional antipsychotics for the treatment of schizophrenia and that agranulocytosis is more likely to occur in children, adolescents and elderly people (Wahlbeck *et al* 1999).
- Changing to an atypical antipsychotic is not appropriate if symptoms are controlled and side effects are mild and acceptable.

As commented above, olanzapine and risperidone are associated with a greater risk of stroke in elderly patients.

Table 27.2   Examples of common side effects produced by antipsychotics

Side effect	Drugs implicated	Drugs least likely to cause the ADR
Extrapyramidal effects	Haloperidol, phenothiazines (see Table 27.1 for comparison), depot preparations	Atypical antipsychotics, including amisulpiride, sulpiride and particularly clozapine, olanzapine, quetiapine and risperidone
Antimuscarinic effects	Phenothiazines (see Table 27.1), clozapine	Haloperidol, amisulpiride, olanzapine, quetiapine, risperidone, sulpiride
Cardiac arrhythmias	Sertindole, phenothiazines, pimozide, clozapine	Amisulpiride, flupentixol, sulpiride, olanzapine, risperidone
Galactorrhoea	Sulpiride	Atypical antipsychotics
Parkinsonism	Fluphenazine, perphenazine, trifluoperazine, prochlorperazine	Atypical antipsychotics
Photosensitivity	Chlorpromazine	
Jaundice	Conventional antipsychotics, particularly phenothiazines (Chapter 5)	
Hypotension	Haloperidol, phenothiazines, sertindole	Amisulpiride, sulpiride, clozapine, risperidone, flupentixol, olanzapine, quetiapine
Drowsiness	Chlorpromazine (Table 27.1)	Amisulpiride, haloperidol, flupentixol, pimozide, quetiapine, sulpiride or zotepine
Sexual dysfunction (Chapter 5)	Phenothiazines, pimozide and sulpiride	
Weight gain	Chlorpromazine, sertindole, risperidone, olanzapine, clozapine	Pimozide
Agranulocytosis	Clozapine	All antipsychotics, except clozapine

ADR, adverse drug reaction.

Aggressive symptoms

Haloperidol is the common choice for violent or aggressive patients and often first choice for acute treatment of psychosis, prescribed 'when required' alongside other antipsychotics. Drugs such as lorazepam or haloperidol may be administered by intramuscular injection. It should be noted that haloperidol is often the choice for elderly patients because it has a lower incidence of hypotension. For further information about the management of acute schizophrenia, including rapid tranquillization, the reader is referred to guidelines issued by the NICE (2002).

Depot preparations

Depot preparations may be used for maintenance therapy, given every 1–4 weeks, particularly when compliance is a problem, and may benefit people who exhibit considerable first-pass metabolism. A test dose may be given initially (see *British National Formulary* or summary of product characteristics). There may, however, be an increased risk of extrapyramidal side effects compared with oral agents. Problems include difficulty in titrating doses, pain on injection and variable pharmacokinetics according to muscle mass and rate of metabolism. Side effects may take weeks to dissipate following the last dose. A depot preparation of the atypical antipsychotic, risperidone, is now licensed and available and may be associated with fewer side effects, as discussed above.

Duration of maintenance treatment

Treatment with antipsychotics is often long term. However, patients who appear to be in remission may withdraw gradually from treatment with regular monitoring for signs of relapse for at least 2 years after the last acute episode (NICE 2002). These patients include those who have suffered only one acute psychotic episode over 1–2 years of treatment and have responded well to treatment. Patients who have suffered two or more psychotic episodes are continued on medication for at least 5 years.

Non-pharmacological interventions

Cognitive–behavioural therapy (CBT) is recommended alongside drug treatment, to help patients to understand their symptoms and develop coping mechanisms in order to control them. It is particularly beneficial for persistent psychotic symptoms: longer courses of more than 6 months and at least 10 sessions are recommended (NICE 2002). Shorter courses may benefit only depressive symptoms. Carers may also benefit from support in the form of CBT or counselling and supportive psychotherapy. These interventions are beneficial for the patient and aim to prevent relapse, reduce symptoms,

Table 27.3   Concurrent disease and the prescribing of antipsychotics

Disease	Comment
Cardiovascular disease, e.g. angina, arrhythmias, chronic heart failure, stroke	• Increased risk of arrhythmias, particularly with sertindole and pimozide • Increased risk of hypotension in susceptible patients, e.g. elderly people or those prescribed antihypertensives. Reduced doses of antipsychotics may be recommended • Increased risk of stroke with olanzapine and risperidone in elderly patients
Closed-angle glaucoma	• Antimuscarinic drugs reduce drainage, therefore worsening this condition. Prochlorperazine and chlorpromazine use should be avoided • Patients at increased risk include those with diabetes mellitus and/or a family history of glaucoma
Prostatic hypertrophy	Antimuscarinic effects may lead to urinary retention
Depression	• There is currently no evidence for the benefit of antidepressants in patients with schizophrenia (Whitehead et al 2002) • See also drug interactions (Table 27.4)
Diabetes mellitus	• Risk of type 2 diabetes due to weight gain with antipsychotics and particularly chlorpromazine, sertindole, risperidone, clozapine and olanzapine • Risk of exacerbation or ketoacidosis (olanzapine)
Dementia and elderly people	• Drugs with antimuscarinic effects may cause or worsen dementia • Risperidone and olanzapine are associated with increased risk of stroke in elderly patients
Epilepsy	• The convulsive threshold is lowered by antipsychotics. Reduced doses may be indicated (e.g. clozapine) • Additional risk factors for convulsions are listed in Chapter 23
Parkinson's disease	Antipsychotics may exacerbate symptoms, mainly as a result of dopamine receptor antagonism
Severe respiratory disease	Use with caution, particularly in combination with other CNS depressants such as alcohol

CNS, central nervous system; NICE, National Institute for Health and Clinical Excellence.

increase insight and improve compliance with medication (NICE 2002). It should therefore be possible for patients to live a fairly normal life and this should be emphasized at the start of treatment.

The effect of environmental factors on patients with schizophrenia is recognized and benefit may be gained from moving patients to a low-stress environment. Social, group and physical activities are also beneficial.

Concurrent disease

Table 27.3 summarizes possible influences on the choice of antipsychotic drugs.

Drug interactions

Some of the older antipsychotic agents may cause Q–T prolongation and increase the risk of torsade de pointes arrhythmias. Accordingly, these drugs should be used with caution in elderly people, those with pre-existing arrhythmias and with other drugs that may prolong the Q–T interval. Atypical antipsychotics do not normally alter the Q–T interval but should be used with caution with drugs that do. Additional interactions are summarized in Table 27.4.

Monitoring

General

Monitoring for patients prescribed antipsychotics may include blood pressure due to the risk of hypotension, electrocardiogram (ECG), weight, urinary glucose and temperature. Temperature monitoring is useful for the early diagnosis of neuroleptic malignant syndrome, although this is rare.

Cardiovascular

An ECG should be performed for patients at risk of cardiotoxicity such as those with pre-existing cardiovascular disease, elderly patients, those taking medication associated with prolongation

of the Q–T interval and those prescribed high doses of antipsychotics.

Elderly

Drugs used in the treatment of schizophrenia may increase the risk of falls due to postural hypotension. Accordingly, lower doses are indicated. As commented above, olanzapine and risperidone are associated with an increased risk of stroke in elderly patients and should be avoided where possible.

Renal impairment

Lower doses of antipsychotics may be required in severe renal impairment, due to increased cerebral sensitivity. Lower doses of clozapine, quetiapine, risperidone or olanzapine are required in mild-to-moderate renal impairment with avoidance of clozapine in severe impairment. Sulpiride should be avoided in moderate renal impairment or lower doses used if essential.

Hepatic impairment

All antipsychotics have the potential to precipitate coma in patients with hepatic disease (see Chapter 10). Phenothiazines are hepatotoxic. Lower doses of clozapine, risperidone, quetiapine or olanzapine may be appropriate with regular monitoring of liver function.

Pregnancy and breast-feeding

Phenothiazines and butyrophenones tend to be preferred and in particular chlorpromazine, trifluoperazine or haloperidol, due to greater experience of use during pregnancy. Depot preparations are avoided unless compliance is a significant problem. Treatment is assessed according to risk versus benefit. There is evidence of neonatal toxicity during the third trimester. Symptoms observed in the fetus include tremor, increased muscle tone, abnormal movements and feeding difficulties. Antipsychotics such as chlorpromazine, trifluoperazine, haloperidol or possibly flupentixol may be continued with caution during breast-feeding as necessary but

Table 27.4 Examples of drug interactions involving antipsychotics

Drugs	Consequences	Comments
Clozapine with anticonvulsants (carbamazepine, phenytoin)	• Clozapine levels are reduced • Risk of additive bone marrow suppression (carbamazepine) • Risk of neuroleptic malignant syndrome (Chapter 5)	• Dose of clozapine may need to be doubled when used with carbamazepine or phenytoin • Monitor for signs of infection or neuroleptic malignant syndrome
Haloperidol and anticonvulsants (phenobarbital, carbamazepine, phenytoin) or rifampicin	Reduced levels of haloperidol	• Note that haloperidol may also increase carbamazepine levels • Sodium valproate appears not to interact • Isoniazid may increase haloperidol levels
Clozapine with benzodiazepines	Risk of severe hypotension and respiratory depression	• Monitor closely for signs of these adverse effects • Lorazepam may be prescribed 'when required' during acute schizophrenia
Clozapine with SSRIs (fluoxetine, fluvoxamine, paroxetine, sertraline)	Increased levels of clozapine and also increased risk of serotonin syndrome as both drugs increase serotoninergic neurotransmission	• Dose of clozapine may require adjustment • This combination may be beneficial and is used commonly • Citalopram does not appear to interact
Haloperidol with fluvoxamine or quinidine	Risk of increased haloperidol levels	The dose of haloperidol may require adjustment
Haloperidol with indometacin	Severe drowsiness and confusion	Avoid combination or monitor closely
Haloperidol or phenothiazines with tobacco or cannabis smoke	Reduced levels	Smokers may require an increased dose of haloperidol and chlorpromazine or a reduced dose on cessation of smoking
Conventional antipsychotics (butyrophenones, phenothiazines and thioxanthenes) with antimuscarinics	Additive antimuscarinic effects (Chapter 5) with the risk of rare but serious effects including: • heat stroke • severe constipation • paralytic ileus • psychosis • reduced efficacy of antipsychotic treatment due to reduced plasma levels	• Concurrent use may be beneficial • Monitor for signs of antimuscarinic effects (see text) and consider risk factors such as exposure to hot and humid conditions, polypharmacy, high doses and/or impaired renal or hepatic function
Chlorpromazine and other antipsychotics with lithium	• Reduced levels of chlorpromazine • Risk of severe extrapyramidal effects and neurotoxicity	• Dose adjustment of chlorpromazine may be required • Severe side effects are rare but monitoring for these is important
Phenothiazines with trazodone	Severe hypotension	Additive hypotensive effects. Consider patients at increased risk such as those taking antihypertensive medication

Continued

Table 27.4   (Continued)

Drugs	Consequences	Comments
Phenothiazines with TCAs	• Increased TCA levels and possibly phenothiazine levels • Increased risk of tardive dyskinesia, which may be caused and masked by elevated levels of either or both drugs	• This combination is often used but the safety of co-prescribing is not certain • For a discussion of effects on the Q–T interval, see text • Additional risk factors include high doses and polypharmacy
Pimozide with clarithromycin	Increased levels of pimozide	Increased risk of cardiotoxicity. Consider also use with other drugs known to prolong the Q–T interval (Chapter 5)
Sertindole interactions (e.g. cimetidine, fluoxetine, paroxetine or Q–T interval-prolonging drugs: see text)	Risk of cardiotoxicity with increased levels and/or those that prolong the Q–T interval	Sertindole was withdrawn in 1998 as a result of cardiotoxicity but has recently been reintroduced for restricted indications (see text)
Sertindole with carbamazepine or phenytoin	Reduced levels of sertindole	Increased dose may be required.

SSRIs, selective serotonin reuptake inhibitors; TCAs, tricyclic antidepressants.

the infant should be monitored for adverse effects such as oversedation.

Over-the-counter considerations

Patients may request supplements of poly-unsaturated fatty acids for the symptoms of schizophrenia. Preliminary evidence supports the use of fish oil or evening primrose oil, which may improve symptoms and do not appear to cause adverse effects, although more studies are needed (Joy *et al* 2006).

Counselling

Guidance issued by the NICE (2002) emphasizes the importance of providing 'an atmosphere of hope and optimism' for patients and carers, and forming 'a supportive and empathic relationship' with them. Reassurance should be given that drug treatment is effective and, with adequate support, the patient should be given the opportunity to return to employment if desired.

Pharmacists have key roles in empathic support and the provision of information relating to treatment as necessary.

General lifestyle advice (see Chapter 3) should be given due to the risk of weight gain, diabetes mellitus and cardiac effects with antipsychotics. Alcohol or drug misuse may exacerbate schizophrenia and should therefore be avoided, and patients referred for additional support if necessary.

Compliance with antipsychotic medication is a common problem due to side effects as described above and there may initially be a lack of insight, resulting in patients not recognizing that they are ill. The importance of maintenance treatment in preventing relapse should be emphasized and patients or carers informed that intermittent therapy is not recommended. The side effects and particularly movement disorders should also be explained when treatment is initiated. Patients should be advised that treatment requires gradual withdrawal and should therefore not be stopped without the advice of their doctor.

Changing treatment

Patients should be warned about the risk of relapse and a transient worsening of side effects when changing to an alternative antipsychotic. It is important to reinforce that adherence to treatment should improve symptoms with fewer side effects over time. However, if symptoms persist, an alternative antipsychotic may be tried.

Blood dyscrasias

Patients should be advised to report symptoms of infection such as sore throat and pyrexia, particularly when prescribed clozapine.

Weight gain

Weight gain and the onset of type 2 diabetes should be monitored, particularly in patients prescribed olanzapine, clozapine, chlorpromazine, sertindole or risperidone, and also in patients at risk, such as those with obesity. When initiating treatment, it is useful to reinforce a healthy diet and exercise (see Chapter 3). Urinary glucose should be monitored.

Sexual effects

Counselling at the onset of treatment may help reduce the effect on relationships and quality of life. The importance of compliance should be stressed due to the risk of relapse, and the patient encouraged to discuss problematic effects as they occur. Patients should also be advised to discuss a planned pregnancy.

Antimuscarinic effects

Patients should be warned of antimuscarinic effects, including dry mouth and eyes, blurred vision and constipation. Artificial saliva (e.g. Luborant) or sugar-free boiled sweets, artificial tears or laxatives should be prescribed as necessary. Co-prescribing with other drugs that have antimuscarinic activity may increase the risk of these effects and particularly severe constipation (risk of paralytic ileus and obstruction, particularly with clozapine), heat stroke (see Chapter 5) and psychosis. Patients should be advised of the importance of maintaining regular fluid intake, particularly in hot or humid conditions, due to the increased risk of heat stroke. There is also a risk of hypothermia during cold weather, due to poor temperature regulation.

Cardiovascular effects

Symptoms suggestive of arrhythmias should be explained and reporting encouraged, e.g. patients may become aware of palpitations and/or an altered pulse rate. Prescribers should monitor patients for these symptoms, particularly those at risk (discussed above). Blood pressure should be monitored as hypotension may occur, particularly when treatment is initiated. Also the risk of stroke should be taken into account when using olanzapine and risperidone.

Drowsiness (all antipsychotics and particularly chlorpromazine)

General counselling should be to warn the patient about drowsiness and the effect on driving and operating machinery. This may be particularly prevalent when treatment is initiated.

Photosensitivity

Photosensitivity may occur, particularly with chlorpromazine and therefore exposure to the sun or sunlamps should be avoided. High-factor sunscreen should be applied when exposure to ultraviolet light is unavoidable.

Extrapyramidal symptoms

Patients should be advised about the risk of extrapyramidal symptoms, because these can be frightening (see above).

Tardive dyskinesia

Patients should be advised to consult their doctor urgently if they develop fine involuntary movements of the tongue, because this adverse effect is often irreversible.

Self-assessment

Consider whether the following statements are true or false concerning the use of atypical antipsychotic drugs in the management of schizophrenia:

1. They should be used only once a patient has failed to respond to conventional antipsychotics.
2. Clozapine is associated with agranulocytosis.
3. They are associated with causing weight loss.
4. They are devoid of extrapyramidal side effects.
5. They do not bind to dopamine receptors.

Practice points

General
- Prompt diagnosis of patients with psychosis may improve the clinical outcome.
- Lifestyle changes are important in the management of schizophrenia (see Monitoring and Counselling sections).
- Regular screening for side effects and particularly weight gain, sexual dysfunction, drowsiness and extrapyramidal effects (e.g. tardive dyskinesia) is important.

Antipsychotics
- Starting treatment at a low dose and increasing gradually (ideally once a week or longer) reduces side effects.
- Patients should be maintained on the lowest effective dose.
- Concurrent use of antipsychotics should be used only in the short term, e.g. when changing to an alternative antipsychotic.
- The dose for intramuscular injection is lower than the oral dose, due to the absence of first-pass metabolism by hepatic enzymes.
- Withdrawal should be gradual after long-term treatment with antipsychotics, because of the risk of withdrawal symptoms and possible relapse.
- Treatment should be withdrawn in the presence of early symptoms suggestive of tardive dyskinesia, because this is usually irreversible.
- When the patient is stabilized on an antipsychotic, the dosage interval may be reduced to once-daily administration because these drugs have a long half-life.
- It should be noted that the use of antipsychotic doses greater than the recommended limit constitutes use outside the product licence and increases the risk of side effects without any improvement in symptom control. Alternatives include switching to another antipsychotic. The duration of use of high doses should be limited and reviewed regularly. It is recommended that the dose be reduced if no improvement is observed after 3 months (advice from The Royal College of Psychiatrists reported in the *British National Formulary*, vol. 55).

 CASE STUDIES

Case 1

A 40-year-old male patient presents with worsening auditory hallucinations associated with messages he feels are being given to him by characters in a television soap opera. He recognizes these symptoms and consults his GP urgently according to previous advice. He is currently taking trifluoperazine 5 mg daily. He has been stable on this treatment for 20 years.

continued

CASE STUDIES (continued)

What action do you take?

- A short-term increase in his dose to 15 mg daily may control his symptoms until the period of stress has passed. Further increases (consider divided dosing) can be made at intervals of 3 days according to response. The dose can then be reviewed, particularly if side effects become troublesome. It may be useful to remind him about possible side effects and to discuss these if they become problematic. This case represents the benefits of education as the patient has control of his condition, helped by the support of his GP.

Case 2
The police arrest a 22-year-old man because of his involvement in a fight. He becomes uncommunicative and fails to cooperate. A friend at the scene comments that he has been concerned about his friend for some time as he recently lost his job and became uninterested in his appearance. He mentioned that aliens were laughing at him and told him that a group of men were planning to attack him before he started the fight. He was not provoked.

Which symptoms are typical of schizophrenia?

- This patient has negative symptoms, including lack of communication and loss of interest in his appearance. These may be the first symptoms to occur in schizophrenia and may also include a loss of interest in previous activities and relationships. Positive symptoms include hallucinations, paranoia and thought disorder.

What is the likely treatment for this patient?

- If the patient continues to be aggressive, he may be given haloperidol in the short term, possibly with an antimuscarinic agent 'when required' for the short-term prevention of extrapyramidal effects. He is likely to be prescribed an atypical antipsychotic. The misuse of drugs such as cocaine should be investigated because this may trigger schizophrenia.

References

American Psychiatric Association (1995). *Diagnostic and Statistical Manual of Mental Disorders*, 4th edn (DSM-IV). Washington DC: American Psychiatric Press.

Joy CB, Mumby-Croft R, Joy LA (2006). Polyunsaturated fatty acid supplementation for schizophrenia. *Cochrane Database System Rev* issue 2: CD001257.

Rathbone J, Soares-Weiser K (2006). Anticholinergics for neuroleptic-induced acute akathisia. *Cochrane Database System Rev* issue 3: CD003727.

Martin J, ed. *British National Formulary*, latest edition.

London: British Medical Association and Royal Pharmaceutical Society of Great Britain.

National Institute for Clinical Excellence (2002). *Core Interventions in the Treatment and Management of Schizophrenia in Primary and Secondary Care*. Clinical guideline 1. London: NICE.

Newcomer JW (2007). Antipsychotic medications: metabolic and cardiovascular risk. *J Clin Psychiatry* **68**(suppl 4): 8–13.

Wahlbeck K, Cheine M, Essali MA (1999). Clozapine versus typical neuroleptic medication for schizophrenia. *Cochrane Database System Rev* issue 3: CD000059.

Whitehead C, Moss S, Cardno A *et al* (2002). Antidepressants for people with both schizophrenia and depression. *Cochrane Database System Rev* issue 2: CD002305.

Further reading

Bazire S (2001). *Psychotropic Drug Directory 2001.* Wiltshire: Quay Books.

Glen I (2001). Schizophrenia. Review of antipsychotics. *Hosp Pharm* **8**: 192–4.

McGrath J, Emmerson WB (1999). Treatment of schizophrenia (clinical review). *BMJ* **319**: 1045–8.

Maclean F, Lee A (1999). Drug-induced sexual dysfunction and infertility. *Pharm J* **262**: 780–4.

Parkinson's disease

Characteristics

Parkinson's disease is a relatively common neuro-degenerative disease often, but not always, associated with ageing. Parkinson's disease is a disease of movement and is associated with tremor, rigidity and poverty of movement. Terms used in Parkinson's disease include bradykinesia (slowness of movement), akinesia (lack of movement or rigidity) and dyskinesias (abnormal involuntary movements). The following may be associated with Parkinson's disease: an emotionless facial expression, stooping, autonomic dysfunction (including orthostatic hypotension, constipation and increased urinary frequency), depression, altered handwriting and sleep disturbances.

The underlying cause of the disease is uncertain but may have associations with environmental toxins, a weak genetic link, oxidative stress or, in early onset disease, a relationship with brain trauma as seen in boxers. The disease is characterized by degeneration of dopaminergic neurons in the nigrostriatal pathway in the basal ganglia, and current drug therapy is designed to replace or improve dopaminergic activity. The reduction in dopaminergic activity is also accompanied by increased activity of acetylcholine due to an imbalance. As indicated in Chapter 27, dopamine receptor antagonists (such as antipsychotic agents) may lead to drug-induced parkinsonism, which involves rigidity and problems of movement but tremor is not an important feature.

The diagnosis of Parkinson's disease is generally made by a neurologist, based on symptoms and may involve brain imaging to exclude other pathologies.

Goals of treatment

The central goal of treatment is restoration of dopaminergic function and, ideally, prevention of neurological degeneration. Current therapies aim to restore dopamine but the effects are transient and so the achievable aim is symptomatic relief.

Pharmacological basis of management (Figure 28.1)

Levodopa (L-dopa)

In order to restore function to the dopaminergic system then the 'classic' treatment involves levodopa, which is the precursor of dopamine and so will increase levels of dopamine and provide some relief from the symptoms. Administration of levodopa is associated with widespread side effects, notably nausea and hypotension due to the peripheral conversion of levodopa to dopamine. To reduce these problems, levodopa is given with an inhibitor of dopa decarboxylase such as carbidopa or benserazide and, as these agents do not penetrate the blood–brain barrier, peripheral conversion of levodopa is prevented although levodopa can still lead to central formation of dopamine.

Although levodopa is invaluable in the management of Parkinson's disease, patients often develop 'on–off' effects with rapid fluctuations between rigidity and involuntary movements. Levodopa is also associated with dose-related central nervous system (CNS) side effects such as involuntary movements and psychiatric effects.

Furthermore, its efficacy has a finite period and, after a number of years of usage, the patient may no longer derive benefit. Indeed, this is a reason to delay using levodopa in a patient with Parkinson's disease and this is especially important in younger patients. Treatment with levodopa is also associated with an 'end-of-dose' effect, when its efficacy decreases towards the end of the dose and this is progressive with continued usage. This problem is partly related to the short plasma half-life of levodopa and shortening the dosage interval or using a modified release preparation may help to overcome this problem. Previously patients were temporarily taken off levodopa as a 'dopamine holiday' but this is not advocated in the guidelines produced by the National Institute for Health and Clinical Excellence (NICE 2006).

Dopamine receptor agonists, e.g. bromocriptine, cabergoline, pergolide, ropinirole, rotigotine

These are dopamine D_2-receptor agonists (with variable activity at D_3-, D_4- and D_5-receptors) that increase dopaminergic activity in the basal ganglia and, as the principal peripheral receptor is the dopamine D_1-receptor, they have limited peripheral side effects. Their direct agonist activity circumvents the need for the nigrostriatal pathway to synthesize dopamine. However, they are generally less efficacious compared with levodopa but some practitioners prescribe dopamine receptor agonists, such as rotigotine, to younger patients or in early disease to delay starting levodopa, which has a finite usage (see above). They are also less likely to induce dyskinesias in patients. Dopamine receptor agonists also have a role as an adjunct to levodopa in patients who are inadequately controlled by levodopa alone.

Monoamine oxidase B inhibitors: rasagiline, selegiline

The isoenzyme monoamine oxidase B (MAO-B) is involved in the metabolism of dopamine and so inhibition of this enzyme will increase the concentrations of dopamine. Selegiline is given with

levodopa to enhance its actions and may help to overcome the 'end-of-dose' effect. Rasagiline may also be used in this way or as monotherapy to augment endogenous levels of dopamine.

There had previously been some interest in the use of selegiline and increased mortality (Lee 1995), but it has been shown that, although Parkinson's disease is associated with increased mortality, selegiline does not pose a risk compared with other therapies (Donnan et al 2000; Ives et al 2004). Indeed, the mortality appears related to severity of the disease.

Unlike MAO inhibitors, which are occasionally used in depression, their selectivity for the B type means that their use is not complicated by the 'cheese' reaction with foods containing tyramine and so do not require dietary restrictions. Non-selective MAO inhibitors should not be given at the same time as levodopa because this may lead to a hypertensive crisis.

Catechol-*O*-methyltransferase inhibitors: entacapone, tolcapone

Catechol-*O*-methyltransferase (COMT) is also involved in the breakdown of dopamine, and inhibitors of this enzyme will also increase levels of dopamine, so enhancing dopaminergic function. They are used as adjuncts to levodopa therapy and may smooth out the 'end-of-dose effects'. Indeed, levodopa is also a substrate for COMT and its co-administration will prevent peripheral metabolism of levodopa, so optimizing levels of levodopa for central conversion to dopamine. Some preparations of levodopa are formulated with entacapone in addition to dopa decarboxylase inhibitors.

Amantidine

This is also an antiviral agent, which is thought to act by increasing the release of dopamine.

Muscarinic receptor antagonists, e.g. procyclidine

As commented above, the decreased dopaminergic activity is accompanied by an imbalance of

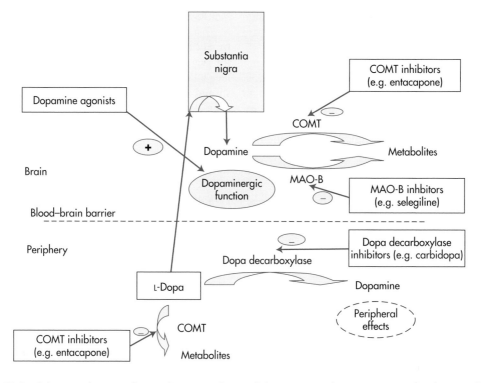

Figure 28.1 Schematic diagram of some the principal sites of drug action in the management of Parkinson's disease with principal drug classes shown in unshaded boxes. COMT, catechol-O-methyltransferase; MAO, monoamine oxidase.

cholinergic activity and so muscarinic antagonists are useful to dampen down the cholinergic system. Muscarinic antagonists are often used where tremor is a leading feature, especially in younger patients. Interestingly, in the older antipsychotic drugs that were found to cause drug-induced Parkinson's disease, it was found that the agents with significant antimuscarinic binding were less likely to cause problems, due to reduced cholinergic activity (Figure 28.1).

Drug choice

The most effective treatment for Parkinson's disease is levodopa in combination with dopa decarboxylase inhibitors and NICE guidance (2006) indicates that most patients will eventually require levodopa. However, as levodopa therapy has a finite period for its effectiveness, it may not always be used as first-line therapy, in which case dopaminergic agonists might be used.

In choosing a dopamine agonist, the non-ergot agents (ropinirole, rotigotine) are preferred because they are not associated with fibrotic reactions (see later), which occur with ergot derivatives. MAO-B inhibitors may also be used as first-line therapy.

If a COMT inhibitor is added to therapy entacapone is the agent of choice as tolcapone is best avoided because it is associated with liver toxicity. The NICE (2006) have indicated that amantidine should be used to manage dyskinesia.

In the case of drug-induced parkinsonism the approach is, where possible, to stop the causative agent. However, this may not be possible in all cases and, for example, in schizophrenia the approach might be to choose an agent less likely to cause the symptoms such as an atypical agent. As drug-induced parkinsonism is essentially due to the agent blocking dopamine receptors levodopa and dopamine receptor agonists are not appropriate for this condition and, where drug treatment is required, antimusarinic agents may be considered.

Neuroleptic malignant syndrome

This is a rare but severe reaction, usually to antipsychotics, but may occur with levodopa. Symptoms include fever, rigidity, altered mental status and autonomic dysfunction (e.g. loss of bladder and bowel control). It is usually managed by dose reduction of levodopa.

Fibrotic reactions

Ergot-derived dopamine receptor agonists (e.g. bromocriptine, cabergoline, lisuride, pergolide) are associated with causing fibrosis that may affect the lungs, heart valves and retroperitoneum. If ergot derivatives are used the Commission for Human Medicines (CHM) has advised that erythrocyte sedimentation rate (ESR), and electrolyte and creatinine levels should be monitored and a chest X-ray taken.

Depression

Parkinson's disease is associated with depression and, where antidepressant therapy is required, selective serotonin reuptake inhibitors (SSRIs) should be used although there are risks of interactions with selegiline (Table 28.1).

Drug interactions

In the context of drugs used in the management of Parkinson's disease, some interactions are summarized in Table 28.1. One key pharmacodynamic interaction is between dopamine receptor antagonists (e.g. antipsychotic agents) and levodopa and dopamine receptor agonists. The other issue, as commented above, is that many of the drug therapies for the management of Parkinson's disease involve positive drug interactions, e.g. levodopa and carbidopa.

Monitoring

In addition to the monitoring mentioned above for ergot derivates (ESR, electrolytes, creatinine levels and chest X-rays), liver function tests should be carried out for the COMT inhibitors (especially tolcapone) in view of the risk of liver dysfunction.

Counselling

Patients with Parkinson's disease should report their condition to the DVLA (Driver and Vehicle Licensing Agency). Levodopa-containing compounds and dopamine receptor agonists can cause the sudden onset of sleep and patients should be warned of this, especially in the context of skilled tasks such as driving. In all cases drug treatment should be adhered to and not stopped abruptly without medical advice.

Levodopa and dopamine receptor agonists

- The beneficial effects may take some time to become fully apparent.
- Levodopa and dopamine receptor agonists are also liable to cause orthostatic hypotension, so patients should be counselled about the possibility of a fall.
- Both levodopa and dopamine receptor agonists can cause abnormal involuntary movements.
- They may cause anxiety, hallucinations and vivid dreams.
- They are occasionally associated with behavioural changes, which may include abnormal gambling and hypersexuality.
- They may cause nausea and domperidone may help as it blocks their peripheral actions.

Levodopa

- If its effects start to wear off at the end of the dose or there are abnormal movements, the patient should consult their doctor.
- High protein diets may reduce the effectiveness of levodopa. This is due to competition of amino acids with levodopa for gastrointestinal absorption.

mine in the brain and so increase its
ration.
ɔa maintains its effectiveness through-
tment of the disease.
idone may be helpful in limiting
a-induced nausea.

4. MAO-B selective inhibitors (such as selegiline) do not give rise to the 'cheese reaction'.
5. Muscarinic antagonists are often used where
tremor is a leading feature.

points

son's disease is a condition requiring specialist diagnosis and treatment.
ent guidelines are set out by the NICE (2006) and should be consulted.
rkinson's Disease Society provides a wealth of patient and professional advice.
ɔpa (with a dopa decarboxylase inhibitor) is the classic treatment but is effective only for a finite period.
(notably older antipsychotic agents) can lead to drug-induced parkinsonism.
of co-careldopa should be checked carefully because confusion can occur between preparations. Note
preparation should be stopped at least 12 hours before another levodopa/dopa decarboxylase inhibitor
ed.

CASE STUDIES

, a 60-year-old man, gives a 6-month history of tremor in the right hand and has some
y in writing; he also complains of dyspepsia. On examination, one can see the tremor at
d there is some slowness of finger movements. The GP suspects Parkinson's disease and
he patient to a neurologist. The neurologist is convinced that the initial diagnosis is correct
escribes:

ne 2 mg patches (daily).

uld a CT or MRI scan help with diagnosis?
, there are no structural lesions but these may be used to exclude other pathologies.
nment on the choice of drugs.
his drug is often used as first line and is appropriate as monotherapy. Dopamine receptor
gonists are also appropriate for relatively young patients with mild symptoms.
y wasn't levodopa prescribed?
he benefits of levodopa may be lost over time, so it might be wise to delay its use.
at are the driving implications for this man?
He should inform the DVLA to judge his fitness to drive.
Dopamine receptor agonists and levodopa are associated with a risk of the sudden onset of
leep and he requires counselling if he is driving.
er a year he still has significant symptoms and the following are prescribed:

emet-Plus (levodopa and carbidopa)
nperidone 20 mg three times daily.

continued

Table 28.1 Summary of important interactions with drugs used in the mc

Interacting drugs	Consequences
Levodopa or dopamine receptor agonists with antipsychotic agents and dopaminergic antiemetics (e.g. metoclopramide)	The dopamine receptor antagonists will oppose the actions and reduce the effectiveness of these anti-parkinsonian drugs (and vice versa)
Levodopa or dopamine receptor agonists with antihypertensives	Increased hypotensive effects
Levodopa and benzodiazepines	Evidence of reduced effectiveness of levodopa
Levodopa and non-selective MAOIs	Risk of hypertensive crisis
SSRIs or TCAs with selegiline	Risk of serotoninergic syndrome
Antimuscarinics with other drugs with antimuscarinic properties	Increased antimuscarinic side effects (e.g. dry mouth, blurred vision, urinary retention and constipation)
Antacids with levodopa	Antacids might reduce the effectiveness of modified-release preparations of levodopa

SSRI, selective serotonin reuptake inhibitor; MAOI, monoamine oxidase inhibitor; TCA, tricyclic antidepre

Dopamine receptor agonists

These are associated with dyspepsia.

Dopamine receptor agonists (ergot derivates)

Patients should be counselled to report cough, breathlessness and abdominal pain because these could indicate a fibrotic reaction.

Antimuscarinic agents

These are likely to cause dry mouth, blurred vision, constipation and urinary retention.

of dop
conce

2. Levod
out tre

3. Domp
levodc

Practic

- Park
- Trea
- The
- Levo
- Drug
- Dose
  that
  is st

Case
Mr A
diffic
rest
refer
and

rotig

1. V
   N
2. C
   T
3. V
   -
4. V
   -

COMT inhibitor

- If patients ar
  vigilant for :
- These may d

Self-assessm

Consider whet
true or false. In
disease:

1. Dopa decarl
   bidopa) are

 CASE STUDIES (continued)

5. Why wasn't levodopa prescribed alone.
   – Carbidopa prevents peripheral conversion of levodopa to dopamine and so limits peripheral side effects.
6. Comment on the choice of domperidone over metoclopramide.
   – Domperidone has poor penetration of the blood–brain barrier, and so will not oppose central actions of dopamine. Metoclopramide penetrates the blood–brain barrier and will oppose the actions of dopamine and could cause drug-induced parkinsonism.
   The patient is severely depressed about having developed this condition.
7. Is drug treatment appropriate for his depression?
   – Yes and an SSRI would be appropriate. TCAs may make the condition worse and the rarely used MAO inhibitors should be avoided with levodopa.

Case 2
Mr AB is a 60-year-old man who shows rigidity with slowness but no tremor. He has a history of hypertension, schizophrenia and vestibular disorder. His current medication is:

bendroflumethiazide 2.5 mg once daily
haloperidol 20 mg daily
temazepam 10 mg every night
cinnarizine 30 mg three times daily.

The GP makes a provisional diagnosis of drug-induced parkinsonism.

1. What action would you recommend?
   Of the drugs that he is prescribed, haloperidol and cinnarizine are both associated with causing drug-induced parkinsonism. The newer atypical antipsychotics (e.g. risperidone, olanzapine) are less likely to cause this and would a sensible alternative to use. If cinnarizine is essential to the management of this patient then it could be changed to betahistine (but not prochlorperazine, because this is also associated with drug-induced parkinsonism).

References

Donnan PT, Steinke DT, Stubbings C *et al* (2000). Selegiline and mortality in subjects with Parkinson's disease. *Neurology* **55**: 1785–9.

Ives NJ, Stowe RL, Marro J *et al* (2004). Monoamine oxidase type B inhibitors in early Parkinson's disease: meta-analysis of 17 randomised trials involving 3525 patients. *BMJ* **329**: 593–9.

Lee AJ (1995). Comparison of the therapeutic effects and mortality data for levodopa combined with selegiline in patients with early, mild Parkinson's disease. *BMJ* **311**: 1602–7.

National Institute for Health and Clinical Excellence (2006). *Parkinson's Disease: Diagnosis and management in adults in primary and secondary care.* Clinical Guideline 35. London: NICE.

Further reading

Clarke CE (2007). Parkinson's disease. *BMJ* **335**: 441–5.

Samili A, Nutt JG, Ranson BR (2004). Parkinson's disease. *Lancet* **363**: 1783–93.

Online resources

www.parkinsons.org.uk
The website of the Parkinson's Disease Society; provides
a wealth of information for both patients and
professionals (accessed April 2008).

Part G
Pain and palliation

Pain management

Pain is one of the most common complaints and impacts greatly on patients' quality of life, possibly leading to reduced mobility, insomnia and depression. Management of pain is complicated, particularly in elderly people, due to side effects such as constipation, and drowsiness with opioids and gastrointestinal bleeding with nonsteroidal anti-inflammatory drugs (NSAIDs), and numerous drug interactions add to this prescribing challenge.

Acute pain is an important protective mechanism preventing or reducing injury by enabling rapid removal from harm. Chronic pain, lasting 6 months or longer, is not beneficial and is widely considered to be a disease.

Physiology of pain

The detection of pain occurs via nociceptive afferent neurons, mechanoreceptors and thermoreceptors, which transmit sensory information to the brain or dorsal horn of the spinal cord. Fast reflex actions involve direct transmission to the dorsal horn of the spinal cord without involving the brain, before the defence or motor response. A detailed description of pain physiology is beyond the scope of this book but terminology in common usage is defined as follows:

- noci: a prefix denoting pain or injury
- nociceptive: describes nerve fibres, endings or pathways concerned with pain
- nociceptors: any receptor that responds to stimuli resulting in the sensation of pain
- thermoreceptors: receptors activated by heat
- mechanoreceptors: receptors activated by light touch

- afferent (sensory) neurons transmit impulses from the sense organs and receptors to the brain or spinal cord
- efferent (motor) neurons transmit impulses from the brain or spinal cord (dorsal horn) to various tissues in response to stimulation by the sensory fibres, leading to defence responses such as muscle contraction to move away from the pain source
- nociceptive afferent (sensory) neurons: afferent fibres directly involved in the detection of pain. These are neurons with sensory endings in peripheral tissues. They are essentially bare nerve endings and are activated by mechanical, thermal or chemical stimuli. They may also set up local reflexes, such that stimulation may elicit a local response, e.g. vasodilatation
- Aδ-, Aβ- and C-fibres describe different types of nerve fibre involved in pain transmission.

Other transmitters of pain (inflammatory mediators, neurotransmitters and neuropeptides)

As described above, physical or chemical insults activate nociceptors resulting in neurotransmission to the brain and/or spinal cord. Inflammatory mediators, including bradykinin, histamine and 5-hydroxytryptamine/serotonin (5HT) produced by injured tissues, may modify the transmission of pain impulses. In addition, prostanoids, which do not produce pain directly, sensitize nociceptors.

Neuropeptides involved in pain transmission include the tachykinins: substance P (neurokinin-1), neurokinin A and calcitonin generelated peptide (CGRP). These are released from sensory neurons and release inflammatory mediators such as histamine, 5HT, leukotrienes and prostaglandins from mast cells. This is known as neurogenic inflammation. These inflammatory mediators sensitize nociceptive nerve endings, lowering the trigger threshold of the nerve to produce hyperalgesia.

Ultimately, the perception of pain occurs in the cerebral cortex. An emotional component from the limbic system is also thought to contribute and explains the subjective response according to psychological characteristics such as anxiety and depression.

Excitatory and inhibitory neurotransmitters

Pharmacological targets include receptors for neurotransmitters involved in complex spinal neural activity. These include N-methyl-D-aspartate (NMDA) receptors for the endogenous excitatory amino acid, glutamate. Anaesthetic agents such as dizocilipine, and the less potent ketamine, are NMDA channel antagonists. The neurotransmitters γ-aminobutyric acid (GABA) and noradrenaline (norepinephrine) produce inhibitory effects. Adenosine is also thought to be involved, indicating a potential target for caffeine, a methylxanthine and adenosine receptor antagonist.

Opioids

Opioid receptors for the endogenous opioids (endorphins, enkephalins and dynorphins) are also involved in pain transmission and perception affecting both the brain and the spinal cord. Activation of these receptors in the spinal cord leads to presynaptic inhibition and blockade of pain transmission.

Gate theory

The gate theory describes the modulation of pain signals either to prevent or to enhance the signal received by the brain. Noxious stimuli activate afferent neurons, invoking a neuronal impulse to the spinal cord. This signal may then be inhibited or enhanced before its transmission to the brain.

Types of pain

Pain is described as somatic, visceral or neuropathic according to its origin.

Somatic

Somatic pain is pain relating to the body wall but excluding the viscera. Pain tends to be localized and follows stimulation of peripheral pain receptors (nociceptors) in the skin and musculoskeletal system. Examples include osteo- or rheumatoid arthritis and myalgia.

Visceral

Visceral pain originates in the viscera, i.e. the internal organs of the body, particularly the abdominal and thorax organs. Visceral pain is usually poorly localized and often referred to peripheral sites, e.g. the pain associated with gallstones, myocardial infarction or appendicitis.

Neuropathic pain

As the name suggests, neuropathic pain results from nerve damage arising in the central or peripheral nerves. Neuropathic pain occurs as a result of disease affecting the sensory pathway and is independent of damage to peripheral tissue. This usually results from damage to neural tissue. Examples include postherpetic neuralgia, phantom limb, peripheral neuropathies (e.g. associated with diabetes), rheumatoid arthritis, trauma, central pain (following a stroke or in multiple sclerosis) and cancer pain due to the tumour impinging on nerves. Neuropathic pain occurs due to a lack of sensory input after sensory nerve damage and is often accompanied by allodynia, i.e. pain caused by non-noxious stimuli (e.g. touch).

The pathophysiology of neuropathic pain is not yet fully elucidated but is thought to involve spontaneous activity in the damaged sensory neurons. The pain is described as burning, shooting or scalding. Sensitivity to noradrenaline due to the expression of α-adrenoceptors may develop, resulting in sympathetically mediated pain.

Goals of treatment

The goals of treatment are to improve the quality of life and to delay disease progress by good pain control but with minimal side effects.

Pharmacological basis of management of non-steroidal anti-inflammatory drugs, e.g. aspirin, diclofenac, diflusinal, flurbiprofen, ibuprofen, naproxen, piroxicam

NSAIDs are among the most widely used drugs for a number of conditions associated with inflammation. In addition to their anti-inflammatory effects, most NSAIDs possess analgesic and antipyretic effects.

Anti-inflammatory effects

When considering anti-inflammatory effects, it is useful to consider the process of inflammation. Important physiological mechanisms combine to produce vasodilatation, increased vascular permeability and cell accumulation. A number of mediators produce these effects to different extents depending on the nature of the inflammation. These mediators include nitric oxide, leukotrienes, prostaglandins and thromboxane; the prostaglandins PGE_2 and PGI_2 (prostacyclin) produce vasodilatation and oedema, in addition to sensitization of nociceptors, as described above. Those mediators produced by cyclo-oxygenase (COX) activity, prostaglandins and thromboxane are the targets for NSAIDs. Production of the inflammatory mediators from membrane phospholipid and COX activity is detailed in Figure 29.1.

The inhibition of cyclo-oxygenase

The predominant mode of action of NSAIDs is inhibition of the COX enzymes, resulting in subsequent inhibition of prostaglandin and

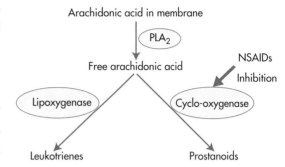

Figure 29.1 Production of the inflammatory mediators from membrane phospholipid, via phospholipase A_2 (PLA$_2$) and cyclo-oxygenase (COX) activity. NSAIDs, non-steroidal anti-inflammatory drugs.

thromboxane production. Most NSAIDs are competitive inhibitors of COX, whereas aspirin irreversibly inactivates COX by acetylation. This action of aspirin is exploited for antiplatelet effects (see Chapter 14).

The anti-inflammatory effects vary between NSAIDs, with ibuprofen being the weakest and indometacin and piroxicam the most potent. Ibuprofen is therefore not considered suitable for the treatment of acute gout. Most NSAIDs are antipyretic due to inhibition of prostaglandin effects, which disrupt the hypothalamic regulation of temperature.

The difference in anti-inflammatory activity of NSAIDs is small compared with tolerability by patients. In the treatment of rheumatoid arthritis, therefore, larger doses of 1.6–2.4 g ibuprofen daily, which possesses only weak anti-inflammatory activity, are required. Longer-acting NSAIDs with more potent anti-inflammatory activity such as naproxen and piroxicam are useful in the treatment of chronic pain.

Analgesic effect

As described above, prostaglandins produced by inflamed tissue sensitize nociceptors to inflammatory mediators such as bradykinin and 5HT. NSAIDs therefore produce an analgesic effect in conditions associated with prostaglandin production. The beneficial effect in headache may result from inhibiting prostaglandin-mediated vasodilatation of the cerebral vasculature. Actions in the spinal cord may also contribute to the central effect.

Adverse effects

NSAIDs are associated with many adverse drug reactions (ADRs: see Chapter 5) but predominantly gastric toxicity with a risk of haemorrhage (see Chapter 7). Other ADRs include diarrhoea, nausea, rashes, urticaria, photosensitivity, sodium and water retention (with worsening of hypertension and chronic heart failure), and renal impairment. Renal toxicity may be due to inhibition of the effects of prostaglandins on renal blood flow or nephropathy. Some NSAIDs may precipitate asthma in certain individuals (see Chapter 21).

Adverse effects due to salicylates

In addition to the adverse effects caused by other NSAIDs, salicylates may also cause 'salicylism' including tinnitus, impaired hearing and vertigo. This usually occurs only after chronic use of larger doses, which may also lead to compensated respiratory alkalosis as a result of increased respiration. Aspirin may also cause encephalitis and liver problems, known as Reye's syndrome, in children aged <12 years and those <15 years with fever and/or viral illness. In view of the wide availability of aspirin through general sale and the Medicines and Healthcare products Regulatory Agency (MHRA) therefore recommended that aspirin should not be taken by any child aged <16 years.

COX-2 inhibitors, e.g. celecoxib, etodolac, meloxicam

There are two subtypes of COX, COX-1 and COX-2, which show some variation in distribution and roles. COX-1 is the constitutive or 'physiological' isoform, found in most tissues and blood platelets. COX-2 is inducible and is produced in activated inflammatory cells; it is, therefore, the COX subtype involved in the production of prostaglandins and thromboxanes that are active in inflammation. The main anti-inflammatory activity of NSAIDs is therefore due to COX-2 inhibition. COX-1 inhibition is thought to produce toxic effects, including gastric irritation (see Chapter 7). Drugs selective for COX-2 have therefore been developed and are thought to be more selective for inhibition of prostanoids associated with inflammation,

rather than those involved in physiological regulation. It is becoming apparent, however, that COX-2 inhibitors may not be as free from gastric toxicity as first thought (Jüni *et al* 2002). A systematic review of the efficacy and safety of celecoxib compared with traditional NSAIDs for the treatment of osteoarthritis and rheumatoid arthritis reported similar efficacy for both treatments and an improvement in gastrointestinal safety and tolerability with celecoxib (Deeks *et al* 2002).

Paracetamol

Paracetamol is the first-choice analgesic for conditions not associated with inflammation. It possesses analgesic and antipyretic activity with similar efficacy to aspirin, but is not thought to exhibit significant anti-inflammatory effects. Its mechanism of action is yet to be elucidated fully but research has suggested that paracetamol inhibits COX-3, a novel COX variant, which is located in the brain (Chandraeskharen *et al* 2002). However, this mechanism of action has yet to be firmly established.

In normal doses, paracetamol is well tolerated; however, hepatotoxicity occurs with doses only two to three times the maximum recommended dose due to saturation of metabolism involving conjugation with glutathione. Toxic metabolites are produced, causing liver necrosis and damage to renal tubules. Early administration of acetylcysteine or methionine increases glutathione formation and therefore prevents liver damage. As few as 20 tablets can produce severe hepatocellular necrosis in the absence of symptoms in the first few days. Nausea and vomiting subside within 24 h but patients should be admitted to hospital urgently. Additional signs of liver toxicity include jaundice, abdominal tenderness (right upper quadrant) and hypoglycaemia. Patients at increased risk of liver damage include those taking concurrent enzyme inducers (carbamazepine, alcohol, phenytoin, rifampicin) and malnourished patients.

Nefopam

Nefopam is used for moderate pain resistant to treatment with non-opioid analgesics. Adverse sympathomimetic and antimuscarinic effects limit its use. These include nervousness, tachycardia, urinary retention, dry mouth and blurred vision.

Opioids

The term 'opioid' applies to morphine-like synthetic and endogenous compounds. Synthetic opioids are used to treat moderate-to-severe pain, often visceral in origin. They are reserved for more severe pain due to their unwanted effects of drowsiness, constipation, nausea and vomiting, tolerance and dependence. High doses may produce respiratory depression and hypotension.

Opioid receptors

The effects of opioids are mediated by opioid receptors. To date, three subtypes have been identified and termed μ-, κ- and δ-receptors. The main pharmacological effects are mediated by μ-receptors and include analgesia, respiratory depression, euphoria, miosis (pupil constriction), physical dependence, constipation and sedation. The κ-receptors are thought to produce dysphoria.

Most morphine-like drugs have a high affinity for μ-receptors with lower affinities for κ- and δ-receptors. The potency of agents such as codeine and methadone is lower than that of morphine, resulting in reduced pharmacological effects even at maximum doses.

Opioid receptors are distributed throughout the brain and spinal cord. The administration of morphine inhibits nociceptive pathways in the brain and dorsal horn of the spinal cord and from the peripheral terminals of nociceptive afferent neurons. Effects on the brain also contribute to the euphoric effect and subsequent reduction in the psychological component of pain.

Weak opioids, e.g. codeine, dihydrocodeine

Dihydrocodeine and codeine have similar moderate potencies, Weak opioids are available in combination with paracetamol (co-codamol, co-dydramol) but are no more effective than aspirin or paracetamol alone when given as single doses.

Strong opioids, e.g. buprenorphine, diamorphine, fentanyl, morphine

Strong opioids form step 3 of the analgesic ladder (described below) and are prescribed for chronic non-malignant pain or in palliative care (see Chapter 31). It should be noted that the risk of psychological dependence is minimal when opioids are used for severe pain and this is not a reason to withhold treatment.

Adverse effects of opioids

The most common adverse effects of opioids are constipation, nausea and vomiting, and drowsiness. Respiratory depression is thought to result from reduced sensitivity of the respiratory centre (in the brain) to carbon dioxide, when higher doses of opioids are administered.

Nausea and vomiting

Nausea and vomiting occur due to the effects of opioids on the chemoreceptor trigger zone in the brain. This is fairly common but usually transient. Antiemetics (see Chapter 8) such as metoclopramide or prochlorperazine are often required when more potent opioids such as morphine are first prescribed. Dystonic (abnormal muscle tone, e.g. muscle spasms) reactions may occur, particularly in young and elderly people.

Constipation

Constipation is common with opioids (see Chapter 9) and co-prescribing of laxatives is required. Bulk-forming laxatives may not be appropriate due to the reduced motility of the colon and, therefore, the reduced reflex effect of increased bulk produced by these agents. Stool softeners combined with stimulants are often used (see Chapter 9). It should be noted that constipation occurs with low doses of codeine, including those used for cough suppression (see Chapter 19).

Tolerance and dependence

Chronic opioid use may result in tolerance, requiring an increase in dosage. Alternatively, another opioid may be administered. Tolerance to analgesia, emetic, euphoria and respiratory effects of opioids occurs but that to constipation and pupil constriction is much less marked.

Table 29.1   A summary of some important properties of opioid analgesics

Opioid analgesic	Comments
Opioids for mild-to-moderate pain	
Codeine	• Constipating when used long term • Laxatives should be prescribed for all patients prescribed regular codeine
Dihydrocodeine	Nausea and vomiting increase with higher doses
Opioids for moderate-to-severe pain	
Alfentanil, fentanyl and remifentanil	• Injections used for intraoperative analgesia • Fentanyl patch used in palliative care (Chapter 31)
Buprenorphine	• Partial agonist at opioid receptors and therefore precipitates withdrawal symptoms in patients dependent on other opioids. This may result in breakthrough pain in patients changing from other opioids during treatment for pain • Longer duration of action, with the sublingual preparation producing analgesia for 6–8 h
Dextromoramide (Palfium)	Shorter duration of action than morphine and less sedating
Diamorphine (heroin)	Less nausea and hypotension than with morphine
Dipipanone (Diconal)	• Contains cyclizine and therefore not recommended in palliative care (see Cyclimorph, Chapter 31) • Less sedating than morphine
Meptazinol (Meptid)	• Lower incidence of respiratory depression • Rapid onset of action, 15 min
Methadone	• Less sedating than morphine • Long half-life and may therefore accumulate with repeated doses
Oxycodone	• Similar to morphine • Used in palliative care (Chapter 31)
Pethidine	• Rapid onset of action but short acting and therefore not recommended for chronic pain • Less constipating than morphine but less potent analgesic
Tramadol	• Fewer opioid side effects, including reduced potential for addiction • May cause adverse psychiatric effects such as hallucinations and confusion • Risk of convulsions, especially when combined with other drugs known to reduce seizure threshold

Dependence may be physical, involving a withdrawal syndrome, or psychological.

Other

Other adverse effects of opioids include bronchoconstriction (induced by morphine due to histamine release from mast cells), hypotension, bradycardia, pruritus and immunosuppression (after long-term opioid misuse). Table 29.1 summarizes some important properties of opioids.

Tramadol

Tramadol exhibits opioid effects and also enhances the effects of 5HT and adrenergic pathways. The use of this drug for moderate-to-severe pain has increased due to reduced opioid side effects. Psychiatric reactions may, however, occur. The response of patients to tramadol varies considerably and the dose is therefore adjusted accordingly.

Local anaesthetics, e.g. lidocaine, bupivacaine, levobupivacaine and prilocaine

Local anaesthetics inhibit reversibly the transmission of nerve impulses via blockade of voltage-sensitive sodium channels. Side effects include agitation, confusion, tremors, convulsions and respiratory depression. Cardiovascular side effects include myocardial depression, vasodilatation and subsequent hypotension.

Tricyclic antidepressants (see Chapter 24)

The pyschotropic effects of antidepressants may be of benefit for pain in patients with anxiety and depression. Tricyclic antidepressants (TCAs) also possess analgesic activity independent of these pyschotropic effects. Indeed, the analgesic effect tends to occur at lower doses than those used for depression. The mechanism is largely unclear but may involve inhibition of spinal neurons in pain pathways by increasing noradrenaline and 5HT concentrations in inhibitory pathways. TCAs may also block sodium channels and they are also NMDA-receptor antagonists.

Anticonvulsants (see Chapter 23)

Anticonvulsants such as carbamazepine, sodium valproate or phenytoin stabilize neuronal membranes. They are particularly useful, therefore, to relieve neuropathic pain. Carbamazepine is widely used for neuropathic pain, including diabetic neuropathy. Its use may be limited by dose-related side effects (see Chapter 23). Phenytoin may be used as an alternative but consideration should be given to zero-order pharmacokinetics (see Chapter 6). It may take 3–4 weeks to reach steady state if loading doses are not used. Lamotrigine is also increasingly being used for neuropathic pain. Although the mechanism of action is unclear, the anticonvulsants are believed to block sodium channels, suppressing neuronal discharge at sites of injury. The anticonvulsant gabapentin also has a role in the management of neuropathic pain but its mechanism of action is less clear and may involve altering GABAergic or calcium channel function.

Caffeine

Caffeine is added to a number of over-the-counter (OTC) preparations with the claim that it increases the analgesic effect of drugs such as paracetamol and aspirin. There is little evidence to support this and the regular use of these preparations may lead to chronic daily headache (see below) and be mildly habit forming. The alerting effect of caffeine may also be a disadvantage.

Counterirritants

Aδ- and C-fibres transmit pain signals to the dorsal horn of the spinal cord. These signals may be modulated by Aβ-fibres, thereby preventing transmission to the brain. This explains the effect of counterirritants such as menthol and capsaicin and/or rubbing, which activate Aβ-fibres and provide relief from pain caused by activation of C-fibres.

Cannabinoids

Although not licensed for pain management, there is good evidence that cannabinoids may exert analgesic effects through inhibition of synaptic transmission at both the spinal level and higher centres. Analogous to the opioid story, endogenous cannabinoids such as anandamide have been identified and may play a role in endogenous pain relief. Patients with certain chronic conditions such as multiple sclerosis appear to gain effective pain relief from cannabinoids. Current aims are to produce routes of administration that do not involve smoking and to identify cannabinoids with analgesic but without psychoactive properties.

Chronic pain and central sensitisation

Dosing 'when required' is not appropriate in the treatment of chronic pain due to the principle of central sensitization. This phenomenon also explains the benefit of administration of opioids before surgery. After damage to peripheral tissue, spinal neurons exhibit hyperresponsiveness to impulses from afferent neurons. This results in an increased perception of a similar intensity of pain. Therefore, if chronic pain recurs, it may be difficult to regain pain control due to the reduced threshold of the spinal neurons. Higher doses may be required to regain pain control. Maintenance treatment also removes the psychological component of fear and a dose reduction may then be possible.

Medication overuse headache

Medication overuse headache (MOH) is a common subtype of chronic daily headache (CDH). It may be caused by a withdrawal effect after the chronic use of analgesic preparations and results in a vicious circle, whereby analgesic administration is continued. It is becoming increasingly recognized as a problem associated with the overuse of analgesics in the treatment of headache. Inappropriate use of OTC analgesia is a particular problem due to the widespread availability of analgesics such as paracetamol, aspirin and ibuprofen from supermarkets and pharmacies.

MOH may follow the regular daily use of simple analgesics such as paracetamol, NSAIDs (more than four times a week), opioids or ergotamine more often than twice a week (Silberstein and Young 1995). Compound preparations containing caffeine or sympathomimetics may also contribute to MOH. Health professionals should be aware of the problem in patients presenting with chronic headache. The suspected causative drug should be withdrawn gradually and the patient monitored for improvement.

A study reported the occurrence of MOH due to excessive use of triptans. A critical number of dosages was reported as 10 single doses per month, above which MOH included a migraine-like daily headache or an increase in frequency of migraine attacks. It was recommended that, on suspicion of triptan-induced MOH, the drug should be withdrawn temporarily (Limmroth et al 2002).

Drug choice

The World Health Organization (1996) recommends that effective analgesia is given 'by the mouth, by the clock and by the ladder', i.e. the oral route is preferred for drug administration if possible and analgesia should be given regularly rather than 'when required'. The analgesic ladder starts with simple analgesics such as paracetamol or ibuprofen and progresses to mild and then strong opioids. Adjuncts including simple analgesics or pyschotropic agents may be added at any stage. Patients are then reviewed regularly and treatment stepped up or down as appropriate (Figure 29.2).

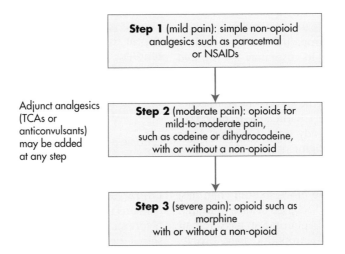

Figure 29.2   A summary of stepped-pain management as advocated by the World Health Organization. NSAIDs, non-steroidal anti-inflammatory drugs. TCAs, tricyclic antidepressants.

Paracetamol

Paracetamol is a common first-line agent, particularly for elderly patients, due to the reduced side-effect profile and fewer drug interactions. The main problem of paracetamol use is life-threatening hepatotoxicity in overdose.

NSAIDs

Aspirin is indicated for the treatment of headache, transient muscle pain, dysmenorrhoea and pyrexia. For inflammatory conditions, safer alternatives include ibuprofen (see Chapter 7).

NSAIDs are indicated for inflammatory conditions such as back pain, soft-tissue inflammation and rheumatoid arthritis. High doses are required to achieve a full anti-inflammatory effect. NSAIDs may also be useful in the treatment of advanced osteoarthritis (see Chapter 30).

It is important to note that it may take up to a week to achieve the full analgesic effect of NSAIDs, while the full anti-inflammatory effect may take up to 3 weeks. A poor response after this time should be followed by an alternative NSAID as their responses vary.

Topical NSAID preparations are widely available but their efficacy is uncertain and the benefit of topical agents over oral preparations has not yet been demonstrated.

Opioids

Mild opioids include codeine and dihydrocodeine and may be prescribed in addition to simple analgesics when these have failed to control pain in sole use. If this fails, more potent opioids may be introduced at step 3. This includes the treatment of chronic pain, which may not always be due to malignancy. For the use of opioids in palliative care see Chapter 31.

Compound preparations

The use of compound preparations containing paracetamol or aspirin with a low dose of opioid (8 mg codeine or 10 mg dihydrocodeine) is discouraged due to the lack of evidence, from single-dose studies, of efficacy compared with paracetamol or aspirin alone (Anon 2000). Coupled to this is the difficulty of titrating individual drug doses and the risk of opioid side effects such as drowsiness and constipation, particularly in elderly patients. Initial prescribing of more than one agent should be for individual drugs, and then fixed doses of combination products should be used once control has been achieved if compliance is a problem. If regular use of higher doses is required, patients may be advised that tolerance to most side effects will develop, with the exception of constipation and pupillary effects. Elderly patients may require a lower dose of codeine such as 15–30 mg daily. The use of combination analgesics for chronic pain may be appropriate for these patients and may improve compliance.

An alternative regimen includes the use of regular paracetamol at 1 g up to four times a day, with a single dose of up to 60 mg codeine when required for more severe pain as a beneficial second step, although opioid side effects may be problematic. This type of regimen limits the development of tolerance to and dependence on opioids (Anon 2000).

Topical preparations

Capsaicin is licensed for neuropathic pain but its use is limited due to an intense burning sensation, occurring when treatment is initiated. Capsaicin is a constituent of chilli powder and acts on vanilloid receptors to release and deplete neurotransmitters from sensory nerves, leading to counterirritation.

Nerve block

This involves the injection of local anaesthetics such as lidocaine close to a sensory nerve or plexus.

Steroids

Corticosteroids are used to treat pain associated with nerve compression, tissue swelling or raised intracranial pressure (see Chapter 31).

Non-pharmacological treatment

Non-pharmacological treatments used in pain management include simple measures such as rest, cooling, compression and elevation, the use of transcutaneous electrical nerve stimulation (TENS), warmth, physiotherapy and/or psychological support. Following a soft-tissue injury, rest, ice, compression and elevation (RICE) are recommended to reduce swelling and inflammation. Subsequent treatment may include the application of warmth, which aims to improve circulation of the affected area.

Transcutaneous electrical nerve stimulation

Current is applied to the painful area via two electrodes placed approximately 2 cm apart, until paraesthesia is experienced. Aβ-fibres are stimulated, closing the gating mechanism in the spinal cord and therefore inhibiting the transmission of A- and C-fibres. The release of endogenous opioids may also be stimulated. TENS machines are battery operated and portable, although not suitable for use while driving. They are used for chronic, postoperative and labour pain but their effectiveness remains to be fully established. Acupuncture is thought to work by a similar mechanism.

Physiotherapy

Physiotherapy may also include the use of warmth or electric currents. This physical technique also encompasses massage, exercises, infrared and ultraviolet rays, and manipulation of the affected joints or muscles.

Psychological support

Depression, insomnia, anxiety, fear, anger, boredom and social isolation all reduce the pain threshold. Conversely, sleep, rest, antidepressants, sympathy, diversion and understanding all raise the pain threshold. Consideration of psychological and lifestyle factors is an important part of pain management.

Specific conditions

The choice of analgesic is determined according to the cause and nature of the pain. The following section deals with specific conditions associated with pain.

Fever

Paracetamol is used first line due to its tolerability. Alternatively, ibuprofen may be used for pyrexia and is often added to paracetamol treatment when pyrexia is difficult to control.

Headache

Treatment should follow the analgesic ladder, with paracetamol being a suitable first-line choice. Diagnosis may include tension, cluster headaches, raised intracranial pressure, chronic daily headache (CDH), arteritis in patients aged >60 years or sinusitis. For a discussion of signs and symptoms and appropriate referral, see Chapters 1 and 22.

Migraine

See Chapter 22.

Dysmenorrhoea

Dysmenorrhoea or painful periods may be relieved by oral contraceptives and may resolve following a pregnancy. First-line analgesia is paracetamol and/or NSAIDs. Treatment is started a few days before a period to improve pain control of severe dysmenorrhoea (see Chronic pain and central sensitization, above). More severe or secondary dysmenorrhoea, often associated with endometriosis, may also lead to vomiting and require treatment with an antiemetic.

Neuropathic pain

Neuropathic pain, including trigeminal neuralgia, postherpetic neuralgia and phantom limb pain, often responds poorly to conventional analgesics. Adjuvant analgesics such as TCAs or anticonvulsants are used. Methadone, tramadol and oxycodone are the most effective opioids and are administered after alternatives have failed. Nerve block or TENS and physiotherapy may be of benefit.

Amitriptyline is commonly the first-choice drug (unlicensed indication), at lower doses compared with those used for the treatment of depression, ranging from 10 mg to 25 mg at night and increasing to a maximum dose of

75 mg if required. Doses rarely need to exceed 75 mg daily and an effect should be observed in 3–7 days. Once again, the sedating properties of amitriptyline would be beneficial if sleep is disturbed. In the absence of a response, other TCAs such as clomipramine or maprotiline may be used. Gabapentin and topical capsaicin are also licensed for neuropathic pain and specialists may prescribe sodium valproate, phenytoin, ketamine or lidocaine. Corticosteroids may help pain associated with compression neuropathy.

Trigeminal neuralgia

Again, only a partial response is observed after treatment with opioids. Carbamazepine is used in acute trigeminal neuralgia and in extreme cases surgery may be required. Plasma levels of carbamazepine should be monitored at higher doses. Alternatives include oxcarbazepine, gabapentin, lamotrigine or phenytoin.

Postherpetic neuralgia

This results from acute herpes zoster (shingles) and is treated with amitriptyline or gabapentin (see Chapter 34). Capsaicin or topical local anaesthetic may be used.

Concurrent disease

The following section summarizes the effect of concurrent disease on the prescribing of analgesics.

Gastrointestinal irritation and ulceration

See Chapter 7.

Cardiovascular disease

As discussed in Chapter 14, low-dose aspirin has a major role in the prevention of myocardial infarction and stroke. However, other COX inhibitors may not be used in place of aspirin for this role. Furthermore, the long-term use of high doses of certain NSAIDs (including ibuprofen and diclofenac, but not naproxen) have been associated with an increased risk of cardiovascular disease and caution should be exercised in patients at risk.

Table 29.2 summarizes these and other considerations, including hypersensitivity reactions to NSAIDs. It should be noted that the cautions highlighted for opioids become less important in palliative care.

Table 29.2   Effects of concurrent conditions on drug choice

Condition	Drug implicated	Comments
Chronic heart failure	NSAIDs, including COX-2 inhibitors	• May cause worsening CHF and fluid overload, due to sodium and water retention (Chapter 15) • An alternative such as paracetamol should be used if possible
Hypertension, oedema, renal failure, ischaemic heart disease and chronic heart failure	Effervescent preparations	• The sodium salt content of six effervescent co-codamol tablets is approximately equal to the recommended daily maximum intake of 6g (2.4 g sodium). These preparations should be avoided, particularly by patients with renal failure or taking diuretics, as increased sodium intake may reduce the efficacy of these drugs • COX-2 inhibitors should not be used with low-dose aspirin, as any benefit of the former will be reduced • The combination of an NSAID and low-dose aspirin should be avoided if possible due to the increased risk of gastrointestinal toxicity

Continued

Table 29.2 (Continued)

Condition	Drug implicated	Comments
Hypotension	Opioids	• Worsening of hypotension
Asthma	NSAIDs (chronic paracetamol), opioids	• NSAIDs are contraindicated if there is a history of asthma, angio-oedema, urticaria or rhinitis induced by previous exposure (Chapter 21)
		• Preliminary evidence indicates that long-term, high-dose paracetamol use may worsen asthma (Shaheen *et al* 2000). However, Levy and Volans (2001) concluded that any deterioration of asthma was short-lived but that practitioners should be alert to the possibility of worsening asthma
		• Opioids should not be used during an acute asthma attack, due to the risk of respiratory depression
Colitis	NSAIDs	May cause or exacerbate inflammatory bowel disease
Female infertility	NSAIDs	Female fertility may be reduced by long-term treatment
Hepatic impairment	Paracetamol, opioids, NSAIDs	• Dose-related toxicity, therefore larger doses of paracetamol should be avoided
		• Avoid or reduce doses of opioids, due to the risk of precipitating coma
		• Risk of fluid retention with NSAIDs, and increased gastrointestinal bleeding (secondary to impaired clotting). Avoid in severe liver disease
Prostatic hypertrophy	Opioids, nefopam	• Increased risk of urinary retention
Renal impairment	NSAIDs (including topical preparations), opioids	• Use with caution, due to the risk of deterioration in renal function as a result of reduced renal perfusion, particularly in elderly patients and those with heart failure and cirrhosis. Additional risk factors include hypertension, diabetes and co-prescribing of drugs excreted renally, such as ACE inhibitors, digoxin and lithium
		• Use the lowest effective dose and monitor renal function (Chapter 2)
		• Avoid NSAIDs in moderate-to-severe renal failure
		• The effects of opioids may be increased and prolonged in moderate-to-severe renal failure, so they should be avoided or their doses reduced
Thyroid dysfunction	Opioids	Use with caution in hypothyroidism due to worsening of symptoms such as bradycardia and hypotension
Epilepsy	Tramadol, nefopam	• The CSM (CHM) recommends the avoidance of tramadol in patients with a history of epilepsy
		• Nefopam should not be used in patients with a history of convulsions

ACE, angiotensin-converting enzyme; CHF, chronic heart failure; CHM, Commission on Human Medicines; CSM, Committee on Safety of Medicines; COX-2, cyclo-oxygenase 2; NSAIDs, non-steroidal anti-inflammatory drugs.

Table 29.3 Some important interactions with analgesics

Interaction	Consequences	Comments
NSAIDs with ACE inhibitors	Reduced antihypertensive effect due to effects on renal prostaglandins. Increased risk of renal damage	Monitor blood pressure and renal function
NSAIDs (except aspirin) with lithium	Increased levels of lithium and possible intoxication	Avoid unless lithium levels are closely monitored and the dose adjusted as necessary
NSAIDs with warfarin	Risk of bleeding due to increased anticoagulant effects and/or stomach irritation	Normal doses of ibuprofen interact only rarely. Careful monitoring, particularly in elderly patients. Azapropazone is contraindicated
NSAIDs with alcohol	Possible increase in gastric irritation	
Paracetamol with warfarin	Paracetamol is the analgesic of choice for patients taking warfarin. However, long-term use of larger doses may increase the anticoagulant effect	
NSAIDs with alendronate	Risk of severe oesophagitis	Avoid concurrent use
NSAIDs with corticosteroids	Increased risk of gastrointestinal bleeding and ulceration	'Steroid-sparing effect' of indometacin and naproxen may allow dose reduction of corticosteroids
NSAIDs with SSRIs	Increased risk of gastrointestinal bleeding and ulceration	
NSAIDs with loop diuretics	Antihypertensive and diuretic effects reduced or abolished	Ibuprofen, meloxicam and ketoprofen may not interact but monitoring is advised with all NSAIDs. Increased doses of diuretics may be required
NSAIDs with ciclosporin	Renal function may be reduced by some NSAIDs, resulting in nephrotoxicity and/or increased ciclosporin levels	Renal function should be monitored. Low doses of diclofenac should be used when newly prescribed
NSAIDs with methotrexate	Excretion of methotrexate may be reduced	Dose of methotrexate should be monitored closely
Colestyramine with diclofenac, ibuprofen, meloxicam, naproxen, piroxicam	• Reduced absorption of diclofenac and ibuprofen • Delayed absorption of naproxen (limited importance) • Increased clearance of meloxicam and piroxicam	• Doses should be separated by at least 2 h • The separation of doses may reduce but not abolish the interaction involving piroxicam and meloxicam
Tramadol with SSRIs/TCAs	Small risk of serotonin syndrome	Monitor
Opioids with alcohol	Enhanced sedation	
Opioids with antibacterials	Rifampicin may reduce the plasma concentrations of methadone and possibly morphine	The dose of methadone or morphine may need to be increased
Opioids with antidepressants	The analgesic effects of morphine may be increased by clomipramine and possibly amitriptyline	This may be an advantageous interaction

Continued

Table 29.3   (Continued)

Interaction	Consequences	Comments
Opioids with antiepilepetic drugs	Enzyme inducers may reduce the concentration of methadone	The dose of methadone may need to be increased
Pethidine with cimetidine	Reduced elimination of pethidine	Proton pump inhibitors or ranitidine are not known to interact
Morphine with metoclopramide	Increased absorption and enhanced effects of morphine	
Nefopam with anticonvulsants, TCAs and MAOIs	Nefopam may cause convulsions in susceptible patients. TCAs may reduce seizure threshold	Nefopam should not be used in patients with a history of convulsions Nefopam may have sympathomimetic activity and should not be given with MAOIs
Pethidine with phenothiazines	Increased analgesia and side effects	This may be used to advantage

ACE, angiotensin-converting enzyme; MAOIs, monoamine oxidase inhibitors; NSAIDs, non-steroidal anti-inflammatory drugs; SSRIs, selective serotonin reuptake inhibitors; TCAs, tricyclic antidepressants.

Drug interactions

Table 29.3 highlights some important drug interactions involving analgesics.

Pregnancy and breast-feeding

If possible, as with all drugs, analgesics should be avoided in the first trimester. If required for headache, pyrexia, musculoskeletal or dental pain, paracetamol is used first line. The use of analgesics during pregnancy and breast-feeding is summarized in Tables 29.4 and 29.5.

OTC considerations

Many analgesic preparations are available over-the-counter and pharmacists are ideally placed to monitor pain control, identify drug interactions (see above) and refer conditions such as suspected rheumatoid arthritis for prompt assessment and prescription of higher doses of anti-inflammatory agents. Misuse and the risk of MOH may also be identified. The provision of lifestyle advice may benefit conditions such as gout, migraine and general painful conditions.

Simple analgesics such as ibuprofen and paracetamol are widely available from many outlets, including supermarkets. Accordingly, health professionals should always enquire about self-medication to ensure the correct use of medicines and avoidance of ADRs, e.g. worsening asthma associated with overuse of NSAIDs (and possibly paracetamol) or the risk of gastro-intestinal toxicity with chronic NSAID use.

Counselling

General counselling should encourage patients to take analgesics if they are in pain. This may sound obvious but many patients are reluctant to take these drugs due to extensive publicity about side effects. Conversely, patients who take chronic analgesia, including OTC preparations, require regular review of treatment and the underlying cause of their pain, e.g. chronic use of co-codamol preparations for headache may be investigated for analgesia-induced headache or migraine.

Elderly patients may often report 'aches and pains' deemed to be an inevitable consequence of old age. Chronic pain is common in elderly people and may coexist with depression. Health professionals have an important role in identifying these patients and advising on appropriate treatment to enable pain control. Education, reassurance, support and patient counselling are

Table 29.4 The use of analgesic drugs in pregnancy

Drug	Trimester of risk	Comment
Paracetamol		• Not known to be harmful • Used first-line, avoiding high doses and chronic use as a precaution
Aspirin	3	• May delay or prolong labour due to COX inhibition • Impaired platelet function and risk of haemorrhage
NSAIDs	3	• Ketorolac is contraindicated • Avoid during pregnancy unless benefit outweighs risk • If necessary, use lowest effective dose (usually ibuprofen first-line) and avoid high-potency NSAIDs such as indometacin • Use in late pregnancy associated with risk of closure of the fetal ductus arteriosus while *in utero* and possibly pulmonary hypertension of the newborn • Delayed onset and increased duration of labour • NSAID use has been associated with increased risk of miscarriage (Nielsen *et al* 2001) • Possible increased incidence and duration of bleeding in fetus and mother during delivery • No NSAID should be used after 32 weeks' gestation
Codeine, dihydrocodeine	3, particularly last few weeks	• Opioids may be used for moderate-to-severe pain • Long-term *in utero* exposure may result in neonatal withdrawal symptoms • Depression of neonatal respiration
Tramadol	Toxic in animal embryo studies	Manufacturer advises avoid in pregnancy

Information derived from the *British National Formulary* and *Therapeutics in Pregnancy and Lactation* by Lee *et al* (2000).
COX, cyclo-oxygenase; NSAIDs, non-steroidal anti-inflammatory drugs.

Table 29.5 Analgesic use during lactation

Drug	Comment
Paracetamol, codeine	Small quantities excreted into breast milk but they appear to be safe. Paracetamol is used first line. Codeine may cause constipation in the mother or baby and colic in the baby
NSAIDs (ibuprofen, naproxen, diclofenac)	Excreted into breast milk in small quantities but appear to be safe
Aspirin	Avoid, due to risk of Reye's syndrome

Information derived from the *British National Formulary* and *Therapeutics in Pregnancy and Lactation* by Lee *et al* (2000).
NSAIDs, non-steroidal anti-inflammatory drugs.

particularly important in achieving good pain control. A pain diary outlining the influence of activity and analgesics may be useful in attaining good pain control. Pharmacists or carers may prepare monitored dosage systems as a memory aid for taking medication. These usually include four compartments per day so that all tablets are taken at the appropriate times.

Drug-specific counselling points are detailed below.

Paracetamol

- Paracetamol is one of the safest drugs at normal doses.
- Liver damage may occur after exceeding recommended doses and may take a few days or more to develop – help should be sought immediately.
- Take care not to exceed the maximum recommended dose by combining with other paracetamol-containing products such as OTC preparations for colds.
- Do not take more than two 500 mg tablets at a time.
- 4–6 h should be left between doses.
- Do not take more than eight 500 mg tablets in 24 h.

NSAIDs

- Patients should report symptoms of indigestion, wheezing or rashes immediately.
- NSAIDs are best taken with or after food and not on an empty stomach.
- Diclofenac and indometacin have a tendency to cause dizziness and patients should be warned that caution is advised when driving.
- Enteric-coated and slow-release preparations should be swallowed whole and not chewed.
- Enteric-coated tablets should not be taken at the same time of day as indigestion preparations.

Tiaprofenic acid
Report urinary symptoms, including increased frequency, nocturia, urgency, pain on urinating or blood in the urine, and stop taking medication immediately.

Indometacin
There is a high incidence of side effects with indometacin, including headache, dizziness and gastrointestinal disturbance.

Topical NSAIDs
- Avoid contact with the eyes, mucous membranes, or inflamed or broken skin.
- Discontinue taking if a rash develops.
- Wash hands immediately after application.
- Do not use with occlusive dressings.
- Avoid excess exposure of the treated area to sunlight as photosensitivity may increase.
- As absorption occurs, the same precautions with hypersensitivity to oral preparations should be observed, particularly when applying large amounts of topical NSAIDs.

Nefopam

- Urine may appear pink.
- Side effects include nervousness, palpitations, dry mouth, blurred vision and other sympathomimetic or antimuscarinic effects.

Gabapentin (see Chapter 23)

- Do not stop taking this medicine without the doctor's advice. Withdrawal should be gradual, over at least 1 week.
- Do not take indigestion remedies at the same time of day as this medicine.

Phenytoin and carbamazepine

See Chapter 23.

Opioids

- Opioids may cause drowsiness, so caution is needed when driving or operating machinery.
- Patients should avoid alcohol.
- Opioids may cause constipation. Laxatives are required with long-term treatment, preferably softeners and stimulants rather than bulk-forming agents.
- They may cause tolerance, requiring increasing doses during chronic treatment.
- Patients should avoid taking opioids regularly unless advised by a doctor or pharmacist, due to the risk of side effects, tolerance and dependence.

Self-assessment

Consider whether the following statements are true or false. In the management of pain:

1. Aspirin is the preferred NSAID.

2. Paracetamol is an effective analgesic but is not an NSAID.
3. Opioids are likely to cause constipation.
4. Amitriptyline is contraindicated in neuropathic pain.
5. Carbamazepine is used for acute pain.

Practice points

General

- Try paracetamol or ibuprofen first for mild-to-moderate pain. Patient counselling regarding the correct dose and effectiveness of paracetamol may help compliance.
- Analgesic combination products are not recommended because these products prevent the titration of individual drug doses. In addition, many combination products containing milder opioids with paracetamol or aspirin are no more effective than either drug alone when given as a single dose. Combination products may, however, be appropriate for the treatment of chronic pain and/or for patients with compliance problems.
- Chronic pain management should be managed 'by the mouth, by the clock and by the ladder', according to World Health Organization (1996) guidelines.

NSAIDs

- The use of two or more NSAIDs is not recommended and this includes low-dose aspirin. Low-dose aspirin should be combined with another NSAID only if absolutely necessary. Gastrointestinal protection with a proton pump inhibitor should be considered, particularly for elderly patients and when prescribing NSAIDs long term.
- Any benefits of COX-2 inhibitors are negated in combination with other NSAIDs, including low-dose aspirin.
- Allow up to a week to achieve the full analgesic effect of NSAIDs. The full anti-inflammatory effect may take up to 3 weeks at full doses.
- Aspirin should not be prescribed for children <16 years due to the risk of Reye's syndrome.
- The use of NSAIDs to treat postoperative pain may reduce the requirement for high doses of opioid analgesics.

Opioids

- Avoid regular use of opioids due to tolerance, dependence, constipation and the risk of falls in elderly people. For severe pain, however, there is little risk of psychological dependence and the use of strong opioids is indicated (see Chapter 31).
- Regular opioid treatment should be accompanied by laxatives.

 CASE STUDIES

Case 1

A patient complains that he is not having much pain relief with the co-codamol that you dispensed for him a week earlier for his osteoarthritis. He has been taking two tablets in the morning, because he doesn't like to take too many. He has not tried paracetamol as he says 'it's not strong enough for this condition'.

continued

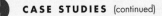

- A common misconception exists that paracetamol is effective to treat a headache or fever but little else. In fact, patients can be reassured that paracetamol is an extremely effective analgesic and relatively free from side effects. This is a suitable first choice in osteoarthritis and should be tried for at least a week of regular dosing. As this patient has not been taking regular co-codamol, it may be appropriate to try paracetamol 1 g four times a day alone for at least a week. He should be advised that he may need to take them regularly to control the pain.

Case 2
While performing a medication review, you come across the following record for an 80-year-old hypertensive female patient with 'painful knees':

dosulepin 75 mg twice daily
co-codamol 8/500 mg two up to four times daily
bendroflumethiazide 5 mg once daily.

How do you respond?

- The first consideration relates to the high risk of constipation with all three drugs. It is very likely that this patient will require treatment with laxatives such as a combination of lactulose solution (up to 15 mL twice daily) and senna tablets (1–2 at night as required). The dose of bendroflume-thiazide is high for hypertension and may increase dehydration and subsequent electrolyte disturbances without a further reduction in blood pressure. Perhaps the addition of an alterna-tive antihypertensive could be considered? The TCA may not be appropriate for this age group and a selective serotonin reuptake inhibitor (SSRI) may be more appropriate (see Chapter 24). Successful treatment of her depression is an important component of her pain management.

Her analgesia should be reviewed, e.g. has she tried paracetamol alone at adequate doses?

Case 3
The following repeat prescription is for a 46-year-old woman:

diclofenac gel 1.16% apply three times daily 100 g
diclofenac sodium enteric-coated tablets 50 mg, take one three times daily
fluoxetine 20 mg capsules take one every morning

What should be the course of action?

- This patient is at risk of gastrotoxicity from the above prescription. SSRIs are associated with increased risk of bleeding events and using two NSAID preparations further increases this risk.
- The nature of her pain should be determined and pain control reviewed. Has paracetamol and/or ibuprofen been used? A proton pump inhibitor should be considered if the diclofenac and fluoxetine are continued. Review the need for both diclofenac tablets and gel due to increased risk of side effects. Check for a history of peptic ulcer disease. Question the patient about signs and symptoms such as dyspepsia, gastric pain, dark stools and symptoms of anaemia.

References

Anon (2000). The use of oral analgesics in primary care. *MeReC Bull* **11**: 1–4.

Chandraeskharen NV, Dai H, Roos KLT *et al* (2002). COX-3, cyclo-oxygenase variant inhibited by acetaminophen and other analgesic/antipyretic drugs: cloning, structure and expression. *Proc Natl Acad Sci USA* **99**: 13926–31.

Committee on Safety of Medicines/Medicines Control Agency (1996). In focus . . . tramadol (Zydol®, Tramake® and Zamadol®). *Curr Probl Pharmacovigilance* **22**: 11.

Deeks JJ, Smith LA, Bradley MD (2002). Efficacy, tolerability, and upper gastrointestinal safety of celecoxib for treatment of osteoarthritis and rheumatoid arthritis: systematic review of randomised controlled trials. *BMJ* **325**: 619–23.

Jüni P, Rutjes AWS, Dieppe PA (2002). Are selective COX 2 inhibitors superior to traditional non steroidal anti-inflammatory drugs? *BMJ* **324**: 1287–8.

Lee A, Inch S, Finnigan D (2000). *Therapeutics in Pregnancy and Lactation*. Oxford: Radcliffe Medical Press.

Levy S, Volans G (2001). The use of analgesics in patients with asthma. *Drug Safety* **24**: 829–41.

Limmroth V, Katsarava Z, Fritsche G *et al* (2002). Features of medication overuse headache following overuse of different headache drugs. *Neurology* **59**: 1011–14.

Martin J, ed. *British National Formulary*, latest edition. London: British Medical Association and Royal Pharmaceutical Society of Great Britain.

Nielsen GL, Sorensen HT, Larsen H *et al* (2001). Risk of adverse birth outcome and miscarriage in pregnant users of non-steroidal anti-inflammatory drugs: population based observational study and case–control study. *BMJ* **322**: 266–70.

Shaheen SO, Sterne JAC, Songhurst CE *et al* (2000). Frequent paracetamol use and asthma in adults. *Thorax* **55**: 266–70.

Silberstein SD, Young WB (1995). Analgesic rebound headache. How great is the problem and what can be done? *Drug Safety* **13**: 133–44.

World Health Organization (1996). *Cancer Pain Relief, With A Guide To Opioid Availability*, 2nd edn. Geneva: WHO.

Further reading

Blenkinsopp J (2002). Over-the-counter analgesics and the treatment of pain. *Pharm J* **268**: 252–6.

Chapman V (2000). *Future Pain Drugs*. London: SMi.

Loeser JD, Melzack R (1999). Pain: an overview. *Lancet* **353**: 1607–9.

Rang HP, Dale M, Ritter JM *et al* (2003). *Pharmacology*, 5th edn. Edinburgh: Churchill Livingstone.

Silverstein FE, Faich G, Goldstein JL *et al* (2000). Gastrointestinal toxicity with celecoxib vs nonsteroidal anti-inflammatory drugs for osteoarthritis and rheumatoid arthritis: the CLASS study: a randomized controlled trial. Celecoxib Long-term Arthritis Safety Study. *JAMA* **284**: 1247–55.

Skelly MM, Hawkey CJ (2002). Potential alternatives to COX 2 inhibitors. *BMJ* **324**: 1289–90.

Van Walraven C, Mamdani MM, Wells PS *et al* (2001). Inhibition of serotonin reuptake by antidepressants and upper gastrointestinal bleeding in elderly patients: retrospective cohort study. *BMJ* **323**: 1–6.

30

Musculoskeletal pain

Disorders of the muscles, joints and bones are a common cause of chronic illness and inability to work and have a considerable impact on quality of life. Musculoskeletal conditions include rheumatoid arthritis (RA), osteoarthritis, gout, muscle cramps and osteoporosis.

Disease characteristics and clinical features

Arthritis

Arthritis, literally inflammation of the joints, includes osteo- or rheumatoid types.

Osteoarthritis

Osteoarthritis is the most common form and is a degenerative disease of the joints due to wearing of articular cartilage with subsequent changes in the underlying bone. This may be secondary to obesity, fractures, dislocation, sports injuries, hyperparathyroidism, haemophilia, RA, gout or Paget's disease.

The pain of osteoarthritis differs from RA in that it usually occurs after exercise and at night. Any stiffness occurring in the morning tends to be transient. The pain may be present at rest and there is often tenderness. Joints of the feet (particularly the big toe), knees, hips, and cervical and lumbar spine are often affected. Diagnosis is usually by X-ray of painful joints, revealing a narrowing of the joint space due to loss of cartilage and the presence of osteosclerosis (increased bone density), osteocytes and cysts in the bone. There are no systemic (extra-articular) features.

Rheumatoid arthritis

RA is a chronic inflammatory condition affecting the synovial lining of the joints. Disease progression leads to ligament damage and erosion of bone: joints become deformed and tendons may rupture. RA tends to follow a relapsing–remitting course and is progressive.

The assessment of presenting symptoms of pain (see Chapter 29) includes the location of affected joints and timing of the pain, which is often worse in the morning and persists for an hour or more. The principal features include inflammation and swelling predominantly affecting the hands, wrists and knees. Symptoms progress to muscle wasting due to joint disuse, joint deformity and joint erosion. Extra-articular symptoms may also be present and include the following (Greene and Harris 2008):

- Non-specific: tiredness, depression and fever.
- Dermatological: nodules, palmar erythema (red palms), sweaty palms.
- Circulatory: Raynaud's syndrome, pericarditis, myocarditis, vasculitis, anaemia.
- Ophthalmic: keratoconjunctivitis sicca (dryness of the cornea and conjunctiva due to reduced production of tears), episcleritis (inflammation of the episclera resulting in painful red eyes sensitive to light) or scleritis (inflammation of the white of the eye).
- Neurological: trapped nerves, peripheral neuropathy.
- Pulmonary: lung nodules, pleurisy and pulmonary fibrosis.

RA is an autoimmune disease with rheumatoid factors (autoantibodies against immunoglobulin G) detected in serum. Radiological changes are also observed. The erythrocyte sedimentation rate (ESR) is elevated (see Chapter 2).

Gout

Gout occurs due to the overproduction of purines, resulting in acute arthritis. The metabolism of purines leads to the production of uric acid, which forms urate crystals in joints, particularly affecting the big toe (podagra). This triggers an inflammatory response. Gout may also occur as an adverse drug reaction (ADR; see Chapter 5), particularly due to thiazides, which impair the excretion of uric acid. Disorders such as heart failure, hypercalcaemia and hypertensive nephropathy are also associated with gout.

Gout presents with inflammation and joint pain affecting the big toe and may also affect the ankles, knees, elbows, wrists and fingers. The skin of the affected joint may flake after the initial onset of pain. The attack may resolve spontaneously after a few days or weeks. Laboratory tests reveal hyperuricaemia, although this is occasionally present with arthritic conditions.

Osteoporosis

Osteoporosis is a disorder of bone structure with a characteristic reduction of bone mass resulting in brittle bones at increased risk of fracture. Bone is constantly being absorbed by osteoclasts and new bone is formed by osteoblasts. In osteoporosis, absorption exceeds formation, with reductions in bone matrix and therefore strength. Causes include oestrogen deficiency, particularly after an early menopause, and age-related degeneration of bone, declining from a peak in the 20s. There are hereditary and lifestyle components and the most common drug cause is corticosteroids.

Osteoporosis may be asymptomatic, being diagnosed after fracture. Patients presenting with a fracture resulting from minimal trauma, also known as 'low trauma' fracture, are treated for osteoporosis and further investigations may not be necessary, because management is the same. Bone-density scans (commonly dual-energy X-ray absorptiometry or DEXA scans) are useful for early diagnosis and are increasingly performed for patients with risk factors for osteoporosis as follows:

- early menopause (<45 years of age, also prolonged secondary amenorrhoea)
- aged >65 years
- family history of osteoporosis or low trauma fractures
- poor diet (lacking in calcium and vitamin D)
- low exposure to sunlight (reduced vitamin D)
- low body weight (body mass index or BMI <20)
- smoking
- excess alcohol intake
- low level of physical activity
- concurrent disease should be considered and treated (hyperthyroidism, hyperparathyroidism, osteomalacia or hypogonadism)
- drugs (corticosteroids: more than the equivalent of 7.5 mg of prednisolone daily for 3 months or more).

Pharmacological basis of management

The management of musculoskeletal conditions predominantly involves the relief of pain and the reduction of inflammation. In treating osteoporosis, lifestyle factors are also important and treatment may include the correction of calcium and vitamin D intake. Additional treatments target the mineralization of bone using bisphosphonates, anti-oestrogens and oestrogens. Bisphosphonates reduce bone turnover and oestrogens and anti-oestrogens target and reduce the resorption of bone.

The pharmacology of analgesics, including non-steroidal anti-inflammatory drugs (NSAIDs), cyclo-oxygenase-2 (COX-2) inhibitors and topical counterirritants, together with non-pharmacological options, is discussed in Chapter 29.

Osteoarthritis

Osteoarthritis involves joint degeneration and may be improved by lifestyle measures such as weight reduction and increased exercise. Paracetamol is used first line, particularly in elderly people, followed by topical then oral NSAIDs with or without paracetamol. Topical capsaicin may provide relief. Advanced osteoarthritis may require full doses of NSAIDs. It should be noted, however, that NSAIDs do not alter the disease process and are mainly used for their analgesic effects. The benefits of NSAIDs are therefore compared with the risks, such as gastrointestinal toxicity (see Chapter 7), and alternative interventions such as lifestyle measures may be preferred (see Chapter 29).

Rheumatoid arthritis

NSAIDs are used for symptomatic treatment of pain associated with inflammation in RA and corticosteroids are occasionally injected locally into the affected joints, providing temporary relief. Disease-modifying antirheumatoid drugs (DMARDs) such as penicillamine, gold salts or antimalarials are used to suppress the disease process. These drugs are given for 4–6 months before a full response is observed. This may allow a subsequent reduction in the dose of NSAID. Sulfasalazine or methotrexate may be tolerated better than alternative DMARDs.

Disease-modifying anti-rheumatoid drugs

NSAIDs control the symptoms associated with RA but do not alter the disease progression and may even make it worse due to the increased availability of arachidonic acid as a substrate for lipoxygenase-mediated production of leukotrienes. DMARDs are therefore used to slow disease progression and include:

- gold compounds
- penicillamine
- sulfasalazine
- methotrexate
- chloroquine
- hydroxychloroquine.

Their mechanisms of action are complex and are yet to be fully elucidated. Immunosuppressants such as azathioprine, ciclosporin and corticosteroids are also used as DMARDs.

Corticosteroids

These drugs are used in the treatment of RA, e.g. when treatment with other anti-inflammatory drugs is unsuccessful. If long-term treatment is required, prophylaxis for the prevention of osteoporosis is required (see below). Courses of corticosteroids should use the lowest effective dose, e.g. 7.5 mg prednisolone. This is sufficient to reduce the rate of joint destruction in patients with moderate-to-severe disease that has been present for <2 years. Prednisolone treatment is required for 2–4 years for beneficial effects on joint destruction, before gradual dose reduction to prevent long-term adverse effects. It should also be noted that the effects of reduced joint destruction persist despite a possible reduction in symptom control, which may occur after 6–12 months, and this does not necessarily indicate a higher dose of prednisolone.

Etanercept, adalimumab and infliximab

These are new immunomodulatory drugs, which have been introduced for severe refractory disease that has not responded to at least two other DMARDs, including methotrexate, and their use is restricted to rheumatologists. Etanercept is a fusion protein which binds to tumour necrosis factor α (TNF-α) and leads to its inactivation. Infliximab and adalimumab are monoclonal antibodies to TNF-α and so reduce its action in inflammation. These agents may be used alongside methotrexate or, in the case of entanercept and adalimumab, as monotherapy.

Osteoporosis

Agents used for the prevention or treatment of osteoporosis include bisphosphonates, vitamin D derivatives, hormone replacement therapy (HRT), calcitonin and selective oestrogen receptor modulators (SERMs). It is also important that concurrent medication and other risk factors for falls are assessed in these patients and that preventive counselling includes advice about diet and exercise (see Counselling, below), e.g. concurrent diseases that may increase the risk of falls include hypothyroidism, epilepsy, diabetes mellitus, Ménière's disease and cardiovascular disease (particularly with a history of transient ischaemic attacks or arrhythmias). Drugs associated with an increased risk of falls, particularly in elderly patients, include:

- diuretics
- other antihypertensives, particularly α-blockers, and the concurrent use of angiotensin-converting enzyme (ACE) inhibitors with diuretics
- antipsychotics
- benzodiazepines, sedating antihistamines and other drugs with sedative properties (see Chapter 5)
- alcohol.

Bisphosphonates (alendronate, etidronate, risedronate)

Bisphosphonates are now considered a first line for osteoporosis. They reduce the risk of vertebral fracture (alendronate and risedronate have been shown to reduce the risk of non-vertebral fractures) by reducing the turnover of bone. These drugs are enzyme-resistant analogues of pyrophosphate and, by binding to hydroxyapatite crystals, slow dissolution. They also inhibit osteoblast-mediated resorption.

Vitamin D and its derivatives

Vitamin D and derivatives, together with parathyroid hormone, cytokines and calcitonin, are involved in the metabolism and mineralization of bone. Vitamin D requirements are met through diet, metabolism in the liver and kidney, and from reactions in the skin occurring in the presence of sunlight. The supplementation of vitamin D is partly dependent on the cause of deficiency, as follows:

1. Poor diet or malabsorption is treated with supplements of vitamin D_2 (ergocalciferol), which is formed in plants, or vitamin D_3 (colecalciferol), formed in the skin in the presence of ultraviolet radiation. High doses (up to 1 mg or 40 000 units daily) of ergocalciferol are required by patients with intestinal malabsorption or chronic liver disease.

2. In renal failure, 1,25-dihydroxyvitamin D_3 (calcitriol) or 1α-hydroxycholecalciferol (alfacalcidol) is given. Deficiency would otherwise result because these hydroxylated compounds are usually formed in the kidney.

Hormone replacement therapy

Both HRT and bisphosphonates are indicated for the treatment of osteoporosis. Oestrogens have a protective effect on bone by preventing bone resorption. Postmenopausal women may benefit from HRT prophylaxis for osteoporosis, particularly after an early menopause. However, their use is limited due to increased cardiovascular risk (notably stroke) and certain cancers when used long term.

Tibolone

Tibolone possesses mixed oestrogenic, progestogenic and androgenic effects, and is used for the prevention of hot flushes and bone loss. This is given for only at least 1 year after the menopause because of problems with irregular bleeding. If the patient is to be changed from cyclical HRT, a withdrawal bleed is induced using progestogens, given until the withdrawal bleed has stopped. This minimizes the risk of irregular bleeding during tibolone therapy.

Calcitonin

Calcitonin may be a useful alternative for the prophylaxis or treatment of postmenopausal osteoporosis when HRT and bisphosphonates are not appropriate. After a vertebral fracture, breakthrough pain resistant to analgesics may respond to calcitonin, given for up to 3 months. Calcitonin is a hormone secreted by the thyroid gland. It acts to inhibit calcium resorption into bone and reduces reabsorption of calcium and phosphate in the kidney. An increased plasma calcium level stimulates endogenous calcitonin secretion.

Raloxifene

Raloxifene is an SERM used to treat osteoporosis. This is an analogue of tamoxifen, developed after the observation that, despite possessing anti-oestrogen activity, tamoxifen produces agonist-like oestrogenic activity in bone, because it is a partial agonist.

Prevention of osteoporosis

The first step in the prevention of osteoporosis is to identify patients who are at risk, as outlined above. Interventions such as lifestyle changes may then be addressed and the need for drug treatment considered, e.g. calcium and vitamin D intake is corrected by supplementation and HRT initiated for female patients particularly after premature menopause. Treatment is continued for up to 5 years. This is a highly effective intervention for the prevention or treatment of osteoporosis. It should also be noted when prescribing HRT that:

- women with an intact uterus should be given HRT containing a progestogen to reduce the risk of endometrial cancer
- after a hysterectomy, a progestogen is not required
- oestrogens are contraindicated for patients with previous oestrogen-receptor-positive breast cancer.

When bisphosphonates are not appropriate (Table 30.1), HRT may be prescribed. It should be noted that disodium etidronate administration is alternated with calcium carbonate (Didronel PMO) because it can increase the risk of fractures due to reduced calcification of bone. Raloxifene is licensed for prophylaxis of postmenopausal osteoporosis. Further lifestyle interventions are outlined below (see Counselling).

Table 30.1   Some considerations of the effects of concurrent conditions on drug choice in musculoskeletal conditions

Disease	Drug(s)	Comments
IHD	Colchicine, sulfinpyrazone, HRT	• Sulfinpyrazone may cause salt and water retention and should therefore be used with caution • The CSM/CHM warns that HRT is not indicated for the prevention of IHD (Chapter 14)
Upper gastrointestinal disorders: dysphagia, oesophagitis, gastritis, duodenitis or ulcers	Alendronic acid and risedronate sodium	May cause or exacerbate these disorders (Chapter 7)
Delayed gastric emptying	Alendronic acid and risedronate sodium	Contraindicated
Peptic ulcer disease	Sulfinpyrazone	Use with caution
Gastrointestinal disease	Colchicine	Use with caution since colchicine may exacerbate all gastrointestinal disease
Hypocalcaemia	Alendronic acid, risedronate sodium	Contraindicated
VTE	HRT, raloxifene	• HRT is contraindicated in patients with a history of confirmed VTE, active or recent arterial thromboembolic disease • Raloxifene also increases the risk of thromboembolism

CHM, Commission on Human Medicines; CSM, Committee on Safety of Medicines; HRT, hormone replacement therapy; IHD, ischaemic heart disease; MCA, Medicines Control Agency; VTE, venous thromboembolism.

Prevention of corticosteroid-induced osteoporosis

It is recognized that treatment with corticosteroids equivalent to more than 7.5 mg prednisolone daily for 3 months or more constitutes a risk factor for the development of osteoporosis. Such patients may benefit from a DEXA scan and may require treatment as indicated above, particularly in the presence of additional risk factors. Drugs with the best evidence to support their use for preventing corticosteroid-induced osteoporosis appear to be the bisphosphonates (Adachi and Papaioannou 2001). The American College of Rheumatism (Buckley *et al* 2001) recommendations include the use of calcium and vitamin D supplements for all patients taking corticosteroids.

Current recommendations by the British Society for Rheumatology (see Online resources, below) are that patients prescribed a 3-month course (or longer) of the equivalent of 7.5 mg prednisolone daily should be offered treatment for the prevention of osteoporosis after the results of a DEXA scan. It is suggested that a DEXA scan revealing a *T*-score (number of standard deviations from the value of peak bone density of a 25- to 30-year-old woman) of –1.5 or less would indicate preventive treatment.

Gout

The treatment of gout involves the use of NSAIDs, with the exception of aspirin, which reduces urate excretion and ibuprofen due to its weak anti-inflammatory activity. Additional treatment may include allopurinol, colchicine, sulfinpyrazone and probenecid.

Acute gout

Acute gout is treated with high doses of NSAIDs including diclofenac, indometacin, ketoprofen, naproxen, piroxicam and sulindac. Allopurinol should not be initiated during or within 1 month of an acute attack because it may prolong the attack. The manufacturers recommend that prophylaxis with an NSAID or colchicine be given for the first month of treatment because allopurinol may precipitate a further attack. Patients already taking allopurinol when suffering an exacerbation should continue treatment.

Weight loss and dietary measures are also important (see Counselling below).

Chronic gout

The long-term management of gout includes prophylaxis with allopurinol or colchicine (short term only during initial treatment with allopurinol) and the reduction of inflammation by NSAIDs during an acute exacerbation.

Allopurinol

Allopurinol is a xanthine oxidase inhibitor and reduces the synthesis of uric acid.

Colchicine

The mechanism of action of colchicine in the treatment of gout involves inhibition of leukocyte migration into the joint by reducing the production of chemotaxins.

Sulfinpyrazone and probenecid

Sulfinpyrazone and probenecid inhibit uric acid reabsorption by the kidneys, thereby increasing excretion.

Nocturnal leg cramps

Quinine salts are used for nocturnal leg cramps but are effective only in a small proportion of patients, e.g. quinine sulphate or quinine bisulphate is given. It should be noted that quinine disulphate 300 mg contains less quinine than 300 mg quinine sulphate.

Concurrent disease

Some considerations are summarized in Table 30.1.

Drug interactions

Table 30.2 highlights some important drug interactions involving drugs used to treat musculoskeletal disorders. For interactions associated with NSAIDs, see Chapter 29.

Table 30.2   Some drug interactions involving drugs used in musculoskeletal conditions

Drugs	Consequences	Comments
Alendronate with antacids and calcium supplements	Reduced absorption	Separate the administration of alendronate from calcium supplements and antacids by at least 30 min
Penicillamine with aluminium or magnesium-containing antacids and iron salts		• Separate the administration of penicillamine by 2 h • Caution if iron is withdrawn when patients are stabilized on penicillamine, due to risk of toxicity
Allopurinol with theophylline	Increased levels of theophylline	There is limited evidence for this interaction but monitoring for signs of theophylline toxicity is recommended
Alendronate with NSAIDs	Risk of severe oesophagitis	Avoid concurrent use
Allopurinol with warfarin	Increased bleeding	This interaction is reported to be uncommon but monitoring is prudent
Calcium and vitamin D supplements or corticosteroids with thiazide diuretics	Increased risk of hypercalcaemia or hypokalaemia	• Thiazides retain calcium and therefore monitoring of plasma calcium may be required (Chapter 2) • Increased risk of hypokalaemia if thiazides are given with corticosteroids (Chapter 2)
Quinine with digoxin	Small risk of increased levels of digoxin	Monitor for signs of digoxin toxicity
Methotrexate with NSAIDs	Reduced excretion and therefore increased risk of methotrexate toxicity	• Increased risk with higher doses of methotrexate and/or impaired renal function • Careful monitoring is recommended
Methotrexate with corticosteroids	• Increased risk of methotrexate toxicity • Possible steroid-sparing effect	Monitor for signs of methotrexate toxicity or reduced efficacy of corticosteroids
Methotrexate with co-trimoxazole or trimethoprim	Risk of severe bone marrow depression	Avoid concurrent use or monitor full blood count closely
Penicillamine with digoxin	Limited reports of reduced levels of digoxin	Monitor for signs of reduced efficacy (Chapter 15)

NSAIDs, non-steroidal anti-inflammatory drugs.

Monitoring requirements

More detailed monitoring information is produced by the British Society for Rheumatology (see Online resources below).

Penicillamine

A full blood count (FBC) and urine (protein) should be monitored before the start of treatment, every 1–2 weeks for 2 months, every 4 weeks, and the week after a dose increase. In the presence of proteinuria, urea and electrolytes and 24-h urine are tested (see Chapter 2).

Sulfasalazine

• Monitor differential white cell, red cell and platelet counts initially and at monthly intervals for the first 3 months.

- Liver function tests (LFTs) should be monitored monthly for the first 3 months.
- Renal function should be monitored at regular intervals.

Methotrexate (advice of Committee on Safety of Medicines)

- Carry out an FBC, renal function tests and LFTs before starting treatment and repeat weekly until therapy is stabilized, then every 2–3 months. See also Counselling below.
- Treatment should not be started or should be discontinued if any abnormality of LFTs or liver biopsy is present or develops during treatment. Abnormalities return to normal after 2 weeks and treatment may be restarted if appropriate.
- Risk factors for haematopoietic suppression include advanced age, renal impairment and concomitant treatment with a second antifolate drug.

Gold

- Urine tests and FBCs (including total and differential white cell and platelet counts) should be performed before treatment is started and before each intramuscular injection.
- During oral treatment, urine and blood tests are carried out monthly.
- The occurrence of blood disorders or proteinuria (repeatedly >300 mg/L and without urinary tract infection) necessitates withdrawal of treatment.

Antimalarials

- Measure renal and liver function before starting treatment.
- Monitor visual changes.

Corticosteroids

Monitoring during treatment with corticosteroids may include blood pressure, urinary glucose, weight gain, bone density, visual changes and lung function.

Sulfinpyrazone

Regular blood counts are recommended.

Etanercept, adalimumab and infliximab

Patients should be tested for tuberculosis before treatment.

Vitamin D supplements (e.g. ergocalciferol, calcitriol)

All patients receiving vitamin D supplements for the prevention and treatment of osteoporosis should have their plasma calcium levels monitored weekly when treatment is initiated, and then at regular intervals and when presenting with nausea and vomiting, which may suggest hypercalcaemia. Breast milk from mothers taking vitamin D supplements may also cause hypercalcaemia in the infant.

Disodium etidronate

Serum phosphate and alkaline phosphatase (and urinary hydroxyproline) should be measured before starting treatment and then every 3 months.

Alendronic acid and risedronate sodium

Hypocalcaemia and vitamin D deficiency should be corrected before initiating treatment.

Renal function

The following points are intended to highlight drugs to be used with caution in renal impairment:

- Allopurinol: dose adjustment is required in moderate-to-severe renal failure. There may be increased toxicity and rashes.
- Methotrexate: dose adjustment is required.
- Penicillamine is nephrotoxic and should be avoided if possible, or the dose reduced.
- Sulfasalazine should be avoided in severe renal failure. In moderate failure, there is an increased risk of toxicity, including crystalluria. A high fluid intake is therefore required.
- Antimalarials: use with caution.

- Alendronic acid or risedronate sodium is not recommended if creatinine clearance is <35 or 30 mL/min, respectively.
- Disodium etidronate should be avoided in moderate-to-severe renal impairment or administered at a reduced dosage in mild impairment.

Hepatic function

The following points are intended to highlight drugs to be used with caution in hepatic disease:

- Methotrexate: dose-related toxicity, avoid in non-malignant conditions.
- Allopurinol: reduce dose.
- Gold: avoid in severe liver disease.
- Antimalarials: use with caution.

Pregnancy

Table 30.3 summarizes examples of issues associated with drug use for musculoskeletal conditions during pregnancy. For information about NSAIDs, the reader is referred to Chapter 29.

Over-the-counter considerations

The availability of analgesic preparations over-the-counter is discussed in Chapter 29. In relation to musculoskeletal disorders, pharmacists are ideally placed to refer conditions such as suspected RA for prompt assessment and prescribing of higher doses of anti-inflammatory agents and/or DMARDs. The provision of lifestyle advice may benefit conditions such as gout, migraine and general painful conditions. Pharmacists may also provide a screening service for osteoporosis as part of the multidisciplinary healthcare team.

Although widely used by patients with osteoarthritis, the supplements chondroitin and glucosamine are not recommended by the National Institute for Health and Clinical Excellence guidelines (NICE 2008).

Counselling

Patient counselling should comprise a combination of lifestyle factors, including advice about diet and exercise, together with information relating to drug treatment. Careful exercise is important to improve joint mobility, muscle strength, aerobic fitness and function, with the aim of promoting both physical and psychological health without worsening any fatigue or joint symptoms. This is also important in elderly people to prevent falls.

Osteoporosis

- Patients with risk factors for developing osteoporosis should maintain a high intake of

---

Table 30.3 Some considerations of drug use in pregnancy

Drug	Trimester of risk	Comment
DMARDs	3	Sulfasalazine is the DMARD of choice in pregnancy
Bisphosphonates	All	Contraindicated
Colchicine	All	Contraindicated
Corticosteroids		• Assess risk of not treating. Commonly used in asthma and inflammatory bowel disease during pregnancy
		• Risk of neonatal adrenal suppression with long-term high-dose treatment
Antimalarials	All	Hydroxychloroquine and chloroquine (except in malaria prophylaxis) should be avoided in pregnancy and breast-feeding

DMARDs, disease-modifying antirheumatic drugs.

calcium and vitamin D (milk, Cheddar cheese, Edam, yogurt, canned sardines and whitebait), e.g. half a litre (1 pint) of semi-skimmed milk or 100 g (4 oz) of Cheddar cheese contains 700–800 mg calcium. Supplements of calcium should be considered when a risk of deficiency is recognized, such as in strict vegetarians. Vitamin D should be included for the housebound and others with low exposure to sunlight.

- Recommended intakes of calcium and vitamin D are as follows:
  - calcium:
    males 11–18: 1000 mg daily
    females 11–18: 800 mg daily
    adults 19+ years: 700 mg daily
  - vitamin D: 400 IU daily.
- Weight-bearing exercise should be emphasized, particularly to women in their 20s, and immobility should be avoided. Exercise programmes are useful for patients with osteoporosis in building muscle strength, general wellbeing and improving posture, thereby reducing the risk of further fractures.
- Patients should stop smoking and avoid excess alcohol intake.
- Excess dieting and vigorous exercise routines, which result in amenorrhoea, should also be avoided by women of all ages.
- Hip protectors may help prevent hip fractures in elderly patients.

Bisphosphonates

- Bisphosphonates may cause gastrointestinal disturbance, oesophagitis (particularly alendronic acid) and occasionally bone pain.
- Premenopausal women initiated on bisphosphonates should be counselled about the appropriate use of contraception.

Alendronic acid

- Alendronic acid may be administered as a weekly dose.
- Patients should stop taking alendronate if they develop symptoms of oesophageal ulceration, e.g. dysphagia, dyspepsia, pain on swallowing or retrosternal pain.

- Tablets should be swallowed whole with a tumbler full of water while standing and not immediately before rising or retiring to bed.
- Tablets should be taken 30 min before breakfast (and other medication) and patients advised to remain standing or to sit upright for at least 30 min. Patients should not lie down until after breakfast.

Risedronate

- Food, particularly calcium-containing food (milk), iron and mineral supplements and antacids should be avoided for at least 2 h before and after tablets are taken.
- Tablets are usually taken 30 min before breakfast (and other medication).
- Patient should remain standing or sit upright for at least 30 min. Patients should not take the tablets before rising or at bedtime.

Disodium etidronate

Should be avoided for at least 2 h before and after tablets are taken.

Vitamin D

Excess intake may lead to hypercalcaemia, including symptoms of constipation, depression, nausea and vomiting, polyuria and polydipsia, weakness and fatigue. These symptoms should be reported to the prescriber.

NSAIDs

See Chapter 29.

Topical counterirritants (capsaicin)

See Chapter 29.

Quinine salts for nocturnal leg cramps

- Stretching the affected muscle regularly may reduce leg cramps.
- Take quinine salts for up to 4 weeks before improvement is observed.
- Reassess every 3 months.

- Caution is required because quinine is extremely toxic and has caused fatalities in children.

Allopurinol

- The affected joint should be rested.
- Avoid purine-rich food, including offal, anchovies, sardines, herring, mackerel, shrimps, crab, fish roes and meat extract.
- Reduce intake of protein.
- Maintain an adequate fluid intake of 2–3 L/day. This reduces plasma urate levels and prevents the formation of renal urate stones.
- Try to limit alcohol intake to 1 unit/day. Alcohol reduces the solubility of urate and beer contains high levels of purines.
- Gradual weight loss may improve symptoms. Avoid overeating.
- Take with or after food with plenty of water.
- Do not stop taking allopurinol unless advised by the prescriber.

Colchicine

- Dietary advice is as for allopurinol.
- Take until either pain is relieved or vomiting and diarrhoea occur, or a maximum dose of 6 mg has been reached (12 tablets of 500 micrograms).

Sulfinpyrazone

- Maintain an adequate fluid intake of 2–3 L/day.
- Take with or after food.
- Do not take with aspirin.

Penicillamine

- Penicillamine may cause nausea, so take 30–60 min before food or on retiring to bed.
- Do not take indigestion remedies or medicines containing iron or zinc at the same time of day as this medicine.
- The dose will be increased gradually.
- Penicillamine may cause loss of taste after 6 weeks' treatment, but taste will then return.
- Mineral supplements are not recommended during penicillamine treatment.

- Report sore throat, fever, infection, unexplained bleeding and bruising, purpura, mouth ulcers, metallic taste or rash to the doctor immediately.
- Penicillamine may cause rashes in the first few months of treatment. These should disappear when the drug is stopped, allowing reintroduction at a lower dose and gradually increasing. Later rashes may require cessation of treatment.
- Patients who are allergic to penicillin may also be hypersensitive to penicillamine, although this is rare.

Sulfasalazine

- Report unexplained bleeding, bruising or purpura, sore throat, fever or malaise. These symptoms are most likely to occur in the first 3–6 months of treatment.
- Sulfasalazine may cause rashes and gastrointestinal intolerance. Upper gastrointestinal intolerance is common at doses >4 g/day.
- Contact lenses may be stained.
- Urine may be coloured orange.

Methotrexate

- Treatment is taken weekly. This is an important safety issue and all prescriptions for methotrexate that are not for a weekly dose should be queried.
- Folic acid supplement 5 mg weekly will reduce side effects resulting from folic acid deficiency.
- Contact the doctor immediately with breathlessness or cough.
- Do not take over-the-counter (OTC) aspirin or ibuprofen without the prescriber's advice.
- Pregnancy: avoid conception (this applies to males and females) for at least 6 months after stopping treatment.

Gold

- Report sore throat, fever, infection, unexplained bleeding and bruising, purpura, mouth ulcers, metallic taste or rash to the doctor immediately.
- Also report breathlessness or cough immediately.

- Rashes with pruritus often occur after 2–6 months of intramuscular treatment and may require cessation of treatment.
- The most common side effect of oral therapy, diarrhoea, with or without nausea or abdominal pain, may respond to bulking agents or temporary dose reduction.
- Stop treatment at least 6 months before conception.

Antimalarials

- Report any visual disturbances.
- Do not take indigestion remedies at the same time of day.

Etanercept, adalimumab and infliximab (an alert card should be provided)

Be vigilant for signs of serious infections (such as tuberculosis)

Etanercept

Report any signs of infection or increased bleeding.

Infliximab

- Its use may be associated with a hypersensitivity reaction.
- Patients should always keep their alert card with them and be aware that hypersensitivity reactions may be delayed.

Corticosteroids

See Chapter 21.

Self-assessment

Consider whether the following statements are true or false. In terms of the management of arthritis:

1. Paracetamol is considered as a first-line treatment for osteoarthritis.
2. Paracetamol should not be combined with NSAIDs.
3. Methotrexate is effective in osteoarthritis.
4. Patients taking methotrexate should be counselled to avoid self-medicating with OTC NSAIDs.
5. Infliximab is now recommended as first-line treatment for rheumatoid arthritis.

Practice points

- For NSAIDs, see Chapter 29.
- Methotrexate is given as a *weekly* dose.
- To reduce the risk of corticosteroid-induced osteoporosis, doses should be low and the course duration as short as possible. Long-term use of inhaled steroids may also reduce bone mineral density.
- Early intervention to prevent osteoporosis is important for patients prescribed corticosteroids because the greatest loss of bone occurs in the first 6–12 months.
- Prophylaxis for the prevention of osteoporosis should be considered alongside additional risk factors in patients prescribed the equivalent of 7.5 mg prednisolone or more daily for 3 months or more, and particularly in patients aged >65 years. Otherwise, a bone scan should be offered if treatment is likely to be continued for 6 months or longer.
- Patients suffering a fracture after relatively low trauma should be treated as for osteoporosis.
- Patients aged >65 years and those with low exposure to sunlight may be advised to take supplements of vitamin D (400 IU daily). Calcium supplements are indicated if requirements are not met by the diet. Calcium and vitamin D supplements are recommended for all frail elderly people, including those at home, in hospital or in nursing or residential homes.
- The effects of calcium are less than HRT or other agents in the prevention and treatment of osteoporosis.
- Exclude vitamin D deficiency and secondary hyperparathyroidism in elderly patients with osteoporosis or osteomalacia.

CASE STUDY

Case study
A 70-year-old woman with RA comes to ask you if you sell sulphur tablets for arthritis. She has just heard a radio programme talking about the benefits of sulphur for arthritis. She asks what you think and if you know of anything that might be better. You check her patient medication record, which shows regular supplies of ibuprofen 200 mg three times daily as required and co-codamol two tablets four times daily as required.

What is the first issue that you should consider?

- The fact that this patient is requesting additional treatment demonstrates poor pain control and this should be reviewed. The dose of ibuprofen is low for arthritis and may not be providing sufficient anti-inflammatory activity (see Chapter 29). Co-codamol may not be appropriate and the patient should be asked about any side effects such as constipation and how often she has been taking her as needed analgesics (see Chapter 29).

Do you recommend sulphur tablets?

- This patient was particularly interested in alternative remedies but, as she is seeking advice from her health professional, information should be evidence based. If she insists on taking alternative products such as sulphur tablets, you could offer to check the literature and/or the manufacturer for any known interactions or problems with her current medication. The opportunity should be taken to recommend a healthy diet as before (see Chapter 3), and particularly a high intake of fish oils. You could recommend a fish oil supplement to help her joint pain and any morning stiffness (providing 1–2 g eicosapentaenoic acid/docosahexanoic acid per dose). This intervention would also benefit patients with concurrent cardiovascular disease (see Chapters 12 and 13).

References

Adachi JD, Papaioannou A (2001). Corticosteroid-induced osteoporosis – detection and management. *Drug Safety* **24**: 607–24.

Greene RJ, Harris ND (2008). *Pathology and Therapeutics for Pharmacists*, 3rd edn London: Pharmaceutical Press.

National Institute for Health and Clinical Excellence (2008). *Osteoarthritis: The care and management of osteoarthritis in adults*. Clinical Guideline 59. London: NICE.

Further reading

American College of Rheumatology (2002). Guidelines for the management of rheumatoid arthritis. *Arthritis Rheum* **46**: 328–46.

Anon (1997). Topical non-steroidal anti-inflammatory drugs: an update. *MeReC Bull* **8**: 29–32.

Anon (1999). Prevention and treatment of osteoporosis. *MeReC Bull* **10**: 25–28.

Buckley L, Greenwald MD, Hochberg M *et al* – Ad Hoc Committee on Glucorticoid-induced Osteoporosis. (2001). Recommendations of the American College of Rheumatology. *Arthr Rheum* **44**: 1496–503.

Cummings SR, Meltin LJ (2002). Epidemiology and outcomes of osteoporotic fractures. *Lancet* **359**: 1761–7.

Delmas PD (2002). Treatment of postmenopausal osteoporosis. *Lancet* **359**: 2018–26.

Kanis JA (2002). Diagnosis of osteoporosis and assessment of fracture risk. *Lancet* **359**: 1929–36.

Medicines Control Agency/Committee on Safety of Medicines (2002). *Curr Probl Pharmacovigilance* **28**: 1–6.

National Institute for Health and Clinical Excellence (2005). *Bisphosphonates (alendronate, etidronate, risedronate), Selective Oestrogen Receptor Modulators (raloxifene) and Parathyroid Hormone (teriparatide) for the Secondary Prevention of Osteoporotic Fragility Fractures in Postmenopausal Wome*n. Technology Appraisal 87. London: NICE.

National Institutes of Health (2001). Osteoporosis prevention, diagnosis, and therapy. *JAMA* **285**: 785–95.

Seeman E (2002). Pathogenesis of bone fragility in women and men. *Lancet* **359**: 1841–50.

Solomon CG (2002). Bisphosphonates and osteoporosis. *N Engl J Med* **346**: 642.

Online resources

www.nos.org.uk
The National Osteoporosis Society is a charity providing information for both patients and healthcare professionals. The main aims are to improve the diagnosis, prevention and treatment of osteoporosis (accessed May 2008).

www.rheumatology.org.uk
The website of the British Society for Rheumatology with access to latest guidelines, including recommendations for monitoring requirements (accessed May 2008).

31

The cancer patient: cancer and palliative care

After cardiovascular disease, neoplastic disease or cancer represents the next largest cause of mortality, with more than one in three people developing cancer in their lifetime and one in four people dying as a result of it. The treatment of cancers is a highly specialized area and as such is beyond the scope of this book. This chapter describes the main pharmaceutical care issues involved in palliative care such as limiting the side effects associated with treatment and optimizing pain relief. In addition, the importance of prevention, screening, diagnosis, treatment and care, as outlined in the *NHS Cancer Plan* (Department of Health 2000), is discussed. This plan aims to lower the cancer death rate and improve survival rates and quality of life for both patients and carers.

Prevention, detection and screening

The primary aim is to reduce the risk of cancer by lifestyle changes such as smoking cessation and a healthy diet (see Chapter 3) and improved screening. Cancers may affect many organs and tissues within the body: cancers of the lungs, skin, breast and gastrointestinal tract are the most common. The outcome of cancer treatment varies between the sites affected and the stage at presentation, e.g. lung cancer has a very poor 5-year survival rate because it often presents at a late stage when it has spread via metastases (in general this means spread to distant sites, including the liver, brain, lungs and bone). By contrast, treatment of testicular cancer often has a high cure rate if detected early. Healthcare professionals therefore have an important role in the education of patients to recognize and report

serious symptoms early (see Chapter 1). This is particularly important for patients with additional risk factors such as a family history of breast or bowel cancer, and these patients should be encouraged to undertake regular screening. Interventions include the following:

- The provision of information relating to the importance of self-examination for lumps of the breast, testicles, neck or arm pits.
- To alleviate fear and encourage early referral to improve outcome.
- To encourage patients to attend screening such as cervical smears and mammograms, and to discuss concerns with healthcare professionals.
- To educate patients about the risk of skin cancer and the importance of protecting skin from the sun, particularly for those with fair skin (see Chapter 34). Vigilance of changes to moles suggestive of melanoma is also important.
- To educate patients to recognize other warning symptoms such as sudden unexplained weight loss, rectal bleeding or haemoptysis (see Chapter 1).
- Future screening may include screening for colorectal and ovarian cancers.

Treatment

Treatment of cancer is usually by hospital specialists and is divided into surgery, chemotherapy and radiotherapy. The aim of surgery is to remove the tumour and, if the tumour is localized, this may be curative. Surgery may also be used palliatively, e.g. to remove obstructions, or even preventively, such as the removal of a second breast in women at very high risk of the recurrence of breast cancer.

Chemotherapy is the use of cytotoxic drugs to kill fast-growing cells. Drugs used in anticancer chemotherapy generally target the synthesis of nucleotides (antimetabolites such as methotrexate and mercaptopurine), may chemically modify the DNA by alkylation (e.g. busulfan, chlorambucil, cyclophosphamide), cause fragmentation (e.g. bleomycin) or interchelation (e.g. dactinomycin), or may destroy mitotic spindle fibres (vinca alkaloids) involved in cell division. Corticosteroids also have a role, although this is poorly understood. In targeting these processes, the agents kill rapidly dividing cells in the tumour but also suppress growth of 'normal' cells with high rates of division, such as bone marrow cells producing blood cells and epithelial cells. Accordingly, the lack of selectivity gives rise to a wide range of side effects, including myelosuppression leading to pancytopenia, which is associated with anaemia, increased susceptibility to infections due to neutropenia and increased bleeding due to thrombocytopenia. Myelosuppression is a common occurrence with many agents and is a reason to carry out chemotherapy in cycles, because this allows the bone marrow to recover between cycles. Colony-stimulating factors may be used under some circumstances to increase the white cell count and reduce the time between cycles. Prophylactic antimicrobial agents may also be required. As a result of the toxic nature of cytotoxic agents they may exhibit a range of side effects which, depending on the agent, may include:

- alopecia
- nausea and vomiting
- mouth ulcers
- renal damage
- bladder damage
- infertility
- lung damage
- cardiotoxicity
- carcinogenic effects.

In the treatment of cancers, chemotherapy may be curative, e.g. in the treatment of testicular cancer, or may be used to kill leukaemia cells before bone marrow transplantation leading to a cure. Chemotherapy may be used in addition to surgery, e.g. after the removal of a solid tumour, courses of anticancer chemotherapy may be used to prevent recurrence or suppress the growth of any metastases. It may also be used in palliation to reduce tumour size or growth and to prolong life. There are a number of chemotherapeutic agents and these are often used in specific combinations, generally involving three agents. The purpose of using combinations is to attack different pharmacological targets and so limit the development of resistance. Aside from the conventional agents mentioned above, newer approaches include the use of monoclonal antibodies, which selectively target certain cell types, e.g. rituximab targets B lymphocytes and is used in non-Hodgkin's lymphomas.

Hormone-based therapy plays a significant role in certain tumours, e.g. the oestrogen receptor antagonist tamoxifen is widely used in oestrogen receptor-positive breast cancer. It is given after surgery, with or without chemotherapy, and is effective at suppressing the growth of oestrogen-sensitive cells, including residual cells and metastases. Other approaches include the use of aromatase inhibitors, such as aminoglutethimide, which prevent the metabolism of androgens to oestrogens.

Radiotherapy also plays a role, whether by radiation from isotopes or from X-rays. By targeting the radiation on the tumour, cancerous cells may be killed. Certain tumours are especially sensitive to irradiation (such as bladder cancers) and radiotherapy may play an important role in localized disease. Radiotherapy is also used when surgery is not possible in vital organs such as the head and neck. In addition, radiotherapy may be used after surgery, in palliation to reduce the size of tumours, to reduce obstruction of the vena cava and for relief from bony metastases. This may allow a reduction in doses of analgesics and/or stepping down the analgesic ladder.

Palliative care

The following section is intended as an introduction to some of the issues encountered during palliative care, particularly relating to common symptoms, the importance of regular monitoring to optimize treatment and the education of patients and carers. Specialist information should be sought from references given at the end of the chapter and local palliative care teams.

What is palliative care?

The term 'palliative' is used to describe treatment that addresses and alleviates symptoms associated with an incurable disease. Palliative care is therefore applied commonly to the treatment of terminal malignancy but may also include conditions such as the end-stages of chronic heart failure, respiratory diseases, acquired immune deficiency syndrome (AIDS) and motor neuron disease. The aim of treatment is to improve the quality of life of both patients and carers, and includes the control of physical symptoms and attention to spiritual, emotional and social needs. A multidisciplinary palliative care team therefore comprises specialist nurses, doctors, pharmacists, counsellors, dieticians, physiotherapists, social workers and ministers of religion. The National Institute for Health and Clinical Excellence (NICE 2004) has issued guidance for the provision of cancer services including supportive and palliative care. The World Health Organization (WHO 1990) also includes the following recommendations as to the role of palliative care:

- Consider dying as a normal process (see Nuland 1997).
- Death should not be hastened or postponed.
- Patients should be offered the support required, enabling them to live as actively as possible until death.
- The quality of life should be enhanced and care may also provide a positive influence throughout the course of the illness.

Types of cancer pain

Pain is one of the most common and feared symptoms of cancer. However, this is not inevitable and approximately a third of patients do not suffer severe pain at any stage of their illness. When treating pain, the first step is to determine the location and likely source because this will determine the choice of treatment, e.g. pain resulting from compression by a tumour may be reduced by chemotherapy or radiotherapy to remove or reduce the size of the tumour. Some types of pain (see Chapter 29) respond to treatment with opioids, but neuropathic or bone pain may be more resistant to opioids. Bone pain is a somatic pain produced by nociceptors in the bone and tends to be localized, described as gnawing or aching, and often results from secondary tumours in the bone. Visceral pain is triggered by infiltration, compression, distension or stretching of the viscera due to the presence of a tumour, and tends to be diffuse and constant.

WHO analgesic ladder

Once the nature and likely cause of pain are assessed, the recommendation of analgesia follows the analgesic ladder, as recommended by the WHO (see Chapter 29). Analgesia is prescribed continually and not 'when required' for optimum pain management and therefore improved quality of life. Additional analgesia is prescribed for pain occurring despite continuous treatment. This is commonly described as breakthrough pain, for which 'when required' analgesia is appropriate. Adjuvants may be added to treatment at any stage and include tricyclic antidepressants, anticonvulsants and corticosteroids (see Chapter 29). Choice is dependent on the nature of the pain, risk of drug interactions and side-effect profile.

Other symptoms

Other common symptoms of advanced cancer may include fatigue, weakness, anorexia, weight loss, lack of energy, dry mouth, constipation, dyspnoea and early satiety. Symptoms may be drug related and may vary according to the nature of the tumour, e.g. cancer of the head and neck often causes dysphagia whereas dyspnoea is associated with lung, breast or other cancers affecting the thorax. The cause and treatment of

Table 31.1 Examples of the causes and treatment of common symptoms encountered in palliative care

Symptom	Treatment	Comments/common causes
Anorexia	Identify and treat the cause. A short course of corticosteroids may be given or high doses of a progestogen such as megestrol acetate or medroxyprogesterone	• Possible causes include dry mouth, nausea, constipation, anxiety, dyspepsia, pain, gastric stasis, hypercalcaemia, uraemia, depression and malodorous tumours • Dietary supplements may be added but do not replace normal meals. The intake of calorific food such as cheese and full-fat milk should be encouraged • The effects of progestogens may be delayed for a few weeks and side effects such as oedema and the risk of thromboembolic disease may prevent their use. They tend only to be used if the prognosis is greater than 3 months
Anxiety	SSRIs, β blockers, benzodiazepines, e.g. lorazepam sublingually	• May be associated with depression and this may worsen pain (Chapter 24) • Benzodiazepines may be appropriate and the risk of dependence may not be relevant
Breathlessness	• Identify cause and treat as appropriate. Breathing techniques may be beneficial, particularly when dyspnoea is worsened by anxiety • Opioids may be of symptomatic benefit due to reduction of the central respiratory drive • Oxygen is required if the patient is hypoxic	Causes include anaemia, bronchospasm, fluid retention, respiratory infection, COPD, pulmonary embolism, congestive heart failure or drugs such as β blockers or aspirin (Chapter 15)
Confusion	Identify cause. Treatment may include haloperidol or chlorpromazine if the patient is agitated or distressed	• Hyponatraemia, hypercalcaemia, uraemia, pain, constipation, infection, urine retention • Drug causes include opioids, hypnotics and antimuscarinics (Chapter 5)
Constipation	A softener and stimulant are required, e.g. regular lactulose and senna or co-danthrusate (Chapter 9). Suppositories or enemas may be required if severe	• Opioids, reduced mobility, dehydration • Laxatives should be given to all patients prescribed regular opioids
Dehydration	Small amounts of fluids may be administered regularly. Causes should be identified and treated	• Causes include diuretics, laxatives, sweating or difficulty swallowing • Dehydration may lead to deterioration of renal function and should therefore be avoided or identified and corrected promptly

Continued

Table 31.1   (Continued)

Symptom	Treatment	Comments/common causes
Depression	Tricyclic or SSRI antidepressants (Chapter 24)	• Consider the prognosis and delayed efficacy before initiating antidepressants • Monitor for hyponatraemia as a cause of confusion and drowsiness • Antimuscarinic effects of tricyclics may be a disadvantage. Review other medications for risk of additive effects and consider problems such as dry mouth and constipation
Diarrhoea	Loperamide (Chapter 9), other opioids, rehydration	Causes include impacted faeces, bowel obstruction or infections. Drug causes include opioid withdrawal, antibiotics, iron salts, laxatives, NSAIDs and magnesium salts (Chapter 5)
Dry mouth and oral candidiasis	• Sugar-free chewing gum or sweets may help to stimulate saliva production (consider sorbitol as a cause of diarrhoea), artificial saliva, ice or unsweetened pineapple chunks and regular sips of water • Candidiasis may be present and is treated with nystatin or miconazole oral gel • Antiseptic mouth washes (e.g. chlorhexidine) may be used if patients are unable to brush their teeth	• Drug causes include opioids, drugs with antimuscarinic effects (sedating antihistamines, TCAs, hyoscine: see Chapter 5) • Reduce the prescribing of antimuscarinic drugs if possible • Glycerol-based mouthwashes are best avoided because they cause drying • Broad-spectrum antibiotics and steroids (particularly inhaled) and general debilitation may cause candidiasis • Asthmatic patients treated with inhaled steroids are at increased risk of developing oral candidiasis and may benefit from using a spacer device and should be advised to rinse their mouth after inhaler use
Hiccup	Antacid with antiflatulent (simeticone) e.g. Asilone suspension or Maalox Plus, metoclopramide or chlorpromazine	• May be caused by gastric distension • Avoid antacids containing aluminium salts alone, which may cause constipation • Avoid bicarbonate salts, which may increase flatulence from carbon dioxide production
Insomnia	Benzodiazepines, e.g. temazepam	• Causes include anxiety, depression, cramps, pain, night sweats, joint stiffness, fear or discomfort • Drug causes include corticosteroids (administer dexamethasone before 6pm), caffeine, alcohol, sympathomimetics (Chapter 26) or withdrawal from benzodiazepines
Intractable cough	Consider changing posture, particularly at night or opioids, e.g. morphine	Gastric distension
Muscle spasm	Diazepam, baclofen or dantrolene	• Pressure or nerve irritation • The efficacy of dantrolene may be delayed by a few weeks

Continued

Table 31.1   (Continued)

Symptom	Treatment	Comments/common causes
Nausea and vomiting	The cause should be determined and treated if appropriate. Antiemetics include domperidone, metoclopramide, haloperidol, cyclizine, levomepromazine, prochlorperazine when required (Chapter 8). Ondansetron may be used for chemotherapy-induced nausea and vomiting	• For example, gastric stasis, constipation, bowel obstruction, hypercalcaemia (stop drugs such as thiazides, which retain calcium), renal failure, raised intracranial pressure, motion sickness, severe pain, cough, severe anxiety, infection, uraemia or chemotherapy • Antimuscarinic drugs may oppose prokinetic drugs (Chapter 5) • Common cause is initial treatment with opioids but this is usually transient, resolving after a few days • Review every 24 h • Many drugs cause nausea and vomiting (Chapter 5) • Note that extrapyramidal effects of metoclopramide are more common in children
Pruritus	Emollients (cool in the fridge) and/or oral antihistamines. Avoid heat and try cotton clothing. Obstructive jaundice may require treatment with colestyramine	Jaundice or drugs such as opioids (Chapter 34). Note that itching due to opioids is more common in children
Sedation	Reduction of opioid dose if pain is controlled. Also review other drugs causing sedation such as antihistamines (chlorphenamine), antidepressants (amitriptyline, dosulepin (dothiepin), trazodone) or benzodiazepines	• Tends to occur when opioid dose is increased and should be transient, resolving after a few days • Patient should not perform skilled tasks such as driving • If sedation persists, consider toxicity and review dose and factors such as deteriorating renal function
Sweating	Paracetamol or NSAIDs, or hyoscine (opioid-induced sweating)	• Malignancy, infection, anxiety, hyperthyroidism, menopause. Drug causes include antidepressants • Monitor for dehydration, e.g. diuretic doses may need to be withheld

COPD, chronic obstructive pulmonary disease; NSAIDs, non-steroidal anti-inflammatory drugs; SSRIs, selective serotonin reuptake inhibitors; TCAs, tricyclic antidepressants.

common symptoms are summarized in Table 31.1.

Pharmacology

The pharmacology of analgesics is described in Chapter 29. The pharmacology of corticosteroids is summarized in Chapter 21.

Drug choice

Treatment is given according to the analgesic ladder, as described in Chapter 29. The following section outlines analgesic choice according to the analgesic ladder, as applied to palliative care.

Step 1

Regular paracetamol is an effective first choice and is often an adequate analgesic used alone for mild pain, with or without a non-steroidal anti-inflammatory drug (NSAID). This should be used regularly and may be continued at all stages of the ladder.

Step 2

Mild opioids such as codeine or dihydrocodeine may be added (see Chapter 29). Each tablet should contain the equivalent of 30 mg codeine or more and combination analgesics containing less than this dose per tablet are not recommended for cancer pain (National Prescribing Centre 2003). It should be noted that constipation is a problem even with low doses of opioid and a laxative will be required with regular treatment.

Tramadol

Tramadol is considered suitable for use at the second step of the analgesic ladder, as it has fewer opioid side effects such as constipation and respiratory depression compared with strong opioids. However, this may not be appropriate for the management of cancer pain in the absence of evidence for an advantage over weak opioids and also recommendations in the summary of product characteristics (SPC) that the maximum dose of 400 mg/day is not exceeded except in special circumstances due to the risk of convulsions at higher doses. It is also unsuitable for patients with epilepsy or those prone to seizures, e.g. patients with cerebral tumours or uraemia. It should be avoided with other drugs known to lower the convulsive threshold, such as antidepressants (see Chapter 5).

Step 3

Strong opioids

The properties of the strong opioids such as fentanyl, morphine, pethidine, oxycodone and buprenorphine are summarized in Table 31.2 and also in Table 29.1. The latest *British National Formulary* (BNF) should be consulted for equivalent doses of opioids when calculating doses of strong opioids after treatment with milder agents, e.g. codeine and dihydrocodeine are approximately one-tenth the potency of morphine and the use of these opioids is considered when calculating the morphine dose. The dose is then titrated against pain because doses higher than those required to control pain lead to respiratory depression.

Despite the introduction of agents such as oxycodone, morphine remains the first-line strong opioid for moderate-to-severe pain. Strong opioids such as morphine cause euphoria and mental detachment, which may be beneficial, as well as reducing respiratory symptoms. However, bone pain and neuropathic pain are often resistant to even strong opioids, although the response is unpredictable and therefore a trial of opioids is recommended (National Prescribing Centre 2003).

Where possible, it is reasonable to give drugs orally, even in advanced cancer. For patients with vomiting or difficulty swallowing, oral suspensions, patches or suppositories may be used. Alternatively syringe drivers provide a useful and continuous method of drug administration (see below).

Syringe drivers

For patients in the final stages of a terminal illness, syringe drivers can provide an extremely useful way of delivering medication. Syringe drivers provide a continuous subcutaneous infusion and therefore allow effective control of symptoms. When converting from oral morphine to a syringe driver, the more soluble opioid diamorphine is used and the equivalent doses of these opioids are tabulated in the BNF. The dose may, however, need to be increased because of worsening pain and/or increased tolerance by patients at the time that a syringe driver is initiated. It should be noted that a misconception exists whereby patients and carers view the administration of opioids via the parenteral route to be more effective than the oral route, and an inevitable part of the treatment of advanced disease. The BNF indications for the parenteral route include patients unable to take medication by mouth, e.g. due to dysphagia or nausea and vomiting and, importantly, when patients request that they receive their medication by this route.

Important roles for pharmacists include the calculation of diamorphine dose required when converting from oral morphine and assessing the compatibility of drugs to be added to

Table 31.2   A summary of some important characteristics of strong opioids in relation to palliative care

Opioid	Comments
Buprenorphine	• Vomiting may be a problem and withdrawal effects may occur if added to high-dose opioid treatment, resulting from its partial agonist activity. It is therefore not often suitable for cancer pain • Patches have recently been introduced
Cyclimorph	• Cyclimorph is a combination product containing both morphine and cyclizine. This is not appropriate for chronic pain because nausea is a transient effect of opioid treatment, so ongoing treatment with cyclizine is not necessary. In addition, dose increases lead to excessive sedation due to cyclizine • Diconal is a combination product of cyclizine and dipipanone and is therefore also unsuitable in palliative care
Dextromoramide	• A short duration of action makes dextromoramide unsuitable for control of continuous pain and this is rarely used • Available as a sublingual tablet
Diamorphine	• More soluble than morphine and therefore used for infusion due to reduced volume • Activity one-quarter to one-third that of oral morphine • Injection is given by the subcutaneous route, which is easier to administer and less painful than other routes
Fentanyl	• The efficacy of fentanyl is comparable with morphine and this is therefore not a suitable alternative when pain is not controlled by morphine (suspect opioid-resistant pain). The time taken for transdermal fentanyl to reach steady state also makes this preparation unsuitable for unstable pain • Patches changed at the same time every 3 days are useful for patients with dysphagia, malabsorption or poor compliance • Less constipating than morphine and more suitable in renal impairment as there are no active metabolites, although dose reduction may be required • Oral transmucosal fentanyl citrate lozenges are now available for breakthrough pain • New preparations should be started 12 h after the last patch is removed. It should also be noted that fentanyl effects remain for up to 72 h after removal of the patch • When starting fentanyl treatment, apply patch at the same time as the last dose of slow-release morphine. The full effect may take 36–48 h and therefore breakthrough pain may occur and should be treated as required • When changing from morphine, withdrawal symptoms such as colic, diarrhoea, nausea, sweating and restlessness may persist for a few days, although pain may be controlled. Doses of short-acting oral morphine may be given • Adjuncts or alternative analgesia should be considered if pain is not controlled by doses >300 micrograms/h
Hydromorphone	• To date, hydromorphine appears to demonstrate efficacy and tolerability comparable to morphine and is reserved for patients with confusion, loss of concentration, vivid dreams or hallucinations occurring with even low doses of morphine • The contents of controlled-release capsules may be sprinkled on cold soft food
Methadone	Useful in renal failure
Morphine	• Remains the first choice for the treatment of chronic cancer pain • Oral slow-release and quick-acting preparations available for good pain control, including breakthrough pain
Oxycodone	• Suppositories offer alternative routes of administration • Role in relation to morphine remains to be established as side-effect profile and efficacy appear similar but may provide an alternative if symptoms such as hallucinations become problematic with morphine
Pentazocine	Avoided due to high risk of confusion and hallucinations
Pethidine	Pethidine is avoided in palliative care due to the short half-life, reduced potency compared with morphine and the accumulation of toxic metabolites during regular use

diamorphine infusions, thereby maintaining the stability of the infusion and preventing adverse effects in the patient. The infusion solution should be checked regularly for discoloration or precipitation. Examples from the BNF of drugs that may be added to diamorphine infusions include:

- cyclizine
- dexamethasone
- haloperidol
- hysoscine butylbromide
- hyoscine hydrobromide
- metoclopramide
- midazolam.

Drugs contraindicated for use in syringe drivers include chlorpromazine, prochlorperazine and diazepam due to irritation at the injection site. The latest BNF and *The Syringe Driver* (Dickman *et al* 2002) should be consulted for further information.

Adjuncts used in the treatment of pain

Adjuncts may be added at any step of the analgesic ladder and include corticosteroids, antidepressants and anticonvulsants. Other treatment includes nerve block, relaxation therapy and the use of transcutaneous electrical nerve stimulation (TENS) machines (see Chapter 29).

Corticosteroids

Corticosteroids such as dexamethasone are particularly useful for treating pain due to nerve compression, tissue swelling or raised intracranial pressure.

Dexamethasone (doses up to 16 mg/day) is used for raised intracranial pressure, severe bone pain, nerve or soft-tissue infiltration by the tumour or oedema, and hepatic capsular pain. The last dose should be given before 6pm to avoid causing insomnia. Additional benefits include increased appetite, energy and general wellbeing. To avoid side effects, the lowest effective dose is prescribed and the course duration is as short as possible. For patients taking corticosteroids and NSAIDs, gastric protection in the form of a proton pump inhibitor is appropriate.

Neuropathic pain

Neuropathic pain (see Chapter 29) results from treatment such as radiotherapy, or from infiltration of a tumour into peripheral nerves or the central nervous system, causing compression or damage. It may be described as burning, stabbing, tingling, a constricting sensation or shooting pains. The skin may feel numb or oversensitive. Neuropathic pain is often unresponsive to opioids, the most effective being methadone, tramadaol and oxycodone, and is managed by a combination of corticosteroids, tricyclic antidepressants and antiepileptic drugs such as gabapentin and pregabalin (see Chapters 23 and 24). Specialists may also consider the use of ketamine or antiarrhythmics such as flecainide, mexiletine or lidocaine.

Bone pain

Bone pain often arises from secondary tumours, which result in either increased or reduced bone density and the release of prostaglandins. NSAIDs are therefore the analgesics of choice. If an NSAID remains ineffective after 1 week, an alternative NSAID is selected (see Chapter 29). The addition of a weak opioid may be considered but is not often beneficial. Bisphosphonates or calcitonin may be used to reduce bone turnover or inhibit calcium resorption into bone, respectively. Corticosteroids are useful for treating bone pain due to anti-inflammatory properties and also by reducing oedema surrounding the tumour. Regular use of paracetamol is useful at each step of the analgesic ladder.

Colicky pain

Pain associated with the gastrointestinal tract and reported as 'colicky' pain may respond to antimuscarinic agents, such as hyoscine, which reduce intestinal transit.

Common symptoms

Table 31.1 summarizes the causes of some common symptoms associated with cancer and their management.

Concurrent disease

Analgesic prescribing decisions complicated by concurrent diseases are outlined in Chapter 29. Key considerations include gastrointestinal toxicity due to NSAIDs and worsening renal function. For patients with effective pain control with NSAIDs, a proton pump inhibitor may be added for gastric protection. Misoprostol may not be suitable due to colic or diarrhoea. It should be noted, however, that respiratory depression in terminal care does not preclude the use of strong opioids and careful dose titration prevents this effect. Signs of opioid overdose include drowsiness, reduced respiratory rate and the presence of hallucinations, and pain tends to be well controlled. Opioid toxicity may be precipitated by renal impairment.

In general, the risks of initiating further treatment are compared with the likely benefits. Unnecessary treatment is withheld to prevent further complications of drug regimens, e.g. the treatment of hyperlipidaemia may not be appropriate in terminal care. Palliative care is one of the exceptions when polypharmacy is often necessary and adverse drug reactions (ADRs) are treated as they arise. Patients and carers should be as involved as possible in treatment choices and the impact on quality of life considered, e.g. the use of drugs with sedative properties may be avoided for as long as possible in patients wishing to retain the independence gained from driving.

Terminal symptoms

Terminal symptoms occur when death is likely to be within days. These include noisy breathing (death rattle), confusion, fever and severe fatigue. Symptoms should be monitored regularly and those considered to be causing distress, such as urinary retention, constipation, pain and dyspepsia, should be identified and treated. It should be noted that restlessness and agitation may occur in the presence of worsening pain but this is not always the case and care should be taken to avoid misinterpretation. Increasing doses of opioids may worsen such symptoms and dose reduction or an alternative opioid should be

considered when other causes, including pain, have been excluded. Any unnecessary treatment such as antihypertensives, diuretics, antiarrhythmics and hypoglycaemics may be stopped. Artificial feeding such as via a nasogastric tube is not appropriate because it may cause distress to both the patient and the carers.

Drug interactions

See Chapter 29.

Monitoring

The impairment of renal or hepatic function may increase side effects, particularly to opioids, and requires dose reduction or less frequent dosing (see Chapter 29).

The role of the community pharmacist

The community pharmacist is an important source of support and information, particularly for carers of cancer patients who are often involved in collecting and administering medication. Pharmacists are an essential part of the palliative care team, being experts on the use and availability of medicines, e.g. pharmacists can advise on alternative preparations such as suspensions, suppositories and patches available for patients with dysphagia.

Perhaps the most important role of the pharmacist is in the education of patients and carers on the best use of medicines because this improves compliance. The needs of the patient and carers should be considered, e.g. a complicated medication regimen is of no benefit if it causes anxiety and poor compliance. Verbal and written information should be provided; an up-to-date list of medication, dosing information and indications for use of each product may help both patients and carers. Advice may need to be repeated. Regular supply of medication should be ensured and patients and carers encouraged to report new or altered symptoms for early recognition of ADRs or new symptoms. Providing a list of contacts and sources of further information is also helpful, particularly in the early stages of the disease. Pharmacist input to medication assessment and review, of a multidisciplinary palliative care team staffing palliative care clinics, is also to be encouraged because this improves pharmaceutical care for patients (Needham and Wong 1999; Austwick *et al* 2002).

General advice for patients and carers

- Key words to consider when providing advice include education, empathy, reassurance, approachability and resourcefulness.
- Good mouth care should be encouraged to prevent problems such as infection.
- Take care not to run out of medicines.
- Pharmacists may consider producing specific information leaflets to cover the use of medicines outside the product licence.

Pain

- Patients and carers may fear the use of morphine, because it is wrongly associated with 'imminent death'. Reassurance should be given that morphine is an extremely safe and useful analgesic, which may be used for years and with little risk of psychological dependence when used for severe pain.
- Drowsiness caused by strong opioids is often transient. Skilled tasks such as driving should be avoided and prolonged drowsiness should be reported to the prescriber.
- Advice should be given as to the timing of morphine doses, e.g. regular administration of a long-acting preparation twice a day means as close to 12 h as practical between doses, with additional doses of an immediate-release preparation (usually morphine solution) given up to every 4 h as required for breakthrough pain. The total amount of oral solution taken during a 24-h period allows the prescriber to calculate the 12-hourly dose required.
- Reassurance should be given that the effectiveness of morphine will persist even if started early in the disease. It is a common misconception by patients that starting morphine treatment too early may leave them without adequate pain control when the pain worsens.

- The control of neuropathic pain may take a week or more but if the pain worsens the prescriber should be contacted. If agents such as antidepressants or anticonvulsants are used, the use of these drugs for neuropathic pain should be explained.

Opioids, NSAIDs and adjuvant counselling

See Chapter 29.

Fentanyl patches

- Patches should be changed at the same time every 3 days.
- A new patch should be applied to a different area of skin, and not applied to inflamed skin, scar tissue, or swollen or broken skin.
- Direct contact of heat such as from hot-water bottles should be avoided.
- There should be good contact between the skin and the patch, and porous adhesive tape (e.g. Micropore) may be used if necessary.
- Used patches should be folded inwards, protecting the side that contained the drug, and disposed of carefully.

Fentanyl lozenges

- For breakthrough pain with a maximum dose of 4 dose units a day.
- No more than 2 dose units for each pain episode.
- The lozenge should be sucked and moved around the mouth over about 15 min, dissolving any lozenge left after pain is relieved, under hot running water.

Co-danthramer

This may colour urine red.

Self-assessment

Consider whether the following statements are true or false. In the management of cancer:

1. Cyclimorph is a good choice for chronic pain.

2. Cyclizine may be added to an infusion of diamorphine though there is a risk of precipitation (see BNF).

3. NSAIDs are effective in bone pain.

4. An oral solution of morphine is sometimes used to determine the required dose of a modified-release preparation.

5. Treatment with morphine should be delayed as efficacy will reduce with time.

Practice points

- Psychosocial and spiritual support for both patient and family are important components of palliative care and may impact on the severity of symptoms.
- The progressive nature of cancer means that the symptoms and patients' needs are constantly changing. Regular review of medication is therefore essential and should identify ADRs and new symptoms and assess the continued benefit from treatment. Palliative care medicine is a balance between symptom control and avoidance of unacceptable ADRs.
- Palliative care is a specialist area though encountered commonly in the community. It is therefore important for community pharmacists to be familiar with the general principles of pain management and liaise with specialist pharmacists.

General pain control

- Pain control should follow the stepped approach recommended by the WHO (see Chapter 29).
- The WHO also recommends that analgesia be provided continually and not 'when required', although additional analgesia is prescribed for use when required for breakthrough pain.
- Frequent review is required for optimum pain control.
- Consider the timing of doses, e.g. before painful changing of dressings.
- It may be useful to ask the patient to indicate the severity of each symptom on a scale of 1–10 to assess treatment outcome and the need for dose changes or further intervention. A list of drugs, including those found to be ineffective, is useful to prevent omissions and unnecessary treatment.

Opioids

- The total daily dose of morphine should be reviewed daily and the regular dose adjusted according to the number of rescue doses required. In practice, a doubling of the rescue dose may be given at night (50% increase for elderly patients) to ensure a pain-free night and prevent the patient waking for a further dose.
- There is no maximum dose for morphine and therefore the dose is titrated according to increased pain relief compared with side effects. A poor response may necessitate the introduction of adjuncts, e.g. the cause of pain should be reassessed if more than 200 mg/day of morphine is required.
- There are now many brands of morphine that are designed for either daily or twice-daily administration. When prescribing, it is good practice to indicate both the generic and brand name to avoid over- or underdosing.
- Patients sensitive to the adverse effects of one strong opioid can be changed to a similar opioid so long as toxicity has been excluded, but note that frequent changes result in poor pain management.
- Softener and stimulant laxatives (see Chapter 9) should be started when any opioid is initiated and the dose increased according to response rather than the opioid dose. When changing from high doses of morphine, however, laxative doses should be halved as severe diarrhoea may occur.
- Note that, unlike stronger opioids, opioids for mild-to-moderate pain produce a maximum analgesic effect, which is not exceeded by further dose increases. At this stage, stronger opioids are substituted according to step 3 of the WHO analgesic ladder. Substituting for an alternative weak opioid is of no benefit.

Syringe drivers

- Check infusion solutions regularly for discoloration or precipitation and ensure the correct rate of infusion.
- Infusion solutions should not be used for longer than 24 h to reduce the risk of infection.
- Breakthrough pain may be treated with subcutaneous (or intramuscular) injections of diamorphine (a sixth of the total 24-h dose being given by subcutaneous infusion).
- Monitor the injection site and consider changing to an alternative site if there is pain or prominent inflammation.

CASE STUDY

An excellent case study and pharmaceutical care plan are discussed in detail by a specialist palliative care pharmacist in the *Pharmaceutical Journal* (Urie 2000). This should be read in conjunction with up-to-date guidelines although most issues are still relevant.

References

Austwick EA, Brown LC, Goddyear KH *et al* (2002). Pharmacist's input into a palliative care clinic. *Pharm J* **268**: 404–6.

Department of Health (2000). *The NHS Cancer Plan.* London: Department of Health.

Dickman D, Littlewood C, Varga J (2002). *The Syringe Driver. continuous infusions in palliative care.* Oxford: Oxford University Press.

Martin J, ed. *British National Formulary*, latest edition. London: British Medical Association and Royal Pharmaceutical Society of Great Britain.

Miles CL, Fellowes D, Goodman ML *et al* (2006). Laxatives for the management of constipation in palliative care patients. *Cochrane Database System Rev* issue 4: CD003448.

National Institute for Health and Clinical Excellence (2004). *Guidance on Cancer Services. Improving supportive and palliative care for adults with cancer.* London: NICE.

National Prescribing Centre (2003). The use of strong opioids in palliative care. *MeReC Briefing* Issue No. 22. Liverpool: National Prescribing Centre.

Needham D, Wong I (1999). An expert panel review to evaluate the effectiveness of community pharmacist's interventions in the palliative care setting. *Pharm J* **263**(suppl): R32–R3.

Nuland SB (1997). *How We Die.* Berkshire: Vintage.

Urie J (2000). Palliative care. *Pharm J* **265**: 603–14.

World Health Organization (1990). *Cancer Pain Relief and Palliative Care: Report of a WHO Expert Committee.* Geneva: WHO.

Further reading

Allen M, Taylor R (1999). Pain control in palliative care. *Pharm J* **262**: 620–4.

Costello P (2001). Palliative care – an introduction. *Hosp Pharm* **8**: 211–14.

Department of Health (2000). *The NHS Cancer Plan.* London: Department of Health.

Montgomery F (2001). Palliative care. Managing chronic cancer pain. *Hosp Pharm* **8**: 215–18.

Montgomery F (2002). Pain management in palliative care. *Pharm J* **268**: 254–6.

Quigley C (2002). Hydromorphone for acute and chronic pain (Cochrane review). *Cochrane Database System Rev* issue 1: CD003447.

Twycross R, Wilcock A (2001). *Symptom Management in Advanced Cancer,* 3rd edn. Oxford: Radcliffe Medical Press.

Twycross R, Wilcock A, Charlesworth S *et al* (2002). *PCF2 – Palliative Care Formulary,* 2nd edn. Oxford: Radcliffe Medical Press.

Urie J, Fielding H, McArthur D *et al* (2000). Palliative care. *Pharm J* **265**: 603–14.

Online resources

www.palliativedrugs.com
Provides access to drug information on the use of drugs in palliative care, access to books such as the *Palliative Care Formulary* and a monthly newsletter (accessed April 2008).

www.who.int/cancer/palliative/en

For WHO cancer information and publications, including the International Agency for Research on Cancer (IARC) (accessed April 2008).

www.helpthehospices.org.uk

Includes education and a useful e-learning facility (accessed April 2008).

www.cancerbacup.org.uk

Cancer BACUP provides information for health professionals, patients and carers, a telephone helpline and access to information centres throughout the UK (accessed April 2008).

www.dh.gov.uk/en/Healthcare/NationalServiceFrameworks/Cancer/index.htm

For the National Health Service (NHS) cancer plan, current information and research, recommendations for good practice and links to cancer services within the NHS (accessed April 2008).

www.endoflifecare.nhs.uk

For the NHS End of Life Care Programme (accessed April 2008).

www.macmillan.org.uk

For Macmillan Cancer Relief, a charity providing information and support to patients with cancer and their carers, including information on access to Macmillan nurses and a telephone helpline (accessed April 2008).

www.mariecurie.org.uk

For access to Marie Curie Cancer Care, providing access to ongoing research, education and Marie Curie Hospices across the UK (accessed April 2008).

www.eapcnet.org/About/about.html

For the European Association for Palliative Care (accessed 24 April 2008)

www.patient.co.uk

For useful information and access to patient information leaflets also included on EMIS clinical computer systems used by GPs

Part H
Infections

Bacterial infections

Bacterial infections comprise a wide range of diseases from simple, troublesome conditions to life-threatening events. The purpose of this chapter is to give a brief overview of common infections and antibacterial agents. In some cases infections such as respiratory tract and skin infections are dealt with elsewhere (see Chapters 19, 21 and 34). The aim is to illustrate common examples and principles; more detailed sources and guidelines should be consulted for specific information relating to bacterial sensitivity to antibiotics.

Disease characteristics

Infection or invasion by foreign, pathogenic organisms may result from those living as commensals on the body or from gut flora, in addition to those present in soil, food or on other animal hosts. Pathophysiological changes may result from bacterial infection of any part of the body, often entering via a wound or mucous membranes, by contact, ingestion or opportunistic infection, e.g. of immunocompromised patients.

Risk factors for infection include reduced immunity in young, elderly, immunocompromised or malnourished individuals, those with diabetes mellitus, or prosthetic valves or joints, or after surgery or as a result of burns. Foreign travel may also result in infection due to exposure to organisms for which immunity has not developed previously. Drugs may increase the risk of infection by immunosuppression (e.g. corticosteroids), and effects on white cell production (e.g. drugs associated with agranulocytosis such as clozapine) and broad-spectrum antibiotics by affecting the gut flora.

Clinical features of common infections (Table 32.1)

Signs and symptoms of infection may include pyrexia, sweating, tachycardia, hypotension, nausea and vomiting, pallor, local pain and inflammation or purulence. A full blood count may indicate white cells elevated to $>12 \times 10^9$/L, with neutrophilia, but reduced due to depletion in chronic infections (such as tuberculosis [TB], although monocytes may be elevated) or in septicaemia. There may also be a raised erythrocyte sedimentation rate (ESR, see Chapter 2).

Gastrointestinal infections

Infections of the gastrointestinal tract include gastroenteritis, campylobacter enteritis, invasive salmonellosis, shigellosis, typhoid fever, antibiotic-associated pseudomembranous colitis, biliary tract infection (cholangitis) and peritonitis. Specific symptoms include diarrhoea, vomiting and abdominal pain. Cholangitis presents as pain in the right upper quadrant of the abdomen and may be associated with jaundice and high fever. Chronic infection of the stomach or duodenum with *Helicobacter pylori* is associated with ulceration and is dealt with in Chapter 7.

Cardiovascular infections

Endocarditis, inflammation of the lining of the heart cavity (endocardium) and valves, may result from rheumatic fever or bacterial infection by streptococci, enterococci or staphylococci. Patients with existing abnormalities of the heart such as valvular disease are at increased risk. Specific clinical features are chest pain, murmur,

Table 32.1   Some common examples of bacteria and their related conditions

Bacterium	Associated disease
Gram-positive cocci	
Staphylococcus aureus	Associated with styes, impetigo, conjunctivitis, sinusitis, food poisoning, endocarditis, meningitis, pneumonia, UTI and osteomyelitis
Streptococcus pyogenes	Causes scarlet fever, acute tonsillitis, erysipelas; dangerous if it affects wounds because it may cause sepsis
Streptococcus pneumoniae	Pneumonia, bronchitis, infections of the ears and sinuses, meningitis
Streptococcus viridans	Endocarditis
Gram-negative cocci	
Neisseria gonorrhoeae	Purulent ophthalmia or gonorrhoea
Neisseria meningitidis	Cerebrospinal fever or meningococcal meningitis
Gram-positive rods	
Bacillus spp. (B. anthracis, B. cereus)	Anthrax, food poisoning
Clostridium spp. (C. botulinum, C. tetani C. difficile)	Dangerous anaerobes causing tissue damage, affecting wounds and leading to gangrene, food poisoning (botulism), tetanus, pseudomembranous colitis (often secondary to use of broad-spectrum antibiotics such as clindamycin)
Gram-negative rods	
Pseudomonas aeruginosa	Dangerous secondary infection of wounds, pneumonia, eye infections, UTI
Helicobacter pylori	Associated with peptic ulcer
Haemophilus influenzae	Infantile meningitis, conjunctivitis, chronic bronchitis, infections of ear and sinuses
Escherichia coli	Enterobacteria (inhabitants of intestines) causing enteritis in young infants, also pyelitis, pyelonephritis and UTIs
Salmonella spp.	Enteric bacteria causing typhoid, food poisoning
Shigella spp.	Enteric bacteria causing dysentery
Proteus spp.	Enteric bacteria infecting the urinary tract and wounds
Klebsiella pneumoniae	Enteric bacteria and cause of acute bronchopneumonia
Campylobacter jejunum	Enteritis due to food poisoning. Anaerobe
Bacteroides fragilis	Oropharyngeal or gastrointestinal infection. Anaerobe
Chlamydia trachomatis	Trachoma, conjunctivitis and non-gonococcal urethritis
Legionella pneumophila	Legionnaires' disease transmitted in water, pneumonia
Acid-fast organisms	
Mycobacterium tuberculosis	Tuberculosis (Mycobacterium spp. also cause leprosy)
Spirochaetes	
Leptospira icterohaemorrhagiae	Weils' disease (jaundice) carried by rats
Borrelia vincenti	Vincent's angina

UTI, urinary tract infection.

tachycardia and palpitations. Patients may be frightened that they are suffering a heart attack, because symptoms are severe and rapid in onset.

Respiratory infections

Respiratory infections include bronchitis and pneumonia, which are discussed in Chapters 19 and 21.

The incidence of TB is increasing, mainly due to the spread of acquired immune deficiency syndrome (AIDS), increased homelessness and the emergence of resistant strains. An initial latent phase may be asymptomatic. Progressive pulmonary TB produces symptoms of fatigue, night sweats, weight loss, cough with haemoptysis and chest pain. Chest radiology reveals abnormalities such as pulmonary infiltration, visible cavities and fibrosis. These abnormalities may occur before the clinical symptoms. The causative organisms are *Mycobacterium tuberculosis* and *M. avium*, of which multidrug-resistant strains are common.

Central nervous system

The most common infection of the central nervous system (CNS) is meningitis, or infection with inflammation of the membrane (meninges) surrounding the brain. *Neisseria meningitidis* (meningococci), *Streptococcus pneumoniae* (pneumococci), *Haemophilus influenzae* and *Listeria monocytogenes* are important causative agents of bacterial meningitis. Clinical features include photophobia, neck stiffness, headache, rash that does not blanch under pressure (the glass test), general malaise and fever. A rash is not always present. Suspected meningitis is treated with 'blind' antibiotic therapy.

Urinary tract

Bacteriuria may indicate genitourinary infection affecting the kidney (pyelonephritis), bladder (cystitis), prostate in men (prostatitis) or urethra (urethritis), collectively known as urinary tract infections (UTIs). Acute pyelonephritis is an acute kidney infection presenting with fever, chills, rigors and pains, and tenderness. Lower UTIs are more common in women due to a shorter urethra and produce symptoms of urgency, frequency and dysuria (painful urination). More serious symptoms indicating renal involvement include haematuria, lower back or loin pain, and fever with diarrhoea and vomiting.

Risk factors for developing a UTI include diabetes mellitus, pregnancy, impaired voiding and catheters. *Escherichia coli* causes most UTIs occurring in the community. UTIs acquired during a stay in hospital may include infection by staphylococci, streptococci or *Pseudomonas* or *Proteus* species. UTIs are also commonly associated with long-term urinary catheters.

Genital infections

Genital infections include gonorrhoea, uncomplicated genital chlamydial infection, nongonococcal urethritis and non-specific genital infections, pelvic inflammatory disease and, rarely, syphilis. *Neisseria gonorrhoeae* can infect the urethra, cervix, rectum, pharynx and conjunctiva. Infection is associated with a purulent discharge and may be otherwise asymptomatic and a cause of infertility. Non-gonococcal infection may produce a thinner discharge but also requires further investigation. Pyrexia and pelvic pain require urgent referral.

Genital infections are often transmitted sexually and partners should be referred for screening even in the absence of symptoms. Recurrent requests for cystitis or thrush treatment, particularly when previous treatment has been unsuccessful, should be referred to the general practitioner (GP) or genitourinary clinic for further investigation. This is particularly important due to the risk of complications such as infertility.

Blood

Septicaemia (blood poisoning) often results from an existing infection and in susceptible patients such as elderly or immunocompromised individuals. It may be caused by any of a number of pathogens. Treatment is therefore dependent on the nature of the initial infection. Symptoms include chills, diarrhoea, fever and vomiting. Urgent treatment is required to prevent spread, leading to secondary infection of organs and ultimately life-threatening septic shock, which involves severe hypotension and may lead to multiorgan failure.

Musculoskeletal system

Prompt treatment of osteomyelitis (infection and inflammation of bone marrow) and septic arthritis is imperative to prevent bone or joint damage. Alerting symptoms of infection include red, hot and painful swelling of the affected site with difficult movement. Septic arthritis most often involves *Staphylococcus aureus* and occasionally *H. influenzae* or *N. gonorrhoeae* (gonococci). Patients with existing damage to joints, such as those with rheumatoid arthritis and patients taking corticosteroids, are at increased risk of developing septic arthritis. This may also follow osteomyelitis affecting a nearby bone. Osteomyelitis in turn may follow a fracture or bone surgery. Treatment includes high doses of antibiotics, aspiration, analgesia and support of the affected joint or limb.

Eye

Purulent conjunctivitis may indicate bacterial infection requiring antibiotic eye drops such as chloramphenicol or gentamicin. Fusidic acid is used to treat suspected staphylococcal infections. Gonococcal conjunctivitis requires both topical and systemic antibiotics.

Ear, nose and throat

Infections affecting the ear, nose and throat include dental infections, sinusitis, otitis externa, otitis media and throat infections, which are covered in Chapter 19.

Acute otitis media

Acute otitis media is dealt with in Chapter 19.

Skin

Infections of the skin produce the conditions impetigo, erysipelas (*Streptococcus pyogenes* infection of the skin and underlying tissue of the face and scalp), cellulitis and acne (see Chapter 34).

Goals of treatment

The aims of antibacterial treatment are to:

- eradicate the infection
- prevent spread
- prevent complications such as septicaemia and secondary infection.

The appropriate antibiotic is chosen with the spectrum of activity to cover the specific infection while avoiding the development of resistance. Symptomatic treatment may include the use of analgesics such as paracetamol and/or ibuprofen.

Prophylaxis

The use of antimicrobial agents to prevent infection plays an important role in patients at risk due to concurrent disease, surgery or contact with infection. Important examples where prophylaxis is appropriate include the following:

- Patients with rheumatic fever who receive antibiotic prophylaxis until the age of 25 years of age and for subsequent surgery and dental surgery.
- Patients who have had a splenectomy.
- Patients with sickle cell anaemia.
- Patients with a history of endocarditis and/or those with prosthetic heart valves who require antibiotic prophylaxis before dental surgery.
- Patients in contact with meningitis or TB.
- Patients undergoing surgery.

Pharmacological basis of management

The aim of pharmacological treatment is the selective destruction of pathogens without harming human cells. Possible targets are mechanisms unique to pathogens and include protein synthesis and disruption of the unique construction and presence of a cell wall.

β-Lactam antibiotics (penicillins, cephalosporins)

Penicillins: amoxicillin, ampicillin, benzylpenicillin, flucloxacillin, phenoxymethylpenicillin

Penicillins target bacterial cell wall synthesis, by inhibiting cross-linking of peptide side chains, and so are effective only against dividing organisms. Penicillins are thus bactericidal, causing lysis of the bacteria. Some penicillins are inactivated by β-lactamases secreted by resistant bacteria (see below). Benzylpenicillin is active only after parenteral administration.

Cephalosporins, e.g. cefaclor, cefalexin, cefotaxime, cefradine, cefuroxime

Cephalosporins exhibit similar pharmacology to penicillins, binding to β-lactam-binding sites and inhibiting cell wall synthesis. They show cross-reactivity with penicillins and approximately 10% of penicillin-allergic patients will also be allergic to cephalosporins.

Glycopeptides: teicoplanin, vancomycin

These also inhibit bacterial cell wall synthesis by inhibiting the growth of the peptidoglycan chain.

Antibiotics that target bacterial protein synthesis

Tetracyclines, e.g. doxycycline, minocycline, oxytetracycline, tetracycline

Tetracyclines are bacteriostatic following inhibition of protein synthesis, through interference with tRNA binding. They are broad-spectrum antibiotics taken up into bacteria by active transport. Resistance has reduced the clinical indications for tetracyclines (Table 32.2).

Aminoglycosides: amikacin, gentamicin, neomycin, tobramycin

Aminoglycosides bind irreversibly to the bacterial ribosomes, leading to an inhibition of protein synthesis. They enter the bacterial cells via an oxygen-dependent active transport process and are therefore less effective against anaerobes. The bactericidal activity of aminoglycosides is enhanced when they are used with agents that target cell wall synthesis such as penicillins and vancomycin.

Macrolides, e.g. azithromycin, clarithromycin, erythromycin

Macrolides prevent the translocation movement of the bacterial ribosome along the mRNA and so prevent protein synthesis, resulting in bacteriostatic actions. In some organisms they are bactericidal.

Quinolones, e.g. ciprofloxacin, norfloxacin, ofloxacin

These are bacterial DNA gyrase inhibitors, which inhibit the supercoiling of the bacterial DNA that is essential for DNA repair and replication. This group of agents is bactericidal.

Others

- Clindamycin inhibits protein synthesis by a similar mechanism to the macrolide antibiotics (see above).
- Chloramphenicol inhibits protein synthesis by binding to the bacterial ribosome and inhibiting the formation of peptide bonds.
- Fusidic acid is a narrow-spectrum antibiotic inhibiting predominantly protein synthesis by Gram-positive bacteria.

Sulphonamides and trimethoprim

Sulphonamides inhibit the growth of bacteria (bacteriostatic) by inhibiting the enzyme dihydropteroate synthase involved in the synthesis of folate from *p*-aminobenzoic acid. The availability of DNA and RNA precursors is therefore reduced. Human folate synthesis is also reduced, although it may be obtained from the diet. The presence of thymidine and purines from pus and tissue breakdown bypass the need for folic acid, thereby reducing the effectiveness of these agents in such situations.

Trimethoprim is structurally related to folate, thereby acting as a folate antagonist and inhibiting dihydrofolate reductase, which converts folate to tetrahydrofolate. Previously, trimethoprim was widely used in combination with sulfamethoxazole (co-trimoxazole), but the side effects of sulfamethoxazole are pronounced and therefore trimethoprim tends to be used alone.

Table 32.2 Some antibiotic sensitivities

Antibiotic	Sensitivities	Comments and indications
Penicillins (phenoxymethylpenicillin)	Streptococcal (including *Streptococcus pneumoniae*), *Neisseria gonorrhoea* and *N. meningitidis* infection	• Phenoxymethylpenicillin is less active than benzylpenicillin but may be given orally for respiratory tract infections in children, streptococcal tonsillitis and as prophylaxis against streptococcal infections following rheumatic fever, and against pneumococcal infections after splenectomy or in sickle cell disease • Benzylpenicillin may be given intravenously for bacterial meningitis • See text for note on resistance
Penicillinase-resistant penicillin (flucloxacillin)	Penicillin-resistant staphylococci	Otitis externa, adjunct in pneumonia, impetigo, cellulitis, wound infections, osteomyelitis and endocarditis if infection is known or likely to be caused by staphylococci producing penicillinases
Broad-spectrum penicillins (ampicillin, amoxicillin)	Gram-positive and Gram-negative bacteria but inactivated by penicillinases secreted by common Gram-negative bacilli and *Staphylococcus aureus*	• Indicated for exacerbation of chronic bronchitis, otitis media and UTIs • See text for note on resistance • Co-amoxiclav is used for animal bites
Cephalosporins	Varying sensitivities to Gram-positive and -negative bacteria depending on generation of the cephalosporin	Septicaemia, pneumonia, meningitis, biliary tract infections, peritonitis and UTIs
Glycopeptides	Only Gram-positive bacteria	• Vancomycin and teicoplanin are used against MRSA infections • Vancomycin is effective against *Clostridium difficile*
Macrolides	Similar spectrum to penicillins. Also active against *Chlamydia, Mycoplasma, Campylobacter, Legionella* spp.	• Suitable alternative in patients who are allergic to penicillin • Respiratory infections, whooping cough, Legionnaires' disease, campylobacter enteritis • Poor activity against *Haemophilus influenzae*
Chloramphenicol	Broad-spectrum against mainly Gram-positive cocci and -negative bacteria	• It is associated with aplastic anaemia and systemic use is reserved for life-threatening infections such as *Haemophilus influenzae* • It is widely used for bacterial conjunctivitis
Tetracyclines	Gram-positive and -negative bacteria	• Resistance is a problem • *Chlamydia*, exacerbation of chronic bronchitis (*Haemophilus influenzae*), periodontal disease, acne, respiratory and genital mycoplasma infections

Continued

Table 32.2 (Continued)

Antibiotic	Sensitivities	Comments and indications
Quinolones	Aerobic Gram-negative bacilli, particularly *Pseudomonas aeruginosa*, *Haemophilus influenzae*, *Campylobacter* spp.	• Nalidixic acid and norfloxacin used to treat UTIs • Ciprofloxacin for respiratory infection (except pneumococcal pneumonia), UTIs, gastrointestinal infections (including typhoid), gonorrhoea and septicaemia • Ofloxacin for UTIs, lower respiratory tract infections, gonorrhoea, non-gonococcal urethritis and cervicitis • Many staphylococci are resistant to quinolones, which are therefore avoided for MRSA infections
Metronidazole	Anaerobes and protozoa	• Trichomonal vaginosis (*Gardnerella vaginalis*), giardiasis (*Giardia lamblia*), surgical and gynaecological sepsis (*Bacteroides fragilis*), pseudomembranous colitis, fungating tumours and rosacea • Resistance is common
Sulphonamides and trimethoprim	*Pneumocystis jiroveci*, meticillin-resistant *Staphylococcus* spp., some Gram-negative rods	• Decreased use due to resistance and availability of less toxic alternatives • Trimethoprim is now often used alone in place of sulfamethoxazole plus trimethoprim (co-trimoxazole) • Pneumonia in AIDS patients, toxoplasmosis and nocardosis. Acute exacerbation of chronic bronchitis, acute otitis media in children and UTI if good bacteriological evidence
Aminoglycosides	Some Gram-positive and many Gram-negative	• Gentamicin is administered systemically (thus hospital use) and plays an important role in serious infections such as septicaemia, meningitis, acute pyelonephritis and endocarditis • Inactive against anaerobes and poor activity against haemolytic streptococci and *Streptococcus pneumoniae* • Synergism with agents that target cell wall synthesis such as penicillins and vancomycin • Requires therapeutic drug monitoring (Chapter 6)
Clindamycin	Gram-positive cocci, including penicillin-resistant staphylococci, many anaerobes	• Staphylococcal joint and bone infections, e.g. osteomyelitis and intra-abdominal sepsis • Limited use due to toxic side effects

AIDS, acquired immune deficiency syndrome; MRSA, meticillin-resistant *Staphylococcus aureus*; UTIs, urinary tract infections.

Metronidazole

Metronidazole was originally developed to treat amoebiasis (protozoan infection). The mechanism of action is thought to be via DNA damage due to toxic oxygen products generated from the drug by these parasites. It is also active against anaerobic bacteria, containing nitroreductases, which activate metronidazole. It is useful for the treatment of dental abscesses, fungating tumours, pseudomembranous colitis and sepsis secondary to bowel disease when anaerobic infection is suspected.

Antituberculous drugs: ethambutol, isoniazid, pyrazinamide, rifampicin

First-line agents include a combination of isoniazid, rifampicin, ethambutol (if resistance to isoniazid is likely) and pyrazinamide. Combination therapy is given in two phases to prevent resistance. The initial phase includes the use of at least three drugs for 2 months. A combination of two drugs is then given for the continuation phase lasting 4 months or longer in drug-resistant infection, meningitis or bone/joint involvement. Intermittent regimens are recommended when compliance is a problem.

Isoniazid

Isoniazid possesses selective bacteriostatic activity against mycobacteria, with some bactericidal activity against actively dividing mycobacteria. It is actively taken up: possible inhibition of *Mycobacterium*-specific mycolic acid constituents of the cell wall is the suggested mechanism. Disruption of cell metabolism may also be involved.

Resistance occurs due to reduced penetration of the drug. Side effects include allergic skin eruptions, fever, hepatotoxicity, haematological changes, arthritis and vasculitis (see Chapter 5).

Rifampicin

Rifampicin binds to and inhibits DNA-dependent RNA polymerase in prokaryotic but not eukaryotic cells. It is also active against some Gram-positive and -negative species. Resistance occurs rapidly due to a mutation in the chromosome encoding the DNA-dependent RNA polymerase. Adverse drug reactions (ADRs) include skin eruptions, jaundice, hepatotoxicity, fever and gastrointestinal disturbances.

Ethambutol

Ethambutol inhibits the growth of mycobacteria, although resistance is common if used alone. The development of optic neuritis is dose related, with an increased risk in renal impairment. Colour blindness and reduced visual acuity may occur, so monitoring of visual symptoms is required. Additional ADRs include gastrointestinal disturbance, arthralgia, headache, dizziness and mental disturbances.

Pyrazinamide

This agent becomes tuberculostatic at acidic pH. It is effective against intracellular mycobacteria found in macrophages after phagocytosis. Pyrazinamide is most effective against rapidly dividing intracellular organisms and is most effective in the first 2 months. Unwanted effects include gout, gastrointestinal disturbances and hepatotoxicity.

Drug choice

Current guidelines can be found at the start of Section 5 of the *British National Formulary*. Local guidelines may be available from health authorities, primary care trusts or the local infectious diseases centre, and based on local sensitivities these may well differ from those in the *British National Formulary*. Table 32.2 summarizes examples of the main sensitivities of some antibiotics in regular use. Factors for consideration when prescribing antibiotics include:

- the likely causative organism
- risk of pathogen resistance
- age and sex of patient
- history of drug allergy
- tolerance of gastrointestinal side effects
- renal and hepatic function
- concurrent illnesses, e.g. epilepsy (see Table 32.3)

- concurrent drug treatment (see Table 32.4)
- route of elimination (renal excretion of active drugs resulting in therapeutic concentrations in the urinary tract, a distinct advantage in UTIs)
- is the patient pregnant or breast-feeding?
- risk factors, e.g. immunocompromised
- is the patient taking oral contraceptives?

Common organisms causing disease in humans

Bacteria are classified according to a staining method developed by Christian Gram in the nineteenth century. Gram-positive bacteria retain a solution of dye, which can be washed away from Gram-negative bacteria due to differing cell wall structures. Further nomenclature results from additional properties including morphology, the formation of spores and movement. Acid-fast bacteria are also named according to a staining reaction. For examples of disease-causing bacteria see Table 32.1; some sensitivities of antibacterial agents are indicated in Table 32.2.

Resistance

Antibiotic resistance is an increasing problem. It occurs as a result of evolution of the rapidly dividing populations of bacteria. The spread of resistance occurs by the transfer of bacteria between people and the transfer of genetic material encoding resistance properties between bacteria. Mechanisms of resistance include the following:

- Development of pumps to exclude the drug from the bacteria, e.g. resistance to quinolones.
- Impermeability of bacteria to drugs, e.g. resistance to streptomycin.
- Inactivation of the drug, e.g. production of the enzyme β-lactamase by *Staphylococcus* spp. results in the breakdown of both phenoxymethylpenicillin and benzylpenicillin. Flucloxacillin is penicillinase resistant and therefore used for treating infections caused by penicillin-resistant *Staphylococcus* spp. Alternatively, the combination of the broad-spectrum penicillin amoxicillin with clavulanic acid

may be given. Clavulanic acid inhibits β-lactamase.
- Some Gram-negative bacteria have reduced permeability of the cell wall, thereby impeding penetration of hydrophilic antibiotics to the target site.
- Alternative metabolic pathways to bypass blockade, e.g. in resistance to trimethoprim.
- Alteration in the drug target so that it is no longer recognized by the drug, e.g. in resistance to erythromycin, aminoglycosides.

Meticillin-resistant *Staphylococcus aureus*

Resistance of *Staphylococcus aureus* bacteria to the discontinued drug meticillin is known as meticillin-resistant *Staphylococcus aureus* (MRSA). MRSA has received much attention because its incidence is on the increase and is associated with significant mortality. Although the bacterium responsible for these infections may be present innocently on many individuals (e.g. colonizing the nasal passages), it poses a special problem for debilitated patients in hospital. Wounds may become infected leading to infection of major organs (e.g. the lungs), which may proceed to septicaemia.

The mechanism of resistance includes the modification of bacterial penicillin-binding sites. Treatment is indicated according to the infecting strain and currently includes vancomycin and teicoplanin. In addition to treatment, carriers may require eradication of the bacterium by using topical antiseptics such as mupirocin. New antibiotics effective against MRSA are reserved for strains resistant to conventional antibiotics and as such are currently beyond the scope of this book. These agents include linezolid (an oxazolidinone) and a combination of the streptogramin antibiotics quinupristin and dalfopristin.

Measures to limit resistance include the following:

- The use of short courses of antibiotics such as a 3-day course to treat uncomplicated UTI.
- A reduction in unnecessary use of antibiotics in the treatment of viral infections and other self-limiting infections.
- The avoidance of antibiotics on repeat prescriptions.

- The avoidance of inappropriate prescribing of broad-spectrum agents (see Table 32.2).
- Ensuring that patients complete courses of antibiotics, so that more resilient strains do not survive.
- In the case of TB, the use of combination therapy

Clostridium difficile

This 'superbug' infection is also receiving interest because it is associated with significant mortality, largely in debilitated hospital patients. Once again this bacterium is present in the gastro-intestinal tracts of many otherwise healthy individuals. Broad-spectrum antibiotic treatment may alter the normal gut flora, killing off many harmless bacterial that normally keep patho-genic bacteria in check and this may lead to an outgrowth of *Clostridium difficile*, resulting in pseudomembranous colitis, which may present as severe bloody diarrhoea. To confound the problem, the spores of this bacterium are resist-ant to heat and some disinfectants, and so the spores are widespread in hospitals and may lead to severe outbreaks.

Penicillin allergy

Reports of penicillin allergy are common and it is often difficult to distinguish between true peni-cillin allergy (see Chapter 20) and less serious ADRs. A high proportion of patients reporting penicillin allergy may lack immunoglobulin E (IgE) antibodies specific for penicillin. It has been suggested that the unnecessary use of broad-spectrum antibiotics may be avoided by perform-ing penicillin skin tests (Solensky *et al* 2002). This study revealed that patients with a previous history of true penicillin allergy might safely receive subsequent courses of penicillin after a negative skin test result.

Concurrent conditions

Although bacterial sensitivity of the causative organisms is a prime factor in the choice of appropriate antibacterial agents, concurrent con-ditions should also be taken into account. Some considerations are detailed in Table 32.3.

Children aged <12 years should not receive tetracyclines due to deposition in the teeth, leading to discoloration.

Pregnancy

The safest antibiotics for use during pregnancy are considered to be the penicillins, erythro-mycin and cephalosporins. The following drugs should be avoided or used with caution:

- Ciprofloxacin and other quinolones: adverse effects on developing cartilage have been reported in animal studies, even though there is no evidence of teratogenicity in humans.
- Co-trimoxazole: this is a folate antagonist, so there is a possible teratogenic risk.
- Fusidic acid: not known to be harmful; consider risk versus benefit.
- Gentamicin: there is a risk of auditory damage to the fetus.
- Metronidazole: avoid high doses if possible but this is an important treatment of tricho-moniasis and giardiasis infections.
- Nitrofurantoin may cause nausea.
- Tetracycline: there is a risk of deposition in growing bones and teeth and the resultant risk of fetal abnormalities if given during preg-nancy.

Breast-feeding

Amoxicillin, erythromycin or cephalosporins are appropriate for use during breast-feeding. Peni-cillins may in theory produce hypersensitivity in the infant and therefore mothers should be vigilant for signs of allergy such as a rash. Tetracyclines are not recommended, although calcium should prevent the infant from absorb-ing the small amounts present in breast milk.

Chloramphenicol eye drops as an OTC medicine

Recently, chloramphenicol eye drops were reclas-sified as an over-the-counter (OTC) medicine and may be recommended to patients aged >2 years for the treatment of bacterial conjunctivitis for a maximum of 5 days. This move is clearly to be

Table 32.3   Concurrent disease and antibiotic prescribing

Concurrent disease	Drugs to avoid or use with caution	Comments
Arrhythmias	Macrolides	Prolongation of Q–T interval
History of allergy	Penicillins (phenoxymethylpenicillin, flucloxacillin, amoxicillin, pivmecillinam)	Increased risk of penicillin hypersensitivity including urticaria, fever, joint pains, rashes, angio-oedema
Penicillin allergy	Penicillins and cephalosporins	• If possible, penicillin side effects should be differentiated from true penicillin allergy (see text) • Usually occurs within 72 h of starting treatment • Penicillin allergy is a contraindication to using penicillins and a reason not to use cephalosporins
Asthma (see also above)	Co-trimoxazole	May cause shortness of breath or pulmonary infiltrates
Epilepsy	Quinolones	May induce convulsions
Immunocompromised	All antibiotics	Higher doses are often required, as infections may be severe
Porphyria (hereditary disorder of haem biosynthesis)	Flucloxacillin, cephalosporins, erythromycin, isoniazid, sulphonamides, chloramphenicol, co-trimoxazole, trimethoprim, nitrofurantoin, nalidixic acid, tinidazole, oxytetracycline	For complete list see *British National Formulary*, Section 9.8.2
Sore throat	Broad-spectrum penicillins (ampicillin, amoxicillin)	Due to a rash with glandular fever
Psychiatric disorders	Quinolones	Discontinue if there is a psychotic reaction
Diabetes mellitus	Cephalosporins, nitrofurantoin	False-positive urinary glucose (test for reducing substances)
Myasthenia gravis	Aminoglycosides	Impairment of neuromuscular transmission
Diarrhoea	Clindamycin	Contraindicated
History of deafness	Vancomycin, gentamicin	Ototoxic

welcomed because it utilizes the pharmacist's expertise and makes readily available an effective treatment for this condition without the need to visit a doctor. However, this raises a number of issues because it requires the pharmacist to differentiate bacterial conjunctivitis from a range of other eye conditions, some of which could be potentially serious. Therefore, the pharmacist should be cautious and seek the advice of a specialist if there are any uncertainties. Indeed The Royal Pharmaceutical Society (2005) has produced detailed guidance as to when referral is essential and circumstances include: contact lenses, eye trauma, when vision is affected, con-current glaucoma and pregnancy. Furthermore, if there is treatment failure after 48 hours or the condition gets worse the patient should visit their doctor.

Despite the introduction of chloramphenicol as the first OTC antibiotic, a recent study has indicated that its use in otherwise healthy children results only in a very modest improvement in outcome (Rose *et al* 2005). Therefore, the use of chloramphenicol for most children offers little in the way of benefit as the infection usually resolves in a similar time frame. Simple measure such as bathing the eye in cotton wool soaked in sterile physiological (0.9%) saline may be helpful.

Table 32.4 Examples of drug interactions involving antibiotics

Drugs	Consequences	Comments
Aminoglycosides with furosemide	Increased risk of aminoglycoside toxicity	• Monitor carefully for signs of nephrotoxicity and/or ototoxicity • Bumetanide does not appear to interact
Aminoglycosides with vancomycin	Increased risk of nephrotoxicity due to both drugs	Monitor for signs of nephrotoxicity
Broad-spectrum antibacterials (penicillins, trimethoprim and co-trimoxazole, tetracyclines, erythromycin, metronidazole) with oral contraceptives	Rarely, contraceptive failure and pregnancy	• Additional precautions should be taken during treatment and for at least 7 days thereafter • During long-term antibiotic treatment, with oral contraceptives additional precautions are recommended for the first 3 weeks of treatment • This rare interaction is thought to be due to alterations in gut bacteria, which are involved in the enterohepatic cycling of oestrogens
Quinolones with oral contraceptives	No reports of an interaction	This combination is included in view of confusion about the interaction of antibiotics with oral contraceptives
Rifampicin with oral contraceptives	Risk of contraceptive failure and pregnancy	Additional precautions are required during treatment and for 4–8 weeks after withdrawal due to enzyme induction and accelerated metabolism of oestrogens
Quinolones (ciprofloxacin, ofloxacin) with NSAIDs and drugs lowering seizure threshold (Chapter 5)	Increased risk of seizures	• Rare and limited evidence • These drugs should not be used in combination in patients with epilepsy
Quinolones with antacids	Reduced absorption of quinolones	• Aluminium and magnesium antacids particularly may reduce serum levels to below therapeutic concentrations • Separate administration by 2–6 h
Ciprofloxacin with theophylline	Increased serum levels of theophylline	• Dose reduction (by half) is required with ciprofloxacin, enoxacin, and possibly norfloxacin • Monitor for signs of theophylline toxicity (Chapter 6)
Metronidazole, tinidazole, the cephalosporin cefamandole with alcohol	Risk of disulfiram-like reaction	• Most antibiotics do not interact with alcohol • Avoid alcohol with the drugs listed, as reaction may be frightening, although not serious
Erythromycin with alcohol	Erythromycin may increase the plasma concentrations of alcohol	• Some reports have also shown that alcohol reduces the absorption of erythromycin ethyl succinate • Drivers should be advised of this potential interaction

Continued

Table 32.4   Examples of drug interactions involving antibiotics

Drugs	Consequences	Comments
Antibiotics with warfarin	Effects of warfarin may be increased	See Chapter 16
Isoniazid with phenytoin, carbamazepine	Increased levels of anticonvulsants	Isoniazid inhibits cytochrome P450
Rifampicin with corticosteroids, oestrogens, phenytoin, carbamazepine, sulphonylureas, anticoagulants	Reduced levels	Rifampicin induces cytochrome P450, therefore increasing metabolism
Macrolides with ciclosporin	Increased levels	• Reduced ciclosporin dosage is usually required (approximately 60% with erythromycin). Monitor levels • Azithromycin appears not to interact
Erythromycin, clarithromycin, with other drugs which prolong the Q–T interval (Chapter 5)	Risk of potentially life-threatening cardiac arrhythmias	The CSM advises that the concurrent use of two or more drugs that prolong the Q–T interval should be avoided because of the risk of additive effects (CSM/MCA 1996)
Erythromycin with various drugs: alfentanil, theophylline, warfarin, atorvastatin, some benzodiazepines, nadolol, carbamazepine (may become toxic), ciclosporin, digoxin (occasionally), felodipine, omeprazole	Inhibition of metabolism and therefore increased levels	Erythromycin inhibits cytochrome P450 enzymes
Erythromycin with zafirlukast	Reduced plasma concentrations	Monitor treatment outcome with zafirlukast

CSM, Committee on Safety of Medicines; MCA, Medicines Control Agency; NSAIDs, non-steroidal anti-inflammatory drugs.

Drug interactions

Antibacterial agents comprise a diverse group of drugs and can be expected to exhibit a range of interactions. In particular, the macrolides are inhibitors and rifampacin an inducer of cytochrome P450 with the ability to alter the metabolism of a range of other drugs. An important consideration is the interaction with oral contraceptives and broad-spectrum antibiotics, which, although rare, should always be borne in mind. Some important interactions are detailed in Table 32.4.

General counselling

- Antimicrobials should be taken regularly, at evenly spaced intervals, and the prescribed course should be completed to prevent recurrence and resistance. Explaining that more resistant bacteria may survive if the course is not completed, creating an increased risk of resistance to subsequent treatment, may aid compliance.
- Women of child-bearing age should be counselled about the possible interaction between antibiotics and oral contraceptives (Table 32.4).
- Patients should be advised that antibacterial agents will take several days for an effect but,

if the condition does not resolve by the end of the course, patients should visit their GP.

- Patients should be advised not to hoard antibacterials or allow them to be used by others.
- A key point to reinforce is that colds and most sore throats are viral in origin and will not respond to antibacterial agents (see Chapter 19).
- An important point is that taking broad-spectrum antibiotics is associated with super-infection, which may lead to candidiasis and diarrhoea. If the diarrhoea is severe (possibly accompanied by pain and pyrexia), this may indicate pseudomembranous colitis and patients should contact their GP urgently. This is particularly associated with clinda-mycin treatment (see Chapters 5 and 9).
- Many antibacterial agents are associated with rashes and this is particularly true of penicillin allergy. In the case of penicillin allergy, anti-histamines may relieve the rash. However, as with any drug, if there is itching, angio-oedema or breathing difficulties, then medical attention should be sought immediately because this may be due to anaphylaxis (see Chapter 20).
- A prominent record of penicillin allergy should be made on all medical records and patients should also be advised to inform GPs, dentists, pharmacists and nurses.

Penicillins

- Penicillins should be taken an hour before food or on an empty stomach for improved absorption, with the exception of amoxicillin.
- Penicillins should not be taken by patients with a history of penicillin allergy.
- Side effects are mild and may include diarrhoea and indigestion.
- Flucloxacillin may rarely cause jaundice.

Cephalosporins

Report increased bruising or signs of bleeding, due to possible interference with blood-clotting factors.

Quinolones

- Separate administration of antacids, particularly aluminium- and magnesium-containing preparations, by 2–6 h because these antacids may reduce serum levels to below therapeutic concentrations.
- Quinolones may impair performance of skilled tasks such as driving. Advice given in the *British National Formulary* suggests that these effects are enhanced by alcohol, but evidence presented in *Stockley's Drug Inter-actions* by Baxter (2008) suggests that quinolones do not interact with alcohol.
- Due to risk of tendon damage, the former Committee on Safety of Medicines (CSM; now know as the Commission on Human Medicines or CHM) warned that treatment should be withdrawn at the first sign of pain or inflammation (CSM/MCA 1995). The affected limb should be rested until tendon symptoms have resolved. Contact the GP immediately.

Macrolides

- Macrolides may cause nausea, so should be taken with or after food.
- Macrolides and erythromycin in particular are associated with a high incidence of nausea and vomiting.

Tetracyclines

- Do not take at the same time as milk, iron or zinc supplements, calcium supplements or indigestion remedies that may hinder absorption. Separate doses by at least 2 h.
- Swallow whole with plenty of water while sitting or standing.
- Doxycycline may cause photosensitivity, so avoid exposure to the sun or use high-factor sun cream. Avoid using sun beds and sun showers.

Metronidazole and tinidazole

- Do not take these with alcohol due to very unpleasant effects such as flushing.
- Take with or after food.
- Swallow whole and do not chew.

- Take with plenty of water.
- For treatment exceeding 10 days, consider providing advice about the increased risk of adverse effects such as peripheral neuropathy (see Monitoring below).

Trimethoprim

- Contact the GP if a rash and/or itching develop.
- If taking trimethoprim long term, report signs of bruising, bleeding, mouth ulcers or sore throat due to rare effects of this antibiotic on the blood.

Clindamycin

- Capsules should be swallowed whole with plenty of water.
- See comments above regarding diarrhoea.

Antituberculous drugs

- Soft contact lenses should not be worn during treatment with rifampicin. Gas-permeable or hard lenses are appropriate.
- The patient should report any signs of liver disease such as persistent nausea, vomiting, malaise or jaundice immediately.
- Rifampicin may colour the patient's urine orange–red.
- Isoniazid should be taken 30–60 min before food.
- The patient should report visual deterioration with ethambutol immediately. This may be irreversible if treatment is continued.
- The importance of compliance should be explained.
- Pyridoxine (vitamin B_6) should be taken with isoniazid to prevent peripheral neuropathy. Increased risk factors include diabetes mellitus, alcohol misuse, renal failure and malnutrition.

Eye drops and ointments

- Eye drops should be applied at least every 2 h and then the frequency reduced as the infection is controlled.
- Treatment should be continued for 48 h after symptoms have cleared.

- Patients should not share eye drops.
- Eye ointment may be used at night or three to four times a day if used alone.
- Remaining drops or ointment should be discarded.
- Sterile saline solution may help soothe the eyes and remove discharge.

Chloramphenicol

The introduction of chloramphenicol requires clear counselling once it is established that its use is appropriate. The following are additional counselling points:

- If there is deterioration or no improvement after 48 h then the patient should consult a doctor.
- The course is for 5 days.
- Although contact lens wearers should consult an optometrist, patients prescribed choramphenicol should not wear their contact lenses until 24 h after completing treatment.

Monitoring

Metronidazole

Laboratory and clinical monitoring is advised if treatment with metronidazole exceeds 10 days. This is due to an increased risk of adverse effects, particularly peripheral neuropathy, and possibly transient seizures, cholestatic hepatitis, jaundice and leukopenia. Full blood counts and liver function tests may be required (see Chapter 2).

Renal impairment

Many drugs require dose reduction, particularly in severe renal impairment. The following are some general considerations:

- Piperacillin: dose adjustment is required.
- Aminoglycosides: dose reduction and monitoring are required with even mild renal impairment. Plasma concentrations should be monitored due to renal and ototoxicity.
- Ethambutol: dose reduction and monitoring are required.
- Isoniazid: maximum dose recommended in severe impairment is 200 mg/day.

- Sulphonamides: maintain a high fluid intake with moderate impairment due to the risk of crystalluria.
- Tetracyclines: other than doxycycline and minocycline, may exacerbate renal failure and should not be given to patients with renal disease.
- Trimethoprim: dose reduction is required in moderate renal failure. Avoid if creatinine clearance is <10 mL/min unless plasma trimethoprim levels are monitored.

Hepatic function

Many antibiotics may cause hepatic disease see (Chapter 5) and therefore monitoring for suspected ADRs is important:

- Clindamycin: dose reduction is required.
- Co-amoxiclav: CSM warns of risk of cholestatic jaundice. Treatment should not normally exceed 14 days.
- Erythromycin may cause idiosyncratic hepatotoxicity.
- Flucloxacillin: CSM warns of a risk of cholestatic jaundice.
- Fusidic acid: impaired biliary excretion and increased risk of hepatotoxicity. A reduced dose is used if treatment is necessary.
- Isoniazid: monitor liver function tests regularly and particularly during the first 2 months of treatment.
- Metronidazole: in severe hepatic disease, the dose of metronidazole is reduced by a third and given once a day.
- Minocycline: monitor liver function tests if treatment exceeds 6 months.
- Pyrazinamide: avoid in liver disease.
- Rifampicin: monitor for toxicity.
- Tetracyclines should be avoided or used with caution in liver disease.

Over-the-counter considerations

Pharmacists are ideally placed to reassure patients and recommend symptomatic relief of infections that do not require antibiotics. Consultations about infections are particularly important in the identification of underlying disease. Patient counselling on the appropriate use of anti-infective agents and preventive measures is important, particularly in preventing drug resistance and treatment failure. General lifestyle advice (see Chapter 3) may also be appropriate.

Genitourinary infection

Recurrent UTIs or candida infections may indicate diabetes mellitus, recent antibiotic treatment or undiagnosed sexually transmitted infection (STI). Appropriate referral including the first UTI in men, pregnant women, abdominal or lower back pain, resistance to treatment and haematuria is warranted.

The following advice is important in the prevention of recurrent infection:

- The avoidance of nylon underwear (cotton is preferable).
- The importance of sexual hygiene, including urination after sexual intercourse.
- Drink plenty of water.
- Urinate frequently with double voiding (go again after 5 min).
- Cranberry juice has been shown to be effective at preventing bacteria adhering to bladder epithelial cells and may be helpful in the treatment of UTIs.
- Consider treating partners.

ADRs

Requests for antidiarrhoeal agents should be dealt with carefully to exclude possible antibiotic-associated colitis, e.g. the severity and duration of diarrhoea should be determined. Throat preparations containing local anaesthetics may cause hypersensitivity.

Drug interactions

For interactions between non-steroidal anti-inflammatory drugs or antacids and antibiotics, see Table 32.4.

Products for cystitis containing sodium are inappropriate for patients with hypertension or those prescribed lithium. Alternative products containing potassium salts should not be given to patients taking angiotensin-converting enzyme inhibitors or potassium-sparing diuretics such as spironolactone or amiloride.

Practice points

- Broad-spectrum antibiotics are more likely to result in fungal infections (vaginitis or pruritus ani) or ADRs such as pseudomembranous colitis.
- Viral infections such as simple coughs and colds and viral sore throats should not be treated with antibacterials.
- Whenever possible, an accurate diagnosis and clear documentation of penicillin hypersensitivity should be made.
- Chloramphenicol eye drops are now available as an OTC medicine and patients should be identified and counselled as appropriate. If there is any doubt as to the diagnosis the patient should be referred to his or her doctor.
- In prescribing chloramphenicol, community pharmacists might consider developing links with local opticians for assistance in diagnosis.

Self-assessment

Consider whether the following statements are true or false. In the management of bacterial infections:

1. It is important to complete the course to reduce the chances of resistance developing.
2. The use of broad-spectrum antibiotics is associated with causing diarrhoea.
3. Cephalosporins are a safe alternative in patients with a penicillin allergy.
4. Macrolides have a significant number of drug interactions through inhibition of cytochrome P450.
5. Chloramphenicol eye drops are available as an OTC medicine only for adults.

CASE STUDIES

Case 1

A 60-year-old woman requests loperamide for acute diarrhoea. On further questioning you discover that she is taking clindamycin.

Do you give loperamide?

- No! Clindamycin is associated with antibiotic-associated colitis, which is potentially fatal. This is most common in middle-aged and elderly women and particularly postoperatively. The antibiotic should be stopped immediately.

Case 2

A 65-year-old man presents at the accident and emergency department complaining of a persistent productive cough with haemoptysis and general ill health. A chest X-ray reveals a lesion.

How would TB be confirmed?

- TB is becoming more prevalent. A positive Mantoux (tuberculin test) confirms TB together with the above symptoms and possibly a sputum sample culture, although the former is the quickest means of diagnosis.

continued

CASE STUDIES (continued)

What tests would be carried out before starting drug treatment?

- Liver function tests are required, because isoniazid, rifampicin and pyrazinamide are all associated with liver toxicity. Renal function would be determined because doses of ethambutol and isoniazid may need to be adjusted. Visual acuity is monitored with ethambutol because this can cause loss of acuity, colour blindness or restriction of visual fields.

Is it necessary to treat contacts?

- Yes. Chemoprophylaxis with isoniazid for 6 months is the current recommendation.

What are the possible causes of treatment failure?

- Treatment failure may result from incorrect prescribing, poor compliance or drug resistance. Taking a sample of urine, which is orange–red when taking rifampicin, may be a useful method to monitor compliance.

Case 3
A 55-year-old male patient presents with an acute exacerbation of chronic bronchitis. He has seen adverts about overuse of antibiotics and is reluctant to take them. He reports purulent green sputum.

What is the appropriate treatment?

- Amoxicillin is an appropriate first-line treatment, assuming that this patient is not allergic to penicillin. His symptoms and history indicate the use of antibiotics and he should be advised accordingly. Amoxicillin is a broad-spectrum antibiotic covering the main organisms causing community-acquired infection, such as *Streptococcus pneumoniae*, *Haemophilus influenzae* or *Staphylococcus aureus*. Erythromycin is a suitable alternative in penicillin allergy, though drug interactions should be considered. Smoking cessation advice should be reinforced if necessary.

References

Baxter (2008). *Stockley's Drug Interactions*, 8th edn. London: Pharmaceutical Press.

Committee on Safety of Medicines/Medicines Control Agency (1995). Tendon damage associated with quinolone antibiotics. *Curr Probl Pharmacovigilance* **21**: 8.

Martin J, ed. *British National Formulary*, latest edition. London: British Medical Association and Royal Pharmaceutical Society of Great Britain.

Rose PW, Harnden A, Brueggemann AB *et al* (2005). Chloramphenicol treatment for acute infective conjunctivitis in children in primary care: a randomised double-blind placebo-controlled trial. *Lancet* **366**: 37–43.

Royal Pharmaceutical Society of Great Britain, Practice Division (2005). Practice guidance: OTC chloramphenicol eye drops. Available at: www.rpsgb.org/pdf/otcchloramphenicoleyedropsguid.pdf (accessed July 2008).

Solensky R, Earl HS, Gruchala RS (2002). Lack of penicillin resensitization in patients with a history of penicillin allergy after receiving repeated penicillin courses. *Arch Intern Med* **162**: 822–6.

Further reading

Hugo WB, Russell AD, eds (1987). *Pharmaceutical Microbiology*, 4th edn. Oxford: Blackwell Scientific Publications.

Standing Medical Advisory Committee (SMAC), subgroup on antimicrobial resistance (1998). *The Path of Least Resistance*. London: HMSO.

Online resources

www.hpa.org.uk
The website of the Health Protection Agency; provides the latest information relating to infectious diseases (accessed May 2008).

www.rpsgb.org.uk
The website of The Royal Pharmaceutical Society of Great Britain and has produced clinical guidelines on the use of a range of OTC medicines, including chloramphenicol (accessed April 2008).

33

Non-bacterial infections

The term 'parasite' describes organisms that rely on another organism or host for food and shelter without providing a positive contribution to the host. Parasitic infections therefore include bacteria, fungi, worms, viruses and protozoa. Non-bacterial infections include:

- fungal: *Candida albicans* and tinea (see Chapter 34)
- viral: herpes simplex and varicella-zoster (see Chapter 34), influenza (see Chapter 19)
- protozoan: *Plasmodium* spp. (malaria)
- helminthic: roundworms (ascariasis), thread worms (enterobiasis)
- ectoparasitic infections: head lice (*Pediculus humanus capitis*), crab lice (*Phthirus pubis*) and scabies (*Sarcoptes scabiei*).

Goals of treatment

The main aims of treatment are to:

- prevent or treat infections such as malaria
- prevent spread of lice or scabies
- prevent reinfection by implementing hygiene measures and contact tracing.

Malaria

Malaria is a potentially fatal mosquito-borne infection of red blood cells (erythrocytes) caused by the protozoan parasites *Plasmodium falciparum, P. vivax, P. ovale* and *P. malariae*. Red blood cells are destroyed by the parasites, resulting in haemolytic anaemia. Other symptoms include shivering, fever and sweating. The parasites live and reproduce inside the liver, being re-released into the bloodstream in a continuous cycle.

Drug treatment for prophylaxis of malaria

The choice of antimalarial agent depends largely on the destination of travel and the presence of resistance. Recommendations for effective prophylaxis are reviewed regularly and therefore the latest guidelines should be sought from organizations such as the National Pharmaceutical Association (NPA), the Health Protection Agency, Schools of Tropical Medicine, the Department of Health or the World Health Organization (see *British National Formulary* [BNF], Section 5.4 and Online resources at end of chapter).

4-Aminoquinolines (chloroquine)

Chloroquine is a disease-modifying antirheumatoid drug (DMARD, see Chapter 30). In protozoal infections, chloroquine becomes concentrated in infected erythrocytes as it binds to a breakdown product of haemoglobin. It then inhibits haem polymerase, an enzyme produced by *Plasmodium* spp., which prevents the parasite from digesting haemoglobin. It is therefore effective against the erythrocytic forms *P. malariae, P. ovale* and *P. vivax*. It is not, however, effective against latent forms of *P. ovale* and *P. vivax*, which reside in the liver. The resistance of *P. falciparum* to chloroquine tends to result from increased efflux of the drug and/or reduced uptake.

Quinoline methanols (quinine, mefloquine)

Quinine is active against all erythrocytic forms of *Plasmodium* spp. but is mainly used to treat

P. falciparum infections. In view of its adverse effects, it is not appropriate for prophylaxis. Quinine is an alkaloid with negative inotropic effects on the heart, a mild oxytocic effect on the uterus in pregnancy (although use is appropriate for malaria treatment) and a weak antipyretic effect. Mefloquine has no effect on hepatic forms of the parasites but is often used for prophylaxis or treatment of *P. falciparum* infection, particularly against chloroquine-resistant forms. Quinine resistance occurs after increased expression of an efflux transporter.

Drugs affecting the synthesis or utilization of folate (pyrimethamine, proguanil)

These agents exhibit activity similar to that of sulphonamides (see Chapter 32) in that they inhibit the utilization of folate by inhibiting dihydrofolate reductase. Combinations of folate antagonists with drugs targeting folate synthesis are used to produce a synergistic action resulting from blockade of different parts of the synthetic pathway.

8-Aminoquinolones (primaquine)

Primaquine is active against the latent phase of *P. ovale* and *P. vivax* and may be used in combination with other drugs such as chloroquine. It enters the parasites in the liver and is thought to inhibit mitochondrial respiration. Active metabolites may also bind to parasitic DNA. Resistance is currently rare.

Doxycycline

Doxycycline may be used as an alternative when antimalarials are contraindicated (see Chapter 32).

Artemether with lumefantrine

This combination is a relatively recent introduction for the treatment of acute uncomplicated falciparum malaria. These drugs target the conversion by the parasites of toxic haem to haemozoin in red blood cells during active infection. This stops the re-infection cycle at the blood stage.

Future developments

Work is continuing into a malaria vaccine, the first of which is expected to be licensed by approximately 2012. New antimalarial drugs are also being developed.

Drug choice

Local guidelines may be available from health authorities, primary care trusts or on the advice of the local infectious disease centre. Factors for consideration when prescribing include:

- risk of pathogen resistance
- age and sex of patient
- history of drug allergy
- concurrent disease (Table 33.1)
- is the patient pregnant or breast-feeding?
- time and destination of travel.

Patient counselling

Patients should be encouraged to consult health-care professionals at least 2 months before foreign travel to ensure time for immunizations.

Antimalarials

- Preventive measures are extremely important, even during prophylaxis with antimalarials.
- The application of repellents containing diethyltoluamide (DEET, now called diethylmethylbenzamide), with increasing concentration (up to 50%) or frequency of applications, offers greatest protection (Fradin and Day 2002). These products are suitable for children aged >2 months and during pregnancy and breast-feeding.
- Mosquito nets should be used at night. Nets impregnated with permethrin and vaporized insecticides are also effective.
- Protective clothing should be worn in the evening, after dusk.
- Patients may be concerned about side effects from antimalarials and should be advised of the importance of taking these drugs because malaria is life threatening, e.g. many people are worried about the psychiatric effects of mefloquine (see Chapter 5).

Table 33.1 The effects of concurrent disease on drug choice

Concurrent disease	Drugs to avoid or use with caution	Comments
Arrhythmias	Mefloquine, quinine, artemether with lumefantrine	Prolongation of Q–T interval (Chapter 5)
Asthma and/or eczema	Pesticides and particularly those containing alcohol	Some pesticide preparations may trigger an allergic response. All pesticides should be applied in a well-ventilated room Dimeticone or wet combing is preferred
Epilepsy	Chloroquine, mefloquine, piperazine	May induce convulsions and should therefore be avoided
Gastrointestinal disease (severe)	Chloroquine	Use with caution
Glucose-6-phosphate dehydrogenase (G6PD) deficiency	Primaquine	• G6PD activity should be assessed before starting treatment • Patients with G6PD deficiency may suffer haemolysis if given standard doses • Reduced doses are appropriate
Hepatic disease	All antimalarials with the possible exception of proguanil and atovaquone (HPA)	Avoid in severe liver disease Mefloquine may also be used in moderate impairment Chloroquine and doxycycline (with caution) are additional choices in mild impairment (HPA)
Psychiatric disorders	Mefloquine	Contraindicated for patients with a history of psychiatric disorders including depression
Psoriasis	Chloroquine	May exacerbate psoriasis
Renal impairment	Proguanil (avoid or reduce dose), piperazine	• Chloroquine, mefloquine or doxycycline are appropriate for malaria prophylaxis • The dose of chloroquine may require reduction in severe impairment • Malarone should not be used for prophylaxis in patients with creatinine clearance <30 mL/min • Piperazine should be avoided in severe renal impairment

HPA, Health Protection Agency.

- Prophylaxis is recommended for 1 week before travel (2–3 weeks for mefloquine to identify psychiatric adverse drug reactions before travel), during the stay and for 4 weeks after return with the exception of Malarone, which should be stopped 1 week after leaving.
- Any illness within 1 year of travel to an area associated with risk of malaria should be reported, particularly within the first 3 months.

Helminthic and ectoparasitic infections

Pruritus is the most common feature of the presence of worms, head lice, crabs or scabies. These parasites may then be observed, e.g. head lice on the hair or worms in the faeces. Scabies are more difficult to diagnose because they burrow under the skin, but close examination will reveal 'tracks' along the skin and a magnifying glass may be used to view the mites. Suspicion of scabies is aroused if more than one patient living in the same house is affected and often the wrists are the first sites of infection.

Pharmacological basis of management

Anthelmintics: mebendazole, piperazine

Anthelmintics target the formation of intracellular microtubules in helminths (parasitic worms). They must penetrate the cuticle of the worm or be eaten by the worm. The resultant effects are paralysis, partial digestion or an immune response to the damaged cuticle. Alternatively, helminth metabolism may be targeted. This is a species-dependent effect, explaining the varied activity of some anthelmintics.

Mebendazole is a broad-spectrum agent and may take several days to expel worms by targeting intracellular organelle function such as microtubules.

Piperazine is used to treat the common roundworm (*Ascaris lumbricoides*) and threadworm (*Enterobius vermicularis*). It inhibits neuromuscular transmission in the worm, possibly by activation of γ-aminobutyric acid (GABA)-gated chloride channels in nematode muscle, leading to muscle relaxation. The paralysed worms are passed alive. Side effects include gastrointestinal disturbance and urticaria.

Malathion, carbaryl, phenothrin, permethrin, dimeticone

Malathion and carbaryl are organophosphorous inhibitors of acetylcholinesterase, and so prevent the breakdown of acetylcholine, which causes paralysis and kills the louse. The use of carbaryl is, however, restricted to prescription use when lice are resistant to other agents. Phenothrin and permethrin are pyrethroid compounds, which also produce death by paralysis after activation of sodium channels on peripheral nerves. Dimeticone is a silicone-based substance and is used as an alternative choice to insecticidal neurotoxins; it probably acts by coating the louse and disrupting its function. Dimeticone has the advantage that it does not readily cause skin irritation

and resistance that develops to neurotoxins is not a problem.

Drug choice

Anthelmintics

These are combined with hygiene measures to prevent reinfection. Mebendazole is used to treat threadworms in patients aged >2 years. This is available over-the-counter but not for use during pregnancy. A fatty meal aids the absorption of mebendazole, which is given as a single dose for threadworm infection, or twice a day for 3 days to treat hookworms or roundworms, and repeated after 2 weeks. Mebendazole is the most commonly used benzimidazole; gastrointestinal disturbances are the main side effect.

Piperazine is an alternative, e.g. given to children aged from 3 months by a GP, as a single dose, and repeated after 14 days for threadworm infections or monthly for up to 3 months for roundworms.

Levamisole is available on a named-patient basis and is the drug of choice for the common roundworm *Ascaris lumbricoides*.

Head lice preparations

The choice of preparation depends upon previous treatment and the presence of asthma or skin sensitivity such as eczema (see Table 33.1). Dimeticone and wet combing are suitable first-line choices. Alternatively, products with an aqueous base, such as Derbac M, are preferred for people with asthma or sensitive skin, and young children. Lotions or liquid formulations are recommended rather than shampoos, mousses and cream rinses because the contact time is too short for the latter products to be effective and some preparations may be too dilute. If a previous treatment has failed, an alternative agent should be used, once the reason for treatment failure has been established, e.g. failure to apply a second application after 7 days. The presence of live head lice 7–9 days after treatment indicates the survival of eggs and therefore is not treatment failure. The same treatment should be repeated. Resistance is also becoming a problem, and this is most marked with pyrethroids but less of a problem with carbaryl (Clark 2007). Other causes of treatment failure include the following:

- Re-infection due to the lack of treatment of close contacts including parents and grand-parents.
- The product not being left on the hair for sufficient time.
- The application of conditioner before the product, which should be applied to dry hair.
- Application of too low a concentration of active ingredient.

Carbaryl

It should be noted that carbaryl preparations have been restricted to prescription-only use due to the observation that carbaryl is carcinogenic in rodents. The risk to humans is reported to be theoretical, especially if use is intermittent. Carbaryl and malathion can irritate the skin and should not be used in damaged skin or where there is infection.

Alternative treatments for head lice

A new product containing isopropyl myristate and cyclomethicone is available but reliable evidence for efficacy is not yet available (Clark 2007). Evidence is also lacking for alternatives such as tea tree oil, quassia and delphinine. Electric combs are also marketed but evidence is limited and conflicting.

Crab lice

Permethrin, phenothrin and malathion are licensed for the eradication of crab lice. Aqueous preparations are applied to all parts of the body for 12 h.

Patient counselling

Head lice preparations

Prevention

- Parents should be reassured that head lice have no preference for dirty or clean hair. Long hair may, however, be more accessible as

head lice 'walk' from head to head. They do not hop, jump or fly. Long hair should therefore be braided close to the head if possible. Shaving the hair is not an effective method because lice only need 1 mm of hair to cling to. Head lice are not harmful but may cause an itchy scalp with the risk of secondary bacterial infection after chronic scratching.
- Regular checking for lice is advisable using a fine nit comb when the hair is wet, going through a small section at a time. This will help to remove lice, aid early diagnosis and prevent the spread of head lice. The excessive use of pesticides may then be prevented. The use of conditioner may help the manual removal of lice. The eggs may appear similar to dandruff but are differentiated by their ability to stick to the hair.
- The presence of lice should be confirmed before treating, because infection is not prevented by treatment. The hair may be combed over white paper to identify live lice.
- Contact tracing is important to prevent spread of the infection. This includes all close contacts such as grandparents who should be treated if infected.

Wet combing

Wet combing is useful for detection and treatment of head lice infestation and some products for this method can be prescribed. However, this is not necessarily an easy option because to fully wet comb the hair can take a significant amount of time. The *British National Formulary* recommends an interval of 4 days and a minimum of 2 weeks with hair conditioner or vegetable oil used to make combing and removal of eggs and lice easier. An appropriate comb should be used from the scalp to the ends of the hair and lice removed after each stroke. Conditioner can then be washed off. Information leaflets with detailed instructions about wet combing should be provided. Weekly wet combing is recommended for detection if head lice are present in a school or nursery (Clark 2007). Note that metal combs are not appropriate for wet combing but can be useful for removing noticeable nits.

Table 33.2   Examples of drug interactions with antiparasitic agents

Drugs	Consequences	Comments
Antimalarials with antacids or antidiarrhoeals	Reduced absorption of chloroquine and proguanil	Doses of antimalarials and antacids (particularly magnesium trisilicate or kaolin) should be separated by at least 2–3 h
Antimalarials with warfarin	Increased effects of warfarin and other anticoagulants	• Chloroquine does not appear to interact and interactions with proguanil are rare • A baseline INR should be checked and then re-checked 1 week after taking malaria prophylaxis (HPA)
Mefloquine or quinine with drugs which prolong the Q–T interval (Chapter 5)	Increased risk of arrhythmias	• Mefloquine and quinine prolong the Q–T interval • The WHO has warned that mefloquine should be used with caution with concurrent antiarrhythmics, β blockers, calcium channel blockers, antihistamines or phenothiazines
Mefloquine or chloroquine with other drugs which lower the convulsive threshold (Chapter 5)	Increased risk of convulsions	Consider patient with increased risk (Chapter 5)
Chloroquine with cimetidine	Increased effects of chloroquine due to reduced hepatic metabolism	• Risk of increased adverse effects of chloroquine • Ranitidine may be a suitable alternative
Mebendazole with cimetidine	Increased levels of mebendazole	Monitor for adverse effects of mebendazole
Mebendazole with phenytoin or carbamazepine	Reduced levels of mebendazole	Increased doses of mebendazole may be required but not when treating infections of the gut
Mefloquine with β blockers, calcium channel blockers, digoxin or antidepressants	Increased risk of bradycardia	Concurrent use should be avoided if possible, particularly for patients considered to be at increased risk of developing bradycardia, until more is known about these interactions
Quinine with cimetidine	Increased levels of quinine	• Monitor for adverse effects of quinine • Ranitidine is a suitable alternative

INR, international normalized ratio; HPA, Health Protection Agency; WHO, World Health Organization.

Treatment

- Treatment is most likely to be successful if patients understand the mode of action of preparations for head lice and the life-cycle of lice. This enforces the likelihood of a second application being required after 7 days. A leaflet should be provided alongside verbal advice.
- Most products require a 12-h application and should be applied to dry hair at night, in a well-ventilated room. The hair and scalp should be soaked in the product and then allowed to dry naturally. The hair may then be washed the following morning.
- A second application is required after 7 days, after which time any eggs not eradicated by the initial treatment may begin to hatch. This should not be confused with treatment failure or reinfestation.

- Repeat applications should be avoided within a week and for more than 3 consecutive weeks. The manufacturers suggest that not more than five applications of head lice preparations be used per year. The likelihood of eradication is not increased.
- It should be noted that Full Marks mousse contains alcohol and may not be suitable for patients with asthma or eczema.

Crab lice

Apply aqueous lotion to all parts of the body, including scalp, neck, ears and face, for 12 h. A second treatment is recommended after 7 days to kill lice hatching from eggs, which may have survived the initial treatment (BNF).

Anthelmintics

- Combine with hygiene measures to break the cycle of reinfection. Hands should be washed and nails scrubbed before each meal and after each visit to the toilet. A bath immediately after rising will remove ova laid during the night. Fingernails should be kept short.
- A second dose may be required to prevent reinfection.
- Infected patients should use separate towels.
- Avoid using dirty towels in public toilets.
- All members of the same household should be treated, even if asymptomatic.

Concurrent conditions

Table 33.1 provides examples of the influence of concurrent disease on the choice of non-antibiotic anti-infective drugs.

Pregnancy

Antimalarials

Ideally, travel to areas with malaria should be avoided during pregnancy but proguanil and chloroquine may be used. Folic acid 5 mg supplementation is required with proguanil. Mefloquine is considered for areas of chloroquine resistance but the manufacturer recommends that it should be avoided. Malarone is used only if there is no alternative. Doxycycline is contraindicated.

Anthelmintics

Mebendazole should be avoided during the first trimester. The *British National Formulary* reports a lack of evidence of harm with piperazine but the manufacturer advises avoidance of use during the first trimester.

Head lice

Dimeticone or wet combing is preferred. Malathion products were used before the introduction of dimeticone.

Drug interactions

Table 33.2 summarizes examples of drug interactions with antimalarial and anthelmintic drugs.

Self-assessment

Consider whether the following statements are true or false. In the management of non-bacterial infections:

1. Insecticides are a useful prophylactic treatment for recurrent head lice.
2. Doxycycline is a suitable choice for a pregnant woman travelling to an area with malaria.
3. Doxycycline is a suitable choice for a patient with epilepsy.
4. Proguanil, atovaquone, doxycycline and mefloquine do not exacerbate psoriasis.
5. Doxycycline can affect progestogen-only contraception.

Practice points

Malaria

- The latest guidelines should always be consulted when recommending malaria prophylaxis due to increased resistance and the potentially fatal nature of this disease.
- Pharmacists should be vigilant of flu-like symptoms in patients who have recently returned from abroad, particularly from regions associated with malaria.

Helminthic and ectoparasitic infections

- Contact tracing should be encouraged when eliminating head lice.
- Hygiene measures are important when recommending treatment for worms and head lice.
- Repeat applications of pesticides are generally recommended after 7–9 days for head lice.
- The mosaic approach to head lice treatment is no longer used. Current recommendations consist of using a different insecticide for a second application after treatment failure.
- A leaflet should be provided alongside verbal information, e.g. *The Prevention and Treatment of Head Lice* is available from the Department of Health (www.dh.gov.uk).
- Pharmacists should refer treatment failure and infants aged <6 months for assessment of scabies. Pharmacists may wish to refer to a GP patients exceeding five applications of pesticide per year and when counselling has failed.

References

Clark C (2007). Head lice treatments and advice. *Pharm J* **279**:185–8.

Fradin MS, Day JF (2002). Comparative efficacy of insect repellents against mosquito bites. *N Engl J Med* **347**: 13–18.

Martin J, ed. *British National Formulary*, latest edition. London: British Medical Association and Royal Pharmaceutical Society of Great Britain.

Further reading

Marshall S (2008). Malaria: the issues and advice. *Pharm J* **280**: 603–6.

Online resources

www.hpa.org.uk
The Health Protection Agency for information on infectious diseases including an informative section on malaria with answers to commons questions (accessed April 2008).

www.fitfortravel.scot.nhs.uk
The website for National Health Service (Scotland) travel and health information (accessed April 2008).

www.chc.org
For Community Hygiene Concern, a charity providing information on parasitic infections such as head lice, including *Bug busting* product information (accessed April 2008).

www.who.int/ith
The website for World Health Organization travel and health information (accessed April 2008).

Part I
Dermatology

34

Dermatology

Dermatology is a relatively specialized area but the pharmacist has important roles, which include:

- identifying and treating common skin diseases or advising appropriate referral
- recognizing skin conditions caused by an adverse drug reaction (ADR), including topical preparations (see *British National Formulary*, Section 13.1.3 for excipients associated with sensitization)
- dispensing and monitoring treatment in more complicated cases
- identifying and referring serious skin diseases or serious diseases presenting with skin changes.

Dermatology encompasses common conditions such as eczema and skin infections and serious (such as skin cancers) and rare conditions, which are only likely to be dealt with by hospital specialists. In addition, ADRs may manifest as dermatological changes, which are considered in Chapter 5. This chapter concentrates on common skin conditions including eczema, psoriasis, acne, fungal infections and some cancers. In order to aid recognition of dermatological conditions the reader is referred to the many textbooks and atlases of dermatology, such as *Dermatology in Focus* by Wilkinson *et al* (2005).

Eczema

Disease characteristics

This is a common inflammatory skin condition, which has many forms. Within dermatology, the terms 'eczema' and 'dermatitis' are both used but eczema should be used for the endogenous inflammatory conditions and dermatitis for reactive changes, e.g. to allergens. Examples of eczema/dermatitis include:

- atopic or infantile eczema
- irritant contact dermatitis
- allergic contact dermatitis
- seborrhoeic eczema: cradle cap in infants and a dry and itchy scalp in older children and adults.

In addition, rarer forms include pompholyx (vesicles on hands or feet, which may be related to heat, stress or a reaction to fungal foot infections, or may be cryptogenic), hyperkeratotic palmar eczema (typically occurring in middle age and presenting with fissured eczema on hands), asteatotic eczema (reduced lipids in the skin, drying and cracking, which give rise to a 'crazy paving' appearance) and discoid eczema (rare, discoid lesions, perhaps related to alcohol abuse).

Atopic eczema

Atopic or infantile eczema is the most common form of eczema and is associated with an inherited tendency for asthma and hayfever. It often appears in babies at around 3 months of age and, by the age of 5, almost a third of children will have been diagnosed as having atopic eczema at some stage. Fortunately, most children grow out of the condition. It is characterized by the following:

- Prominent pruritus: this is a central feature and its absence may suggest another condition.
- Itchy papules on the cheeks.

- The skin is often dry or inflamed and licheni-fied, especially around the flexures of the elbows and knees.
- There may be sensitivity to allergens. The dry and inflamed skin may be aggravated by cold, heat, hard water, infections and clothes (especially wool).
- The affected area is often scratched and may become infected, particularly with staphylo-cocci or streptococci, and this may lead to a flare of eczema and, sometimes, impetigo. Viral infection with herpes simplex (eczema herpeticum) leads to painful vesicles and is a serious complication requiring immediate antiviral treatment.

Management

Guidelines for the management of eczema have been produced on behalf of the British Association of Dermatologists (and for children, by the National Institute for Health and Clinical Excellence or NICE 2007) and these should be consulted.

The initial treatment is regular use of emollients, which hydrate the skin and prevent drying. Emollients have a range of constituents that may include liquid and soft paraffins and cetomacrogol. The most effective are the oily emollients but these may be cosmetically less acceptable. To prevent dehydration of the skin, soap and bubble bath should be avoided, and bathing should be with emollient bath oils and use of emollient creams as a soap substitute. Other lifestyle measures include keeping the house cool (to reduce itchiness), limiting allergens such as house-dust mite (see Chapter 20) and cutting the child's nails to reduce scratching.

Pharmacological management

Topical steroids

When emollients are not sufficient, topical steroids should be considered for treatment, especially in inflamed eczema. Topical 1% hydrocortisone is the first-line agent and is the only agent suitable for infants aged <1 year. It is very effective at reducing the inflammatory response and should be used for short bursts of aggressive treatment rather than occasional 'dabbing'.

Ointments give better skin penetration for the steroid than creams, although creams are less greasy and may be more acceptable to patients. Topical 1% hydrocortisone is a mild corticosteroid and is rarely associated with side effects. However, failure of treatment may lead to the short-term use of more potent corticosteroids such as hydrocortisone butyrate, betamethasone and clobetasol propionate to bring the condition under control. These are, however, more likely to be associated with side effects, especially if used for prolonged periods or excessively, and these include:

- secondary infections due to immunosuppression
- thinning of the skin
- telangiectasia (appearance of dilated arterioles in the skin due to thinning)
- acneiform lesions
- glaucoma which may be caused by application near to the eyes or on the eyelids; use with caution
- mild depigmentation
- pituitary–adrenal axis suppression
- Cushing's syndrome.

If oral steroids (e.g. prednisolone) are used in severe disease, height suppression is an important side effect in children and this should be monitored. However, it may be appropriate to use 'steroid-sparing' approaches as described below in preference.

The steroid creams may also be combined with topical antibacterial agents or antifungal agents to prevent infection. Oral antibacterial agents may also be required occasionally to bring any infections under control.

Topical calcineurin inhibitors: tacrolimus and pimecrolimus

These are a relatively new addition to therapy and have immunosuppressant actions similar to ciclosporin. They act indirectly by interfering with the induction of interleukin-2 (which is involved in cell growth and differentiation) in T lymphocytes and so dampen down the immune response. These agents are now available for use as topical agents by dermatologists for patients with moderate-to-severe disease who are unsuitable for or who do not respond to topical steroid treatment. In the case of pimecrolimus, it is recommended for use on the face and neck of children (>2 years).

Oral antihistamines

Non-sedating antihistamines may be of benefit where there is marked itching. Some practitioners might use sedating agents where scratching interferes with sleep.

Additional treatments

Ultraviolet phototherapy is used by hospital dermatologists in some patients.

Counselling

Lifestyle measures are the first step and are detailed earlier.

Emollients

- These are best applied after bathing when the skin is hydrated.
- They may sting on application.
- They should be applied liberally at least twice daily.
- They should be used even after the condition has improved.
- Paraffin-based emollients are associated with a fire hazard and patients should be advised not to smoke when using large amounts of these products, and to keep away from flames.

Topical steroids

The use of topical steroids requires clear counselling:

- They are very effective and safe in the treatment of eczema if they are used correctly.
- Steroids have different potencies and mildly potent agents such as topical hydrocortisone have few side effects. More potent steroids may be used to bring the eczema under control.
- Apply the cream or ointment thinly.
- The steroid should be applied once or twice daily as directed.
- Avoid application to the face (unless specifically prescribed). This is to limit systemic absorption, facial telangiectasia and acne.

- Avoid application to the anogenital region (unless specifically prescribed) to limit systemic absorption.
- Over-the-counter (OTC) use of hydrocortisone is appropriate only for children aged >10 years for 7 days. Longer treatment or application to the face or anogenital region requires referral to the GP.
- Clobetasone cream is available over the counter for short-term symptomatic control of eczema and dermatitis (except seborrhoeic dermatitis) for adults and children aged >12 years.
- Avoid application to infected areas including cold sores, acne and fungal infections (in the absence of a concomitant antifungal agent).
- The preparation is applied in 'fingertip units' in adults:
  - hand: 1 unit
  - face: 2.5 units
  - arm: 3 units
  - leg: 6 units
  - foot: 2 units
  - front of trunk: 7 units
  - back of trunk: 7 units.

Contact dermatitis

This is also a common form of eczema, which is either an irritant reaction to chemicals such as detergents or an allergic reaction to chemicals such as nickel, cosmetics and creams (e.g. some constituents such as lanolin, sodium stearate). It is characterized by inflammation with dryness and chapping after exposure to the irritant or allergen. The initial management is to remove or avoid the cause, coupled with emollients, barrier creams, topical steroids or oral antihistamines as appropriate. Occupational causes should be referred for patch testing to identify the irritant.

Napkin dermatitis

This form of contact dermatitis is due to the irritant effects of ammonia from faeces and urine in the nappy region and may often coexist with fungal infection. In napkin rash that results solely from irritation, the skin folds are relatively spared, because there is less contact in these areas. Treatment should include improved hygiene, such as frequent nappy changes, leaving the nappy off for a time and washing, with the application of barrier creams (e.g. dimeticone) to prevent contact and emollients to hydrate the skin. In more severe dermatitis not responding to these measures 1% hydrocortisone cream may be prescribed for up to a week. Fungal infection should be suspected if the skin folds are affected or there are small red dots, because the fungi may spread. Accordingly, antifungal treatment with a topical imidazole, clotrimazole (see later), is appropriate, often with hydrocortisone to reduce the inflammation. Bacterial infections may present as pustules.

Seborrhoeic eczema

In infants this manifests on the scalp as cradle cap, for which there are a number of preparations, some of which include oils to soften the skin and facilitate removal.

In children and adults seborrhoeic eczema may present as a dry and flaky scalp for which corticosteroid lotions are effective. The condition may be related to a hypersensitivity to yeast infection due to *Pityrosporum* spp. and ketoconazole shampoo is effective.

Other forms

In relation to the rarer forms of eczema, pompholyx may be managed by potent topical steroids and potassium permanganate. Oral antihistamines may provide symptomatic relief and, if the condition is a reaction to a fungal infection, this should be treated with antifungal agents (see later). Hyperkeratotic palmar eczema is treated with emollients, topical steroids, keratolytics and, in severe disease, immunosuppressants. Asteatotic eczema is treated with emollients, emollient bath oils and weak topical steroids. Discoid eczema is treated with emollients and steroids.

Psoriasis

This is a reasonably common inflammatory skin condition that affects 2–3% of the population and is due to rapid epidermal transit caused by increased cell division and increased passage of keratinocytes through the epidermis. As part of the inflammatory response, there is infiltration of the dermis with lymphocytes and the epidermis with neutrophils. The release of cytokines and lymphokines stimulates keratinocyte proliferation and alters their maturation.

The most common form is plaque psoriasis, which presents as a well-demarcated, erythematous region with thick silvery scales, and is associated with pruritus. The plaques may be localized to a few areas or are extensively distributed. Less common forms include guttate psoriasis ('raindrop' lesions that may follow a streptococcal throat infection in younger patients), pustular psoriasis (a rare and serious condition, which presents as sterile pustules) and flexural psoriasis (well-demarcated erythematous regions). Decreased levels of cAMP (adenosine cyclic 3':5'-monophosphate) are found in lesions and β blockers may exacerbate the condition. In addition, lithium may exacerbate psoriasis.

Pharmacological management

There are a number of pharmacological approaches to psoriasis that may be tried and used according to their response. A central theme of the agents used is to reduce the proliferation of dermal cells and the inflammatory response, which contribute to the condition.

Emollients

As with eczema, emollients play an important role in hydrating the skin and should be used widely.

Topical steroids

Their anti-inflammatory actions may be of benefit but they may become less effective on continued use and there may be rebound effects on withdrawal.

Topical dithranol

This is often used first line in plaque psoriasis and has antiproliferative properties by inhibiting mitotic activity. It may lead to hypersensitivity and so patch testing is sometimes used before treatment. The ability of this agent to stain skin and clothes may limit its acceptability with patients.

Topical vitamin D₃ analogues: calcipotriol, tacalcitol

Vitamin D₃ analogues act on keratinocyte vitamin D receptors, with antiproliferative actions, and reduce epidermal proliferation. They are also anti-inflammatory through their interference with the release of cytokines and suppression of both lymphocyte proliferation and neutrophil accumulation. Calcipotriol has now been formulated with betamethasone (in Dovobet) and appears to give good control of stable plaque psoriasis.

Coal tar

The keratolytic, antipruritic and anti-inflammatory actions of coal tar provide relief.

Phototherapy

Phototherapy with ultraviolet A (UVA) reduces dermal cell proliferation by interfering with DNA synthesis and reduces lymphocyte infiltration of the psoriatic epidermis. In extensive disease, the patients are treated with oral or topical methoxsalen (a psoralen) as a photosensitizing agent, to enhance the effects of UVA, and this is known as PUVA (psoralen UVA). Alternatively, the patient may receive narrow-band UVB treatment, which does not require a photosensitizing agent.

Oral retinoids: acitretin

Acitretin (a metabolite of etretinate) binds to nuclear retinoic acid receptors and affects gene transcription, resulting in antiproliferative actions and normal keratinocyte maturation. It should be avoided in pregnancy and in females of child-bearing age; adequate contraception should be used and conception should be delayed for 2 years after stopping treatment. Acitretin may also alter the lipid profile by increasing plasma triglycerides and cholesterol, so this should be monitored along with liver function tests. Tazarotene is available as a topical retinoid.

Other treatments

Low-dose methotrexate is used by dermatologists for its cytotoxic actions, which reduce cellular turnover. Ciclosporin is also used by dermatologists for its immunosuppressant actions. In addition, etanercept and infliximab are now used by specialists in severe and refractory disease (see Chapter 30).

Counselling

Emollients and steroids

See earlier.

Dithranol

- This should be applied for 30–60 min and then washed off.
- It should be applied only to the lesions.
- It may stain skin and clothes.
- Patients should wash their hands thoroughly after application.

Oral acitretin

- This agent is teratogenic and should not be used during pregnancy. In females, conception should be delayed for at least 2 years after the patient has stopped taking the drug.
- Acitretin may also cause cracked and dried lips, which may be helped by the application of Vaseline.
- It may cause a drying of mucous membranes.
- It may cause thinning of the skin.
- The effects may be delayed for 2–4 weeks.
- The patient should not donate blood for at least 1 year after stopping treatment.
- Excessive exposure to sunlight should be avoided.

Acne

Acne vulgaris is a common condition, typically affecting teenagers, but in a few patients it may persist beyond these years. It is due to excessive sebum production in response to androgens, and results in the formation of comedones and pustules. Closed comedones are white cysts and open comedones are blackheads.

The bacterium *Propionibacterium acnes* is present in the skin and can lead to inflammatory lesions. The lipid-rich sebum favours the growth of *P. acnes,* which produces lipases that act on the sebum to release fatty acids, favouring comedone formation. The *P. acnes* also activates the complement system, leading to the release of proteases, which cause inflammation. Pustules form as part of the inflammatory lesions.

Management

In the mild form of the disease, general cleansing may provide relief. There is no evidence that altering the diet will bring about an improvement. The treatments for acne are directed against the comedones and/or the infected lesions and the following are used.

Topical agents

Topical benzoyl peroxide
Topical benzoyl peroxide is used for its keratolytic and bactericidal properties and is used in all forms of acne.

Azelaic acid
This may be used as an alternative to benzoyl peroxide and is less irritating.

Topical retinoids
If topical benzoyl peroxide fails, then topical applications of retinoids (tretinoin and isotretinoin) are used for their keratolytic actions by reducing adhesion between epidermal cells. The main adverse effect is skin irritation. Retinoids are teratogenic and are used only in patients who are not pregnant.

Topical antibiotics
The topical antibiotics erythromycin, tetracycline or clindamycin are prescribed. When used alone they are ineffective against comedones but in pustular disease they are as effective as tretinoin and benzoyl peroxide. However, resistance may develop and this may be partly overcome by combining either zinc (such as Zineryt, which is erythromycin plus zinc acetate) or benzoyl peroxide with the antibiotic. They are often used for a 10- to 12-week trial.

Systemic treatments

Oral antibiotics
In moderate-to-severe acne or when there is a poor response to topical treatments, oral antibiotics are used. Tetracycline is used first line, with oxytetracycline, minocycline, erythromycin, clindamycin or trimethoprim as alternatives. The penetration of the antibiotics into the sebaceous glands is low and so treatment can take up to 3–4 months for an effect; maximal effects may take up to 2 years. Tetracycline and erythromycin may exert additional anti-inflammatory actions, independent of their antibacterial activity.

When minocycline is used for more than 6 months the *British National Formulary* recommends that hepatotoxicity, skin pigmentation and signs of systemic lupus erythematosus are monitored every 3 months.

Oral retinoids (tretinoin and isotretinoin)
A failure of oral antibiotics or severe acne may lead to referral to a dermatologist, who may prescribe the oral retinoid isotretinoin. This inhibits sebum production by reducing the number and activity of sebaceous glands. It can be highly effective but is associated with depression. It may also alter the lipid profile by increasing plasma triglycerides and cholesterol, so this should be monitored along with liver function tests. It is teratogenic and used only in patients who are not pregnant and who should be advised to avoid conception for at least 1 month after stopping treatment.

Hormonal therapy

In females only, co-cyprindiol (oral cyproterone, a testosterone receptor antagonist, plus ethinylestradiol) may be used because it will alter the hormonal balance away from androgens.

Counselling

General counselling should include hygiene advice and emphasize the importance of not touching lesions, to reduce the spread of infection.

Benzoyl peroxide

- It may bleach hair and clothes.
- It may irritate the skin and cause dryness.
- Apply once daily in the evening to begin with, in case there is redness or peeling.
- If there is irritation, reduce the frequency or stop and consider reintroducing gradually.
- Apply to the affected area, not just the spots.

Topical retinoids

- These are a photoirritant: patients should avoid UV sun beds and may need to wear sunscreen in the sunshine.
- Topical retinoids are teratogenic and females should take adequate contraceptive measures.

Oral antibiotics

- See Chapter 32.
- Broad-spectrum antibiotics may reduce the effectiveness of combined oral contraceptives containing ethinylestradiol (by altering the gastrointestinal flora), so alternative barrier contraceptive measures should be used. This reduction in effectiveness lasts for only 3 weeks because resistance within the gastrointestinal flora develops, so additional measures need be taken only for this time.
- Patients developing severe diarrhoea while taking antibiotics (especially clindamycin) should stop taking them and consult their GP urgently.
- An improvement may take 3–4 months.

Oral isotretinoin

- This is teratogenic and females must not become pregnant during treatment and for at least 1 month after treatment.
- Patients should not donate blood during treatment and for 1 month afterwards.
- This drug may cause depression.
- Patients should not exceed the daily allowance of vitamin A and should not take supplements containing vitamin A without consulting their pharmacist or GP.
- Patients should not take other products for acne unless advised to by their GP or dermatologist.
- Isotretinoin may cause thinning of the skin: patients should not wax or epilate their skin for 5–6 months after stopping treatment. Vaseline may be helpful in preventing dry and cracked lips. Dry eyes may also affect vision and hypromellose eye drops may be helpful.
- Patients should avoid strong sunlight and UV light and wear sunblock if exposed.

Co-cyprindiol

- As with other oestrogen-containing contraceptives, there is a risk of thromboembolism, which is compounded by other risk factors such as smoking and increased age (see Chapter 3).
- An improvement may take several months.
- This should be used as a contraceptive only for patients with severe acne or hirsutism because there is an increased risk of thromboembolism compared with other hormonal contraceptives. Treatment should be stopped 3–4 months after complete resolution of symptoms (Medicines and Healthcare products Regulatory Agency or MHRA).

Rosacea

Rosacea is an inflammatory condition with acneiform lesions, and telangiectasia (prominent and dilated arterioles) but without comedones. It is more common in women with fair skin, especially around the menopause. It may be precipitated by sunshine, alcohol and spicy foods.

Hypertrophy of sebaceous glands around the nose may lead to an enlargement, rhinophyma, which is more common in men.

Management

The first active treatment is topical metronidazole gel (0.75%) and this may be followed by oral erythromycin or tetracycline. β Blockers or clonidine may be used to help the symptoms of flushing. Sunscreen should be used to reduce the effects of the sun.

Fungal infections

The skin is a common site of fungal infection due to tinea (dermatophyte) or *Candida* spp., and is commonly encountered in primary care. Common forms are as follows.

Ringworm (tinea infections)

This may occur at different sites on the body, as shown in Table 34.1.

Pityriasis versicolor

This is a relatively common condition, which presents as hypo- or hyperpigmented macules. It is due to infection by the yeast *Pityrosporum* spp.

Candidiasis

This is a common yeast infection due to *Candida albicans* and is known as thrush. It commonly affects the skin and mucous membranes. Skin infections tend to present as moist, inflamed regions, which are less well demarcated than in tinea infection, presenting with pain and itching. The infections are favoured by warm and moist skin folds, such as the groin, breasts, armpits and buttocks, especially in obese individuals (intertrigo). Mouth infections present as white patches and vaginal infections as pruritus with a creamy discharge, which is sometimes described as being like cottage cheese in appearance although it is sometimes watery. Candidiasis is favoured by the use of antibiotics and corticosteroids in diabetes mellitus, eczema and immunocompromised patients. Patients who have recurrent candidiasis should be investigated to exclude diabetes mellitus. It may also present as angular stomatitis at the corner of the mouth. Nails may be affected and become discoloured.

Management

In superficial infections, simple hygiene measures should be advocated and these may involve thorough drying after washing, not sharing towels and avoiding occlusive clothing (e.g. nylon). In athlete's foot, more frequent changes of socks and shoes may help.

Topical imidazoles: clotrimazole, miconazole, tioconazole

These act to inhibit a cytochrome P450-dependent demethylase which converts lanosterol to ergosterol, a fungal membrane lipid. This results in the accumulation of lanosterol which disrupts the membrane phospholipids. The imidazoles are fungistatic and so must be used for about

Table 34.1   The different forms, sites and features of tinea infection

Form	Site	Features
Tinea corporis	Trunk and limbs	Discoid, erythematous scaly plaques
Tinea capitis	Scalp	Bald, scaly patches
Tinea pedis (athlete's foot)	Between the toes	May present as scaling or inflammation between the toes
Tinea unguium	Nails	Nails become yellow and crumbly
Tinea cruris	Groin	Reddened and scaly groin.

2 weeks after healing to prevent a relapse. They are widely used in superficial skin infections and are effective against both tinea and candidal infections.

Oral imidazoles and triazoles ('azoles')

The imidazole ketoconazole and the triazoles itraconazole and fluconazole are orally active and act via inhibition of cytochrome P450-dependent demethylase, as described above. The azoles are associated with hepatotoxicity. The prescribing of oral ketoconazole has been restricted because of this risk and increased monitoring of liver function is recommended during treatment (MHRA).

Polyenes: nystatin

This polyene macrolide binds to fungal ergosterol in the cell membrane. It disrupts the cells and is effective in candidiasis but not tinea.

Allylamines: terbinafine

Terbinafine inhibits the conversion of squalene to lanosterol, with the accumulation of squalene causing cell death. This fungicidal action has the advantage that shorter treatment courses are required. Terbinafine is available as a cream, spray or gel for superficial infections or orally for deeper infections, such as those affecting the nails. It is available over-the-counter for the treatment of tinea pedis, cruris and corporis. The indication varies according to the preparation.

Griseofulvin

This interferes with fungal microtubules and nucleic acid synthesis but has largely been replaced by oral terbinafine and azoles. It is suitable for tinea infections but not candidiasis, because it is ineffective against the yeast.

Topical steroids

These may be used in addition to antifungal agents to relieve the symptoms due to irritation and are especially useful in concomitant eczema.

In terms of the use of antifungal agents, topical agents are used in more superficial infections and oral agents for deeper infections. The agents are chosen according to the spectrum of activity; some recommendations are given in Table 34.2.

Counselling

A long course is often required and should be completed.

Imidazole creams

- For cutaneous infections, these should be applied two to three times daily and for 2 weeks after the infection has healed.
- For vaginal infections, hygiene advice should be given and sexual partners treated if they are symptomatic. Other sources of infection may include fingernails, umbilicus, gastrointestinal tract and bladder.
- Vaginal preparations (excluding nystatin pessaries) may damage latex condoms and diaphragms.
- Vaginal preparations should be administered high into the vagina and may be used during menstruation.
- They may cause a burning sensation on application.

Oral azoles and oral terbinafine

- These may cause gastrointestinal side effects. Itraconazole capsules (but not liquid) and ketoconazole should be taken with food.
- Patients taking oral antifungal agents should report signs of liver toxicity such as nausea, vomiting, dark urine or jaundice (see Chapters 5 and 10).

Nystatin

The cream may stain clothes yellow.

Griseofulvin

- Avoid during pregnancy.
- Males should avoid fathering children for 6 months after stopping treatment.

Table 34.2   Treatment for fungal infections

Condition	Possible primary treatments
Tinea corporis	• Topical imidazole, continued for 2 weeks after healing • Topical terbinafine: 1–2 weeks • Topical imidazole is first-line while terbinafine is reserved for resistance
Tinea capitis	• Oral griseofulvin: 8 weeks • Oral terbinafine: 4 weeks (unlicensed) • Oral itraconazole (unlicensed)
Tinea pedis (athlete's foot)	• Topical imidazole, continued for 2 weeks after healing • Topical terbinafine: 1 week
Tinea unguium	• Oral terbinafine: 6 weeks to 3 months, sometimes longer in toenail infections • Oral itraconazole: 3 months or 2 pulses (fingernails) or 3 pulses (toenails)[a] • Oral griseofulvin for 6 months (fingernails) or 12 months (toenails) • In mild infection limited to 1–2 nails, local therapy with amorolfine or tioconazole may be used
Tinea cruris	• Topical imidazole, continued for 2 weeks after healing • Topical terbinafine: 1–2 weeks • Topical imidazole is first line whereas terbinafine is reserved for resistance
Pityriasis versicolor	• Selenium sulphide shampoo daily for 1 week • Topical imidazole for 10 days • Itraconazole for 1 week
Candidiasis – cutaneous	• Topical imidazole continued for 2 weeks after healing • Topical terbinafine: 2 weeks • Topical nystatin, continued for 7 days after healing
Candidiasis – nail	Oral itraconazole: 3 months or 2 pulses (fingernails) or 3 pulses (toenails)
Vaginal candidiasis	Either clotrimazole pessaries (single dose) or cream (10% clotrimazole is available for single application); oral fluconazole (150 mg as a single dose); may also be used for candidal balanitis

Failure of topical treatment or extensive infection should be treated with oral agents, such as terbinafine or itraconazole. The recommended agents and duration of the above therapies are largely derived from the *British National Formulary*.

[a] A pulse is a twice-daily dose for 7 days followed by 21 days without the drug.

Other infections affecting the skin

In addition to fungal infections, the skin is also the site of a wide range of bacterial and viral infections, which vary from benign to potentially serious. Some of the infections may be related to increased susceptibility due to chronic skin conditions, e.g. impetigo (as a complication of eczema) or as a result of manifestations of viral infections with both skin and systemic symptoms. A summary of the features and management of a range of common skin infections is given in Table 34.3.

Pruritus

This is a symptom of a range of conditions and presents as itchiness. Possible causes include (Greene and Harris 2008):

- dermatological inflammatory conditions:
  - eczema
  - psoriasis
- skin infections:
  - lice/scabies
  - viral infection – chickenpox, herpes
  - fungal infection

Table 34.3   Additional skin infections and their treatment

Condition	Comments	Management
Impetigo	Usually a staphylococcal or occasionally streptococcal infection of the skin. Reddening with a golden crust. Contagious and may complicate eczema	• Limited infection may be treated with topical fusidic acid or mupirocin (use limited to 10 days to prevent the emergence of resistance). More extensive infections require oral flucloxacillin (or phenoxymethylpenicillin if there is streptococcal infection) or erythromycin if penicillin allergic • Antiseptic bath oils may reduce colonization
Cellulitis	Deep streptococcal or staphylococcal infection, often following trauma. There may be a red, oedematous rash which may be accompanied by pyrexia	Phenoxymethylpenicillin plus flucloxacillin or erythromycin if penicillin allergic
Erysipelas	Superficial cellulitis of the skin, often due to *Streptococcus pyogenes*. Often affects the face or legs	Phenoxymethylpenicillin in mild infections. Flucloxacillin is added if staphylococcal infection is suspected
Herpes simplex	Painful vesicles on mucous membranes and skin due to herpes simplex virus. Tingling precedes the lesions	Analgesics provide symptomatic relief. Topical aciclovir and penciclovir reduce the length of symptoms if started at the first signs of an attack. Oral aciclovir may be less effective
Chickenpox	• Varicella infection leading to fever and vesicular rash. Usually uncomplicated in children but in adults may be complicated by pneumonia, hepatitis, encephalitis and myocarditis • Smoking increases the chances of complications of pneumonia • Chickenpox is especially severe in patients taking systemic steroids	• Antihistamines may provide symptomatic relief • Emollients may be soothing • Older remedies such as calamine lotion may be ineffective • Aciclovir is indicated for high-risk patients who develop the infection and should be started in the first 24 h • Immunoglobulin is appropriate for pregnant contacts and those taking steroids who do not have immunity
Shingles	Reactivation of varicella-zoster virus leading to pain, with red papules that become vesicular. Shingles cannot be caught from contact with chickenpox but contact of patients with shingles may lead to chickenpox in patients who are not immune	• Aciclovir is indicated for patients aged >60 years or immunocompromised. It should be started within 72 h of the appearance of the rash • Neuralgic pain after infection may require low doses of tricyclic antidepressants such as amitriptyline or carbamazepine, which are routinely used in older patients as a preventive measure
Warts and verrucae (plantar warts)	Warts are hyperkeratotic papules and verrucae are deep lesions on the soles. They are caused by the human papillomavirus	• Warts generally resolve but may be treated with salicylic acid, glutaraldehyde or cryotherapy with liquid nitrogen or dry ice • Verrucae may be treated with salicylic acid plasters or podophyllin/salicylic acid ointment or cryotherapy

Continued

Table 34.3   (Continued)

Condition	Comments	Management
Molluscum contagiosum (water blisters)	Drop-like papules affecting infants and children due to a virus	None indicated and reassurance is all that may be required
Hand, foot and mouth disease	Coxsackie viral infection in children with vesicles around the mouth, palms and soles	None
Scabies	Severe pruritus due to scabies mite infestation	• Malathion or permethrin as aqueous preparations as alcohol may irritate damaged skin (Chapter 33) • All members of the family should be treated • Treatment should be applied to the whole body, particularly to the web of digits and fingernails • Two applications, 1 week apart ,are recommended • Crotamiton and/or sedating antihistamines may be used for pruritus

• reactions:
 – drug reactions
 – urticaria
• psychogenic
• ageing
• manifestations of systemic changes:
 – diabetes
 – pregnancy
 – liver failure
 – renal failure
 – malignancy.

The treatment should be directed at the cause, but additional symptomatic measures include the use of crotamiton cream or lotion and oral antihistamines. Colestyramine is used in pruritus associated with liver failure, because it will bind bile salts and so reduce plasma bilirubin, which causes pruritus (see Chapter 10). Anogenital pruritus may be due to fungal infection, haemorrhoids or contact dermatitis caused by irritation from poor hygiene. It should be treated with hygiene measures, antifungal agents, emollients if due to dry skin or short-term hydrocortisone as appropriate, but topical local anaesthetics are best avoided because they may lead to hypersensitivity.

Manifestations of systemic disease

In addition to pruritus as a symptom, systemic diseases may manifest as changes in the skin. Examples of this include the following:

• Pigmentation that may be yellow in jaundice (due to increased bilirubin in liver disease), a lemon tinge in renal failure or vitiligo in Addison's disease.
• Spider naevi are dilated central arterioles with spidery arterioles feeding from them, and are present, especially above the nipple line, in liver cirrhosis, frequently due to alcohol.
• Fungal infections that recur may suggest that the patient has impaired immunity. Frequent candidiasis occurs in diabetes mellitus.

Skin cancers

The incidence of skin cancers is on the increase and they are dealt with by specialists in dermatology. However, recognition of potential skin cancers in primary care is clearly important and the pharmacist should be vigilant for changes in the skin that require referral.

Table 34.4 Some important drug interactions for drugs used in dermatology

Interacting drugs	Consequences	Comments
Methoxsalen with phenytoin	Phenytoin may, by enzyme induction, reduce concentrations of methoxsalen	This combination should be avoided
Acitretin with ciclosporin	An increase in ciclosporin concentration may occur	
Acitretin with methotrexate	Increased toxicity of methotrexate	BNF recommends avoiding concomitant use of acitretin and methotrexate
Isotretinoin with carbamazepine	The plasma concentration of carbamazepine may be reduced	Epileptic control should be monitored
Isotretinoin with tetracycline/minocycline	Increased risk of benign intracranial hypertension	Their concomitant use should be avoided
Methotrexate	Toxicity of methotrexate is known to be enhanced by NSAIDs and so extreme caution should be exercised, although this is less likely to occur at the lower doses used for psoriasis	Methotrexate exhibits a wide range of interactions and *Stockley's Drug Interactions* (Baxter 2008) should be consulted
Ciclosporin		Ciclosporin exhibits a wide range of interactions and *Stockley's Drug Interactions* (Baxter 2008) should be consulted
Oral cyproterone plus ethinylestradiol (co-cyprindiol)	Efficacy may be reduced by broad-spectrum antibiotics and enzyme inducers. When used with minocycline there may be an enhancement of facial pigmentation	
Oral imidazoles and triazoles	• Phenytoin reduces the plasma concentrations of itraconazole and ketoconazole but fluconazole may increase the concentrations of phenytoin • Carbamazepine may reduce the plasma concentrations of itraconazole • Rifampicin reduces the plasma concentrations of itraconazole, fluconazole and ketoconazole. • Additional interactions include reduced absorption of ketoconazole and itraconazole (but not fluconazole) by antacids and H_2-receptor antagonists	• These are inhibitors of cytochrome P450 and will inhibit the metabolism of a range of drugs, increasing their plasma concentrations (Chapter 5) • Similarly, inducers of cytochrome P450 may accelerate the metabolism of the azoles, reducing their plasma concentrations • Inhibitors of cytochrome P450 may inhibit the metabolism of azoles and increase their concentrations
Antifungals (fluconazole, itraconazole, ketoconazole and miconazole) with warfarin	Increased anticoagulant effect	Includes oral and vaginal preparations of miconazole
Griseofulvin with warfarin	In some patients, griseofulvin decreases the plasma concentration of warfarin	Monitoring is recommended

Continued

Table 34.4   (Continued)

Interacting drugs	Consequences	Comments
Itraconazole with clarithromycin	Itraconazole levels doubled	Monitoring and possible dose reductions are recommended
Ketoconazole with omeprazole	Reduced antifungal effects	• Fluconazole is a suitable alternative for patients prescribed omeprazole • Alternative proton pump inhibitors such as lansoprazole may also interact and an alternative such as H_2-receptor antagonists is recommended
Oral terbinafine	• Plasma concentrations are decreased by concomitant rifampicin and its dose may need to be increased • Terbinafine may increase plasma levels of theophylline but this is unclear	
Amphotericin with corticosteroids	Adverse cardiac effects due to potassium loss and water and sodium retention	Electrolytes should be monitored, particularly in patients at risk (e.g. elderly people)
Oral aciclovir	• There is a report of aciclovir reducing plasma concentrations of phenytoin and sodium valproate • Aciclovir can increase plasma concentrations of theophylline, which may lead to toxicity	Monitoring may be appropriate

BNF, *British National Formulary*; NSAIDs, non-steroidal anti-inflammatory drugs.

Basal cell carcinoma (rodent ulcer)

This is the most common skin cancer and presents as a colourless lump with pearly edges, but may become ulcerated and crusty in the centre and is often on the edge of the ear, temple or side of the nose. It is very slow growing and may have been present for several years. Although it is a malignant tumour, it has only very limited local invasion and is cured by surgical removal. Extensive invasion may require radiotherapy or cryotherapy. Topical 5-fluorouracil is also used. Prevention of occurrence or recurrence (which is common) should be stressed by advising sun protection measures, such as wearing a hat in the sun and using a high-factor sun block.

Solar keratosis

These are common, premalignant lesions with crusts on an erythematous base. Solar keratosis is associated with exposure to the sun and occurs more often on fair-skinned patients on the forehead, scalp, face or hands. It may be managed by cryotherapy and topical 5-fluorouracil.

Squamous cell carcinoma

This is a relatively common malignancy, often appearing on sun-damaged skin on the hand and face, especially the ear and lip. It is removed surgically but metastases may occur if it is untreated.

Malignant melanoma

This involves evolution and possibly malignant transformation in a large mole. This is more likely in larger moles and in sun-exposed skin. The following features may be seen:

Asymmetry
Border irregular
Colour irregular
Diameter >0.5 cm
Elevation irregular.

Any change in a mole requires referral for an expert opinion. In malignant melanoma, surgical excision has a good outlook in small lesions that are caught early. Chemotherapy is palliative in disease that has spread.

Drug interactions involving drugs widely used in dermatology

In drugs used in dermatology there are a wide range of potential drug interactions, generally affecting the oral azoles, and also ciclosporin and methotrexate, which are initiated only by specialists. Table 34.4 contains a summary of some important interactions.

Self-assessment

Consider whether the following statements are true or false. In the management of skin diseases.

1. The regular use of emollients is both the initial and mainstay of therapy in eczema.
2. Hydrocortisone 1% cream should not be used in children aged <12.
3. Topical tacrolimus is used by specialists in moderate-to-severe eczema.
4. Retinoids used in psoriasis and acne are highly teratogenic.
5. The use of terbinafine is complicated by many drug interactions.

 CASE STUDIES

Case 1
Toddler TR is 2 years old and has scaly inflamed skin on her back and on the back of her knees. A diagnosis of atopic eczema has been made.

1. How might the parents manage this condition using lifestyle changes and OTC treatments?
   - Simple lifestyle measures should involve regular but not excessive washing, and using emollients in place of soap. After bathing, emollient should be applied liberally and reapplied throughout the day. Keeping the house cool may help reduce the discomfort of itching. Limiting allergens in the house is controversial and may or may not help. The child's nails should be kept short to avoid scratching and a sedative oral antihistamine given at night might help her sleep and reduce scratching at night.
2. Might the toddler benefit from topical antihistamines?
   - These are of no benefit in eczema and they may actually sensitize the skin.
3. What are the treatment options open to her GP?
   - For poorly controlled and inflamed eczema, topical corticosteroids (1% hydrocortisone preferred in infants) may be prescribed (not over-the-counter at this age) for short periods to bring the condition under control.

continued

4. What other conditions will she be susceptible to?
   – Atopic individuals are more susceptible to asthma and hayfever.
   Toddler TR's skin condition deteriorates and becomes covered with a golden crusty coat over a red and inflamed surface. The GP decides that she has an impetigo-like infection.
5. What is impetigo?
   A staphylococcal or streptococcal infection of the skin leading to reddening with a golden crust, which may complicate eczema.
6. How would this be treated?
   – In limited infection, topical fusidic acid 2% is used. If widespread, either oral flucloxacillin 125 mg four times daily or erythromycin 250 mg four times daily is appropriate. If streptococcal infection is suspected, then phenoxymethylpenicillin 125 mg four times daily may be prescribed.

Case 2
Ms GS is a 16-year-old (50 kg) girl with acne vulgaris.

1. What are the goals of treatment?
   – eradication of acne, which is important both cosmetically and psychologically
   – reduction in sebum production
   – to limit the growth of the bacteria involved
   – to prevent recurrence
   – to prevent scarring.
2. What would the ladder of treatment be in her case?
   – Step 1: mild acne – general cleansing.
   – Step 2: topical benzoyl peroxide for its keratolytic and bactericidal actions.
   – Step 3: if there is a poor response to the above, then topical tretinoin or topical antibiotics (not effective against comedones).
   – Step 4: if there is a poor response to the above, then oral antibiotics.
   – Step 5: if there is a poor response to the above, then oral isotretinoin.
   – Any stage: co-cyprindiol may be used. Severe acne should be referred to a dermatologist.
At one stage she is prescribed tetracycline 500 mg twice daily.
3. How would you counsel her?
   – Do not take at the same time as milk and antacids: take at least 30 min before food or on an empty stomach. Calcium in milk and antacids will bind tetracycline and prevent it from being absorbed.
   – Complete the course.
   – Avoid direct sunlight/UV due to photosensitivity.
   – An improvement may take 3–4 months.
4. What might be tried if there is no improvement?
   – Oral erythromycin or trimethoprim might be tried.
   Later her dermatologist prescribes isotretinoin orally
5. Suggest an appropriate dosage.
   – 500 micrograms/kg daily, so her dose is 25 mg daily.

continued

CASE STUDIES (continued)

6. How would she be counselled?
   – Isotretinoin is teratogenic and she will require a pregnancy test and must not become pregnant until at least 1 month after stopping treatment. She should use effective contraception.
   – Her skin may become thin.
   – She should avoid waxing or epilation, because this will strip skin.
   – Her lips may become dry and Vaseline may help.

Case 3
An elderly man presents a prescription for metronidazole 0.75% gel 30 g for his wife. You notice from her patient medication record (PMR) that she is receiving medication for palliative care. How do you proceed?

Confusion can arise when prescribing topical metronidazole preparations. A product providing 0.75% metronidazole gel in a 30 g pack size is indicated for acne rosacea. It is important to check the indication because it is possible that the above prescription is for a malodorous fungating tumour. An appropriately licensed product should be supplied.

References

Baxter K, ed. (2008). *Stockley's Drug Interaction*, 8th edn. London: Pharmaceutical Press.

Greene RJ, Harris ND (2008). *Pathology and Therapeutics for Pharmacists*. London: Pharmaceutical Press.

Martin J, ed. *British National Formulary*, latest edition. London: British Medical Association and Royal Pharmaceutical Society of Great Britain.

National Institute for Health and Clinical Excellence (2007). *Atopic Eczema in Children*. Clinical Guideline 57. London: NICE.

Wilkinson JD, Shaw S, Orton D (2005). *Dermatology in Focus*. Edinburgh: Elsevier Churchill Livingstone.

Further reading

Brown SK, Shalita AR (1998). Acne vulgaris. *Lancet* **351**: 1871–6.

Cunliffe W (2002). A rational approach to acne management. *Prescriber* **13**: 46–67.

Hindle E (2001). Eczema: first- and second-line drug treatments. *Prescriber* **12**: 49–71.

Rudikoff D, Lebwohl M (1998). Atopic dermatitis. *Lancet* **351**: 1715–21

Stern RS (1997). Psoriasis. *Lancet* **350**: 349–53.

Online resources

www.eczema.org
The website of the UK National Eczema Society (accessed May 2008).

www.bad.org.uk
The website of the British Association of Dermatologists providing professional guidance and patient information (accessed April 2008).

Part J
Endocrine disorders

Diabetes mellitus

Diabetes mellitus is a serious condition associated with a considerable disruption to a patient's life and potentially serious long-term consequences. In particular, diabetes mellitus is a major risk factor for cardiovascular disease, comparable to hypertension and hypercholesterolaemia. Diabetes mellitus is broadly classed as either type 1 (previously known as insulin-dependent) or type 2 (non-insulin-dependent) diabetes mellitus. Both conditions are characterized by impaired glucose metabolism. In type 1, there is an inability to produce insulin whereas in type 2 there is reduced production and/or a reduced sensitivity to its actions. Type 1 is generally associated with onset at an early age, whereas type 2, previously termed 'maturity-onset diabetes', presents later in life and is strongly associated with obesity. A small subset of type 2 diabetes is maturity-onset diabetes of the young (MODY), a genetic condition, with onset at an earlier age. It is now recognized that the incidence of type 2 diabetes mellitus is increasing, with many cases remaining undiagnosed, and it is believed that we are on the edge of a hidden epidemic. Type 2 diabetes represents 90% of patients who have diabetes.

Common clinical features of diabetes are:

- increased thirst (secondary to increased plasma osmolality)
- increased urination (due to osmotic diuresis secondary to glucose in the urine)
- glycosuria
- increased superficial infections such as genital candidiasis due to glucose in the urine
- tiredness
- weight loss in type 1
- ketoacidosis (in the form of dehydration, nausea, vomiting, thirst, weight loss, hyperventilation, ketone breath) in type 1, rarely in type 2.

Diagnosis may be secondary to complications of diabetes, such as hypertension, myocardial infarction, retinal damage, peripheral vascular disease and renal damage. Diabetes can be induced in certain conditions such as pregnancy (gestational diabetes), endocrine conditions associated with the increased production of counter-regulatory hormones (such as corticosteroids in Cushing's syndrome and growth hormone in acromegaly), diseases of the pancreas such as chronic pancreatitis, and by certain drugs (e.g. thiazides, corticosteroids).

Diagnosis is based on elevated plasma glucose levels of >7.0 mmol/L in the fasting state or 11.1 mmol/L on a random test on two occasions. An oral glucose tolerance test may also be carried out and involves measuring plasma glucose levels before and 2 h after a challenge with a glucose-rich drink (75 g). In this test, a diagnosis is made if the fasting glucose is >7.0 mmol/L or the 2-h glucose is >11.1 mmol/L. A fasting value of 6–7 mmol/L is consistent with impaired glucose tolerance. Diabetes may be suggested by detection of glucose in the urine, but this is a less valuable test as individuals vary in their renal threshold (about 7–15 mmol/L) for the appearance of glycosuria.

Type 1 diabetes mellitus

This form is generally associated with onset at a young age (<40 years) but may occur at any age. It may be caused by destruction of β cells of the islets of Langerhans after certain viral infections or due to an autoimmune process. It is characterized by an inability of the β cells to produce insulin and is fatal if not treated.

Pharmacological management

Treatment is directed towards replacing the insulin in an attempt to return blood glucose to normal and preventing diabetic complications. The insulin used is now generally the human peptide derived from recombinant DNA technology, although insulin derived from porcine and bovine (rarely) pancreases is used. The insulin is given by injection (sometimes initially by slow intravenous infusion) and in the maintenance phase by subcutaneous injection. Insulin acts on insulin receptors on target tissues of the body to enable blood glucose to be controlled. This follows the insertion of glucose transporters to promote glucose uptake into muscle, liver and adipose tissue, and by stimulation of glycogen, triglyceride and fatty acid synthesis.

Insulin preparations

As insulin has a short plasma half-life, it may be complexed with various agents to retard its absorption, so prolonging its action.

Human insulin analogues
These are modified insulin peptides (insulin lispro and insulin aspart) which have a rapid onset but short duration of action and may be injected just before a meal or when necessary just after a meal. These preparations increase flexibility and are particularly useful for patients prone to pre-lunch hypoglycaemia and those who tend to eat late in the evening and may therefore be at risk of nocturnal hypoglycaemia.

Short-acting insulins
Soluble insulins have relatively short-lived effects of 6–8 h, with peak effects at 2–5 h. These are given approximately 15–30 min before meals.

Intermediate and long-acting insulins
Combination of insulin with protamine gives rise to intermediate-acting insulin (isophane insulin), binding to zinc gives intermediate-to long-acting insulin and combination with protamine plus zinc gives long-acting insulin. Crystalline insulin zinc suspensions are also long acting. Biphasic preparations contain both an intermediate-acting agent (e.g. isophane insulin) and a shorter-acting form (e.g. soluble insulin).

The aim of insulin therapy is to maintain a plasma glucose level as close to 7.5 mmol/L as possible to prevent future complications, but also to avoid hypoglycaemia. The ideal situation is to match the physiological changes in insulin profile in non-diabetic patients. One method of achieving good glycaemic control is by multiple insulin injections of differing durations of action in an attempt to mimic physiological responses. The aim is to give a long-acting agent to achieve a basal level and to add short-acting preparations in relation to a meal; this is termed 'basal bolus dosing'. The disadvantage here can be one of compliance, because patients are required to monitor blood glucose frequently and administer multiple injections per day. This can be difficult to achieve.

There are no fixed rules and regimens can be adopted to suit the individual needs of the patient. Here are some of the regimens that are commonly used:

- Twice-daily regimens: two daily injections, one 30 min before breakfast and one before the evening meal of short- and longer-acting insulins in combination, with two-thirds of the insulin given as the morning dose. This is the most common regimen.
- Multiple dosing regimens: a single dose of medium-acting insulin is given at bedtime and doses of short-acting insulin are given 30 min before each meal. This allows more flexibility with the timing of meals.

  Alternatively, a short-acting insulin mixed with intermediate-acting insulin is given before breakfast; short-acting insulin is given before the evening meal and an intermediate-acting insulin is given at bedtime.
- Single daily regimens: these are rarely used but involve one daily injection before breakfast or at bedtime of intermediate-acting insulin, with or without a short-acting insulin. They are generally for patients with type 2 diabetes who are unable to control their blood glucose with antidiabetic drugs.

Insulin requirement is increased by stress, infection, accidental or surgical trauma, puberty (effects of growth hormone) and during the latter two trimesters of pregnancy. Reduced insulin requirements may occur in coeliac disease, renal or hepatic impairment, and endocrine disorders such as untreated Addison's disease.

Insulin administration

Intravenous infusion of soluble insulin is a reliable route of administration and may be used in hospital in an acute setting, to bring the diabetes under control. The amount required to control blood glucose may give an indication of daily requirements for future treatment. In the early stages, patients may encounter what is termed a 'honeymoon period', during which time less insulin is required (due to residual β-cell function). The most conventional route is via subcutaneous injection using a disposable syringe, in which the different insulins may be mixed to achieve the desired combination. This method has largely been superseded by the introduction of more convenient injection pens and biphasic insulins.

Insulin pumps may be used that allow continuous subcutaneous administration. These are particularly useful in diabetes that is difficult to control. They have the advantage of providing a continuous infusion, which may be increased at meal times.

Complications of insulin therapy

As the role of insulin is to reduce blood glucose levels, excessive dosing in relation to food intake can lead to hypoglycaemia. Patients may become aware of this through autonomic (anxiety, sweating, trembling, tachycardia and hunger) and neuroglycaemic (confusion, drowsiness, and problems with concentration, speech and co-ordination) symptoms. Awareness of these symptoms is important so that action may be taken, such as intake of 10–20 g glucose in lumps or in glucose-rich drinks to prevent a hypoglycaemic coma, e.g. 10 g glucose is provided by two teaspoons of sugar, three sugar lumps, 200 mL milk, 50–55 mL Lucozade, 90 mL Coca-Cola or

15 mL Ribena original (to be diluted). If this is not sufficient, the same dose may be repeated in 10–15 min. Hypostop gel may be easier to administer with a reduced risk of choking and it contains 10 g/23 g ampoule. Glucagon may be given by subcutaneous, intramuscular or intravenous injection for acute insulin-induced hypoglycaemia resulting in unconsciousness.

Strict glycaemic control and the use of human insulin may also impair hypoglycaemic awareness, and it is for this reason that some patients prefer to be maintained on porcine or bovine insulin. Hypoglycaemia is also common at night, because the evening insulin injection may have peak effects at this time, even if the patient has an evening snack (see insulin regimens).

Exercise not only reduces insulin requirements because glucose is used, but also accelerates the absorption of insulin from the subcutaneous sites. Accordingly, patients may need to reduce the dose of insulin before and after exercise and also to take a snack before exercise. In highly trained patients, multiple daily insulin injections may be the best approach to attain glycaemic control, and avoid hypoglycaemia.

Subcutaneous injection of insulin may lead to changes in the skin. At a site of repeated injections, there may be lipohypertrophy, leading to unpredictable insulin absorption. It is for this reason that patients should rotate the sites used.

Inhaled insulin

Delivery of insulin by inhalation was introduced to therapy. Although this represented an advance in delivery of insulin, it was relatively expensive and was subsequently withdrawn from the market.

Drug interactions and effects on concurrent diseases

A number of drugs may alter glucose control and hence the effects of insulin (Table 35.1). By altering glucose metabolism they will also affect control in diabetes and in some cases uncover diabetes.

Table 35.1   Examples of the effects of some important drugs on glucose control and insulin activity

Drug	Effects on diabetes	Comments
Alcohol	May mask the signs of hypoglycaemia	Alcohol should not be consumed in excess and should be taken with food The carbohydrate content of the drink should also be taken into account (see Counselling in text)
ACE inhibitors	These can sometimes lead to hypoglycaemia	The dose of insulin or antidiabetic drug may need to be reduced
β Blockers	These may mask the awareness of hypoglycaemia by reducing the tremor and tachycardia, although sweating is not affected (as this is cholinergic)	This is most marked with propranolol. This is a reason to choose alternative agents or favour the use of β_1-adrenoceptor antagonists
Corticosteroids	These oppose the actions of insulin and cause hyperglycaemia	The dose of insulin may need to be increased
Isoniazid	Variable effects	Monitoring is appropriate
Lithium	May reduce glucose tolerance	May induce diabetes. Monitoring is appropriate
MAOIs	These may enhance the hypoglycaemic actions of insulin	Monitoring is appropriate
Oral contraceptives	Insulin requirements may be altered	
Thiazides	May increase blood glucose	This is a reason to avoid using thiazides in diabetes
Tobacco smoking	This increases the insulin requirements	Smoking substantially enhances the cardiovascular damage in diabetes

ACE, angiotensin-converting enzyme; MAOIs, monoamine oxidase inhibitors.

Intercurrent illnesses and conditions

As commented in Chapter 1, patients with diabetes are a special group who should have a lower threshold for GP referral during illness. In addition, during an illness there may be a loss of appetite but patients should not reduce their insulin intake. In fact, the illness itself may increase blood glucose levels. Carbohydrate 10 g (see Complications of insulin therapy above) should be taken every hour or sips every 20 min if nauseated. It is also important to allow for the glucose content in rehydration solutions, e.g. Dioralyte powder contains 3.56 g glucose per sachet. Pregnancy is a major issue in patients with diabetes and requires specialist supervision.

Type 2 diabetes mellitus

This is generally associated with increased insulin resistance, in which the body's tissues become less responsive to insulin, leading to increased blood glucose levels. There is also a strong family association. The β cells of the islets of Langerhans still produce insulin but there is sometimes a loss of cells or reduced glucose sensitivity. The patient may also have other associated diseases such as obesity, hypertension and hyperlipidaemia. Type 2 diabetes generally presents after the age of 40 years and may have a gradual onset, such that the patient may have the condition for several years (the prediabetic phase) before recognition. This is a persuasive reason for routine blood glucose testing.

Pharmacological basis of management

In mild or initial disease, all that may be required is dietary modification to reduce the amount of simple carbohydrates in the diet, weight loss in obesity and increased exercise to achieve control of blood glucose. The alteration of diet should limit the intake of mono- and disaccharides, increase non-starch polysaccharides, and reduce the intake of saturated fat to minimize the risk of atherosclerosis, such that fat is 30–35% of the calorific intake and carbohydrate is 50–55%. If dietary changes alone are insufficient after 3 months, antidiabetic drugs are used. If these fail to achieve control at maximum doses and optimal combinations insulin injections may be required. Indeed, type 2 diabetes should be viewed as a progressive disease.

Sulphonylureas, e.g. chlorpropamide, glibenclamide, gliclazide, glimepiride, glipizide, tolbutamide

The sulphonylureas rely on the fact that the β cells can still produce insulin. These drugs act to increase insulin secretion. Pharmacologically, they are inhibitors of adenosine triphosphate (ATP)-sensitive potassium (K_{ATP}) channels. Subtypes of K_{ATP}-channels are present on many cell types such as β cells, smooth muscle cells, cardiac muscle cells and neuronal cells. In β cells, they regulate insulin release. When glucose is present, the production of ATP and the reduction in adenosine diphosphate (ADP) inactivate these channels, leading to cellular depolarization, which results in calcium influx and insulin secretion. When glucose is low, ATP levels fall and ADP rises, channels open, with membrane hyperpolarization, and this decreases insulin release. Sulphonylureas bind to a receptor associated with these channels, resulting in channel closure, which leads to insulin release.

Meglitinide analogues: nateglinide, repaglinide

These also act on β cells but at a site distinct from the sulphonylurea receptor, causing closure of the K_{ATP} channels, leading to depolarization and insulin release. They have a rapid rate of onset and are given at mealtimes to stimulate post-prandial insulin secretion, which is relatively short-lived. Their effects may be enhanced by patients having a meal and they are referred to as prandial glucose regulators (PGRs), which may be regarded as producing a more physiological rise in insulin than that produced by sulphonylureas.

Biguanides: metformin

The action of metformin is less clear but may involve AMP-kinase activation. There are several proposed mechanisms of action, including: (1) increased glucose uptake into muscle; (2) reduced uptake of glucose from the gastrointestinal tract; and (3) reduced output of glucose from the liver. Obviously these proposed mechanisms will lead to either reduced entry of glucose in the blood or increased utilization.

Thiazolidinediones (glitazones): pioglitazone, rosiglitazone

These new agents are 'insulin sensitizers' which work by enhancing glucose utilization in tissues, and so reduce insulin resistance. They activate the γ nuclear peroxisome proliferator-activated receptors (PPAR-γ), which alter gene expression and result in insulin-like effects. These include reduced hepatic glucose output, increased glucose transporters (GLUT) in skeletal muscle with increased peripheral glucose utilization, and the promotion of fatty acid uptake into adipose cells.

Glucosidase inhibitors: acarbose

Acarbose competitively inhibits the α-glucosidases, which metabolize oligosaccharides to monosaccharides in the small intestines. This reduces the production of glucose in the gastrointestinal tract, thereby preventing sharp rises in blood glucose after a meal. The subsequent increased presence of carbohydrates in the gastrointestinal tract may lead to flatulence and osmotic diarrhoea as side effects.

Modulation of incretins: exenatide, sitagliptin

Incretins are endogenous hormones that regulate the endocrine function of the pancreas.

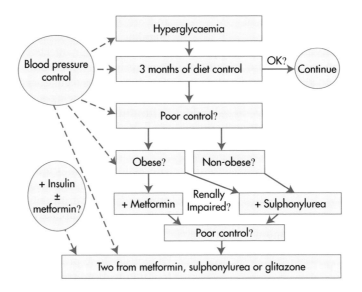

Figure 35.1   A flow diagram summarizing current approaches to the management of type 2 diabetes, which incorporates National Institute for Clinical Excellence (NICE 2003) guidance on the use of glitazones. Updated guidance favours metformin as first-line where possible.

Exenatide is an incretin mimetic that acts on β cells of the islets of Langerhans to stimulate the release of insulin and it also acts to reduce glucagon release. Sitagliptin is a dipeptidyl peptidase-4 inhibitor, which means that it inhibits the breakdown of incretins, so enhancing their action, which promotes insulin secretion and suppresses glucagon release. Both of these agents are add-on therapies to a sulphonylurea and/or metformin, with exenatide being given by subcutaneous injection and sitagliptin being available as tablets.

Drug choice

The initial choice is generally between a sulphonylurea and metformin, with the latter being favoured especially in overweight and obese patients, because it causes weight loss. In choosing a sulphonylurea, age is a consideration. Specifically, elderly patients are more susceptible to the hypoglycaemic effects of sulphonylureas and this may be reduced by using a short-acting agent such as gliclazide or tolbutamide. Chlorpropamide is not widely used because it is long acting and may enhance antidiuretic

hormone release, leading to hyponatraemia. If monotherapy is inadequate, a sulphonylurea and metformin are used in combination.

The glitazones are currently licensed as 'add-on' therapies to either a sulphonylurea or metformin but they should not be used in triple combinations. The National Institute for Health and Clinical Excellence guidelines (NICE 2003) indicate that rosiglitazone or pioglitazone should be added only once the combination of a sulphonylurea plus metformin has proved inadequate (or not tolerated) (Figure 35.1). In adding a glitazone, the combination of the glitazone and metformin is preferred, especially in obese patients. This use of a glitazone would be an alternative to adding insulin therapy. Nateglinide is currently licensed as add-on therapy with metformin, and repaglinide is licensed for both monotherapy and in combination with metformin.

Other considerations are detailed in Table 35.2.

Concerns over glitazones and cardiovascular disease

It is established that glitazones may cause fluid retention and are contraindicated in chronic

Table 35.2   The effects of concurrent conditions on drug choice in type 2 diabetes mellitus

Condition	Effect on drug choice	Comments
Renal impairment	Avoid metformin. Tolbutamide or gliclazide is preferred	The shorter-acting sulphonylureas should be used at a reduced dose
Heart failure	Avoid metformin in severe heart failure. Avoid glitazones in heart failure	
Liver disease	Avoid metformin. Avoid glitazones	Risk of lactic acidosis
Hyperlipidaemia	Glitazones may cause modest reductions in triglycerides and increases in HDL	Fibrates may also be chosen to manage hyperlipidaemia (Chapter 12)
Porphyria	Sulphonylureas should be avoided	
Pregnancy	Insulin therapy is generally used in place of oral antidiabetic drugs	

HDL, high-density lipoprotein.

heart failure. There is now evidence that rosiglitazone, but not pioglitazone, is associated with an increase in cardiovascular mortality (Nissen and Wolski 2007). In view of the fact that many patients with diabetes have concurrent cardiovascular disease, this should be taken into account when using rosiglitazone.

Concerns over fracture risk and glitazones

There is recent evidence that glitazones may impair bone formation and this has been identified as a risk factor for bone fractures (Meier *et al* 2008).

Drug interactions

In addition to the effects of drugs on glucose control described above, Table 35.3 gives some important interactions with antidiabetic agents.

Complications of antidiabetic drug therapy

The main complication of treatment with the sulphonylureas and, to a lesser extent, meglitinide analogues is hypoglycaemia because they stimulate insulin release. This is most problematic at high doses or in the case of sulphonylureas with long half-lives. Incidents of hypoglycaemia may be managed by sugary drinks (see above)

and may require a change in the drug used. The glitazones and metformin are far less likely to cause hypoglycaemia.

The insulin-stimulating effects of sulphonylureas and insulin-sensitizing effects of glitazones may lead to weight gain, whereas metformin leads to weight loss.

Monitoring

In view of hepatotoxicity to the prototypic glitazone troglitazone (which has been withdrawn), NICE (2003) recommends that liver function tests are carried out in patients receiving rosiglitazone or pioglitazone before treatment, then every 2 months for the first year and periodically thereafter.

Diabetic complications and their prevention

Diabetic complications have serious consequences for both morbidity and mortality. The complications are macrovascular, microvascular and neuropathy.

Macrovascular complications

Diabetes is associated with a substantial increase in the risk of cardiovascular mortality through

Table 35.3 Examples of some important interactions with antidiabetic drugs

Drugs	Consequences	Comments
Insulin with glitazones	Enhanced actions	This combination is contraindicated but would be a logical insulin-sparing combination
Acarbose with insulin/sulphonylureas	Acarbose may enhance the hypoglycaemic effects of these drugs	Dose reduction of insulin or sulphonylurea may be needed
Chlorpropamide with alcohol	Facial flushing	This does not occur with other sulphonylureas
Glipizide with colestyramine	The absorption of glipizide may be delayed	Glipizide should be taken 1–2 h before colestyramine
Sulphonylureas with fibrates	Enhanced effects of the sulphonylureas	This may be an advantage in poor glucose control or dose reduction of the sulphonylurea may be needed
Tolbutamide/glibenclamide with rifampicin	Rifampicin may increase the metabolism of these agents	The dose of the sulphonylurea may need to be increased
Sulphonylureas with sulphonamides	Enhanced hypoglycaemic effects	This applies to some but not all sulphonamides
Repaglinide with erythromycin, fluconazole, itraconazole, ketoconazole, phenytoin or rifampicin	These drugs may alter the actions of repaglinide	The manufacturer contraindicates these combinations
Metformin/sulphonylureas with cimetidine	Cimetidine has been reported to increase the activity of sulphonylureas (especially glipizide). Cimetidine may inhibit the renal excretion of metformin	Patients may be advised of the possibility of hypoglycaemia while taking cimetidine and a sulphonylurea. A dose reduction with metformin may be appropriate. Ranitidine does not appear to interact with these antidiabetic drugs

ischaemic heart disease and stroke. Furthermore, the risk is substantially enhanced by other cardiovascular risks such as hypertension, hyperlipidaemia, obesity and smoking. Cardiovascular disease occurs prematurely in patients with diabetes, even if they have had good control, and accounts for 70% of deaths in these patients. Strict regulation of blood pressure is essential in diabetes: the British Hypertension Society recommends a target of <140/80 mmHg. Evidence from trials indicates that lowering blood pressure in itself is important and reduces both macrovascular and microvascular complications. Trials with antihypertensive drugs have also focused on specific agents in patients with diabetes. In this respect, the Losartan Intervention for Endpoint

Reduction in Hypertension (LIFE) trial (2002) has reported that the angiotensin receptor antagonist losartan is more effective than atenolol at reducing morbidity and mortality in hypertensive patients who have diabetes and/or left ventricular hypertrophy. The Heart Outcomes Prevention Evaluation (HOPE) trial (2000) found that treatment of patients with a high risk for cardiovascular disease with the angiotensin-converting enzyme (ACE) inhibitor ramipril reduced the complications associated with diabetes and also the development of diabetes. Accordingly, ACE inhibitors are often first-choice antihypertensives in patients with diabetes. The Heart Protection Study Collaborative Group (2002) has demonstrated, in patients with diabetes, that simvastatin protects against cardio-vascular events, irrespective of their cholesterol levels.

Microvascular complications

Pathological changes in the microcirculation lead to nephropathy and retinopathy. The mechanism of damage is thought to be due to hyperglycaemia leading to glycation of structural proteins and the toxic effects of free radicals and glycation end-products. Accordingly, there is good evidence that good glycaemic control may limit these complications.

Diabetic nephropathy is a long-term consequence of diabetes and may result in end-stage renal failure. In the early stages of diabetes, there is hyperfiltration in the glomeruli. There are subsequent changes in the basement membranes, including glycation, and these lead to microalbuminuria, a marker of renal deterioration. This may be followed by hypertension and proteinuria. Microvascular damage in the retinal circulation may lead to retinopathy, which is associated with angiogenesis, haemorrhages and detachment of the retina. Retinopathy is a major cause of blindness.

All patients with type 1 diabetes who have microalbuminuria should receive an ACE inhibitor, regardless of whether they have hypertension. NICE guidance (2002) on renal disease in type 2 diabetes indicated that diabetic nephropathy is likely in patients who have albumin in the urine and/or increased plasma creatinine levels, accompanied by retinopathy. In these patients, glycaemic control should aim to achieve levels of glycated haemoglobin (HbA1c) <6.5–7.5%, blood pressure should be <135/75 mmHg and an ACE inhibitor should be given for renal and cardiovascular protection. The CALM study group (2000) demonstrated, in type 2 diabetes, that the angiotensin II receptor antagonist candesartan was as effective as lisinopril at controlling both blood pressure and microalbuminuria. Furthermore, the combination of candesartan and lisinopril was even more effective. The sartan irbesartan has also been shown to be effective at reducing the incidence of diabetic nephropathy and is licensed for

use in type 2 diabetes. This may be an alternative to ACE inhibitors when they are not tolerated, e.g. due to their associated cough.

The Diabetes Control and Complications Trial (DCCT 1993) reported that, in type 1 diabetes, intensive insulin therapy to maintain blood glucose as close to normal as possible delayed the onset and progression of nephropathy, retinopathy and neuropathy. Evidence from the UK Prospective Diabetes Study (UKPDS) (1998a, 1998b) indicated that intensive glycaemic control in type 2 diabetes lowers the risk of microvascular but not macrovascular complications. Furthermore, in overweight individuals metformin was more effective than sulphonylureas in reducing diabetic complications.

Peripheral vascular disease

The vascular damage associated with diabetes is a major risk factor for the development of peripheral vascular disease, leading to ischaemia, and is a major reason for limb amputation.

Neuropathy

Damage to nerves occurs through glycation and the production of polyols. This may lead to impaired nervous conduction and is referred to as neuropathy. The neuropathy may be peripheral, leading to loss of peripheral sensation and ulceration, or autonomic, which may lead to postural hypotension and impotence.

Monitoring

Monitoring of glycaemic control is important in the management of diabetes but is especially important in patients who use insulin and alter their dose according to the level of control. Monitoring is best achieved by measuring blood glucose levels using a reagent stick and simple meter, so that the levels of control may be assessed and the dose of insulin or antidiabetic drugs adjusted accordingly. Long-term monitoring of control is by measuring the levels of HbA1c in the blood. This gives a measure of the long-term control (previous 2 months): a value of 7% or less is associated with reduced diabetic complications. In addition, blood pressure, cholesterol, renal and visual function are routinely monitored.

Over-the-counter considerations

Many medicines, including many over-the-counter (OTC) preparations for coughs and colds, contain sugar and patients should be made aware of this in relation to their daily intake. Sugar-free alternatives are available but may be more expensive and often contain sorbitol, which may cause diarrhoea.

Cornplasters that contain salicylic acid should not be used in patients with diabetes, because patients with diabetic neuropathy may have less sensation in the feet and the corrosive effects of cornplasters may go unnoticed, leading to ulceration. All foot problems affecting patients with diabetes warrant prompt referral.

Decongestants should be used with caution in patients with diabetes because the β-adrenoceptor agonist activity may alter glucose control via anti-insulin affects.

Dietary supplements

Insulin therapy or antidiabetic drugs are the only appropriate treatments for diabetes. However, a number of dietary supplements, in addition to a balanced diet, may play some role in the management of diabetes. Examples of these include aloe vera, which has been shown to exert hypoglycaemic actions and may have a potential role as an adjunct to conventional treatment; carnitine may increase glucose utilization. Other herbal preparations with potential hypoglycaemic activity include burdock, celery, dandelion, eucalyptus, garlic, ginger, ispaghula, juniper, marshmallow, nettle and sage. Studies on animal models of diabetes suggest that evening primrose oil may be of benefit in neuropathy. Hyperglycaemic effects are associated with hydrocotyle, liquorice and rosemary. For a more detailed discussion of this topic, the reader is referred to *Dietary Supplements* by Mason (2007).

Counselling

Diabetes mellitus is a lifelong condition and patients will receive a range of counselling from doctors, specialist nurses and dieticians. Patients may also be directed to organizations such as Diabetes UK for further information and advice. The key to counselling is to ensure good glycaemic control, which is associated with the prevention of diabetic complications. In addition, practical advice that may be given includes the following.

Diabetes in general

- Give advice about the regimen.
- The patient should be made aware of the signs of hypo- and hyperglycaemia and how to respond to them.
- Patients with diabetes should inform the DVLA (Driver and Vehicle Licensing Agency) of their condition.
- Patients should be warned to avoid hypoglycaemia while driving.
- Patients prescribed insulin and those at risk of hypoglycaemia should carry glucose tablets or similar at all times.
- In addition to dietary advice, special diabetic foods are expensive and of little value.
- It is a misconception that natural fruit juice, honey and reduced-sugar products are low in sugar.
- Patients with diabetes represent a risk group (see Chapter 1) and the importance of consulting their GP should be emphasized.
- Patients with diabetes should consult their GP if they experience problems with their feet, including fungal infections.
- Patients with type 1 and type 2 diabetes (treated with drugs) are exempt from prescription charges.
- Lifestyle advice to reduce cardiovascular risk, including cessation of smoking, should be emphasized.
- Alcohol should be consumed only in moderation and it may mask the signs of hypoglycaemia.
- Alcoholic drinks will also contribute towards the carbohydrate load.

- Low-dose aspirin should be considered for patients with a significant risk of cardiovascular disease.
- Exercise improves insulin sensitivity and reduces cardiovascular risk.
- Advice should be sought before becoming pregnant.
- A MedicAlert chain or card should be carried if possible to alert doctors that the patient is prescribed insulin. A service is available whereby patients register their insulin regimen and a number is available for emergency doctors to contact if needed.

Type 1 diabetes

- Patients should be advised to maintain adequate supplies of insulin.
- Patients should not stop taking insulin.
- Give advice about injection technique.
- Insulins should be stored in a refrigerator but not frozen.
- Different injection sites should be used, although the rate of absorption may differ between sites.
- The dispensed container of insulin should be shown to the patient for confirmation that it is expected by the patient.
- The size of the pen needle should be checked carefully when prescribing and dispensing due to the increasing variety of sizes, which reflect different injection techniques.

- Sugary food may be eaten but preferably as part of a meal.
- Needles should be disposed of correctly.

Type 2 diabetes

- Metformin should be taken with or after food.
- Diarrhoea is a common side effect with metformin and acarbose.
- Nateglinide and repaglinide should be taken just before meals.
- Alcohol should be avoided with chlorpropamide.

Self-assessment

Consider whether the following statements are true or false. In the management of diabetes:

1. Dietary measures alone usually control type 1 diabetes.
2. Sulphonylureas do not usually promote weight gain.
3. Metformin is contraindicated in renal impairment.
4. Glitazones are PPAR-γ agonists.
5. ACE inhibitors are regarded as renoprotective.

Practice points

- Diabetes is a major risk factor for cardiovascular disease, so a healthy lifestyle (including avoidance of obesity and cessation of smoking) is essential.
- Blood pressure should be adequately controlled and ACE inhibitors are effective at reducing diabetic nephropathy.
- The risk of developing type 2 diabetes may be reduced by a lifelong healthy diet, weight control and exercise.
- Type 2 diabetes continues to be underdiagnosed.
- Good glycaemic control may prevent future complications.

CASE STUDY

A 65-year-old woman visits her pharmacist for her third tube of clotrimazole for vaginal thrush in as many weeks and also complains that she is always thirsty. This time her pharmacist refers her to her GP.

Why was a referral made?

- Both recurrent genital thrush and thirst are symptoms of diabetes and should raise suspicion for referral.

  On visiting her GP an examination reveals a blood pressure of 160/100 mmHg and biochemistry reveals:

  random glucose: 14.0 mmol/L (<11.1 mmol/L)
  creatinine: 100 micromoles/L (60–120 micromoles/L)
  cholesterol: 6 mmol/L (ideal <5.2 mmol/L)
  haematology: normal.

  She was referred for further glucose tests and then to a dietician.

Why was she referred for dietary advice?

- The random glucose level is consistent with diabetes and in type 2 diabetes dietary control should be tried for 3 months to determine whether this alone controls the condition.

  Three months later she presents you with a prescription:

  atenolol 50 mg once daily
  glibenclamide 5 mg daily.

  Comment on this prescription.

- The atenolol is for blood pressure control, which is essential in diabetes. Although atenolol is effective, it may impair warning signs of hypoglycaemia. Atenolol is no longer recommended as a first-line antihypertensive and an ACE inhibitor would be a better choice in diabetes. Glibenclamide is relatively long acting and is associated with hypoglycaemia. A shorter-acting agent such as gliclazide or tolbutamide might have been more appropriate, especially in older patients. If the woman were obese then metformin would be more appropriate.

How does glibenclamide act?

- It inhibits K_{ATP} channels on the ß cells of the islets of Langerhans, leading to cellular depolarization and insulin release.

After several weeks she complains to her pharmacist of feeling weak and confused and once again is referred to her GP. This time her random glucose was measured as 3 mmol/L and her blood pressure was 140/90 mmHg. Her GP advised her to drink a sugary cup of tea immediately and her prescription was changed to:

atenolol 50 mg once daily
tolbutamide 1 g daily in divided doses.

continued

CASE STUDY (continued)

Why was this change made?

• The confusion and low glucose levels are indicative of hypoglycaemia, which is probably due to glibenclamide. She was changed to tolbutamide, which is less likely to cause hypoglycaemia. A year later she is under the care of a consultant diabetologist and her prescription was changed to:

> ramipril 2.5 mg daily (with a view to increments over several weeks up to 10 mg)
> tolbutamide 1 g daily in divided doses
> simvastatin 10 mg every night.

What was the rationale behind these changes?

• The ACE inhibitor is a more logical antihypertensive in patients with diabetes. The HOPE trial indicates that ramipril is protective against diabetic nephropathy and reduces complications of diabetes. The simvastatin has been used to reduce plasma cholesterol and so reduce her overall cardiovascular risk.

How would you counsel the patient with respect to these changes?

• She should initially take the ramipril on retiring to bed at night in case of profound first-dose hypotension.
• Simvastatin should be taken at night when endogenous cholesterol synthesis is greatest.

On changing her medication, she complained of a racing heart.

What is the possible explanation for this?

• Abrupt withdrawal of atenolol is associated with tachyarrhythmias due to upregulation of β-adrenoceptors on the heart. Withdrawal should be gradual or under close supervision.

References

CALM study group (2000). Randomised controlled trial of dual blockade of the renin–angiotensin system in patients with hypertension, microalbuminuria, and non-insulin dependent diabetes: the candesartan and lisinopril microalbuminuria (CALM) study. *BMJ* **321**: 1440–4.

DCCT (Diabetes Control and Complications Trial Research Group) (1993). The effect of intensive treatment of diabetes on the development and progression of long-term complications in insulin-dependent diabetes mellitus. *N Engl J Med* **329**: 977–86.

Heart Protection Study Collaborative Group (2002). MRC/BHF Heart Protection Study of cholesterol lowering with simvastatin in 20 536 high-risk individuals: randomised placebo-controlled trial. *Lancet* **360**: 7–22.

HOPE (Heart Outcomes Prevention Evaluation) study investigators (2000). Effects of an angiotensin-converting-enzyme inhibitor, ramipril, on cardiovascular events in high-risk patients. *N Engl J Med* **342**: 145–53.

LIFE (Losartan Intervention for Endpoint Reduction in Hypertension) study investigators (2002). Cardiovascular morbidity and mortality in patients with diabetes in the Losartan Intervention for Endpoint

Reduction in Hypertension study (LIFE): a randomised trial against atenolol. *Lancet* **359**: 1004–10.

Mason P (2007). *Dietary Supplements*, 3rd edn. London: Pharmaceutical Press.

Meier C, Kraenzlin ME, Bodmer M *et al* (2008). Use of thiazolidinediones and fracture risk. *Arch Intern Med* **168**: 820–5.

National Institute for Clinical Excellence (2002). *Management of Type 2 Diabetes: Renal disease – prevention and early management*. London: NICE.

National Institute for Clinical Excellence (2003). *Glitazones for the Treatment of Type 2 Diabetes Mellitus*. Technology Appraisal Guidance no. 63. London: NICE.

Nissen SE, Wolski K (2007). Effect of rosiglitazone on the risk of myocardial infarction and death from cardiovascular causes. *N Engl J Med* **356**: 2457–73.

UKPDS (UK Prospective Diabetes Study) Group (1998a). Intensive blood-glucose control with sulphonylurea or insulin compared with conventional treatment and the risk of complications in patients with type 2 diabetes (UKPDS 33). *Lancet* **352**: 837–53.

UKPDS Group (1998b). Effects of intensive blood-glucose control with metformin on the complications in overweight patients with type 2 diabetes (UKPDS 34). *Lancet* **352**: 854–65.

Further reading

Berger J, Moller D E (2002). The mechanisms of action of PPARs. *Annu Rev Med* **53**: 409–35.

Simpson H (2001). Insulin regimens in type 1 diabetes management. *Prescriber* **12**: 43–57.

Online resource

www.diabetes.org.uk
The website of Diabetes UK, the current name of the British Diabetic Association, which provides both patient and professional information (accessed May 2008).

36

Thyroid disorders

The thyroid gland releases predominantly thyroxine (T_4), but also triiodothyronine (T_3), which is the more active hormone; indeed, T_4 may undergo peripheral conversion to T_3. Both of these hormones play important roles in the regulation of cellular metabolism and growth, while also influencing activity of the sympathetic nervous system. Clinically there may be excessive activity (hyperthyroidism) or underactivity (hypothyroidism), both of which have widespread pathophysiological effects. Detailed guidance on thyroid disorders and their treatment may be found in Vanderpump *et al* (1996), which is published on behalf of The Royal College of Physicians (London) and the Society for Endocrinology.

Hyperthyroidism

This is also known as thyrotoxicosis and is generally characterized by elevated levels of T_3 and T_4. The most common form is Graves' disease, which is due to antibodies against the thyroid-stimulating hormone (TSH) receptor, responsible for stimulating the release of T_3 and T_4. The antibodies activate the receptor and lead to the increased production of thyroid hormone, and there is usually an increase in the size of the thyroid gland (goitre). Other less common causes include toxic multinodular goitre, toxic adenoma and iatrogenic causes. In the last case, drugs that have a high iodine content such as amiodarone and radiological contrast agents may lead to increased thyroid activity; lithium may rarely cause hyperthyroidism.

Clinical features

Hyperthyroidism is especially common in women and occurs most often between the ages of 20 and 40 years. There may be widespread changes, which include:

- weight loss
- increased appetite
- diarrhoea
- nervousness and irritability
- fatigue
- tremor
- increased sweating
- heat intolerance
- pruritus
- exophthalmos (bulging eyes, seen in Graves' disease only)
- eyelid retraction
- goitre
- cardiac arrhythmias, including palpitations and atrial fibrillation
- angina
- precipitation of heart failure
- shortness of breath on exertion
- nausea and vomiting in pregnancy
- palmar erythema.

Many of these symptoms may be attributable to the increased action of catecholamines.

Diagnosis

In addition to the above symptoms, biochemistry will reveal increased levels of thyroid hormones but undetectable levels of TSH. This latter finding is due to increased levels of thyroid hormone causing negative-feedback inhibition of TSH release from the pituitary gland. Thyroid function tests may be complicated by concurrent drug treatment, including the use of amiodarone, aspirin, β blockers, carbamazepine, corticosteroids, heparin, oestrogens, phenytoin, rifampicin and radiological contrast agents. In this respect, the enzyme inducers carbamazepine, phenytoin and rifampicin may accelerate the metabolism of T_4 and T_3, leading to reduced levels. Corticosteroids may inhibit TSH release, lowering T_4 and T_3. By contrast, heparin may give a rapid but short-lived increase in T_4 and radiological contrast agents may elevate T_4 due to their high iodine content.

Given the non-specific nature of some of the symptoms, thyroid function is often routinely measured in patients presenting with a range of symptoms, e.g. palpitations in young adults.

Goals of treatment

These are to achieve a euthyroid state (normal levels of thyroid hormones), and to provide symptomatic relief from the increased sympathetic activity.

Management

To achieve euthyroidism the choice is from the use of antithyroid drugs (thionamides), radioactive iodine to irradiate and destroy part of the thyroid gland, and a partial or subtotal thyroidectomy.

Pharmacological basis of management

Thionamides: carbimazole and propylthiouracil

These decrease the production of thyroid hormones by inhibiting the iodination of thyroglobulin, which occurs via inhibition of thyroperoxidase. The thyroid hormones have long plasma half-lives, so inhibiting their synthesis will take several weeks for an effect to occur. Thionamides may also suppress the immune response, but whether this contributes to their action in hyperthyroidism is unclear.

β Blockers: atenolol, nadolol, propranolol

These are dealt with extensively in Chapter 11. In the context of hyperthyroidism, they will reduce the actions of catecholamines at β-adrenoceptors, which are augmented in this condition, and will provide relief from symptoms such as tremor, anxiety and palpitations. Non-selective β blockers (e.g. propranolol) are required to relieve the tremor. It should also be noted that hyperthyroidism accelerates the metabolism of propranolol.

Treatment (Figure 36.1)

Thionamides are indicated for the first episode of Graves' disease with a view to achieving a remission. It is also used in subsequent episodes of Graves' disease, in more elderly patients and those with toxic nodular hyperthyroidism, to achieve euthyroidism before surgery or with radioactive iodine for a definitive cure. In the case of drug-induced hyperthyroidism, the causative drug should be stopped and a β blocker used to control the symptoms.

Carbimazole is the thionamide of choice, with once-daily administration. It is initially given at higher doses, known as reducing doses, to achieve a euthyroid state, which takes about 1–2 months to achieve. During this time, unless contraindicated (asthma, chronic obstructive pulmonary disease, uncontrolled heart failure), a β blocker is given to control symptoms. Once the euthyroid state is achieved, maintenance therapy with the thionamide at a lower dose may be used, typically for 18 months, and the β blocker withdrawn gradually. Alternatively, a high dose of carbimazole may be maintained to suppress thyroid activity completely and combined with replacement T_4, and this is known as the blocking-replacement regimen. This has the advantage of avoiding hypothyroidism, which may be induced by antithyroid drugs, and a reduced requirement for monitoring of thyroid function. Block-and-replace regimens might be most appropriate for patients in whom it is difficult to achieve a euthyroid state on antithyroid drugs alone. Despite the use of antithyroid drugs, the relapse rate is around 50% on discontinuation of

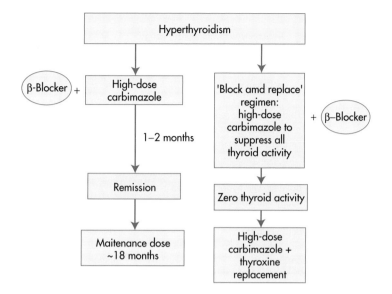

Figure 36.1   A summary of approaches to the management of hyperthyroidism.

treatment, although it is unclear whether blocking-replacement regimens have a higher success rate.

Other considerations

Pregnancy and breast-feeding

Carbimazole may cause hypothyroidism in the fetus but is generally considered safe in pregnancy under specialist care, with the lowest effective dose used, and this may be stopped before birth. Propylthiouracil is sometimes preferred because carbimazole may induce fetal aplasia cutis (a localized absence of skin at birth). A blocking-replacement regimen is contraindicated in pregnancy, because the antithyroid drugs more readily cross the placenta than T_4 and this may lead to fetal hypothyroidism.

Carbimazole at doses of <20 mg is considered safe during lactation, because the amounts in the milk are low. Once again, propylthiouracil is sometimes preferred because it enters the breast milk to a lesser extent.

Asthma

Hyperthyroidism may sometimes lead to a worsening of asthma. β_2 Agonists should be used with caution as bronchodilators because they may be expected to have enhanced systemic actions in uncontrolled hyperthyroidism. Indeed,

the symptoms of toxicity with β_2 agonists may also be confused with those of hyperthyroidism. As commented above, asthma is a contraindication to using β blockers in the management of hyperthyroidism. In patients who cannot receive a β blocker, calcium channel blockers such as diltiazem may be useful in controlling tachycardia.

Monitoring

No specific monitoring, except thyroid function, is required for treatment with thionamides. However, carbimazole and propylthiouracil may both cause agranulocytosis leading to leukopenia. If patients report with sore throats, mouth ulcers, bruising or non-specific illness, a full blood count should be carried out and the drug withdrawn if there is leukopenia. Although an alternative thionamide may be used as a replacement, there is a high degree of cross-reactivity between agents.

Drug interactions

Drug interactions with antithyroid drugs are limited and detailed in Table 36.1.

Table 36.1   Some important drug interactions with antithyroid drugs

Drugs	Consequences	Comments
Corticosteroids with carbimazole	Increased elimination of prednisolone	The dose of prednisolone may need to be increased
Digoxin with carbimazole	Carbimazole may reduce the plasma levels of digoxin. Patients with hyperthyroidism may be resistant to the actions of digoxin, such that digoxin may be less effective in atrial fibrillation in patients with hyperthyroidism	Higher doses of digoxin may be required initially and then reduced as thyroid levels fall
Theophylline with thionamides	Theophylline levels may rise in patients treated with thionamides for hyperthyroidism	Monitoring may be required and the dose of theophylline may need to be reduced
Warfarin with thionamides	The actions of warfarin may be decreased	The dose of warfarin may need to be increased

Counselling

Lifestyle advice may be helpful in relieving symptoms such as heat intolerance. Caffeine consumption should be reduced, because this may exacerbate symptoms. Ophthalmopathy in Graves' disease, presenting as photophobia and grittiness, may be relieved by sunglasses and artificial tears. Drug-specific counselling points are detailed:

- If carbimazole or propylthiouracil is taken without a β blocker, it will take several weeks for an improvement in symptoms to be noticed.
- If a β blocker is used, it is worth explaining its role to the patient, and that it is not being used for hypertension or angina, which may be indicated on the patient information leaflets. General counselling for β blockers is found in Chapter 11.
- Both carbimazole and propylthiouracil may cause agranulocytosis, leading to leukopenia. Patients should report urgently to their GP with sore throats, mouth ulcers, bruising or non-specific illness.
- Both carbimazole and propylthiouracil may cause mild gastrointestinal disturbances and urticarial rashes. Pruritus may be managed with antihistamines and treatment continued. If this fails, an alternative agent may be tried because cross-sensitivity may not occur.

- Patients should be advised to report symptoms of hypothyroidism, which may indicate overtreatment.

Hypothyroidism

This is simply failure of the thyroid gland to produce sufficient thyroid hormone, leading to reduced circulating levels. The most common form (90%) is Hashimoto's thyroiditis, which is an autoimmune destruction of the thyroid gland. Hypothyroidism may also be induced by antithyroid drug treatment with thionamides, lithium, amiodarone and also radioactive iodine.

Clinical features

As with hyperthyroidism, there is an increased incidence of hypothyroidism in women and this increases with age. There are widespread changes in hypothyroidism, which include:

- tiredness
- weight gain
- hypothermia
- cold intolerance
- hoarseness
- bradycardia (rarely angina and heart failure)
- mental slowness

- delayed reflexes
- depression
- anaemia
- dry skin and hair
- goitre
- oedema, leading to puffiness around the eyes
- constipation.

Diagnosis

Hypothyroidism is identified on a thyroid function test, which reveals elevated TSH and reduced T_4 levels. In addition there may be macrocytosis and hypercholesterolaemia. In secondary failure due to pituitary or hypothalamic disease, TSH levels will be reduced. Other causes should be considered before starting treatment.

Goals of treatment

These are to achieve a euthyroid state.

Management

Restoring thyroid hormone levels is achieved by administration of levothyroxine (T_4). In young patients the starting dose is usually 50–100 micrograms/day, which may be increased after 6 weeks by 25–50 micrograms, and thereafter until maintenance levels are achieved. The dose required is the one that leads to correct TSH levels. In elderly patients, and those with ischaemic heart disease, the starting dose used is 25 micrograms, which is increased every 3–4 weeks by 25 micrograms, until TSH levels are normalized. The reason to exercise caution in patients with ischaemic heart disease is that T_4 may lead to worsening or uncovering of angina (there is also an increased risk of myocardial infarction and death) by increasing the metabolic rate and sympathetic activity. In patients who experience angina, a β blocker may be prescribed. If the TSH levels are suppressed by overtreatment, there is a significant risk of atrial fibrillation. Once established, T_4 therapy will need to be used lifelong.

Diabetes mellitus

An increased dose of antidiabetic agents, including insulin, may be required.

Pregnancy

T_4 treatment is continued during pregnancy but the dose may need to be increased to normalize TSH levels.

Drug interactions

Some important interactions with T_4 are detailed in Table 36.2. The interactions relate to altering the effects of T_4 or interacting drugs.

Counselling

Aside from guidance on the regimen, a key counselling point should be to advise patients to consult their GP if they start to suffer from angina or pre-existing angina deteriorates. Additional points:

- It is difficult to distinguish between the strengths of T_4 tablets, because they are all small and white. Patients should make sure that they take tablets of the correct strength.
- If a dose is missed, the missed dose may be taken the next day with the next dose (as T_4 has a long half-life of 7 days).
- Patients should be encouraged to report symptoms of overtreatment, particularly when treatment is initiated. These include diarrhoea, nervousness, rapid pulse, insomnia, tremors or anginal pain. These symptoms may necessitate a reduced dose or the omission of a dose for 1–2 days before restarting at a lower dose.

OTC medicines in patients with thyroid disorders

Topical or oral sympathomimetic drugs should be avoided in patients with hyperthyroidism, due to the enhancement of catecholamines.

Table 36.2   Drugs interacting with levothyroxine

Drug	Consequences	Comments
Amiodarone	Reduced effects of levothyroxine	Contraindicated by manufacturers. The *British National Formulary* indicates that, if amiodarone causes hyperthyroidism, amiodarone should be withdrawn and antithyroid drugs may be required. If hypothyroidism is induced then replacement therapy may be needed
Antiepileptic drugs (carbamazepine and phenytoin)	These enzyme inducers have been reported to lower thyroid hormone levels occasionally	Monitoring may be appropriate
Colestyramine	This may reduce the absorption of levothyroxine	Their use should be separated by 4–6 h
Ferrous sulphate	This may reduce the absorption of levothyroxine	Their doses should be separated by 2 h
Digoxin	Hypothyroid patients are relatively more sensitive to digoxin	The dose of digoxin may need to be reduced as levothyroxine treatment is established
Sertraline	The effects of levothyroxine have been reported to be reduced	The dose of levothyroxine may need to be increased
Lofepramine		Its use with levothyroxine is contraindicated by the manufacturers
Theophylline	Reduced effects of theophylline	The dose of theophylline may need to be increased
Tricyclic antidepressants	Levothyroxine may accelerate the responses to imipramine and amitriptyline	The manufacturers of lofepramine contraindicate its use with levothyroxine
Warfarin	Increased anticoagulant effects of warfarin	The dose of warfarin may need to be reduced

Pharmacists can help to remind patients of the need for prompt referral when presenting with signs of infection on being prescribed antithyroid medication. Pharmacists may also help to identify patients presenting with symptoms suggestive of thyroid disorder and encourage referral for further investigation, e.g. the common request for over-the-counter (OTC) products for fatigue and/or slimming advice may prompt further questioning to identify the possibility of an underlying thyroid disorder.

Herbal medicines in patients with thyroid disorders

Kelp is used as herbal treatment for thyroid disorders. However, it has a high iodine content that may lead to hyper- or hypothyroidism, and it should be avoided. Preparations of ephedra should be avoided due to the ephedrine content. Shepherd's purse also has the potential to cause hypothyroidism and should therefore be avoided by patients prescribed thyroid treatment.

Other supplements

Many multivitamin and mineral preparation contain approximately 50–100% of the recommended daily intake of iodine. This is generally provided in the diet, with the possible exception of the vegan diet. Toxicity is rare at these doses but patients prescribed thyroid treatment should be careful to avoid excess doses, which may interfere with their treatment.

Practice points

- Both hyperthyroidism and hypothyroidism may present with relatively non-specific symptoms.
- Both may be readily diagnosed by thyroid function tests.
- Both may be managed by drugs; β blockers provide symptomatic relief in hyperthyroidism.
- Be alert for leukopenia in patients taking carbimazole and propylthiouracil.

Self-assessment

Consider whether the following statements are true or false. In the management of thyroid disorders:

1. In hyperthyroidism, β blockers are used to reduce the release of T_4.
2. Carbimazole is occasionally associated with agranulocytosis.
3. Amiodarone may cause thyroid dysfunction.
4. Block-and-replace regimens are used to manage hypothyroidism.
5. Levothyroxine may worsen ischaemic heart disease.

 CASE STUDY

A 35-year-old woman with a history of mild asthma developed anxiety, palpitations, rapid pulse and feelings of panic not long after a fall down a full flight of stairs. She put the symptoms down to the fall. Her symptoms worsened until she lost 10 kg (1.5 stone) in a week, developed a tremor, had broken vessels in the eye and the back of the knee, and a pulse of 150 beats/min, at which time she visited her GP. She was hyperthyroid and was prescribed propranolol and carbimazole. The pharmacist picked up a history of asthma and she was changed to atenolol. She developed a rash on her hands and feet but continued treatment for 2 years, at which point treatment was withdrawn.

- In this case it is possible that the initial palpitations and tachycardia may, in part, have been due to overuse of a β_2-adrenoceptor agonist or its increased sensitivity in hyperthyroidism. The pharmacist was correct to question the use of propranolol and atenolol was appropriate only if symptomatic control was considered absolutely essential because β_1-adrenoceptor antagonists may still lead to bronchospasm in patients with asthma. The rash would have been viewed as an acceptable side effect of carbimazole.

References

Martin J, ed. *British National Formulary*, latest edition. London: British Medical Association and Royal Pharmaceutical Society of Great Britain.

Vanderpump MPJ, Ahlquist JAO, Franklyn JA *et al* (1996). Consensus statement for good practice and audit measures in the management of hypothyroidism and hyperthyroidism. *BMJ* **313**: 539–44.

Further reading

Dale J, Franklyn J (2002). The drug treatment of thyroid disorders. *Prescriber* **13**: 50–71.

Online resource

www.british-thyroid-association.org
The website of the British Thyroid Association providing professional and patient advice (accessed May 2008).

Feedback on self-assessments

Chapter 3

1. False: this is the recommendation for general health. Long sessions of 45–60 minutes are recommended to prevent obesity.
2. False: norethisterone and other progestogens interact with antibacterials that are enzyme inducers but not all antibiotics, unlike oral oestrogens whose absorption is reduced by broad-spectrum antibiotics.
3. True: although it should be noted that this interaction may not be clinically significant with all calcium channel blockers.
4. True: warfarin is a vitamin K antagonist and its actions may be reduced by foods rich in vitamin K.
5. True: there is a risk of symptoms of depression, including suicidal thoughts and behaviour in patients taking varenicline to help them stop smoking.

Chapter 4

1. False: they contain pharmacologically active components and may therefore produce adverse effects, particularly in concentrated form as supplements.
2. False: not many products currently have a THR number as this system is still in its infancy. However, these products should be supplied in preference to those without as more become available.
3. False: all serious adverse reactions to herbal preparations should be reported.

4. False: those with cardioactive activity or which alter clotting should be discontinued before surgery (see Table 4.1).
5. True.

Chapter 7

1. True: they inhibit the final common pathway
2. False: proton pump inhibitors (PPIs) inhibit the H^+/K^+ pump.
3. True: newer H_2-receptor antagonists that do not interact are preferred.
4. True: these have a major role.
5. True: they will promote emptying of the stomach.
6. False: PPIs (and H_2-receptor antagonists) should be avoided for 2 weeks before the test because they may mask the disease.
7. True: this is the leading cause of ulceration.
8. False: it involves two antibiotics (from amoxicillin, clarithromycin and metronidazole) plus a PPI.
9. True: chronic bleeding may lead to iron deficiency anaemia.
10. True: see Chapter 5.

Chapter 9

1. False: loperamide will not reduce the time course but does reduce the need to pass stools. Loperamide reduces motility and so may reduce the washout of the causative agent, potentially increasing the length of infection.
2. True and requires immediate investigation.

3. True and is a reason to co-prescribe laxatives.
4. False: selective serotonin reuptake inhibitors (SSRIs) do cause some degree of gastro-intestinal dysfunction (especially nausea) but it is the tricylic antidepressants that are constipating.
5. False: irritable bowel syndrome may be diagnosed in long-standing bowel disorder with pain, bloating and episodes of diarrhoea and/or constipation. Bloody diarrhoea is not a feature and is an alerting symptom for referral.

Chapter 11

1. True: they are initially taken on retiring to bed to limit the impact of this.
2. False: they become less effective in renal impairment as they are normally excreted in the proximal convoluted tubules to reach their site of action.
3. False: they are used in ischaemic heart disease and are suitable for concurrent hypertension.
4. True.
5. False: although dual blockade is sometimes used, their major role is in patients who cannot tolerate ACE inhibitors.

Chapter 12

1. False: it is taken at night when cholesterol synthesis is greatest.
2. False: it may be used for moderate risk male patients aged >45 years and patients aged >55 years who are either male or females with moderate risk factors.
3. True: although statins may be used.
4. True: a significant adverse drug reaction.
5. True: statins are now recognized as reducing mortality in patients with cardiovascular disease.

Chapter 13

1. False: rimonabant is a cannabinoid receptor antagonist.
2. False: there may be a clinical need for an antipsychotic. A risk vs benefit assessment is needed.
3. True: monitoring is required particularly during the first 4 weeks of treatment.
4. True: close monitoring is required.
5. False: SSRIs are less likely to cause weight gain and are therefore preferred.

Chapter 14

1. False: there is a risk of a serious interaction between β blockers and verapamil with a risk of asystole.
2. True: if this fails to provide relief help should be sought as the patient may be experiencing a heart attack.
3. False: antiplatelet drugs are used such as low-dose aspirin or clopidogrel because arterial thrombosis is largely a platelet-dependent event.
4. True.
5. True: a standard and effective regimen for secondary prevention.

Chapter 15

1. True: this may exceed the maximum licensed dose.
2. True.
3. False: they provide symptomatic relief from oedema but are not established at improving outcome.
4. False: metoprolol, bisoprolol and carvedilol are now recognized as playing a major role in CHF.
5. False: patients should be counselled to report to the doctor if the pulse rate falls below 60 beats/min.

Chapter 16

1. True: heparin causes rapid anticoagulation and is often used when this is required immediately and when warfarin is being initiated.
2. False: INR is measured to monitor the actions of warfarin.
3. False: warfarin inhibits the production of functional coagulation by the liver and acts only *in vivo*.
4. False: warfarin is a vitamin K antagonist and its actions may be reversed or opposed by vitamin K.
5. True: this is a common interaction.

Chapter 17

1. False: it is microcytic.
2. False: it is commonly associated with chronic bleeding and rarely due to a poor diet.
3. True: due to the breakdown of the red blood cells.
4. False: it is managed with folic acid and/or vitamin B_{12} as hydroxocobalamin.
5. False: pregnancy is commonly associated with anaemia and iron tablets are often given for prophylaxis.

Chapter 18

1. False: they are increased.
2. True: due to reduced production of EPO.
3. False: phosphate binders are used to reduce intake of phosphate from the diet.
4. True: this limits further renal damage.
5. True: ACE inhibitors have a major role in the prevention of diabetic nephropathy.

Chapter 19

1. True: simple analgesia plays a major role. Antibiotics are rarely indicated as most infections are viral.

2. False: prolonged use often leads to rebound secretion.
3. True: be alert for this in patients taking drugs associated with causing neutropenia.
4. True: requires urgent referral to exclude serious lung disease.
5. True: a common first-line drug.

Chapter 21

1. True: indeed if it is required more than three times a week then the patient's therapy should be moved up a step.
2. True: this is an important counselling point.
3. False: they are preventive and should not be used to relieve an attack.
4. False: this used to the case but β_2 agonists and then inhaled steroids are the initial measure.
5. True: leukotrienes are likely to be involved in NSAID-induced asthma.
6. False: only about 15% of patients will respond to steroid therapy and this may be because they actually have undiagnosed asthma.
7. False: but a controversial issue. β Blockers should be avoided in asthma but in COPD one has to balance the advantages (e.g. in heart failure) against the drawbacks (bronchoconstriction). Some clinicians might cautiously use a cardioselective agent at a low dose.
8. True: an important cause of exacerbations.
9. False: they are the mainstay of therapy.
10. False: in severe disease oxygen up to 28% is used.

Chapter 22

1. True: migraine may reduce gastric emptying.
2. False: they are actually full $5HT_{1D}$ agonists and may also activate $5HT_{1B}$- and $5HT_{1F}$-receptors.
3. False: they should be taken at the start of an attack when pain is mild.

4. False: rotation may identify a triptan to which the patient may respond.
5. True.

Chapter 23

1. False: monotherapy is preferred and combination therapy is used only once different drugs alone have failed to control the condition.
2. False: enzyme-inducing antiepileptic drugs reduce the effectiveness of oral contraceptives.
3. True: due to risk of teratogenesis and weight gain may also be unacceptable.
4. True: patients should be counselled to report signs and symptoms of infection.
5. False: when seizures have been absent for prolonged periods it may be appropriate to consider the gradual withdrawal of drugs.

Chapter 24

1. False: on average they are equally effective but SSRIs have a superior side-effect profile.
2. False: antidepressants are best avoided in patients aged <18 years but, if one is indicated, fluoxetine is preferred and paroxetine should be avoided.
3. False: the response should occur after 2–3 weeks.
4. True: an important side effect due to antimuscarinic binding.
5. False: this combination should be avoided because it may lead to serotoninergic syndrome.

Chapter 25

1. False: benzodiazepines enhance the inhibitory actions of the GABA system.
2. False: their effects are quick in onset but they should not be used for prolonged periods (>2–4 weeks).

3. False: they may relieve the somatic symptoms of anxiety.
4. True: these include citalopram, escitalopram, paroxetine.
5. True.

Chapter 26

1. True: diuretics may be associated with insomnia indirectly if diuresis occurs at night.
2. False: temazepam is a short-acting benzodiazepine and therefore suitable for short-term treatment of insomnia, having reduced hangover effects compared with longer-acting drugs.
3. True: excess caffeine and alcohol consumption and eating a large meal late at night are all associated with insomnia.
4. False: promethazine is an antihistamine available over-the-counter but should be used only occasionally due to the risk of adverse effects, e.g. antimuscarinic effects, and also reduced effectiveness after a few days of treatment.
5. True: establishing the pattern of insomnia is important so that an appropriate referral can be made and the underlying cause treated.

Chapter 27

1. False: the NICE considers them as first-line agents, except clozapine which is restricted to patients who have failed to respond to at least two other agents, including an atypical antipsychotic.
2. True: white blood cell counts require monitoring and patients should be counselled to report signs of infection.
3. False: they are associated with weight gain.
4. False: although they have a lower incidence.
5. False: they are dopamine receptor antagonists.

Chapter 28

1. False: they inhibit the peripheral conversion of levodopa to dopamine which is associated with side effects.
2. False: the usefulness of levodopa has a finite period.
3. True: domperidone does not penetrate the blood–brain barrier and so will not antagonize the central effects of dopamine.
4. True: they do not require dietary restrictions.
5. True.

Chapter 29

1. False: aspirin is generally avoided now due to gastric side effects and its use being prohibited in children.
2. True: it is devoid of anti-inflammatory actions.
3. True: a common side effect and laxatives are co-prescribed when they are used long term.
4. False: it is widely used in neuropathic pain.
5. False: it is appropriate for chronic neuropathic pain.

Chapter 30

1. True.
2. False: this is a safe and effective combination for pain relief.
3. False: it is used in rheumatoid arthritis.
4. True: risk of an interaction leading to methotrexate toxicity.
5. False: it is used by specialists when two other DMARDs have failed to control the condition.

Chapter 31

1. False: combined preparations of antiemetic and opioid are not recommended because opioid-induced nausea usually resolves after

4–5 days and therefore long-term use of the antiemetic is not necessary.
2. True.
3. True as this may be associated with the release of prostaglandins.
4. True: a 24-hour dose is calculated and divided by 2 for modified-release preparations given twice a day.
5. False: this is a common misconception and patients should be encouraged to discuss their concerns about morphine.

Chapter 32

1. True: this is an important counselling point and patients should complete the course even if their infection appears to have resolved.
2. True: this is a common adverse effect,
3. False: patients who experience hypersensitivity to penicillins may also be hypersensitive to cephalosporins, which precludes their use in patients with a penicillin allergy unless there is no alternative.
4. True.
5. False: chloramphenicol is available as an OTC medicine for patients aged 2 years and above.

Chapter 33

1. False: they should be used only during an infestation.
2. False: it is unsuitable for use in pregnancy.
3. True.
4. True: chloroquine exacerbates psoriasis.
5. False: combined oral contraception may be affected due to reduced enterohepatic circulation of the oestrogen ethinylestradiol.

Chapter 34

1. True: it should be used at all stages.
2. False: it is available as a prescription-only medicine for children and is available as an OTC medicine for patients aged >10 years.

3. True: when topical steroids are unsuitable or fail to control the condition.
4. True: they are highly teratogenic and patients must ensure adequate contraception.
5. False: it has relatively few drug interactions, which contrasts with some 'azoles' that have widespread interactions.

Chapter 35

1. False: dietary measures may control type 2 diabetes but insulin therapy is required in type 1.
2. False: because they increase insulin release they tend to cause weight gain.
3. True.
4. True: this leads to insulin sensitization.
5. True: they are used to prevent nephropathy and are often regarded as the antihypertensives of choice in patients with diabetes.

Chapter 36

1. False: they are used to oppose increased sympathetic activity and so provide symptomatic relief.
2. True: a significant adverse reaction and patients should be counselled to be vigilant of increased infections (e.g. sore throats, mouth ulcers).
3. True: in a significant proportion of patients it can lead to hyper- and hypothyroidism, as well as alterations in thyroid function tests.
4. False: it may be used in hyperthyroidism.
5. True: it should be used with caution as it may worsen the symptoms of angina.

Appendix 1

Formulary of some important classes of drugs, commonly used examples, mechanisms of action and uses

Class	Examples	Actions	Common uses
Gastrointestinal			
Proton pump inhibitors (PPIs)	Omeprazole,[a] lansoprazole, rabeprazole	Irreversible proton pump inhibition	Acid suppression – peptic ulceration, GORD, prophylaxis against NSAID-induced damage
Histamine H_2-receptor antagonists	Ranitidine,[a] cimetidine[a]	Antagonism of histamine H_2-receptor	Acid suppression – peptic ulceration, GORD, dyspepsia
Cytoprotective prostaglandin analogue	Misoprostol	Analogue of PGE_1, reduces H^+ secretion and stimulates bicarbonate and mucus secretion	Prophylaxis against NSAID-induced damage
Triple therapy for *Helicobacter pylori* eradication	PPI plus two from amoxicillin, clarithromycin and metronidazole	Acid suppression and *H. pylori* eradication	*H. pylori* eradication in peptic ulceration
Prokinetic drugs	Domperidone,[a] metoclopramide	Increase gastric emptying	Bloating and nausea
Laxative	Lactulose,[a] senna,[a] ispaghula[a]	Lactulose: osmotic. Senna: stimulant. Ispaghula: bulk	Constipation, constipation due to drugs, IBS. Lactulose: also in liver failure to prevent encephalopathy
Antidiarrhoeal agents	Loperamide[a]	Opioid: reduces colonic motility via presynaptic inhibition	Diarrhoea
Antispasmodic agents	Mebeverine[a]	Phosphodiesterase inhibitor?	IBS
Cardiovascular			
Cardiac glycosides	Digoxin	Inhibition of Na^+/K^+ ATPase	AF, positive inotrope in CHF
Class I antiarrhythmics	Lidocaine	Inhibition of Na^+ channels	Ventricular tachycardia
Class II antiarrhythmics	β Blockers (including sotalol)	Antagonism of β-adrenoceptors	Paroxysmal AF
Class III antiarrhythmics	Amiodarone, sotalol	Blockade of K^+ channels leading to action potential prolongation	AF
Class IV antiarrhythmics	Verapamil	Blockade of Ca^{2+} channels	Supraventricular tachycardia

Class	Examples	Actions	Common uses
Thiazide diuretics	Bendroflumethiazide	Inhibition of Na^+/Cl^- transporter in DCT	Hypertension, mild CHF (especially elderly people)
Loop diuretics	Furosemide, bumetanide	Inhibition of $Na^+/K^+/Cl^-$ transporter in loop of Henle; vasodilatation	CHF and LVF, renal failure
Potassium-sparing diuretics	Amiloride	Inhibition of aldosterone-sensitive Na^+ channels in DCT	Weak diuresis, especially in combination with K^+-losing diuretics (thiazides and loops)
Potassium-sparing diuretic, aldosterone antagonist	Spironolactone	Aldosterone receptor antagonist	Weak diuresis, especially in combination with K^+-losing diuretics (thiazides and loops), CHF and liver failure (ascites); Conn's syndrome
β Blockers (non-selective)	Propranolol	Antagonism of β-adrenoceptors	Hypertension, angina, post-MI, anxiety, migraine prophylaxis, hyperthyroidism.
$β_1$ Blockers	Atenolol, metoprolol, bisoprolol	Antagonism of $β_1$-adrenoceptors	Hypertension, angina, post-MI; stable CHF (with caution)
ACE inhibitors	Captopril, enalapril, ramipril, lisinopril, perindopril	Inhibition of ACE, reducing synthesis of angiotensin II	Hypertension, post-MI, CHF, diabetic nephropathy
Angiotensin (AT_1) receptor antagonist (sartans)	Losartan, candesartan, valsartan	Antagonism of AT_1-receptors	Hypertension, CHF diabetic nephropathy?
Calcium channel blockers	Verapamil, amlodipine, nifedipine, diltiazem	Inhibition of VSM Ca^{2+} channels and cardiac Ca^{2+} channels (diltiazem, verapamil)	Hypertension, angina. Diltiazem and verapamil: antiarrhythmic
Nitrates	Glyceryl trinitrate,[a] isosorbide mononitrate[a]	Act via nitric oxide to increase cGMP	Angina, CHF
K^+ channel activators	Nicorandil	Activation of ATP-sensitive K^+ channels and release of nitric oxide	Angina
α Blockers	Prazosin, doxazosin, indoramin	Antagonism of α-adrenoceptors	Resistant hypertension, prostatic hypertrophy
Centrally acting antihypertensives	Clonidine, moxonidine, α-methyldopa	Clonidine: central $α_2$-adrenoceptors. Moxonidine: central imidazoline receptors	Resistant hypertension
HMG-CoA reductase inhibitors (statins)	Simvastatin,[a] pravastatin, atorvastatin, fluvastatin	HMG-CoA reductase inhibition in cholesterol synthesis	Reduction of cholesterol in hypercholesterolaemia and in patients with a high CV risk
Fibrates	Bezafibrate, gemifibrozil	Activates α-peroxisome proliferator-activated receptors (PPAR-α)	Hypercholesterolaemia and hypertriglyceridaemia

Class	Examples	Actions	Common uses
Bile binding agents	Colestyramine	Binds bile in gastrointestinal tract	Hypercholesterolaemia
Fibrinolytics	Streptokinase	Activates plasminogen to form plasmin	Clot busting in MI, PE
Antiplatelet drugs	Low-dose aspirin,[a] clopidogrel	Aspirin: inhibition of platelet COX. Clopidogrel: ADP (P2Y$_{12}$) receptor antagonist	Prevention of MI and CVA. Prophylaxis for CVA in low-risk patients with AF
Injectable anticoagulants	Low-molecular-weight heparins (dalteparin, enoxaparin, tinzaparin), unfractionated heparin	Activates antithrombin III	Immediate anticoagulation
Oral anticoagulants	Warfarin	Vitamin K antagonist	Prophylaxis against thrombosis e.g. DVT, PE, CVA in AF, thrombosis on mechanical heart valves
Respiratory			
β$_2$ Agonists	Salbutamol, terbutaline	Activation of β$_2$-adrenoceptors	Relief in asthma, COPD
β$_2$ Agonists, long acting	Salmeterol, formoterol	Long-lasting activation of β$_2$-adrenoceptors	Long-term control in asthma, COPD
Corticosteroids	Beclometasone, budesonide	Anti-inflammatory	Prevention in asthma; 15% of COPD patients also benefit. Nasal use in hayfever[a]
Muscarinic antagonists	Ipratropium	Blockade of vagal bronchoconstriction	Relief in asthma, COPD
Cromones	Sodium cromoglicate	Unclear – may stabilize mast cells/sensory nerves	Prevention in asthma. Nasal and ocular use in hayfever[a]
Xanthines	Theophylline	Phosphodiesterase inhibition, adenosine receptor antagonist	Relief in asthma
Leukotriene receptor antagonist	Montelukast, zafirlukast	Leukotriene receptor antagonist	Prevention in asthma; NSAID-induced bronchospasm
Antihistamines	Loratadine,[a] chlorphenamine,[a] cetirizine[a]	Antagonism of H$_1$-receptors	Allergy, older sedating agents (diphenhydramine, chlorphenamine, promethazine) for insomnia
Central nervous system			
Benzodiazepines	Diazepam, temazepam	Enhancement of GABA at GABA-A receptors	Anxiety, insomnia. Short-term only
Z-drugs	Zopiclone, zolpidem	Enhancement of GABA at GABA-A receptors	Insomnia
Antipsychotics	Haloperidol, chlorpromazine, fluphenazine	Dopamine (D$_2$)-receptor antagonists	Schizophrenia
Atypical antipsychotics	Clozapine, olanzapine, risperidone	Dopamine and 5HT receptor antagonists	Schizophrenia

Class	Examples	Actions	Common uses
Antimanic drugs	Lithium	Uncertain	Bipolar affective disorder
Tricyclic antidepressants (TCAs)	Amitriptyline, lofepramine, dosulepin	Inhibition of noradrenaline (norepinephrine) and 5HT reuptake	Depression. Amitriptyline: neuropathic pain; prophylaxis in migraine, IBS
Serotonin selective reuptake inhibitors (SSRIs)	Fluoxetine, paroxetine, citalopram, sertraline	Inhibition of 5HT reuptake	Depression, anxiety, panic disorder
Monoamine oxidase inhibitors (MAOIs)	Phenelzine, moclobemide	Inhibition of MAO enzymes (moclobemide is reversible) and catecholamine metabolism	Resistant depression
Other antidepressants	Venlafaxine, reboxetine, mirtazapine	Reboxetine: noradrenaline reuptake inhibitor. Venlafaxine: serotonin–noradrenaline reuptake inhibitor. Mirtazapine α_2-antagonist and $5HT_2$ and $5HT_3$ antagonist	Depression. Venlafaxine also for anxiety
Antiobesity	Sibutramine, orlistat	Sibutramine: amine reauptake inhibitor. Orlistat: pancreatic lipase inhibitor	Obesity
Antiemetics	Promethazine,[a] cyclizine,[a] hyoscine,[a] metoclopramide, ondansetron	Promethazine and cyclizine: H_1-receptor antagonists. Hyoscine: M-receptor antagonist. Metoclopramide: dopamine D_2-receptor antagonist. Ondansetron: $5HT_3$-receptor antagonist	Promethazine, hyoscine and cyclizine: motion sickness. Metoclopramide: emesis due to anticancer drugs. Ondansetron: emesis due to anticancer drugs; postoperative nausea and vomiting
Non-opioid analgesics	Paracetamol,[a] NSAIDs (ibuprofen,[a] diclofenac, naproxen, mefenamic acid)	COX inhibition. Paracetamol may inhibit the putative COX-3?	Pain, antipyretic and NSAIDs in inflammation
COX-2 inhibitors	'Coxibs' (celecoxib, rofecoxib). Etodolac and meloxicam	Inhibition of COX-2	Inflammation
Opioid analgesics	Morphine, tramadol, codeine,[a] dihydrocodeine[a]	Opioid receptors	Pain
Opioid antagonist	Naloxone	Opioid receptor antagonist	Reversal of opioids
Antimigraine (triptans)	Sumatriptan,[a] naratriptan	$5HT_{1D}$-receptor agonists	Treatment of a migraine attack
Antimigraine, prophylaxis	Pizotifen	$5HT_2$-receptor antagonist	Prevention of migraine

Class	Examples	Actions	Common uses
Antiepileptic drugs	Sodium valproate, carbamazepine, phenytoin	Valproate: potentiation of GABA. Carbamazepine and phenytoin: use-dependent inhibition of Na+ channels, inhibiting propagation of excitation	Forms of epilepsy: all for tonic–clonic and partial seizures; valproate for absences and myoclonic seizures. Carbamazepine is also used in neuropathic pain and for bipolar affective disorder
Newer antiepileptic drugs	Lamotrigine, gabapentin	Lamotrigine: blockade of Na+ channels and decreased release of glutamate. Gabapentin: unknown	Certain forms of epilepsy (gabapentin in combination), neuropathic pain
Antiparkinsonian drugs	Levodopa with carbidopa, ropinirole, rotigotine, procyclidine, selegiline	Levodopa: conversion to dopamine. Ropinirole, rotigotine: dopamine D_2 agonists. Procyclidine: muscarinic antagonist. Selegiline: MAO-B inhibitor	Parkinson's disease
Alzheimer's disease	Donepezil, galantamine, rivastigmine	Acetylcholine esterase inhibitors	Alzheimer's disease
Antimicrobial agents			
Penicillin	Amoxicillin, phenoxymethyl-penicillin, flucloxacillin	Inhibition of cross-linking of peptide side chains	Phenoxymethylpenicillin: tonsillitis. Flucloxacillin: impetigo, cellulitis. Amoxicillin: chest infections, otitis media, UTIs
Cephalosporins	Cefalexin, cefotaxime, cefaclor	Binding to β-lactam-binding sites and inhibiting cell wall synthesis	Septicaemia, pneumonia, meningitis, biliary tract infections, peritonitis, and UTIs
Tetracylines	Tetracycline, doxycycline.	Inhibition of protein synthesis, through interfering with tRNA binding	Chlamydia infection, exacerbation of chronic bronchitis (*Haemophilus influenzae*), periodontal disease, acne, respiratory and genital mycoplasma infections. Doxycycline in malaria prophylaxis
Macrolides	Erythromycin, clarithromycin	Prevent the translocation movement of the bacterial ribosome along the mRNA and prevent protein synthesis	Suitable alternative in patients who are allergic to penicillin. Respiratory infections, whooping cough, Legionnaires' disease, campylobacter enteritis

Class	Examples	Actions	Common uses
Aminoglycosides	Gentamicin	Irreversibly bind to the bacterial ribosomes leading to an inhibition of protein synthesis	Gentamicin is used in various infections such as septicaemia, meningitis, acute pyelonephritis and endocarditis
Sulphonamides and trimethoprim	Trimethoprim	Inhibition of folate synthesis and reduces the precursors of DNA and RNA	Pneumonia in AIDS patients, toxoplasmosis and nocardiosis. Acute exacerbation of chronic bronchitis, otitis media and UTIs
Antituberculous	Rifampicin, isoniazid, pyrazinamide, ethambutol	Isoniazid and rifampicin most effective versus continually growing bacteria. Rifampicin versus intermittently dividing bacteria. Pyrazinamide versus rapidly dividing intracellular organisms hence most effective in first 2 months	Tuberculosis
Quinolones	Ciprofloxacin, ofloxacin	Inhibition of bacterial DNA gyrase	*Pseudomonas aeruginosa, Haemophilus influenzae, Campylobacter* spp.
Others	Metronidazole	DNA damage due to toxic oxygen products	Trichomonal vaginosis, giardiasis, pseudomembranous colitis, tumours and rosacea
	Chloramphenicol[a]	Binds to bacterial ribosomes and inhibits protein synthesis	Eye drops used in bacterial conjunctivitis
Antiviral	Aciclovir,[a] famciclovir, zanamivir	Aciclovir: inhibition of herpesvirus DNA polymerase. Zanamivir: a neuramidase inhibitor which prevents the entry and release of the viral particles from the host cells	Aciclovir: herpes simplex and herpes varicella. Zanamivir: influenza
Imidazoles	Clotrimazole[a]	Inhibition of cytochrome P450-dependent demethylase which converts lanosterol to ergosterol; accumulation of lanosterol disrupts fungal membrane	Fungal infections
Triazoles	Itraconazole, fluconazole[a]	As for imidazoles	Fungal infections

Class	Examples	Actions	Common uses
Other antifungal agents	Griseofulvin, terbinafine,[a] amphotericin	Terbinafine inhibits the conversion of squalene to lanosterol, with the accumulation of squalene causing cell death. Griseofulvin: interferes with fungal microtubules and nucleic acid synthesis	Griseofulvin: suitable for tinea infections but not candidiasis
Endocrine			
Sulphonylureas	Glibenclamide, tolbutamide, gliclazide, glipizide, glimepiride	Inhibition of ATP-sensitive K^+ channels, leading to insulin release	Type 2 diabetes
Biguanides	Metformin	Activation of AMP kinase? This may increase glucose uptake and reduce glucose production by the liver. It may also suppress lipid synthesis and promote fatty acid oxidation	Type 2 diabetes with obesity
Thiazolidinediones	Rosiglitazone, pioglitazone	'Insulin sensitizers', which work by enhancing glucose utilization in tissues, and so reduce insulin resistance. They activate the nuclear peroxisome proliferator-activated receptors γ (PPAR-γ)	Type 2 diabetes in combination with sulphonylurea or metformin
Antithyroid	Carbimazole	Decreases the production of thyroid hormones by inhibiting the iodination of thyroglobulin	Hyperthyroidism
Corticosteroids	Prednisolone, hydrocortisone,[a] dexamethasone	A range of immunosuppressant actions, including production of lipocortin, which inhibits phospholipase A_2	Anti-inflammatory. Topical hydrocortisone for eczema. Dexamethasone for nerve compression in palliative care
Others			
Topical vitamin D_3 analogues	Calcipotriol	Acts on keratinocyte vitamin D receptors, and has antiproliferative actions and reduces epidermal proliferation	Psoriasis
Oral retinoids	Acitretin, tretinoin and isotretinoin	Binds to nuclear retinoic acid receptors and affects gene transcription, resulting in antiproliferative actions and normal keratinocyte maturation	Acitretin: psoriasis. Tretinoin and isotretinoin: acne

Class	Examples	Actions	Common uses
Folate antagonist	Methotrexate	Inhibits dihydrofolate reductase	Anticancer chemotherapy; immunosuppressant for psoriasis, asthma, Crohn's disease
Immunosuppressants	Azathioprine, ciclosporin	Azathioprine: inhibits nucleic acid synthesis and prevents lymphocyte production. Ciclosporin: prevents activation of T lymphocytes	Immunosuppression including prevention of transplant rejection
5-Aminosalicylates	Mesalazine, sulfasalazine	Yield 5-aminosalicylic acid, leading to inhibition of leukotriene and prostanoid formation, scavenging free radicals, and decreasing neutrophil chemotaxis	Ulcerative colitis, Crohn's disease

[a] Certain preparations of these drugs are available over-the-counter for certain indications.

5HT, 5-hydroxytryptamine; AIDS, acquired immune deficiency syndrome; AF, atrial fibrillation; AMP, adenosine monophosphate; ATP, adenosine triphosphate; cGMP, guanosine cyclic 3':5'-monophosphate; CHF, chronic heart failure; CoA, coenzyme A; COPD, chronic obstructive pulmonary disease; COX, cyclo-oxygenase; CV, cerebrovascular; CVA, cerebrovascular accident; DCT, distal convoluted tubule; DVT, deep venous thrombosis; GABA, γ-aminobutyric acid; GORD, gastro-oesophageal reflux disease; HMG, hydroxymethylglutaryl; IBS, irritable bowel syndrome; LVF, left ventricular failure; MI, myocardial infarction; NSAID, non-steroidal anti-inflammatory drug; PE, pulmonary embolism; PGE_1, prostaglandin E_1; UTIs, urinary tract infections; VSM, vascular smooth muscle.

Appendix 2

Some important clinical measurements and therapeutic drug monitoring

Table A2.1 Biochemical measurements

Biochemical parameter	Reference ranges	Comments
Sodium (Na+)	135–145 mmol/L >155–160 mmol/L confusion and coma <120 mmol/L weakness and confusion	Sodium controls the volume of extracellular fluid. Sodium is involved in neuronal action potentials and is therefore important for excitable tissues
Potassium (K+)	3.5–5.3 mmol/L >6.5 mmol/L or <2.5 mmol/L are medical emergencies	• Potassium levels determine membrane potential and influence the functioning of excitable tissues such as muscles and neurons • Hypokalaemia increases toxicity with digoxin therapy
Calcium (Ca^{2+})	2.25–2.6 mmol/L >3.50 mmol/L danger of cardiac arrest <1.6 mmol/L tetany (muscle spasm/twitching)	Calcitonin and parathyroid hormones maintain calcium blood plasma levels. As well as its role as a component of bone and teeth, calcium is essential for many metabolic processes, including nerve function, muscle contraction and blood clotting
Magnesium (Mg^{2+})	0.7–1.2 mmol/L	Magnesium is found in bones and is essential for the functioning of nerves and muscles. It is also a cofactor for many enzymes
Creatinine (plasma)	60–120 micromoles/L	When calculating creatinine clearance as an indication of renal function, creatinine levels are adjusted according to age, weight and sex
Creatinine clearance	97–140 mL/min males 85–125 mL/min females	Used to estimate GFR
eGFR	>90 mL/min per 1.73 m^2	Used to indicate renal function
Urea	2.0–6.5 mmol/L	May be elevated in renal disease or high protein intake
Uric acid	0.15–0.47 mmol/L	• Elevated by thiazide diuretics • Excess may present as gouty arthritis due to deposits of uric acid crystals in joints
Bicarbonate (HCO$_3^-$)	22–29 mmol/L	• Important for acid–base balance • Reflects renal and metabolic function

Continued

Table A2.1   (Continued)

Biochemical parameter	Reference ranges	Comments
HbA1c	4–5% (non-diabetic); in diabetes the aim is to keep it <7%	• Glycated haemoglobin • Measured to assess the glycaemic control by patients with diabetes over the previous 2 months
Cholesterol	Ideal <5.2 mmol/L	A risk factor for cardiovascular disease. Should be considered as the ratio of LDL:HDL (ideally <3)
Triglycerides	<2.1 mmol/L males <1.7 mmol/L females	A mild risk factor for cardiovascular disease. Associated with obesity and alcohol abuse

(e) GFR, (estimated) glomerular filtration rate; HDL, high-density lipoprotein; LDL, low-density lipoprotein.

Table A2.2   Summary of liver function tests

Parameter	Reference range (check local ranges)	Comment
Aspartate transaminase (AST)	<50 IU/L	Elevated in acute hepatocyte damage but considered to be a non-specific parameter
Alanine transaminase (ALT)	<45 IU/L	Elevated following hepatocyte damage and tends to indicate acute damage
Alkaline phosphatase (ALP)	39–117 IU/L	Indicator of cholestasis but non-specific as it is also found in bone, placenta and intestine. Consider also the level of GGT as levels of ALP may be increased in other types of liver disease
γ-Glutamyl transferase (transpeptidase) (GGT)	Up to 70 IU/L (males) Up to 40 IU/L (females)	Often used in the diagnosis of cholestasis but may also be elevated in acute or chronic hepatitis, alcoholism and in patients taking inducers such as anticonvulsants
Unconjugated (free) bilirubin	5–17 micromoles/L (>35 micromoles/L produces jaundice)	Increased levels indicate impaired liver function
Prothrombin time	10–14 s	Prolonged when clotting factor synthesis is reduced, e.g. chronic hepatitis and/or malabsorption of vitamins, warfarin treatment
INR	1–1.2	Ratio of prothrombin time compared with a control
Albumin	30–48 g/L	Reduced levels are associated with reduced synthetic activity of the liver

INR, international normalized ratio.

Table A2.3   Haematological parameters

Haematological parameter	Reference value(s)	Comments
White blood cells (leukocytes: WBC): Differential	$4–11 \times 10^9/L$	Increased levels (leukocytosis) during infection or malignancy
Neutrophils	$2.5–7.5 \times 10^9/L$	Reduced levels (leukopenia) due to drugs (Chapter 5), viral infections, chronic infections or hypersensitivity reaction
Lymphocytes	$1.5–3.5 \times 10^9/L$	
Monocytes	$0.2–0.8 \times 10^9/L$	
Eosinophils	$0.04–0.4 \times 10^9/L$	
Basophils	$0.01–0.1 \times 10^9/L$	
Erythrocyte sedimentation rate (ESR)	0–9 mm/h male 0–20 mm/h female	Elevated with increasing age, during pregnancy, chronic infection, dysproteinaemias, cancer and inflammatory diseases (e.g. giant cell arteritis, rheumatoid arthritis)
Serum ferritin	15–300 micrograms/L male 15–200 micrograms/L female	A measure of iron stores
Haemoglobin (Hb) (Chapter 17)	13.5–17.5 g/dL male 11.5–15.5 g/dL female	Symptoms of anaemia appear at levels <9–10 g/dL
Platelets	$140–400 \times 10^9/L$	Low due to infections, drug-induced thrombocytopenia (Chapter 17), bone marrow hypoplasia, uraemia, liver disease, severe megaloblastic anaemia and alcohol abuse
Mean corpuscular volume (MCV)	76–95 fL	• Raised in vitamin B_{12} or folate deficiency, excess alcohol consumption or liver disease • Reduced in iron-deficient anaemia or chronic blood loss or thalassaemia • May be normal during acute blood loss or anaemia of chronic disease (e.g. renal anaemia)
Red blood cells (RBCs, erythrocytes)	$4.5–6.5 \times 10^{12}/L$ male $3.8–5.8 \times 10^{12}/L$ female	
Haematocrit (Hct) or packed cell volume (PCV)	37–54 % male 35–47% female	PCV of anticoagulated blood The Hct gives a crude indication of red cell volume but the RBC and MCV reveal more specific details
Mean corpuscular haemoglobin (MCH)	27–33 pg	• Consider with other red cell parameters • Raised in vitamin B_{12} or folate deficiency • Lowered due to chronic blood loss, iron deficiency, thalassaemia or megaloblastic anaemia
Vitamin B_{12}	211–911 ng/L	• Deficiency may result in macrocytic anaemia (Chapter 17) • Vitamin B_{12} deficiency may be due to low dietary intake (vegans)
Folate (serum)	2.9–18 micrograms/L	• Deficiency may result in macrocytic anaemia (Chapter 17) • Folate deficiency may be due to malabsorption or drug causes (Chapter 17)

Table A2.4 Some important examples in therapeutic drug monitoring

Drug	Concentration range	Comments
Digoxin	0.8–2.0 micrograms/L	The risk of toxicity is increased in renal impairment Sample >6 hours after the dose Toxicity may present as visual disturbances, arrhythmias, vomiting, gastrointestinal disturbances, confusion Patients should be counselled to ensure that their pulse does not drop <60 beats/min
Theophylline	10–20 mg/L	Risk of toxicity is increased by drug interactions Smoking reduces plasma concentrations Toxicity may present as nausea, vomiting, arrhythmias, convulsions
Lithium	0.4–1 mmol/L	Plasma levels influenced by renal function Patients should be hydrated and not greatly alter sodium intake Sample 12 hours after dose A failure of treatment might be due to subtherapeutic levels Toxicity may present as tremor, visual disturbances, gastrointestinal disturbances, weakness, CNS disturbances
Phenytoin	10–20 mg/L	Zero order kinetics (Chapter 6) mean that therapeutic concentrations are difficult to achieve. Patients vary considerably. Therapeutic drug monitoring guides the dosage Toxicity may present as nystagmus, nausea, vomiting, CNS disturbances Low therapeutic levels may lead to failure to control seizures

CNS, central nervous system.

Index

Note: page numbers in *italics* refer to information in Figures and Tables.

4S trial (Scandinavian Simvastatin Survival Study) 137
A/CD guidelines, hypertension *123*, 130
absences (epilepsy) 249, *252*
absorption (drug) 73
  drug interactions 64, 66
acarbose 431
  adverse reactions 103, 437
  interactions *152*, *434*
acebutolol 121, *122*
acetylcholine, effect on gastric acid production *86*
aciclovir *417*, *460*
  interactions *231*, *420*
acid secretion control 87–88
acid suppression, effect on drug absorption 64
acid-fast bacteria 385
acitretin 411, *419*, *461*
acne 412–413
  case study 422–423
  referral points *12*
acrivastine 218, *220*, 224
activated partial thromboplastin time (APTT) 187
acute bronchitis *6*, 212, 215
acute dystonia 306
acute renal failure 199
acute stress disorder 288
adalimumab 349, 354, 358
Addison's disease 271
adrenal insufficiency 60
adrenal suppression, inhaled corticosteroids 231
adrenaline
  interactions 223, 280
  use in anaphylaxis 222–223
adverse drug reactions (ADRs) 49, *50–51*, 304, *305–307*, 308
  anti-obesity drugs 153
  antidepressants 277–278
  antiepileptic drugs *250–251*, 255
  antihypertensive drugs *122*
  in asthma therapy 230–231
  in cancer treatment 362
  case studies 68–70
  corticosteroids 228
  dermatological *61–62*

endocrine 60–61
gastrointestinal 55–56
  non-steroidal anti-inflammatory drugs 86–87
haematological 58, *59*
hepatic 56
hypokalaemia 173
in iron therapy 195
in lipid-lowering therapy 140, 141, 142
mechanisms 52–54
monitoring 62
musculoskeletal 62
neurological 60
NSAIDs 86–87, 330
opioids 331–332
psychiatric 58, 60
renal 57–58
reporting 62
respiratory 58
risk factors 51–52
rofecoxib 63
types A and B 51
see also interactions
affective disorders 259–262
  see also bipolar affective disorder; depression
aggression, management in schizophrenia 308, 315
agoraphobia 287
agranulocytosis 307, *308*
airway resistance, asthma 226–227
akathisia 306
akinesia 306, 317
alanine transferase (ALT) 17, 18, *464*
albumin levels 17, 18, *464*
alcohol consumption 24–25
  association with hypertension 121
  in diabetes *430*, 436
  drug interactions *26*, 65, *92*, *93*, *125*, 221, 255, *273*, 275, *339*, *388*, *434*
  withdrawal responses 54
alcohol misuse
  as cause of anaemia 195
  food supplements *28*
  use of antidepressants *267*
alcoholic liver disease 115

alendronate 350, 354
    contraindications *351*, 355
    counselling 356
    interactions *339*, *353*
alfacalcidol 202
alfentanil *332*
alginates 87, 91
alimemazine 218
aliphatic phenothiazines 304
alkaline phosphatase (ALP) 18, *464*
allergic rhinitis 217–19
    case study 223–224
    choice of drugs *219*, *220*
    counselling 221–222
    drug interactions 220–*221*
allergy 217
    anaphylaxis 222–223
    drug-induced 222
    effect of concurrent conditions *220*
ALLHAT trial 120
allopurinol 352, 354
    counselling 357
    interactions *353*
almotriptan 242
aloe vera 436
alpha blockers *456*
    counselling 179
    in heart failure *172*, 175
    in hypertension 121, 126
alprazolam, use in anxiety 289
alteplase *163*
alternative remedies
    in heart failure 180
    in hypertension 127–128
    for migraine 246
    see also herbal medicines
aluminium hydroxide 87
    interactions *245*
    as phosphate binder 202, 205
amantadine 318
    in influenza prophylaxis 212
amenorrhoea, as side effect of antipsychotics 305
amiloride *456*
    in heart failure *172*
    in liver disease 114
aminoglutethimide 362
aminoglycosides 381, *383*, *387*, 391, *460*
    interactions *388*
aminophylline 227–228
5-aminosalicylates 108
    adverse reactions 110
amiodarone 441, *455*
    interactions 68, *231*, *446*
    pulmonary fibrosis 58
amisulpiride 307
amitriptyline 262, *458*
    interactions 281
    in irritable bowel syndrome 106
    in migraine 242, *244*
    in neuropathic pain 336–337

amlodipine 121, 158, *456*
amobarbital, use in insomnia 296
amoebic dysentery 103, 104
amoxicillin *382*, 394, *459*
    in sore throat 213, 216
amphetamines, adverse reactions 303
amphotericin *420*, *461*
ampicillin *382*
    interactions 108
    in sore throat 213, 216
anaemia *10*, 86, 193
    aplastic 58, *59*, 197
    in chronic renal failure 196, 200, 202
    haemolytic 58, 197
    iron-deficiency 193–195
    megaloblastic 58, 195–196
    pernicious 195
analgesic ladder *334*, 363, 366–367
analgesic nephropathy 68
analgesics 333–334, *458*
    in cancer pain 363
    counselling 340–342
    COX-2 inhibitors 330
    drug choice 334–335
    during pregnancy and breast-feeding 340, *341*
    effects of concurrent disease *337–338*
    interactions *273*, *274*, *339–340*
    medication overuse headache 334
    in migraine 241–242, 242–243, 246
    nefopam 330–331
    over-the-counter preparations 340
    see also non-steroidal anti-inflammatory drugs
        (NSAIDs); opioids; paracetamol
anaphylaxis *220*, 222–223
angina pectoris *7*, 157–158
    choice of drugs 159–*160*, *161*
    counselling 160–161
    drug interactions 160
    pharmacological basis of management 158–159
angiotensin II receptor antagonists *456*
    adverse reactions 49
    in chronic renal failure 202
    in diabetes 435
    in heart failure 173
    in hypertension 120, *124*
angiotensin-converting enzyme (ACE) inhibitors *456*
    adverse reactions 49, *50*
    in angina 158
    in chronic renal failure 201–202
    counselling 178, 182
    in diabetes 434, 435
    in heart failure 171–173, 175, 179, 181–182
    in hypertension 120, 123, *124*, 125, 126, 130, 154
    interactions 68, *125*, *178*, *273*, *339*, *430*
    in MI *163*
    in secondary prevention of MI 164
anion-exchange resins 136, 138, *139*
    counselling 142
ankle swelling *10*
anorexia, cancer patients *364*

antacids 87
  counselling 91
  in heart failure *177*
  interactions *92, 128, 194, 275, 321, 353, 388, 402*
anti-inflammatory activity, NSAIDs 329
antiarrhythmics *455*
  in acute MI *163*
  in secondary prevention of MI 164
antibiotic prophylaxis 380
antibiotic resistance 385–386
antibiotics 380–381, 384, *459–460*
  in acne 412, 413
  in acute bronchitis 212, 215
  in acute sinusitis 212–213
  adverse reactions *51, 59*
    diarrhoea 103, 104, 105
  concurrent conditions 386, *387*
  counselling 389–391
  in diarrhoea 104
  drug choice 384–386
  in exacerbations of COPD 235–236, 237
  interactions 66, *388–389*
  monitoring 391–392
  in otitis media 213
  in pneumonia 212
  sensitivities *382–383*
  for sore throats 213, 215–216
anticancer drug therapy, nausea and vomiting *99*
anticoagulants 185–186, *457*
  clinical use 186–187
  contraindication 187, 188–189
  in haemodialysis 203
  in MI *163*
  in secondary prevention of MI 164
antidepressants 262–264, *458*
  adverse reactions 49, *50, 59*
  in anxiety 288, *289*, 291
  choice of drugs 265–267
  concurrent conditions 270–271
    Parkinson's disease 320
  counselling 277–278
  effectiveness 268
  interactions *152*, 271–272, *273–274, 321, 339, 402, 446*
  monitoring 272
  use after MI 164–165
  withdrawal 54, 274, 277, 279
antidiuretic hormone (ADH), inappropriate secretion 61
antiemetics *458*
  choice of drugs 98–100
  interactions 101
  pharmacological basis 97–98
  use in cancer patients *366*
  use in migraine 241–242, 243
  use with opioids 331
antiepileptics *250–251, 459*
  adverse reactions *59*, 255
  in bipolar affective disorder 269, 270
  drug choice 251–253

interactions 253–254, *311, 312, 340, 402, 446*
  monitoring 254
  in pain management 333, 336, 337
  use during pregnancy 252–253
  withdrawal 254
antifungal treatment *414–416, 460–461*
  interactions *419–420*
  in napkin dermatitis 410
antihelmintics 400, 403
antihistamines *457*
  in allergic rhinitis 217–218, 219, *220*, 224
  antiemetic use 97–98, 101
  counselling 101, 221
  dependence 32
  in insomnia 296, 299
  interactions *220–221*
  masking of anaphylaxis 222
  in pruritus 114, 409
  side effects 100
antihypertensives 120–121
  adverse reactions 56–57, *122*
  interactions *26, 38, 40, 65*, 68, 69, *125, 321*
antimalarials 349, 354, *355*, 358, 397–398
  counselling 398–399
  effects of concurrent disease *399*
  interactions *402*
  use during pregnancy 403
antimotility agents 104
antimuscarinic agents 98, 100
  adverse reactions 105
  counselling 321
  in diarrhoea 104
  interactions *321*
  in irritable bowel syndrome 106
  in Parkinson's disease 318–319
antimuscarinic effects, antipsychotics 306, *307, 308, 311*, 313
antioxidants 136–137
antiplatelet drugs 159, 162, 186, *457*
  gastrotoxicity 55, *90*
  interaction with herbal remedies *38*
antipsychotics 304–305, *457*
  adverse reactions 65, *305–307, 308*
  in bipolar affective disorder 269
  caution in liver disease 114, 270
  depot preparations 308
  drug choice 307–308
  duration of use 309
  interactions *273*, 310, *311–312*, 320, *321*
  malignant neuroleptic syndrome 320
  monitoring 310
  and obesity *150*
  withdrawal 54
antithyroid drugs, adverse reaction *59*
antituberculous drugs 384, 394
  counselling 391
antitussives 210, 211
anxiety *266*, 285
  in cancer patients *364*
  case study 292–293

classification 286–288
clinical features 285–286
concurrent disease 290
counselling 291–292
drug choice *289*–290
drug interactions 290
herbal medicines 290–291
pharmacological management 288–289
aplastic anaemia 58, *59*, 197
arachidonic acid metabolism *329*
aromatase inhibitors 362
arrhythmias
   antianginal agents *161*
   use of antidepressants *266*
   use of antimalarials *399*
artemether 398, *399*
arthritis 347
ascites 113
   management 114
ASCOT trial 121
aspartate transaminase (AST) 17, 18, *464*
aspirin 335
   in acute myocardial infarction *163*
   adverse effects 90, 330
   combination with warfarin 190
   interaction with vitamin C *23*
   low-dose 127, *128*, *457*
      in atrial fibrillation 188
      in prevention of MI 159, 162, 165
   in migraine 241, 242
   use during pregnancy and breast-feeding *341*
asteatotic eczema 407, 410
ASTEROID trial 138
asthma *6*, 225–226, *387*
   acute severe attacks 233
   adverse drug reactions 230–231
   analgesic use *338*
   antianginal agents *161*
   choice of drugs 228–230
   choice of inhaler 230
   clinical features 226–227
   counselling 232–233
   drug interactions 231–232
   drug-induced 226
   exercise-induced 230
   management of allergic rhinitis *220*
   management of heart failure 175
   management of hypertension *124*
   management of hyperthyroidism 443
   management of migraine *244*
   over-the-counter considerations 232
   pharmacological basis of management 227–228
   stepped-care approach *229*
   use of antimalarials *399*
atenolol 121, *122*, *456*
   in hyperthyroidism 442
   in MI *163*, 165
atherogenesis *134*–135
atopic eczema 407–409
   case study 421–422

atorvastatin 135, 138, 141, *456*
atrial fibrillation 171
   management of heart failure 175
   target INR *186*
   thromboembolic prophylaxis 188, 191–192
   thrombosis risk 185
atropine, use in diarrhoea 104
atypical antipsychotics 305, 307
augmented drug responses *see* type A ADRs
autoantibodies 19
autoinduction 67
azathioprine *204*, 205, *462*
   in inflammatory bowel disease 109
   interactions *108*
   in rheumatoid arthritis 349
azelaic acid 412
azelastine 218

Bacillus species *378*
baclofen 54, *274*
bacterial infections 377
   case studies 393–394
   clinical features 377–380
   concurrent conditions 386, *387*
   over-the-counter considerations 392
   pharmacological basis of management 380–381,
      384
   prophylaxis 380
   of the skin 416, *417*
   see also antibiotics
Bacteroides fragilis 378
balance disturbance *12*
balsalazide 108, 110
barbiturates
   interactions *231*, 298
   use in insomnia 296
Barrett's oesophagus 85
basal bolus insulin regimen 428
basal cell carcinoma (rodent ulcer) 420
beclometasone *457*
   inhaled 228
   intranasal 218, 224
bendroflumethiazide 120, 130, 173, 344, *456*
benserazide 317
benzodiazepines *457*
   in anxiety 289, 290, *364*
   caution in liver disease 114
   counselling 255, 291
   in depression 264
   in epilepsy *251*, 252
   in insomnia 296, 297
   interactions 298, *311*, *321*
   withdrawal 54
benzoyl peroxide 412, 413
benzylpenicillin *382*
bereavement 261
beta blockers *455*, *456*
   in acute MI *163*
   adverse reactions 49, *50*, 57, 58, *122*
      asthma provocation 226

in angina 158, 159, *160, 161*
in anxiety 288, 290, 291–292, 293, *364*
in bleeding oesophageal varices 115
contraindications 175–176, 443
counselling 161, 179
in heart failure *172*, 174, 175, 182
in hypertension 121, 123, *124*, 125, 126, 154
in hyperthyroidism 442
interactions *65*, 68, *125*, 160, 166, *210*, 223, *245*, *430*
migraine prophylaxis 242, *244*
pharmacological activity *122*
in secondary prevention of MI 162, 164
beta-adrenoceptor agonists *457*
adverse reactions 230, 443
in asthma 227, 229
in COPD 234, 235, 237
counselling 232
interactions *402*
use during pregnancy 230
use in young children 229–230
beta$_2$-adrenoceptors 225, 232
beta-lactam antibiotics 380–381
beta-lactamase 385
betahistine 98, *99*, 101
contraindications 100
betamethasone, topical 408
bezafibrate 135–136, 138, *456*
bicarbonate *463*
bile acid-binding resins 136, 138, 139, 142
bilirubin 17, 18, *464*
binding, co-prescribed drugs 66
bioavailability 73
biochemical measurements *463–464*
bipolar affective disorder 268
case studies 281, 301
insomnia 301
treatment 268–270
during pregnancy 271
use of antidepressants *266*
bismuth chelate 88, 93
bisoprolol 121, *456*
in heart failure 174, 182
bisphosphonates 350, 356
avoidance of oesophagitis 55
interactions *23, 353*
in management of bone pain 369
biventricular heart failure 170
bloating 106
blood pressure
control in diabetes 434, 438
measurement 126–127
target levels 119
see also hypertension
blood sugar monitoring 435–436
body mass index (BMI) 147–*148*
bone marrow suppression 58, *59*
bone metabolism
effect of antiepileptics 255
effect of chronic renal failure 200

effect of glitazones 433
bone pain 363, 367, 369
Borrelia vincenti 378
bowel habits, referral points *9*
bradykinesia 317
breakthrough pain 363
breast-feeding
analgesics 340, *341*
antibiotics 386
antiepileptic drugs 253
antipsychotics 310, 312
benefits 228
management of dyspepsia *90*
management of hyperthyroidism 443
management of insomnia 297
breathing control, in management of hypertension 128
breathlessness 6–7
in cancer patients *364*
referral points *10*
broad-spectrum antibiotics *382*, 394
bromocriptine 304, 318
adverse reactions 320
bronchial smooth muscle, autonomic control *225*
bronchiectasis 6
bronchitis *see* acute bronchitis; chronic bronchitis
bronchodilators
use in asthma 227–228, 229–230
use in COPD 234–235
buclizine *99*
budesonide *457*
in inflammatory bowel disease 108
inhaled 228
intranasal 218
bumetanide *456*
bupivacaine 333
buprenorphine 331, *332, 368*
bupropion 29, 32, 264
cautions and contraindication *30–31*
burns, referral points *12*
buspirone 288–289, 290, 292
butobarbital, use in insomnia 296
butyrophenones 305
interactions *311*

C-reactive protein (CRP) 19
cabergoline 318
adverse reactions 320
caffeine 25–27, 32
addition to analgesics 333
caution in heart failure *180*
effects in depression 275
interaction with sympathomimetics *210*
calcipotriol 411, *461*
calcitonin 350
in management of bone pain 369
calcitriol 202
calcium, reference ranges *463*
calcium balance, role of kidneys 200

calcium channel blockers *456*
  adverse reactions 105, *122*
  in angina 158, 159, *160*, *161*
  in bipolar affective disorder 269
  cautions in heart failure *177*
  in hypertension 120–121, 123, *124*, 126
  interactions *125*, *402*
  pharmacological activity *122*
  in secondary prevention of MI 164
calcium salts, as phosphate binders 202, 205
calcium supplements, interactions *353*
calf pain and swelling *10*
CALM study 435
camomile 299
cAMP response element-binding protein (CREB)
  259–260
Campylobacter jejunum 378, 382
cancer 361
  pain management 363
    adjuncts 369
    analgesic ladder 366–367
    concurrent disease 370
    syringe drivers 367, 369
  palliative care 362–363
    common symptoms 363, *364–366*
  of the skin 418, 420–421
  terminal symptoms 370
  treatment 361–362
candesartan 120, 173, 435, *456*
candidiasis 414, *416*
  during antibiotic treatment 390
  oral *365*
  recurrent 392, 418, 438
cannabinoids 33
'Can't Wait' cards 109
capsaicin 333, 335, 337
captopril 120, 171–173, *456*
carbamazepine *250, 252*, 253, *459*
  in bipolar affective disorder 269, 270
  counselling 255, 256
  interactions *231*, 253, 254, *273*, *311*, *312*, 389, *402*,
    419, *446*
  in pain management 333, 337
  use during pregnancy 253, 271
carbaryl 400, 401
carbidopa 317, 323, *459*
  interactions *194*
carbimazole 442, 443, 444, *461*
  interactions *231*, *444*
cardiomyopathies 169
cardiovascular ADRs 56–57
cardiovascular disease
  risk in diabetes 433–435
  use of antidepressants *266*
  use of antipsychotics 309
cardiovascular effects, antipsychotics 306, *308*, 313
carvedilol, in management of heart failure *172*, 174
case studies
  adverse drug reactions 68–70
  allergic rhinitis 223–224

anxiety 292–293
bacterial infections 393–394
constipation 110
COPD 237
coughs and colds 13–14, 215–216
depression 279–281
diabetes mellitus 438–439
dyspepsia 94
epilepsy 256
heart failure 181–182
herbal remedies 43–44
hormonal contraception 35
hyperlipidaemia 143–144
hypertension 129–130
insomnia 301
migraine 247–248
myocardial infarction 165–166
obesity 154–155
pain 343–344
Parkinson's disease 322–323
rheumatoid arthritis 359
schizophrenia 314–315
skin conditions 421–423
thromboembolic prophylaxis 191–192
catamenial epilepsy 252
catatonic states 303
catechol-*O*-methyltrasferase (COMT) inhibitors 318,
  319, 320
cefamandole *388*
celecoxib 330, *458*
cellulitis *417*
centesimal system, homeopathy 41
central sensitization 333–334
centrally acting antihypertensives 121, *122*, 126
cephalosporins 381, *382*, 387, 390, *459*
cerivastatin *140*
cetirizine 218, *457*
CFC-free inhalers 230
chemoreceptor trigger zone (CTZ) 97, *98*
chemotherapy 362
  management of nausea and vomiting *366*
chest pains 6, *7*
  angina 157
  myocardial infarction 162
  referral points *10*
chickenpox *12*, *417*
children
  antiepileptic drugs 253
  asthma 229–230
  avoidance of aspirin 330
  avoidance of tetracyclines 386
  choice of inhaler 230
  depression 261–262
  dysthymic disorder 260
  insomnia 298
  obesity 152
  phobias 287
  post-traumatic stress disorder 288
  use of cold preparations 211
  use of inhaled corticosteroids 231

Chlamydia species *382*
  C. pneumoniae, implication in atherogenesis 135
  as cause of pneumonia 212
  C. trachomatis 378
chloral hydrate 297, *298*
chloramphenicol 381, *382, 460*
  eye drops 380, 386–387, 391
chlordiazepoxide, use in anxiety 289
chloroquine 349, 354, *355*, 358, 397, *399, 402*, 403
chlorphenamine 97–98, 218, *220, 457*
chlorpromazine 304, *364, 457*
  adverse reactions 306, 307, *308*, 313
  in bipolar affective disorder 269
  contraindications *309*
  interactions *311*
chlorpropamide 431, 432, 437
  interactions *434*
cholangitis 377
cholecystokinin 106
cholestasis, liver function tests 18
cholesterol *464*
  synthesis in liver *136*
cholesterol absorption inhibitors 136
chondroitin 355
chronic asthma 227
  see also asthma
chronic bronchitis *6*, 234, 394
  see also chronic obstructive pulmonary disease
    (COPD)
chronic liver disease, liver function tests 17, 18
chronic obstructive pulmonary disease (COPD) 13,
    234
  antianginal agents *161*
  case study 237
  counselling 236
  exacerbations 212, 235–236
  management 234–236
  management of heart failure 175–176
  management of hypertension *124*
  management of insomnia *298*
chronic pain, central sensitization 333–334
chronic renal failure 199–200
  complications 200
  counselling 205
  impaired drug excretion 200–201
  management 201–204
  over-the-counter considerations 204
  use of herbal remedies 204
  see also renal impairment
chylomicrons 133
ciclosporin *204*, 205, *462*
  in asthma 229
  in inflammatory bowel disease 109
  interactions *141, 152, 339, 389, 419*
  in psoriasis 411
  in rheumatoid arthritis 349
cimetidine 87, *455*
  adverse effects 92
  interactions 91, *92, 128, 231*, 254, *275*, 298, *312,*
    340, 402, 434

cinnarizine 97–98, *99*, 100, 323
ciprofloxacin *383, 460*
  cautions 386
  interactions *23, 231, 388*
  in travellers' diarrhoea 104
cirrhosis of the liver 17, 25
citalopram 262, 265, *458*
  interactions 290
  use in anxiety *289*
citrate, interaction with aluminium hydroxide 202
CLARICOR trial 135
clarithromycin *459*
  caution in heart failure *177*
  interactions 254, *312, 389, 420*
clavulinic acid 385
clearance 74
clindamycin 381, *383*, 387
  counselling 391, 393
clinical biochemistry
  lipid screen 18
  liver function tests 17–18, *464*
  renal function tests 15, 17
  thyroid function tests 19
  urea and electrolytes 15, *463*
clobazam *251*, 252
clobetasone, use in eczema 408, 409
clomethiazole 297
clomipramine
  in anxiety *289*
  in neuropathic pain 337
clonazepam *251*, 252
  in anxiety 289, *289*
  interactions *273*
clonidine 121, *124*, *456*
  migraine prophylaxis 242, *244*
clopidogrel 159, 162, *457*
  gastrotoxicity 55
Clostridium species *378*
  C. difficile 103, 104, 386
clotrimazole 414, *416, 460*
clotting impairment, liver disease 113, 114, 115
clozapine 304, 305, 307, *457*
  adverse reactions *308, 309*, 313
  interactions *311*
clubbing, digital 5, 113
co-amoxiclav 392
co-cyprindiol 413
co-danthramer 371
co-trimoxazole 381
  cautions 386, *387*
  interactions *196, 353*
coal tar 411
Cockcroft–Gault equation 15
codeine 331, *332*, 367, *458*
  as antitussive 211
  in diarrhoea 104
  in migraine 242
  use during pregnancy *341*
cognitive–behavioural therapy
  in anxiety 290

in depression 264–265
in insomnia 296
in obesity 148
in schizophrenia 309–310
colchicine *351*, 352
counselling 357
colds (coryza) *6*, 209–211
colecalciferol (vitamin D$_3$) activation 200
colestyramine 136, *457*
counselling 115
in Crohn's disease 109
in hyperbilirubinaemia 114, 418
interactions *23*, 66, *140*, *194*, *339*, *434*, *446*
colicky pain 369
colony-stimulating factors 362
combined oral contraceptives (COCs) 32–34
see also hormonal contraception
compulsions 287
confusion, management in cancer patients *364*
congestive heart failure *6*
conjunctivitis 380
chloramphenicol eye drops 386–387
CONSENSUS (Cooperative North Scandinavian
Enalapril Survival Study) 172
constipation 105, *364*
and antidepressants *267*
case study 110
in chronic renal failure 202
counselling 106
in irritable bowel syndrome 106
management 105–106
opioids as cause 331
consultations 3–5
contact dermatitis 409
contact oesophagitis 55, 85
prevention 91
continuous ambulatory peritoneal dialysis 203
contraception 32–34
and use of antiepileptic drugs 253
cor pulmonale 235
cornplasters, caution in patients with diabetes 436
coronary artery bypass grafting (CABG) 158
coronary artery disease (CHD) *see* ischaemic heart
disease
corticosteroids *457*, *461*
adverse reactions 49, 60, 85, 231, 352
in allergic rhinitis 218, 219, 224
in anorexia *364*
antiemetic use 98
in asthma 228, 229, 230, 232–233
in cancer treatment 362
in COPD 235, 237
counselling 205
in eczema 408, 409
in immunosuppression *204*
in inflammatory bowel disease 108
interactions 253, *339*, *353*, *389*, *420*, *430*, *444*
monitoring requirements 354
in pain management 335, 337, 369
in psoriasis 410

in rheumatoid arthritis 349
use during pregnancy *355*
withdrawal 54
cough 214
ACE-inhibitor associated 120
in asthma 232
case studies 13–14, 215
causes *6*
management in cancer patients *365*
referral points *10*
cough mixtures 210–211
counterirritants 333, 335
cowslip 290
COX inhibition, NSAIDs 329
COX-2 inhibitors 87, 330, *458*
gastrointestinal side effects 93, 94
crab lice 401, 403
cradle cap 410
cranberry juice 392
creatine kinase levels 142
creatinine 15, *463*
Crohn's disease 107–10
cromones 233
in allergic rhinitis 218, 221, 224
in asthma 228
Cushingoid symptoms *11*
Cushing's syndrome 60
cyclimorph *368*
cyclizine 97–98, *99*, *458*
use in MI *163*, 165
cyproterone *419*
cytochrome P450 isoenzymes 52–53, 66
cytotoxic agents, adverse reactions *51*

dabigatran 186
dalfopristin 385
dalteparin 185–186, *457*
damiana 290
dantrolene *365*
dantron 106
decimal system, homeopathy 41–42
decongestants 209–210
in allergic rhinitis 218
caution in heart failure *180*
counselling 221
interactions *128*, *275*
deep vein thrombosis 188
target INR *186*
DEET (diethylmethylbenzamide), in malaria
prophylaxis 398
dehydration *9*, *364*
delusions 303
dementia 261, *459*
management of hyperlipidaemia *139*
management of insomnia *298*
use of antipsychotics 309
depression 259–260
after MI 164–165
in cancer patients *365*
choice of drugs 265–267

classification 260–262
concurrent conditions 270–271
counselling 276–278
dietary supplements 276
drug interactions 271–272, *273–274*
drug-induced 58
duration of treatment 267
effect of alcohol 275
electroconvulsive therapy (ECT) 264
in heart failure 177
herbal medicines 276
management of hypertension *124*
management of insomnia *298*
management of migraine *244*
management of obesity *150*
management of epilepsy 252
monitoring 272
non-pharmacological therapy 264–265
oral contraception *33*
over-the-counter considerations *275–276*
in Parkinson's disease 320
pharmacological basis of management 262–265
SSRIs *90*
suicide risk 267
treatment failure 267–268
withdrawal of medication 274, 277, 279
dermatitis 409–410
see also eczema
dermatological adverse drug reactions *61–62*
dermatology 407
see also skin conditions
desloratadine 218
DEXA (dual-energy X-ray absorptiometry) scans 348, 352
dexamethasone *461*
antiemetic use 98, *99*
in pain management 369
dextromethorphan, interactions *152, 275*
dextromoramide *332, 368*
Diabetes Control and Complications Trial (DCCT) 435
diabetes mellitus 427
antianginal agents *161*
antibiotic treatment *387*
case study 438–439
complications 433–435
counselling 436–437
herbal remedies *39, 44*
intercurrent illness 430
levothyroxine therapy 445
management of heart failure 176, *177*
management of hyperlipidaemia *139*, 140
management of hypertension *124*, 125
management of obesity *150*
monitoring 435–436
over-the-counter considerations 436
rimonabant therapy 149
suggestive symptoms *11*
type 1 427–430
type 2 430–433

use of antidepressants 270
use of antipsychotics *309*
dialysis 203
diamorphine 331, *332, 368*
in MI *163*, 165
in pulmonary oedema 182
use in syringe drivers 367, 369
diarrhoea *9*, 103
in cancer patients *365*
in chronic renal failure 204
counselling 104–105, 392
during antibiotic treatment 390, 393
in inflammatory bowel disease 109
in irritable bowel syndrome 106
pharmacological basis of management 103–104
diazepam *251, 457*
in anxiety 289
in insomnia 297
diclofenac *458*
counselling 342, 344
in migraine 242, 243, 246
dicycloverine, use in irritable bowel syndrome 106
diet 21–22
drug–food interactions 22, *23–24*
effect on mental health 22, 24
food supplements 27, *28*
in depression 276
in hyperlipidaemia 140–141
iron-rich foods 195
low-protein diet 201
in obesity 148
osteoporosis prevention 355–356
and warfarin therapy 191
digital clubbing 5, 113
digoxin *455*
adverse reactions 49, 57, 103
counselling 178–179
in heart failure *172*, 174, 175
interactions 66, 68, *108, 178, 353, 402, 444, 446*
monitoring *466*
pharmacokinetics 74, 76, *77, 79*, 80
use in renal impairment 52, 201
dihydrocodeine 331, *332, 367, 458*
use during pregnancy *341*
dihydropyridines 120–121, *122, 124*
interactions 253
diltiazem 121, *122, 456*
in angina 158, 159
interactions 254, 290
in secondary prevention of MI 164
dimeticone 400, 403
diphenhydramine *275, 296*
diphenylbutylpiperidines 305
dipipanone *332*
dipyridamole 186
discoid eczema 407, 410
disease-modifying anti-rheumatoid drugs (DMARDs) 349
use during pregnancy 355
disulfiram, interactions 66, 68, *152, 231*

dithranol 411
diuretics *456*
    adverse reactions 49, *50*, *59*, 105, *122*, 179
    in chronic renal failure 201
    in COPD 235
    counselling 178
    dehydration risk 100
    in heart failure *172*, 173–174, 175
    in hypertension 120, 123, *124*, 126
    interactions *65*, *68*, *178*, *273*, *339*, *353*, *430*
    in liver disease 114
    salt intake *23*
    in secondary prevention of MI 164
dizocilipine 328
dobutamine 175
domperidone 88, 98, *99*, *455*
    in migraine 242, 243
    in Parkinson's disease 323
donepezil *459*
dopa decarboxylase inhibitors 317, *319*
dopamine receptor agonists 318, *319*, *321*
    counselling 320, 321
    fibrotic reactions 320
dopamine receptor antagonists 98, *99*
    interactions 320
dosage interval 77–78
dosulepin (dothiepin) 262, *458*
doxazosin 121, *456*
doxycycline *459*
    interactions 253
    in malaria prophylaxis 398
driving regulations, epilepsy 255
droperidol 305
drowsiness
    antidepressants as cause 277, 278
    antipsychotics as cause *307*, *308*, 313
drug excretion, impairment in chronic renal failure
        200–201
drug history 4–5
drug interactions *see* interactions
drug overdoses *12*
drug–food interactions 22, *23–24*
drug-induced allergy 222
drug-induced asthma 226
dry mouth, management in cancer patients *365*
dyskinesias 317
dysmenorrhoea 336
dyspepsia 85
    choice of drugs 88–91
    counselling of patients 91–93
    management in chronic renal failure 204
    over-the-counter drugs 91
    pharmacological basis of management 87–88
    referral points *9*
dysphagia *9*, 85
dyspnoea *see* breathlessness
dysthymic disorder 260

eating disorders *267*
echinacea *39*, 43, 211

'economy-class syndrome' 188
eczema 407
    atopic 407–409
    case study 421–422
    referral points *12*
    seborrhoeic 410
    use of antimalarials *399*
eformoterol 227
elderly people
    chronic pain 340–341
    depression 261
    hypertension *124*
    insomnia 297–298
    risk of falls 349–350
    schizophrenia 310
electrocardiography (ECG)
    in angina 157
    in atrial fibrillation 171
    in myocardial infarction 162
electroconvulsive therapy (ECT) 264
electrolyte disturbances, symptoms and drug causes *16*
electrolytes 15, *463*
    monitoring in heart failure 179
    monitoring in heparin therapy 189
eletriptan 242
elimination of drugs 74–75
    zero-order kinetics 79–*81*
ELITE II trial 173
emollients
    use in eczema 408, 409
    use in psoriasis 410
emphysema 234
    see also chronic obstructive pulmonary disease
        (COPD)
enalapril 120, 171–173, *456*
encephalopathy, hepatic 113, 114
end-of-dose effect, L-dopa 318
endocarditis 377, 380
endocrine ADRs 60–61
enoxaparin 185–186, *457*
entacapone 318, 319
enterotoxins 103
enzyme induction and inhibition 66–67
ephedra 446
ephedrine 32, *275*
epilepsy 8, 249, *387*
    analgesics *338*
    case study 256
    counselling 254–255
    drug choice 251–253
    drug interactions 253–254
    management of allergy *220*
    monitoring 254
    over-the-counter medicines 254
    pharmacological management *250–251*
    use of antidepressants *266*
    use of antimalarials *399*
    use of antipsychotics *309*
    vagal nerve stimulation 251
    withdrawal of medication 254

episodic asthma 227
ergotamine 242, 243
    contraindications *164, 244*
    counselling 246
    interactions *245*
erysipelas *417*
erythromycin 392, 394, *459*
    caution in heart failure *177*
    counselling 390
    interactions 66, 67, 68, *152, 231, 245*, 254, 290, *388, 389, 434*
    use in acne 412
erythropoietin 196, 200
    use in chronic renal failure 202
Escherichia coli 378, 379
    benefits in ulcerative colitis 109
escitalopram 262, *289*
ESR (erythrocyte sedimentation rate) *465*
estimated GFR (eGFR) 17, *463*
etanercept 349, 354
    counselling 358
    use in psoriasis 411
ethambutol 384, 391, 394, *460*
ethosuximide *251, 252*, 255
etidronate 350, 351, 354, 355, 356
etodolac 330, *458*
evening primrose oil 436, 254
exenatide 432
exercise 27, 148–149, 151
exercise-induced asthma 230
expectorants 211
extrapyramidal effects, antipsychotics 305–306, *307, 308*, 313
eye drops 391
    chloramphenicol 380, 386–387, 391
eye problems *12*
ezetimibe 136

fainting 8
falls risk, elderly people 349–350
famciclovir *460*
familial hypercholesterolaemia 134, 137, 141
famotidine 87
fear 285
felodipine 158
fenofibrate 135–136
fentanyl 331, *332*, 367, *368*, 371
ferritin *465*
ferrous salts 194–195, *446*
fertility, effect of NSAIDs *338*
fever 336
feverfew 246
fexofenadine 218
fibrates 135–136, 138, *139, 456*
    as cause of myopathy 62
    counselling 141–142
    interactions *140, 141, 434*
    safety 140
first-order kinetics *74–75*
first-pass metabolism 73

fish oils
    counselling 142, 143, 359
    effect on blood pressure 127
    interactions *141*
    levels in depression 276
    in hyperlipidaemia 136, 138
    in inflammatory bowel disease 109
flecainide 369
flucloxacillin *382*, 392, *459*
fluconazole 415, *416, 460*
    interactions *231, 419, 434*
5-fluorouracil 420
fluoxetine 262, 265, 268, *458*
    in anxiety *289*
    interactions *271, 273*, 280, 290, *311, 312*
    use in children 261, 262
    use during pregnancy 270–271
flupentixol 264, 305
    counselling 278
fluphenazine *308, 457*
flurazepam, use in insomnia 297
fluticasone
    inhaled 228
    intranasal 218
fluvastatin 135, 202, *456*
fluvoxamine 262
    interactions *231, 271, 273*, 275, 290, *311*
    use in anxiety *289*
folic acid *465*
    drug interactions *196*
    levels in depression 276
folic acid deficiency 195–196
folic acid supplementation 196
    in homocysteinaemia 140
    in pregnancy *28*, 253
food *see* diet
forced expiratory volume (FEV$_1$)
    in asthma 226–227
    in COPD 234
formoterol 227, *457*
fruit and vegetable consumption 21–22
full blood count 19
fungal infections of the skin 414–*416*
    napkin dermatitis 410
'funny turns' 8
furosemide 173, 182, *388, 456*
fusidic acid 380, 381, *417*
    cautions 386, 392
fybogel, interactions *275*

GABA (gamma-aminobutyric acid) 328
gabapentin *250, 252*, 253, 254, *459*
    in bipolar affective disorder 269, 270
    counselling 255, 342
    in neuropathic pain 333, 337
galactorrhoea, as side effect of antipsychotics 304, 305, *308*
galantamine *459*
gall stones, management of hyperlipidaemia *139*
γ-glutamyl transferase (GGT) 18, *464*

gastric acid production *86*
gastric bleeding, management in liver disease 114
gastric motility, role in drug interactions 66
gastrin *86*
gastritis 85
　management of insomnia *298*
gastro-oesophageal reflux disease (GORD) *7*, *8*, 85
　counselling 91
　management 88
gastrointestinal ADRs 55–56
gastrointestinal disease
　case studies 94
　important referral points *9*
　see also dyspepsia; peptic ulceration
gastrointestinal infections 377, *378*
gastrotoxicity, antiplatelet drugs 55
gate theory of pain 328
gemfibrozil 135–136, 138, *456*
general anxiety disorder (GAD) 286, *289*, 290
　see also anxiety
generalized seizures 249
genital infections 379
gentamicin *383*, *460*
　cautions 386, *387*
　eye drops 380
　pharmacokinetics 78
gentian 299
GGT (γ-glutamyl transferase (transpeptidase)) 18, *464*
giardiasis 103, 104
ginger, antiemetic use 101
ginkgo biloba, contraindications 254
ginseng *38*, *39*, *40*, 44, 291, 299
glandular fever 213, 216
glaucoma
　antianginal agents *161*
　management of heart failure 176, *177*
　management of insomnia *298*
　management of allergy *220*
　use of antidepressants *267*
　use of antipsychotics *309*
glibenclamide 431, *434*, 438–439, *461*
glicazide 431, *461*
glimepiride 431, *461*
glipizide 431, *434*, *461*
glitazones (thiazolidinediones) 431, 432–433, *461*
　contraindications *177*
　interactions *434*
glomerular filtration rate (GFR) 15, 17, 199, *463*
glomerulonephritis 213
glucagon 429
glucosamine 355
glucose, blood levels 22, 24, 427
glucose-6-phosphate dehydrogenase (G6PD)
　　deficiency 53, 197
　use of antimalarials *399*
glycaemic index (GI) of foods 24
glyceryl trinitrate (GTN) 157, 158, 159, *456*
　counselling 160–161, 166
　first-pass metabolism 73
glycopeptides 381, *382*

goitre 441
gold compounds 349
　counselling 357–358
　monitoring requirements 354
gonococcal conjunctivitis 380
gonorrhoea 379
gout 348, 352
　counselling 357
　management of hyperlipidaemia *139*
　management of hypertension *124*
Gram staining 385
grapefruit juice, drug interactions 22, 69, *125*, *141*,
　　205
Graves' disease 441, 444
　treatment 442–443
Grazax 219
griseofulvin 415, *416*, *419*, *461*
gut flora, eradication in hepatic encephalopathy 114
gut flora alterations, role in drug interactions 66
gynaecomastia 113

H_1-receptor antagonists, use in nausea and vomiting
　　97–98
H_2-receptor antagonists 87, *455*
　counselling patients 91–92
　interactions *196*
haematemesis *9*
haematocrit (packed cell volume, PCV) *465*
haematological ADRs 58, *59*
haematological monitoring 19, *465*
haemodialysis 203
haemoglobin *465*
haemolytic anaemias 58, 197
　G6PD deficiency 53
Haemophilus influenzae 212, 213, *378*, 379, 380
haemoptysis 13
half-life 75
hallucinations 303, 304, 314
haloperidol 305, 308, 315, *364*, *457*
　adverse reactions *308*, 323
　in bipolar affective disorder 269
　interactions *273*, *274*, *311*
hand, foot and mouth disease *418*
hayfever *see* allergic rhinitis
HbA1c 435, *464*
HDL (high-density lipoprotein) 18, 133, 134
head lice 400–403
head trauma, antiemetics 99
headaches 7–8, 336
　medication overuse headache 334
　referral points *11*
　see also migraine
health promotion campaigns 34
'healthy heart checks' 143
hearing problems 12
heart failure 169
　analgesia *337*
　antianginal agents *161*
　case study 181–182
　classification 169–170

clinical features 170–171
concurrent disease 175–176, *177*
counselling 177–179
drug interactions *178*
management of dyspepsia *90*
management of hypertension *124*, 125
monitoring 179–180
oral hypoglycaemics *433*
over-the-counter considerations *180*
pathophysiological changes *170*
pharmacological basis of management 171–175
treatment goals 171
Heart Outcome Prevention Evaluation (HOPE) trial
    158, 434, 439
Heart Protection Study Collaborative Group 136,
    137–138, 434–435
Helicobacter pylori infection 86, 87, 377, *378*
case study 94
diagnosis 88
triple therapy 89, 93, *455*
helmintic infections 399, 400, 403
heparin 185–186, *457*
clinical use 187
contraindications 188, 189
use after MI *163*
hepatic impairment *see* liver disease
hepatic metabolism of drugs 52–53
hepatitis, liver function tests 18
herbal medicines 37
in anxiety 290–291
case studies 43–44
in chronic renal failure 204
in depression 276
effects on blood sugar levels 436
evidence 37, 40
and heart failure 180
in insomnia 299
interactions *38–40*, 41
for nausea and vomiting 101
safety issues 40–41
for weight loss 151
herpes simplex *417*
hiccup *365*
histamine, effect on gastric acid production *86*
histamine analogues 98
HMG-CoA reductase 135, *136*
HMG-CoA reductase inhibitors *see* statins
homeopathy 41–42
homocysteinaemia 138, 140
hops 290, 299
hormonal contraception 32–34
case study 35
interactions 66, 68, *152, 231, 253, 273, 388, 430*
in patients with migraine 244, 247
hormone-based cancer therapy 362
hormone replacement therapy (HRT)
contraindications *177*
effect on cardiovascular risk 137
in management of osteoporosis 350, 351
housebound individuals, food supplements *28*

human insulin analogues 428
hydralazine *124*
counselling 179
in management of heart failure 175
hydrocortisone *461*
use in eczema 408, 409
hydromorphone *368*
hydroxocobalamin 196
hydroxychloroquine 349, 354, *355*, 358
1α-hydroxycholecalciferol 202
5-hydroxytryptamine receptor antagonists 98, *99*
use in irritable bowel syndrome 106–107
hyoscine 98, *99*, *458*
contraindications 100
counselling 101
in management of colicky pain 369
hypercalcaemia *16*
hypercholesterolaemia 133–135
choice of drugs 137–138
see also hyperlipidaemia
hyperkalaemia *16*, 179
in chronic renal failure 203
heparin as cause 189
hyperkeratotic palmar eczema 407, 410
hyperlipidaemia 123, 133
case study 143–144
choice of drugs 137–140
in chronic renal failure 202
counselling 140–142
drug interactions *140, 141*
drug safety 140
monitoring 142
oral hypoglycaemics *433*
over-the-counter drugs 142–143
pharmacological basis of management 135–137
see also hypercholesterolaemia;
      hypertriglyceridaemia
hypernatraemia *16*
hyperparathyroidism, in chronic renal failure 200
hyperprolactinaemia, drug-induced 60, 304, 305
hypersensitivity reactions to drugs 53
hypertension 119
analgesia *337*
case study 129–130
as cause of heart failure 169
choice of drugs 122–125
in chronic renal failure 200, 201–202
counselling 126
drug interactions *125*
lifestyle modification 121
management of hyperlipidaemia *139*
management of migraine *244*
monitoring 126–127
over-the-counter medicines 127, *128*
pharmacological basis of management 120–121
Hypertension Optimal Treatment (HOT) trial 119, 127
hyperthyroidism 441–442
antianginal agents *161*
counselling 444
drug interactions *444*

management 442–443
over-the-counter medicines 445–446
suggestive symptoms *11*
use of antidepressants *267*
hypertriglyceridaemia 135
choice of drugs 138
see also hyperlipidaemia
hypnotics 296–298
counselling 300
hypocalcaemia *16*
hypoglycaemia 429, 433
in liver disease 113, 115
hypokalaemia *16*
as side effect of diuretics 173, 179
hypomagnesaemia *16*
hypomania 268
hyponatraemia *16*, 272
hypoproteinaemia 113, 114, 199
hyposensitization, in allergic rhinitis 219
hypotension, as side effect of antipsychotics 306, *308*
hypothyroidism 444–445
effect of opioids *338*
management of hyperlipidaemia *139*
over-the-counter medicines 446
suggestive symptoms *11*

ibuprofen 329, *458*
interactions 159, 205
use in fever 336
use in migraine 241–242
idiosyncratic drug reactions (type B ADRs) 51
imidazoles 414–415, *416, 419, 460*
imipramine 262
adverse reactions 69
use in anxiety *289*
immunization
against influenza 212
against malaria 398
against *Streptococcus pneumoniae* 212
immunoglobulin tests 19
immunological responses to drugs 53
immunological tests 19
immunosuppressants *204*
counselling 205
interaction with herbal remedies *39, 43*
use in inflammatory bowel disease 109
Impact of Nicorandil in Angina (IONA) trial 159–160
impetigo *12, 417, 422*
incretins 431
indapamide 173
in secondary stroke prevention 176
indigestion *see* dyspepsia
indinavir, interactions 253
indometacin 329
counselling 342
interactions *311*
indoramin *456*
infection
role in atherogenesis 135
see also bacterial infections

inflammatory bowel disease 107–109
analgesics *338*
cautions with oral contraception *33*
counselling 109–110
infliximab 354
counselling 358
in Crohn's disease 109
in psoriasis 411
in rheumatoid arthritis 349
influenza 211–212
inhaled corticosteroids 228, 229
adverse effects 231
counselling 232–233
inhaled insulin 429
inhaler devices 230
INITIATIVE trial 159
INR (international normalized ratio) 187, *464*
target levels *186*
insomnia *11*, 275, 280, 295–296
in cancer patients *365*
case studies 301
classification *295*
concurrent disease 297–298
counselling 299–300
drug choice 296–297
drug interactions 298
over-the-counter considerations 299
pharmacological basis of management 296
use of antidepressants *266*
insulin 428–429
counselling 436, 437
intensive therapy after MI *163*
interactions 429–430, *434*
in treatment of hyperkalaemia 203
interactions 49, 64
with adrenaline 223
with alcohol 25, *26*
in allergic rhinitis 220–*221*
with 5-aminosalicylates *108*
with analgesics *339–340*
with antibiotics *388–389*
with antidepressants 271–272, *273–274*
with antiemetics 101
with antiepileptic drugs 253–254
with antihistamines 220–*221*
with antihypertensive drugs *125*
with antimigraine drugs *245*
with antiobesity drugs 151, *152*
with antiparasitic agents *402*
with antipsychotics 310, *311–312*
with antithyroid drugs *444*
in asthma therapy 231–232
with caffeine 26–27
with citrate and aluminium hydroxide 202
drugs used in anxiety 290
drugs used in dermatology *419–420*
drugs used in heart failure *178*
drugs used in Parkinson's disease 320, *321*
with food 22, *23–24*
with herbal remedies *38–40, 41*

with hormonal contraceptives 34
with hypnotics 298
with insulin 429–*430*
with iron therapy *194*
with levothyroxine *446*
with lipid-lowering drugs *140, 141*
mechanisms 64–67
with sympathomimetics *210*
with tobacco smoke 29
with vitamin B$_{12}$ and folic acid *196*
with warfarin 189–190
intranasal corticosteroids 218, 219, *220*, 224
counselling 221
intrinsic renal failure 199
ipratropium *457*
adverse reactions 230
in allergic rhinitis 218, *220*
in asthma 228
in COPD 234, 237
irbesartan 120, 173, 435
iron supplements 194–195
adverse reactions 103
indications *28*
iron-deficiency anaemia 193–195
irritable bowel syndrome (IBS) 8, 106–107
ischaemic heart disease (IHD) 157
analgesia *337*
as cause of heart failure 169
management of heart failure 176
management of hypertension *124*
management of migraine *244*
see also angina pectoris; myocardial
infarction
isocarboxazid 262–263
isoniazid 384, 391, 392, 394, *460*
interactions *23, 26, 275, 389, 430*
isophane insulin 428
isosorbide mononitrate 158, 161
isotretinoin 412, 413, 422–423, *461*
interactions *23, 419*
serum lipids monitoring 18
ispaghula 106, 107, *455*
interactions *273*
use in hypercholesterolaemia 137
itraconazole 415, *416, 460*
interactions *141, 290, 419, 420, 434*
ivabradine 159

jaundice *9, 12,* 17, 113, 418
antipsychotics as cause *308*
management 114
jugular venous pressure (JVP) 171

kaolin and morphine mixture 104
karela (*Momordica charantia*) 44
kava 291
kelp tablets *40,* 43–44, 446
ketamine 328, 369
ketoconazole 415
interactions *152, 231, 290, 419, 420, 434*

kinetics of elimination *74–75*
zero-order 79–*81*
Klebsiella pneumoniae 378

labetolol *122*
laboratory tests
clinical biochemistry 15–18, *463–464*
in depression 272
in epilepsy 254
haematology 19, *465*
in heart failure 179–180
in hyperlipidaemia 142
in hypertension 127, 129
microbiology 20
in schizophrenia 310
lacidipine 121
lactulose 105, *455*
use in hepatic encephalopathy 114
lady's slipper 290
lamotrigine *250, 252, 253, 459*
in bipolar affective disorder 269, 270
counselling 255
interactions 253
in neuropathic pain 333
lansoprazole 87–88, *455*
interactions *23,* 91, *92*
laxatives 105–106, 110, *455*
caution in heart failure *180*
misuse 32
LDL (low-density lipoprotein) 18, 133, 134
left ventricular failure 169–170, 171
left ventricular hypertrophy (LVH) *124*
leg cramps, use of quinine salts 352, 356–357
legionnaires' disease *378, 382*
Leptospira icterohaemorrhagiae 378
leukotriene receptor antagonists 228, 229, *457*
adverse reactions 231
counselling 233
use during pregnancy 230
levamisole 400
levetiracetam *251, 252*
levobupivacaine 333
levodopa (L-dopa) 317–318, *319,* 322–323, *459*
counselling 320
interactions *194,* 320, *321*
malignant neuroleptic syndrome 320
levodopa-induced nausea *99*
levothyroxine 445
cautions *164, 177*
interactions *194, 231, 253, 446*
use in bipolar affective disorder 269
lidocaine 333, 369, *455*
LIFE (Losartan Intervention for Endpoint Reduction in
Hypertension) trial 434
lifestyle 21
alcohol consumption 24–25
caffeine consumption 25–27
contraception 32–34
diet 21–24
food supplements 27, *28*

exercise 27
smoking 27–32
stress 27
Lifestyle Intervention for Endpoint Reduction in
    Hypertension (LIFE) trial 120
lifestyle modification
    in angina 158, 160
    in anxiety 291
    in asthma 228
    in COPD 236
    in diabetes 436–437
    in gastro-oesophageal reflux disease 88
    in heart failure 177
    in hyperlipidaemia 140–141
    in hypertension 121, 126, 129
    after myocardial infarction 162
    in obesity 148–149
    in osteoporosis 355–356
linezolid 385
lipid screen 18
lipohypertrophy 429
lipoproteins 133
lisinopril 120, *456*
    in management of heart failure 171–173,
        181–182
Listeria monocytogenes 379
lisuride, adverse reactions 320
lithium 264, 268–269, 270, 272, *458*
    adverse reactions 49, 441
    contraindications 270
    counselling 278
    interactions *26, 152, 177, 232, 245, 252, 271,*
        273–274, 275, 281, *311, 339, 430*
    monitoring 272, *466*
    salt intake 23
    use during pregnancy 271
    use in hyperthyroidism *267*
    withdrawal 274
liver disease 113
    alcoholic 115
    antibiotic treatment 392
    drug-induced 56
    drugs used in musculoskeletal disorders 355
    effects 113–114
    management 114–115
    management of heart failure 175
    management of hyperlipidaemia *139*
    oral hypoglycaemics *433*
    thromboembolic prophylaxis 188
    use of antidepressants 270
    use of antimalarials *399*
    use of antipsychotics 310
    use of hypnotics 297
liver function
    effect of drugs 56
    monitoring in antidepressant therapy 272
    monitoring in hyperlipidaemia 142
liver function tests 17–18, *464*
loading doses 76, 78
local anaesthetics 333, 335

lofepramine 262, *458*
    interactions 280, *446*
long-acting beta-adrenoceptor agonists
    use in asthma 227, 229, 232
    use in COPD 235
loop diuretics 120, *456*
    in chronic renal failure 201
    in heart failure *172,* 173
    hypokalemia 179
    interactions *178, 339*
loperamide 104, 106, *455*
    in inflammatory bowel disease 109
loprazolam, use in insomnia 296, 297
loratadine 218, 224, *457*
lorazepam *99,* 289, *289*
lormetazepam, use in insomnia 296, 297
losartan 120, 173, *456*
loss of consciousness *11*
low-molecular weight heparins 185–187
low-protein diet 201
lumefantrine 398, *399*
lumps, referral points *12*
lung cancer *6*

macrocytic anaemia 195
macrolides 381, *382,* 390, *459*
    interactions *141, 177, 389*
    see also erythromycin
macrovascular complications of diabetes 433–435
magnesium, reference ranges *463*
magnesium hydroxide 87, *245*
magnesium salts 105–106
magnesium trisilicate, interactions *196*
maintenance doses 76–77, 79
malabsorption, drug-induced 55–56, 149
malaria 197, 397
malaria prophylaxis 397–399
malathion 400, 401, 403
malignant melanoma 421
malignant neuroleptic syndrome 320
manic episodes 268
maprotiline 264, *267*
    interactions 275
    use in neuropathic pain 337
MDRD (modification of diet in renal disease) formula,
    eGFR 17
mean corpuscular haemoglobin (MCH) *465*
mean corpuscular volume (MCV) 193, 195, *465*
mebendazole 400, *402,* 403
mebeverine 106, 107, *455*
medication overuse headache (MOH) 334
mefenamic acid *244, 458*
mefloquine 58, 398, *399, 402*
megaloblastic anaemia 58, 195–196
meglitinide analogues 431
melaena *9,* 86
melanocortins, MC4 receptor agonists 153
melatonin 299
meloxicam 330, *458*
Ménière's disease *99*

meningitis 379
menstrual migraine *244*
mental health, effect of diet 22, 24
menthol, use as counterirritant 333
meptazinol *332*
mesalazine 108, 110, *462*
metabolic syndrome 147
metabolism
    causes of ADRs 52–53
    role in drug interactions 66–67
metered dose inhalers 230
metformin *150*, 431, 432, *434*, 437, *461*
    adverse reactions 103
    contraindications *433*
methadone *332*, 336, *368*
methotrexate *462*
    in asthma 229
    counselling 357
    folate antagonism *24*, 58
    in inflammatory bowel disease 109
    interactions *26*, 67, 69, *339*, *353*, *419*
    monitoring requirements 354
    in psoriasis 411
    in rheumatoid arthritis 349
methoxsalen 411, *419*
methyldopa 121, *122*, *124*, *456*
    interactions *273*
methylxanthines 26
methysergide 242, *245*, 247
meticillin-resistant *Staphylococcus aureus* (MRSA) *382*, 385–386
metoclopramide 88, 98, *99*, 100, *455*, *458*
    effect on gastric emptying 66
    interactions *26*, *321*, 323, *340*
    use in migraine 242, 243
metoprolol 121, *122*, *456*
    in acute MI *163*
    in heart failure 174
metronidazole *383*, 384, 423, *460*
    cautions 386, 391, 392
    counselling 390–391
    in hepatic encephalopathy 114
    interactions *26*, *92*, 93, *273*, *388*
metronidazole resistance, *Helicobacter pylori* 89
mexiletine 369
mianserin 264
    blood monitoring *272*
    counselling 278
    interactions 275
Michaelis–Menten enzyme kinetics *80*
miconazole 414–415
microalbuminuria, in diabetes 435
microbiology tests 20
microcytic anaemia 193
microvascular complications of diabetes 435
migraine 241, *458*
    alternative therapies 246
    antianginal agents *161*
    antidepressants *266*
    antiemetics *99*

case study 247–248
cautions with oral contraception *33*
concurrent illness *244*
counselling 246–247
drug choice 242–*243*
drug interactions 243, *245*
management of hypertension *124*
over-the-counter products 243, 246
pharmacological basis of management 241–242
milrinone 175
mineral supplements 27, *28*
    in inflammatory bowel disease 109
    in thyroid disease 446
minocycline 62, *392*, 412, *419*
minoxidil *124*
mirtazapine 263, *267*, *458*
    blood monitoring 272
    counselling 278
misoprostol 88, *90*, 370, *455*
    adverse reactions 103
    counselling 93
mizolastine 220, *221*
moclobemide 262–263, *458*
    use in anxiety *289*
moles, changes in *12*
molluscum contagiosum *418*
monitoring for adverse drug reactions 62
monoamine oxidase B inhibitors 318, *319*
monoamine oxidase inhibitors (MAOIs) 262–263, *458*
    cautions and contraindications *266*, *267*, 270
    counselling 278
    interactions *23*, *210*, *245*, 272, *273*, *274*, *275*, 276, 290, 318, *321*, *340*, *430*
monoamine theory of depression 259
monoclonal antibodies
    immunological responses 53
    omalizumab 228, 229
Monospot test 216
montelukast 228, *457*
morphine 331, 367, *368*, *458*
    in acute myocardial infarction *163*
    counselling 371
    interactions *340*
motion sickness *99*, *100* 101
mouth, adverse drug reactions 55
mouth ulcers, referral points *9*
movement disorders, antipsychotics as cause 305–306
moxonidine 121, *456*
multidisciplinary teams, palliative care 363
mupirocin 385, *417*
mural thrombosis, target INR *186*
muscarinic M-receptor antagonists 218, *220*
    use in asthma 228
    use in COPD 234, 237
muscle spasm, management in cancer patients *365*
muscle weakness, management of insomnia *298*
musculoskeletal adverse drug reactions 62
musculoskeletal chest pains *7*
musculoskeletal problems, referral points *12*
myasthenia gravis *387*

Mycobacterium species *378, 379*
mycophenolate mofetil *204*, 205
Mycoplasma species *382*
myelosuppression, cancer treatment 362
myocardial infarction (MI) *7*, 161–162
  case study 165–166
  effect on co-morbidities 164
  management 162, *163*
  management of hyperlipidaemia *139*
  secondary prevention 162, 164–165
  use of antidepressants *266*
myoclonic epilepsy 249, *252*

nabilone 98, *99*, 101
nadolol 121
  in management of hyperthyroidism 442
nalidixic acid *383*
naloxone *458*
napkin dermatitis 409–410
naproxen *458*
naratriptan 242, *458*
nasal decongestants 209–210
nateglinide 431, 432, 437
National Institute for Health and Clinical Excellence
    (NICE) guidelines
  for COPD *235*
  for depression 265, 267
  for heart failure 175, *176*
  for hypertension *123*
  for obesity 147, 152–153
  for statin therapy 137
  for use of zanamivir 211–212
nausea 97
  in cancer patients *366*
  choice of drugs 98–100
  herbal remedies 101
  interactions with antiemetics 101
  in migraine 241–242
  opioid-induced 331
  pharmacological basis of management 97–98
nedocromil sodium
  use in allergic rhinitis 218
  use in asthma 228
nefazodone 263, 267, 268, 277
nefopam 330–331, *338*
  counselling 342
  interactions *340*
negative symptoms of schizophrenia 303, 315
Neisseria species *378, 379*, 380
  antibiotic sensitivities *382*
nelfinavir, interactions 253
neomycin
  interactions *194*
  in management of hepatic encephalopathy 114
nephropathy, diabetic 435
nerve blocks 335
neurological ADRs 60
neuropathic pain *266*, 328–329, 336–337, 367, 369
  counselling 371
  use of anticonvulsants 333

neuropathy, diabetic 435
neutropenia 58, *59*, 213–214, 256
nicardipine 121
nicorandil 158–159, *159–160, 456*
  counselling 161
nicotine replacement therapy (NRT) 29, 31
  cautions and contraindications *30–31, 164*
nicotinic acid (niacin) 136, *139*
nifedipine 121, 158, *456*
  interactions 69, *125, 231*
night terrors 298
nimodipine, use in bipolar affective disorder 269
nisoldipine 121
nitrates *456*
  in acute MI *163*
  adverse reactions *50*
  in angina 158, *161*
  counselling 160–161, 179
  in heart failure *172*, 175
  interactions *65, 245*
nitrazepam, use in insomnia 297
nitrofurantoin, cautions 386, *387*
NMDA (*N*-methyl-D-aspartate) receptors 328
nociceptors 327
nomifensine 264
non-starch polysaccharides (NSPs) 106
  use in hypercholesterolaemia 137
non-steroidal anti-inflammatory drugs (NSAIDs) 329,
    335, 370, *458*
  adverse reactions 49, *51*, 55, 57, *59*, 63, 103, 330
    asthma provocation 226
    in heart failure *180*
    peptic ulceration 86–87, 89–90, 344
  in bone pain 369
  cautions and contraindications 204, *337, 338*
  counselling 91, 342
  in gout 352
  interactions 67, 69, *177*, 205, *274, 275, 339, 353*
  in migraine 241–242
  in osteoarthritis 348–349
  in rheumatoid arthritis 349
  use during pregnancy and breast-feeding *341*
noradrenaline reuptake inhibitors 263
norfloxacin *23, 383*
nortriptyline 262
nutritional therapy, Crohn's disease 109
nystatin 415, *416*
Nytol 280, 299

obesity 147
  case study 154–155
  counselling 151–153
  drug choice 149–151
  drug interactions 151, *152*
  lifestyle modification 148–149
  over-the-counter drugs 151
  pharmacological management 149, 248
obsessive–compulsive disorder 287, *289*
octreotide 115
odynophagia *9*

oedema
in anaphylaxis 222
in chronic renal failure 199–200
in heart failure 169, 171
oesophageal varices 115
oestrogens, interactions 253, *389*
ofloxacin *383, 460*
olanzapine 272, 305, 307, *457*
adverse reactions 306, *308, 309*, 310, 313
in bipolar affective disorder 269
in diabetes 270
olsalazine 108
omalizumab 228, 229
omega-3 fatty acids *see* fish oils
omeprazole 87, *455*
counselling patients 93
interactions 91, *92, 273, 420*
on-off effects, Parkinson's disease 317
ondansetron 98, 101, *366, 458*
use in pruritus 114
opioid receptors 328, 331
opioids 331–*332*, 335, 367, *368, 458*
addiction, misuse of OTC medicines 32
adverse reactions 49, 105
in breathlessness *364*
cautions and contraindications 114, *337, 338*
counselling 342, 371
in diarrhoea 104, 105
interactions *152, 339–340*
in neuropathic pain 336
in terminal care 370
use during pregnancy *341*
withdrawal 54, 103
oral anticoagulants 186
see also antiplatelet drugs; warfarin
oral hypoglycaemic agents 431–433
adverse reactions 49, *50, 59*
complications of use 433
interactions *152, 434*
oral rehydration therapy 104, 105
avoidance in chronic renal failure 204
orlistat 149, *150*, 154–155, 248, *458*
counselling 153
interactions *23, 141*, 151, *152*
steatorrhoea 103
orthopnoea 171, 177
oseltamivir 211
osteoarthritis 347–349
osteomyelitis 379–380, *383*
osteoporosis 348
counselling 355–356
drug-induced 62
management of hyperlipidaemia *139*
management of insomnia *298*
management of obesity *150*
pharmacological basis of management 349–351
prevention 351–352
otitis media *12*, 213
over-the-counter (OTC) medicines
analgesics 340

in asthma 232
in bacterial infections 392
in chronic renal failure 204
in depression 275–276
in diabetes *436*
in epilepsy 254
in heart failure *180*
in hyperlipidaemia 142–143
in hypertension 127, *128*
in insomnia 299
misuse 32, 101
patients with liver disease 115
in schizophrenia 312
oxazepam 289
oxcarbazepine *250*, 255
oxycodone *332*, 336, 367, *368*
oxygen therapy, long-term 235
oxymetazoline 209, 218–219

pain 7–8
in cancer patients 363, 366–370
case studies 343–344
classification 328–329
counselling 340–342, 371
drug choice 334–335
in irritable bowel syndrome 106
non-pharmacological treatment 335–336
pharmacological basis of management 329–334
physiology 327–328
see also analgesics; chest pains; headaches
palliative care 362–363
common symptoms 363, *364–366*
counselling 371
pain management 363
adjuncts 369
analgesic ladder 366–367
concurrent disease 370
syringe drivers 367, 369
role of community pharmacist 370–371
terminal symptoms 370
pancytopenia 197
panic attacks 286, *289*
pantoprazole 87
paracetamol 330, 335, 343–344, 366–367, *458*
counselling 342
in fever 336
hepatotoxicity 56
interactions *26, 339*
in migraine 241–242
in osteoarthritis 348–349
use during pregnancy and breast-feeding *341*
parasites 397
helmintic and ectoparasitic infections 399–403
malaria 397–399
parkinsonism, as side effect of antipsychotics 306, *308*
Parkinson's disease 317, *459*
antidepressants *267*
case studies 322–323
counselling 320–321
drug choice 319–320

drug interactions 320, *321*
drug-induced 60
levodopa-induced nausea *99*
management of dyspepsia *90*
management of hypertension *124*
monitoring 320
pharmacological basis of management 317–319
sites of drug action *319*
use of antipsychotics *309*
paroxetine 262, 268, *458*
adverse reactions 277
avoidance in children 262
interactions 70, *271, 273, 274, 275, 311, 312*
use in anxiety *289*
withdrawal 279
partial seizures 249, *252*
passionflower 299
Paul–Bunnell test 19, 216
peak expiratory flow (PEF) 226, 234
peak and trough concentrations 77
pelvic inflammatory disease 379
penciclovir *417*
penicillamine 349, 354
counselling 357
interactions *353*
monitoring requirements 353
penicillins 380–381, *382, 459*
allergic reactions 53, 386, *387*, 390
cautions *387*
counselling 390
pentazocine *368*
peppermint oil, use in irritable bowel syndrome 106
peptic ulceration 7, 85, 86–87, *99*
antidepressants *267*
choice of drugs 88–91
goals of treatment 87
management of hyperlipidaemia *139*
management of migraine *244*
NSAID-induced 89–90
pharmacological basis of management 87–88
see also dyspepsia
percutaneous transluminal coronary angioplasty
(PCTA) 158
pergolide 318, 320
perindopril 120, 171–173, *456*
in secondary stroke prevention 176
peripheral oedema 171
peripheral vascular disease
management of migraine *244*
risk in diabetes 435
peritoneal dialysis 203
permethrin 400, 401
pernicious anaemia 195
perphenazine, adverse reactions *308*
pethidine *332, 367, 368*
interactions *274, 340*
pharmacokinetic ADRs 52–53, 64, 66–67
pharmacokinetics 73
absorption and availability 73
dosage interval 77–78

elimination 74–75
loading doses 76
maintenance doses 76–77
population-based equations 78–79
regimens 75–76
salt factor 74
therapeutic drug monitoring 81
volume of distribution 74
zero-order kinetics *79–81*
pharmacological drug interactions 64, *65*
pharyngitis 213–214, 215–216
phenelzine 262–263, *458*
phenobarbital *251*
interactions *24, 196,* 253
use during pregnancy 253
phenothiazines 98, 304–305, *305*
adverse reactions 100, 306, *308*
interactions *311, 312, 340*
phenothrin 400, 401
phenoxymethylpenicillin *382, 459*
phenylephrine 209, *210*
interactions *275*
phenylpropanolamine 209, *210*
interactions *231, 275*
phenytoin *250, 252, 459*
counselling 255
interactions *24, 26, 66, 196,* 253, *273, 311, 312, 389,*
402, 419, 434, 446
monitoring *466*
in neuropathic pain 333
pharmacokinetics 80
use during pregnancy 253
phobias 285, 287, *289*
phosphate binders, use in chronic renal failure 202,
205
phosphatidylserine 276
phosphodiesterase inhibitors 175
photosensitivity, drug-induced *61, 62,* 313
phototherapy 409, 411
physiotherapy, in pain management 336
pimecrolimus 408–409
pimozide 305, *308, 312*
pindolol 121
pioglitazone 431, 432, 433, *461*
piperacillin 391
piperazine *399,* 400, 403
piroxicam 329
pityriasis versicolor 414, *416*
pizotifen 242, *245, 247, 458*
Plasmodium species 397
platelets *465*
pleuritic pain *7*
pneumonia 6, 212
polystyrene sulphonate exchange resins 203
pompholyx 407, 410
population-based equations, pharmacokinetics
78–79
porphyria 53
antibiotic treatment *387*
management of insomnia *298*

management of allergy *220*
   oral hypoglycaemics *433*
portal hypertension 113
post-traumatic stress disorder 287–288, *289*
postherpetic neuralgia 337
postnatal depression 260
postoperative nausea and vomiting *99*
postural hypotension 8, *10*, 56
potassium, reference ranges *463*
potassium channel activators 158–159
potassium-sparing diuretics *456*
   in heart failure *172*, 173–174
pravastatin 135, 137, 138, *456*
   interactions *141*
prazosin 121, *456*
   in heart failure *172*, 175
prednisolone *461*
   in asthma 228
   in inflammatory bowel disease 108
   in rheumatoid arthritis 349
pregnancy 4
   alcohol consumption 25
   analgesics 340, *341*
   antibiotics 386
   antidepressants 270–271, 277
   antihelmintics 403
   antimalarials 403
   asthma 230
   diabetes management *433*
   epilepsy 252–253, 255
   food supplements *28*
   herbal remedies 41
   homeopathic remedies 42
   hyperlipidaemia *139*
   hypertension *124*
   hyperthyroidism 443
   insomnia 297
   iron requirements 193–194
   levothyroxine therapy 445
   nausea and vomiting *99*
   schizophrenia 310
   thromboembolic prophylaxis 187
   treatment of dyspepsia *90*
   vaginal bleeding *11*
prerenal renal failure 199
prilocaine 333
primaqine 398, *399*
primidone *24*, *251*, 253
Prinzmetal's angina 157, 159
PRISM trial *139*
probenecid 352
probiotics 104, 109
prochlorperazine 98, *99*, 100, 305
   contraindications *309*
procyclidine 305, 318–319, *459*
progestogen-only pill (POP) 32, 34
progestogens
   interactions 253
   use in anorexia *364*
PROGRESS Collaborative Group trial 176

proguanil 398, *399*, 403
prokinetic drugs 88
promethazine 97–98, *99*, 100, 218, *275*, *458*
   use in insomnia 296
propranolol 121, *122*, *456*
   in anxiety 288, 289, 292–293
   in hyperthyroidism 442
   interactions *245*
propylthiouracil 442, 443, 444
PROSPER study 138
prostaglandin analogues 88
prostaglandins, effect on gastric acid production *86*
prostate-specific antigen (PSA) 19
prostatic hypertrophy
   analgesics *338*
   management of hypertension *124*
   management of insomnia *298*
   management of allergy *220*
   use of antidepressants *267*
   use of antipsychotics *309*
prosthetic heart valves, target INR *186*
protamine 187, 428
protein-binding, role in drug interactions 66
proteinuria 199, 435
Proteus species *378*
prothrombin time 17, 18, *464*
proton pump inhibitors 87–88, *455*
   adverse reactions 103
   counselling 92–93
pruritus 113, 416, 418
   management 114, 201, *366*
pseudoephedrine 209, *210*
   interactions *275*
   misuse 32
pseudomembranous colitis 103, 104
Pseudomonas species *378*
psoriasis *12*, 410–411
   exacerbation by drugs *61*, 68
   use of antimalarials *399*
psychiatric ADRs 58, 60
psychiatric disorders *11*
   see also affective disorders; schizophrenia
psychotic depression 261
pulmonary embolism, target INR *186*
pulmonary oedema 171
pulsatilla 299
purpura, referral points *12*
pyelonephritis 379
pyloric stenosis 100
pyrazinamide 384, 392, 394, *460*
pyrimethamine 398

Q–T interval prolongation 57, *65*, *220*, 274, *389*, *399*, *402*
   antipsychotics 310, *312*
questioning patients 3–5
quetiapine 307
quinidine, interactions *311*
quinine
   cautions *399*

interactions *353, 402*
in malaria prophylaxis 397–398
use for leg cramps 352, 356–357
quinolones 381, *383, 460*
ADRs 62
cautions 386, *387*
counselling 390
interactions *194, 388*
quinupristin 385

rabeprazole 87–88, *455*
radiotherapy 362
antiemetics *99*
RALES trial 174
raloxifene 350–351
ramipril 120, 439, *456*
in heart failure 171–173
in IHD 158
Ramipril Efficacy in Nephropathy (REIN) trial
201–202
ranitidine 87, *455*
rapid cycling, bipolar affective disorder 268
rasagiline 318
rashes, referral points *12*
rate constant, first-order kinetics 75
reboxetine 263, 267, 277, *458*
red blood cells *465*
referral 8–12
reflux oesophagitis 85
regimens 75–76, 79
relaxation techniques 290, 291, 299–300
remifentanil *332*
remodelling of airways 226
renal ADRs 57–58
renal anaemia 196
renal excretion, role in drug interactions 67
renal failure
chronic *see* chronic renal failure
classification 199
drugs to be used with caution 17
vitamin D supplementation 350
renal function tests 15, 17
in heart failure 179
renal impairment
ACE inhibitors 173
analgesia *337, 338*
antibiotic treatment 391–392
antidepressants 270
antiemetics *99*
antimalarials *399*
antipsychotics 310
diabetic nephropathy 435
drugs used in musculoskeletal disorders 354–355
hypnotics 297
management of allergy *220*
management of dyspepsia *90*
management of heart failure 175
management of hyperlipidaemia *139*
management of hypertension *124*
oral hypoglycaemics *433*

prevention of ADRs 52
thromboembolic prophylaxis 188
see also chronic renal failure
renal osteodystrophy 200, 202
renal transplantation 203
renin inhibitors 128
renin-angiotensin-aldosterone system (RAAS),
activation in heart failure 169, *170*
repaglinide 431, 432, *434*, 437
respiratory ADRs 58
respiratory disease
chest pains *7*
management of insomnia *298*
use of antipsychotics *309*
see also asthma; chronic obstructive pulmonary
disease (COPD)
respiratory infections 378–379
reteplase *163*
retinopathy, diabetic 435
reversibility test, COPD 234
Reye's syndrome 330
rhabdomyloysis, drug-induced 62, *139*, 140, 141
rheumatic fever 213
rheumatoid arthritis 347
case study 359
counselling 357–358
pharmacological basis of management 349
rheumatoid factor 19
rifampicin 384, 391, 392, 394, *460*
interactions *108*, *231*, 290, *311*, *339*, *389*, *419*, *420*,
434
right ventricular failure 170, 171
rimonabant 149, 150, 151, *152*, 153
ringworm (tinea infections) 414
risedronate 350, *351*, 354, 355, 356
risperidone 270, 305, 307, *457*
adverse reactions 306, *308*, *309*, 310, 313
ritonavir, interactions *231*
rivastigmine *459*
rizatriptan 242, *245*
rodent ulcers *12*
rofecoxib 63, *458*
role of pharmacists 3
in palliative care 370–371
ropinirole 318, 319, *459*
rosacea *12*, 413–414
rosiglitazone 431, 432, *461*
effect on cardiovascular risk 57, 432–433
rosuvastatin 135, 138
rotaviruses 103
rotigotine 318, 319, 322, *459*
round worms (*Ascaris lumbricoides*) 400

S-adenosylmethionine 276
St John's wort 37, *39*, 43, 151, 204, 254, 290, 291
value in depression 276
salbutamol *457*
mechanism of action *227*
salicylates, adverse effects 330
salmeterol 227, *457*

Salmonella species infection 104, *378*
salt factor 74
salt restriction, liver disease 114, 115
saquinavir, interactions 253
saw palmetto *38, 40*
scabies 399–400, *418*
schizophrenia 303–304
    adverse effects of antipsychotics 305–*307, 308*
    case studies 314–315
    concurrent disease *309*
    counselling 312–313
    depot preparations 308
    drug choice 307–308
    drug interactions 310, *311–312*
    duration of treatment 309
    monitoring 310
    non-pharmacological interventions 309–310
    obesity management *150*
    over-the-counter considerations 312
    parkinsonism 319, 323
    pathophysiology 304
    pharmacological basis of management 304–305
screening for cancer 361
seasonal affective disorder (SAD) 260
seborrhoeic eczema 410
secobarbital, use in insomnia 296
secondary hypertension 119
sedation 60
    antiemetics 100
    antiepileptic drugs 255
    antihistamines 218
    cancer patients *366*
seizure threshold reduction 60
seizures *11*
selective oestrogen receptor modulators (SERMs)
        350–351
selective serotonin reuptake inhibitors (SSRIs) 247,
        262, 265, 267, *458*
    adverse reactions 58, 60
    in anxiety *289, 364*
    cautions *90, 267,* 270
    counselling 277, 291
    interactions *245,* 254, *273, 274, 311, 321, 339*
    in irritable bowel syndrome 106
    in Parkinson's disease 320
    use in children 261
    use during pregnancy 270–271
selegiline 263, 318, *459*
    interactions *273, 321*
senna 106, 110, *455*
septic arthritis 379–380
septicaemia 379
serotonin receptor modulators 263
serotonin syndrome *65,* 70, *152,* 272
sertindole 305
    adverse reactions 306, *308, 309,* 313
    interactions *312*
sertraline 262, *458*
    interactions *273, 274, 311, 446*
    use in anxiety *289*

sexual dysfunction, as side effect of antipsychotics
        305, *308,* 313
sexual health 32
sexually-transmitted infections 379, 392
shepherd's purse 446
Shigella species 103, *378*
shingles *12, 417*
'shock boxes' 222
SIADH (syndrome of inappropriate secretion of
        antidiuretic hormone) 61
sibutramine 149, 151, *458*
    contraindications *150*
    counselling 153
    interactions *152, 245,* 248
sickle cell anaemia 197
side effects 49
    see also adverse drug reactions (ADRs)
signs 3, 5–8
sildenafil, contraindications *164*
simvastatin 135, 137, 143–144, *456*
    benefits in diabetes 435
    interactions *141*
    over-the-counter provision 142
sinusitis 212–213
    referral points *10*
sirolimus 205
sitagliptin 432
sitostanol 137
skin, adverse drug reactions *61–62*
skin cancers 418, 420–421
skin conditions
    acne 412–413
    bacterial and viral infections 416, *417–418*
    case studies 421–423
    drug interactions *419–420*
    eczema 407–410
    fungal infections 414–*416*
    psoriasis 410–411
    rosacea 413–414
sleep apnoea *298*
sleep clinics 296
sleep diaries 300
smoking 27–28
    association with COPD 234, 237
    effect in diabetes *430*
    interactions 29, *231, 311*
smoking cessation 29
    cautions with use of smoking cessation aids *30–31*
    general counselling 31–32
social phobia 287, *289*
sodium, reference ranges *463*
sodium bicarbonate 87
sodium cromoglicate *457*
    in allergic rhinitis 218, 224
    in asthma 228
sodium nitroprusside *124*
sodium picosulphate 106
sodium valproate *250, 252,* 253, *272, 459*
    in bipolar affective disorder 269, 270
    counselling 255

interactions 66, 253
  migraine prophylaxis 242
  in neuropathic pain 333
solar ketatosis 420
somatic pain 328
sore throats 213–214, *387*, 392
  case studies 215–216, 256
  referral points *10*
sotalol *122*, *455*
spacers, use with inhaler devices 230, 232
spherocytosis 197
spider naevi *12*, 113, 418
spironolactone *456*
  counselling 179
  in heart failure *172*, *174*, 175
  in hypertension 123, 125
  in liver disease 114
squamous cell carcinoma 420
stable angina 157
Staphylococcus aureus 378, 380
  antibiotic resistance 385
  antibiotic sensitivities *382*
statins 123, 125, 135, 137–138, *139*, 143–144, *456*
  as cause of myopathy 62
  in chronic renal failure 202
  counselling 141
  first-pass metabolism 73
  interactions *140*, *141*
  safety 140
  in secondary prevention of MI 164, 166
status asthmaticus 227
steady-state concentration *75–76*, *77*
steatorrhoea *9*
  in orlistat therapy 149
stents 158
stepped approach, asthma management *229*
Sternberg diagnostic criteria 272
steroid sparing, asthma 229
Stevens–Johnson syndrome 61
streptococcal infections *378*
  antibiotic sensitivities *382*
  meningitis 379
  sore throat 213
Streptococcus pneumoniae 212
streptokinase *163*, 165, 166, *457*
  antibody development 53
stress 27, 287–288
stroke
  management of heart failure 176
  management of hypertension *124*
  management of migraine *244*
  use of antidepressants *266*
stroke risk, antipsychotics 306
suicidal ideation 267
  drug-induced 58, 60
sulfapyridine 108
sulfasalazine 108, 110, *462*
  counselling 357
  interactions *196*
  monitoring requirements 353–354

  in rheumatoid arthritis 349
sulfinpyrazone *351*, *352*, *354*, 357
sulphonamides 381, *383*, 392, *434*, *460*
sulphonylureas 431, 432, *461*
  contraindications *433*
  interactions *389*, *434*
sulpiride 305, *308*
sumatriptan 242, *244*, *458*
  interactions *245*, *274*
  over-the-counter supply 243, 246
swallowing problems, referral points *9*
sweating, management in cancer patients *366*
sympathetic nervous system, activation in heart
    failure 169, *170*
sympathomimetics
  avoidance in hyperthyroidism 445
  interactions *210*
  use in asthma 232
  withdrawal 54
symptoms 5–8
syphilis 379
syringe drivers 367, 369
systemic lupus erythematosus, drug-induced 62

tacalcitol 411
tacrolimus *204*, 205
  topical 408–409
tamoxifen 362
  interaction with herbal remedies 38, 44
tardive dyskinesia 305, 306, 313
tazarotene 411
teicoplanin 381, *382*, 385
temazepam 296, 297, *457*
terbinafine 415, *416*, *420*, *461*
terbutaline 227, *457*
terfenadine 220–221
terminal symptoms 370
tetracyclines 381, *382*, 392, *459*
  absorption 66
  cautions 386
  counselling 390, 422
  interactions *24*, *194*, *245*, *419*
  use in acne 412
theophylline 227–228, *457*
  interactions *231–232*, 253, *273*, *353*, *388*, *444*,
    446
  monitoring *466*
  pharmacokinetics *77–78*
therapeutic drug monitoring (TDM) 81, *466*
thiazides 120, *122*, *124*, 125, 130, *456*
  in chronic renal failure 201
  in heart failure *172*, 173
  hypokalaemia 179
  interactions *178*, *273*, *353*, *430*
thiazolidinediones (glitazones) 431, 432–433, *461*
  contraindications *177*
  interactions *434*
thionamides 442, *444*
thioxanthenes 305, *311*
thought disorder 303

threadworms (*Enterobius vermicularis*) 400
thrombin inhibitors 186
thrombocytopenia 58, *59*
thromboembolic prophylaxis 143
   case study 191–192
   concurrent disease 188–189
   counselling 190–191
   drug choice 187–188
   drug interactions 189–190
   monitoring 189
   pharmacological basis 185–187
thrombolytic agents *163*, 165, 166
thrombosis 185
thyroid disorders 441
   hyperthyroidism 441–444
   hypothyroidism 444–445
   over-the-counter considerations 445–446
thyroid function tests 19, 441–442, 445
thyroid gland, effect of lithium 269
thyroid-stimulating hormone (TSH) 441, 442
thyrotoxicosis *see* hyperthyroidism
tiagabine *251*
tiaprofenic acid 342
tibolone 350
timolol *122*
tinea infections *414*, *416*
tinidazole *388*, 390–391
tinzaparin 185–186, *457*
tioconazole 414–415
tiotropium bromide 228
tolbutamide 431, 439, *461*
   interactions *245*, *434*
tolcapone 318, 319, 321
tolfenamic acid 241–242, *245*
tonic seizures 249
tonic-clonic convulsions (grand mal seizures) 249,
   252, 256
tonsillitis 213–214, 215–216
topical antihistamines 218
topical steroids
   in eczema 408, 409
   in fungal infections 415
   in psoriasis 410
topiramate *250*, 255
total cholesterol 18
toxic epidermal necrolysis 61
tracheitis 6
Traditional Herbal Registration (THR) scheme 37
tramadol *332*, 336, *338*, 367, *458*
   avoidance during pregnancy *341*
   interactions *274*, *339*
transcutaneous electrical nerve stimulation (TENS)
   336
tranylcypromine 262–263
travellers' diarrhoea 104
trazodone 263, 277, 280, *289*
   interactions 275, *311*
tremor *11*
tretinoin 412, 413, *461*
triamcinolone, intranasal 218

triazoles 415, *419*
tricyclic antidepressants 262, 265, *458*
   cautions and contraindications *164*, *177*, *266*, *267*,
     270
   counselling 277
   interactions *210*, *223*, *271*, *274*, *275*, *276*, *312*, *321*,
     340, *446*
   migraine prophylaxis 242, *244*
   use during pregnancy 270
   use in irritable bowel syndrome 106, 107
   use in neuropathic pain 333, 336–337
trifluoperazine 305, *308*, 314–315
trigeminal neuralgia 337
triglyceride levels 18, 135, *464*
trimethoprim 381, *383*, 392, *460*
   counselling 391
   interactions *196*, *353*
triple therapy, *Helicobacter pylori* infection 89, 94,
   455
   counselling 93
triptans
   contraindications *164*, *244*
   counselling 246
   interactions *245*
   medication overuse headache 334
   in migraine 242, 243
L-tryptophan 22, 264
tryptophan-containing herbs 276
tuberculosis 6, *378–379*, 393–394
   treatment 384, *460*
type A ADRs *50–51*
tyramine 278
   action of MAOIs 262–263

UK Prospective Diabetes Study (UKPDS) 435
ulcerative colitis 107–110
ultraviolet phototherapy 409, 411
unipolar depression 261
   see also depression
units of alcohol 25
unstable angina 157
uraemia 200
urea breath test 88
urea and electrolytes 15, *463–464*
uric acid *463*
urinary tract infections (UTIs) 379, 392
urination problems *11*
urticaria, drug-induced *61*

vagal nerve stimulation 251
valerian 291, 299
valproic acid 272
valsartan 120, 173, *456*
vancomycin 381, *382*, 385, *387*, *388*
varenicline 29, *30–31*, 32
vasopressin, in management of bleeding oesophageal
     varices 115
vasovagal syncope (fainting) 8
vegan diet, food supplements *28*
venesection, in COPD 235

venlafaxine 263, 268, 271, *458*
  adverse effects *266*, 277
  in anxiety *289*
  cautions 270
  interactions *274*
  use during pregnancy 271
venous thrombosis 185
  risk from oral contraception 33
verapamil 120–121, *122*, *455*, *456*
  in acute MI *163*
  in angina 158, 159, *161*
  in bipolar affective disorder 269
  interactions *26*, *65*, 68, 160, 166, *231*, 254, 290
  in migraine prophylaxis 242
  in secondary prevention of MI 164
verrucae *417*
vestibular disorders *99*
vigabatrin *250*, *252*, 253, 254, 255
VIGOR trial 63
Vincent's angina *378*
viral infections, of the skin *417–418*
viral neuramidase inhibitors 211–212
visceral pain 328, 363
vitamin D$_3$ activation 200
vitamin B$_{12}$ *465*
  drug interactions *196*
vitamin B$_{12}$ deficiency 195
vitamin supplements 27, *28*
  in alcoholic liver disease 115
  in inflammatory bowel disease 109
  interactions *152*, 190, *353*
  in thyroid disease 446
  vitamin D 350, *353*, 354, 356
VLDL (very-low-density lipoprotein) 133
volume of distribution 74
vomiting 97
  in cancer patients *366*
  choice of drugs 98–100
  herbal remedies 101
  interactions with antiemetics 101
  in migraine 241–242, *244*
  opioid-induced 331
  pharmacological basis of management 97–98
  referral points *9*
  stimuli, pathways and receptors *98*
vomiting centre 97, *98*

waist circumference 147, *148*
warfarin 186, 192, *457*
  adverse reactions 49
  contraindications 187, 188–189
  counselling 190–191
  indications in atrial fibrillation 188
  initiation of treatment 187
  interactions *24*, *38*, *65*, 66, 67, *141*, *152*, 189–190, *253*, *273*, *339*, *353*, *389*, *402*, *419*, *444*, *446*
  management of elevated INR 187
  in secondary prevention of MI 164
  use in liver disease 114
warts *417*
weight gain, as side effect of antipsychotics 305, *308*, 313
weight loss *9*
weight reduction 148, 151
  benefits in hypertension 121
Weil's disease *378*
Wernicke's encephalopathy 115
wet combing 401
wheezing *10*, 226, 227
white blood cells *465*
'white-coat' hypertension 127
withdrawal of drugs, adverse reactions 53–54
withdrawal symptoms, smoking cessation 29
Wolff–Parkinson–White syndrome, management of migraine *244*
WOSCOPS trial 137
WWHAM mnemonic 4

xanthines *457*
  adverse effects 231
  in asthma 227–228
  in COPD 235
  counselling 233
  interactions *231–232*
xanthomas *10*, 135
xylometazoline 209, 218–219, *220*, 221

Yellow Card reporting 62

zafirlukast 228, 233, *389*, *457*
zaleplon 296, 297
zanamivir 211–212, *460*
zero-order kinetics 79–*81*
zinc, combination with insulin 428
zinc lozenges 209
Zollinger–Ellison syndrome 85
zolmitriptan 242
zolpidem 296, 297, *457*
zopiclone 296, 297, *457*
zotepine 307